# Child and Adolescent Psychopathology

# Child and Adolescent Psychopathology

Second Edition

Edited by

Theodore P. Beauchaine
Stephen P. Hinshaw

John Wiley & Sons, Inc.

This book is printed on acid-free paper. ⊗

Copyright © 2013 by John Wiley & Sons, Inc. All rights reserved.

Published by John Wiley & Sons, Inc., Hoboken, New Jersey.
Published simultaneously in Canada.

No part of this publication may be reproduced, stored in a retrieval system, or transmitted in any form or by any means, electronic, mechanical, photocopying, recording, scanning, or otherwise, except as permitted under Section 107 or 108 of the 1976 United States Copyright Act, without either the prior written permission of the Publisher, or authorization through payment of the appropriate per-copy fee to the Copyright Clearance Center, Inc., 222 Rosewood Drive, Danvers, MA 01923, (978) 750-8400, fax (978) 646-8600, or on the web at www.copyright.com. Requests to the Publisher for permission should be addressed to the Permissions Department, John Wiley & Sons, Inc., 111 River Street, Hoboken, NJ 07030, (201) 748-6011, fax (201) 748-6008.

Limit of Liability/Disclaimer of Warranty: While the publisher and author have used their best efforts in preparing this book, they make no representations or warranties with respect to the accuracy or completeness of the contents of this book and specifically disclaim any implied warranties of merchantability or fitness for a particular purpose. No warranty may be created or extended by sales representatives or written sales materials. The advice and strategies contained herein may not be suitable for your situation. You should consult with a professional where appropriate. Neither the publisher nor author shall be liable for any loss of profit or any other commercial damages, including but not limited to special, incidental, consequential, or other damages.

This publication is designed to provide accurate and authoritative information in regard to the subject matter covered. It is sold with the understanding that the publisher is not engaged in rendering professional services. If legal, accounting, medical, psychological or any other expert assistance is required, the services of a competent professional person should be sought.

Designations used by companies to distinguish their products are often claimed as trademarks. In all instances where John Wiley & Sons, Inc. is aware of a claim, the product names appear in initial capital or all capital letters. Readers, however, should contact the appropriate companies for more complete information regarding trademarks and registration.

For general information on our other products and services please contact our Customer Care Department within the United States at (800) 762-2974, outside the United States at (317) 572-3993 or fax (317) 572-4002.

Wiley publishes in a variety of print and electronic formats and by print-on-demand. Some material included with standard print versions of this book may not be included in e-books or in print-on-demand. If this book refers to media such as a CD or DVD that is not included in the version you purchased, you may download this material at http://booksupport.wiley.com. For more information about Wiley products, visit www.wiley.com.

*Library of Congress Cataloging-in-Publication Data:*

Child and adolescent psychopathology / edited by Theodore P. Beauchaine,
  Stephen P. Hinshaw.— 2nd ed.
    p. cm.
  Includes bibliographical references and index.
  ISBN 978-1-118-12094-1 (cloth)
  ISBN 978-1-118-43167-2 (e-bk)
  ISBN 978-1-118-41636-5 (e-bk)
  ISBN 978-1-118-41914-4 (e-bk)
  1. Child psychopathology. 2. Adolescent psychopathology. I. Beauchaine, Theodore P. II. Hinshaw,
Stephen P.
RJ499.C48237 2012
  618.92′8905– dc23                                                    2012027165

Printed in the United States of America

10 9 8 7 6 5 4 3 2 1

# Contents

v

# Foreword

THE FIELD OF DEVELOPMENTAL psychopathology first came into ascendance during the 1970s, predominantly by being highlighted as an important perspective by researchers conducting prospective longitudinal studies of children at risk for developing schizophrenia. Epidemiological investigations of families exhibiting discord and disruption (but where there was no parental mental disorder), studies of links between cumulative risk factors and developmental outcome, investigations of children with handicapping conditions, and research on cognitive and socio-emotional development in children with autism were among those areas that were influential in the field's emergence. Conceptualizations of the nature of mental disorder, etiological models of risk and resilience, scientific questions that were posed, and research designs and data analytic strategies were all reexamined, challenged, and cast in a new light by developmental psychopathologists.

The belief that the study of typical developmental processes informs understanding of pathological development and, conversely, that the study of pathological development informs the understanding of normative development, is one of the central tenets of developmental psychopathology—an interdisciplinary science that strives to reduce the schisms that so often separate scientific research from the application of knowledge to clinical populations. The field of developmental psychopathology owes its emergence and coalescence to a number of historically based endeavors in a variety of disciplines, including embryology, genetics, and the neurosciences, as well as psychoanalysis, psychiatry, and psychology. As such, developmental psychopathology provides an example of the synergistic contributions of previously disparate fields that result in the emergence of a new discipline. Somewhat surprisingly, given its historical roots, most of the research conducted on both the development of psychopathology and the processes contributing to resilience focused on relatively narrow domains of variables until the late 1990s and early years of the present millennium.

Over the past several decades, there has been a veritable explosion in our knowledge of developmental neurobiology, that area of neuroscience that focuses on factors regulating the development of neurons, neuronal circuitry, and complex neuronal organization systems, including the brain. Additionally, technological advances in the fields of neuroimaging and molecular genetics have contributed to progress in our understanding of normality, psychopathology, and resilience. Consequently, it has become increasingly acknowledged that the investigation of developmental processes, both normal and abnormal, is an inherently interdisciplinary enterprise.

It is now apparent from the nature of the questions addressed by developmental psychopathologists that progress toward a process-level understanding of mental disorders will require research designs and strategies that call for the assessment of multiple domains and multiple levels of variables, both within and outside the developing person. Likewise, research on the developmental pathways to resilience, the achievement of positive adaptation in the face of significant adversity, must follow these interdisciplinary multiple-levels-of-analysis perspectives. To comprehend typical development, psychopathology, and resilience fully, all levels of analysis must be examined and integrated. Multiple levels of analysis are necessary because no one level is sufficient to explain the complexity inherent in the study of development and psychopathology.

Developmental psychopathology is an exciting and complex field. A major goal of graduate and postdoctoral training in developmental psychopathology is to develop the next generation of scholars so that they can go on and launch their own research careers. An important early step in this process is student access to scholarly volumes that demonstrate the depth and breadth of the field in a clear and accessible way. Thus, this edited volume is a long-awaited, much needed, unique and innovative contribution to the field. It is organized around highlighting the principles and major tenets of developmental psychopathology into a work that does not shy away from presenting students, scholars, and clinicians with our current knowledge regarding the multilevel complexity of typical and atypical development.

The editors of this volume, Ted Beauchaine and Steve Hinshaw, are each leading theorists and researchers in developmental psychopathology. They both subscribe to multilevel research and also have engaged in impressive translational research through developing and implementing preventive interventions for high-risk youth that were influenced by basic research findings.

Ted Beauchaine has made seminal contributions to the understanding of the biological underpinnings of a number of mental and personality disorders in children and adolescents and has conducted exemplary research on the prevention of these conditions. Beauchaine also has utilized numerous psychophysiological measures in his research on attention deficit hyperactivity disorder, conduct problems, disinhibitory psychopathology, depression, and teen self-injury. Importantly, Ted also possesses superb quantitative skills that enable him to conduct data analyses across multiple levels of analysis.

Steve Hinshaw has made classic contributions on the role of the family and peer relationships to typical and atypical development. He also has completed impressive multilevel research on externalizing problems (i.e., conduct disorder, attention deficit disorder) and on behavior problems and psychopathology in girls. Furthermore, Hinshaw has implemented combinations of psychosocial and pharmacologic intervention for children with externalizing expressions of dysfunction. Finally, Steve has been a major advocate and contributor to the importance of destigmatizing mental illness. He has written two powerful volumes on this topic—one a personal account of his father's lifelong struggle with bipolar disorder (*The Years of Silence Are Past: My Father's Life with Bipolar Disorder*, 2002), the other a scholarly account of the history of the stigmatizing treatment of persons with mental illness that also reviews the extant research on stigma from various scientific perspectives and provides recommendations for future research, intervention, and social policy (*The Mark of Shame:Stigma of Mental Illness and an Agenda for Change*, 2007).

In order to have this volume adhere to the tenets of developmental psychopathology, Beauchaine and Hinshaw instructed the contributors to take a multiple-levels-of-analysis approach to their assigned chapter topic. All of the authors in this volume are world-class scholars in their area of expertise. Importantly, each contributor communicates clearly, thus enabling graduate students and professionals from a variety of disciplines to develop a firm grasp of psychopathology and resilience in their multi-system entirety.

Major high-risk conditions and mental disorders are given excellent coverage, as are processes contributing to the development of resilient functioning in individuals experiencing significant adverse experiences. The breadth and depth of each chapter's content provides the reader with a deep appreciation of the complex nature of normality, psychopathology, and resilience. The topics and issues addressed in these chapters are immensely important – not only for the developmental sciences, but also for a number of other scientific fields.

I have been teaching graduate courses in developmental psychopathology for over 30 years. I have often searched for appropriate textbooks on psychopathology to assign to students that were undergirded by the principles of developmental psychopathology. Although there were a number of good textbooks available, few were truly developmental in their organization and content. One of the books that was guided by the tenets of developmental psychopathology was a multi-volume set that Donald Cohen and I co-edited on *Developmental Psychopathology*. These extensive volumes were not practical to assign to graduate students for a semester-long course. Thus, I have never assigned a required textbook for my courses on developmental psychopathology. My course syllabus was composed solely of journal articles and book chapters that the students were required to read.

Now that I have read this excellent volume edited by Ted Beauchaine and Steve Hinshaw, I believe that I have finally found the answer to my 30-plus-year search for a developmental psychopathology textbook. The volume is full of rich and exciting ideas that will help students develop a passion for the field of developmental psychopathology. I fully anticipate that my colleagues across the country will feel similarly and that the Beauchaine and Hinshaw text will play an important role in the training of future generations of developmental psychopathologists.

Dante Cicchetti, Ph.D.
McKnight Presidential Chair
William Harris Professor
and Professor of Child Psychology and Psychiatry
Institute of Child Development
University of Minnesota

# Preface

SOCIETAL COSTS OF mental illness—in terms of both morbidity and mortality—are staggering. In 2002, the most recent year for which data are available, 154 million people worldwide suffered from depression, 106 million suffered an alcohol or drug use disorder, 25 million suffered from schizophrenia, and nearly 1 million died by suicide (World Health Organization, 2012). In low- and middle-income countries, mental disorders account for 25% and 34%, respectively, of total years lived with disability, yet the large majority of those affected receive no form of treatment (WHO World Mental Health Survey Consortium, 2004). Although treatment rates are slightly higher in wealthy countries, mental disorders continue to carry significant stigma. As a result, many avoid seeking help, and a lack of treatment parity remains for mental disorders vs. other health-related conditions (Hinshaw, 2007).

When we wrote the preface to the first edition of this book, we noted how important it is to elucidate the causes of mental illness. After all, the better we understand etiology across all relevant levels of analysis, including genetic, neural, familial, and cultural (to name a few), the better position we are in to formulate effective prevention and intervention programs (Beauchaine, Neuhaus, Brenner, & Gatzke-Kopp, 2008). Thus, even though this is not a text about treatment, we hope readers will keep in mind while digesting each chapter how important it is to identify the causes of mental illness in our efforts to reduce human suffering. In this regard, we live in an exciting and promising time. The Human Genome Project, completed only 10 years ago, sequenced 3 billion chemical base pairs that comprise human DNA. Following from this and major advances in psychiatric genetics, our understanding of molecular genetic vulnerabilities to mental illness continues to improve, even though new paradigms are constantly emerging. Similarly, the application of modern neuroimaging techniques—particularly fMRI—has advanced our understanding of neural vulnerabilities to psychopathology. Especially exciting is recent research demonstrating how neural functioning mediates links between genetic vulnerability and high risk personality traits that predispose individuals to psychopathology (e.g., Buckholtz et al., 2008).

Traditionally, most of what we learned about mental illness was obtained through observation and classification of symptoms (see Chapter 2). Although useful in the early stages of identifying different forms of mental illness, symptom classification often tells us little if anything about underlying causal processes—be they biological or environmental—that lead to a particular disorder. Accordingly, in editing this book we sought authors with expertise in the *developmental psychopathology* perspective, which emerged only about 30 years ago (see Chapter 1). This perspective follows from the observation that human behavioral traits—including those that predispose to psychopathology—almost always arise from complex transactions between biological vulnerabilities and exposure to environmental risks across development. For example, heritable disorders such as depression, schizophrenia, and substance dependence are affected strongly by environmental experiences, and the effects of environmentally-transmitted risks such as child maltreatment are moderated by genes and other biological predispositions. Furthermore, through epigenetic mechanisms, the expression of several genes implicated in behavior regulation can be altered by experience including exposure to stress and trauma—findings that defy anachronistic distinctions between nature and nurture.

This shift in the scientific landscape—from a relatively static view of psychopathology based on specific clusters of behavior to a dynamic view of disorders emerging from complex transactions between vulnerabilities and risks across time—served as the impetus for the first edition of this book. It continues to drive the current second edition, which includes considerable new material. Before the first edition was published, most graduate-level psychopathology texts were organized around symptom-based approaches to classifying mental illness, with limited consideration of the genetic and neural underpinnings of behavior, or of unfolding of interactions between biological vulnerabilities and environmental risk across time. However, in the five years since the first edition was published, appreciation for the complexity of such transactions in the development of psychopathology has increased, and many new and exciting findings have emerged. The timing was therefore right for a second edition.

Some readers will likely note that a few disorders often covered in psychopathology texts are not included in this book. For example, we do not address developmental disabilities or mental retardation. In omitting these disorders, we are not implying that they are unimportant. Rather, the ever expanding literature addressing developmental disabilities makes it difficult to cover the topic adequately in a text that already includes 22 chapters. Thus, we were left with a difficult choice, and we decided not to limit coverage of the conditions contained herein. We refer interested readers to other sources (e.g., Jacobson, Mulick, & Rojahn, 2007) for excellent coverage of developmental disabilities and mental retardation.

We now invite you to join us in the quest for a deepened understanding of mental disorders and conditions that originate in childhood and adolescence. We hope that our emphases on genetic and other biological vulnerabilities, and how these interact with environmental risk factors and contexts, will challenge your preconceived notions as to what is "biological" and what is "environmental" in relation to normal and atypical development and psychopathology. We hope as well that our coverage will prompt a new generation of investigators, clinicians, and policymakers to pursue the daunting but essential goal of explaining, treating, and preventing the devastation that so often accompanies psychopathology.

Theodore P. Beauchaine
Stephen P. Hinshaw

## REFERENCES

Jacobson, J. W., Mulick, J. A., & Rojahn, J. (Eds.) (2007). *Handbook of intellectual and developmental disabilities*. New York: Springer.

Beauchaine, T. P., Neuhaus, E., Brenner, S. L., & Gatzke-Kopp, L. (2008). Ten good reasons to consider biological processes in prevention and intervention research. *Development and Psychopathology, 20*, 745–774.

Buckholtz, J. W., Callicott, J. H., Kolachana, B. K., Hariri, A. R., Goldberg, T. E., Genderson, M., . . . Meyer-Lindenberg, A. (2008). Genetic variation in MAOA modulates ventromedial prefrontal circuitry mediating individual differences in human personality. *Molecular Psychiatry, 13*, 313–324.

Hinshaw, S. P. (2007). *The mark of shame: Stigma of mental illness and an agenda for change*. New York: Oxford University Press.

WHO World Mental Health Survey Consortium (2004). Prevalence, severity, and unmet need for treatment of mental disorders in the World Health Organization World Mental Health Surveys. *Journal of the American Medical Association, 291*, 2581–2590.

World Health Organization (2012). *Mental health*. Retrieved April 17, 2012, www.who.int/en/

# List of Contributors

**Charissa Andreotti**
Vanderbilt University, TN

**Robert F. Asarnow**
UCLA School of Medicine

**Theodore P. Beauchaine**
Washington State University

**Sarah R. Black**
University at Stony Brook, NY

**Joseph C. Blader**
Stony Brook University School of
Medicine, NY

**Cara Bohon**
University of California, Los Angeles

**Katherine Shannon Bowen**
University of Wisconsin

**Sandra A. Brown**
Veterans Affairs San Diego Healthcare
System, CA

**Gabrielle A. Carlson**
Stony Brook University School of
Medicine, NY

**Pamela M. Cole**
Pennsylvania State University

**Bruce E. Compas**
Vanderbilt University, TN

**Nicole A. Crocker**
SDSU/UCSD Joint Doctoral Program
in Clinical Psychology, CA

**Sheila E. Crowell**
University of Utah

**Geraldine Dawson**
Autism Speaks, NY

**Marco Del Giudice**
Center for Cognitive Science,
Department of Psychology, University
of Turin, Italy

**Thomas J. Dishion**
Arizona State University

**Bruce J. Ellis**
John and Doris Norton School of
Family and Consumer Sciences, AZ

**Nora L. Erickson**
Washington State University

**Susan Faja**
University of Washington

**Susanna L. Fryer**
University of California, San Francisco

**Lisa M. Gatzke-Kopp**
Pennsylvania State University

**Nastassia J. Hajal**
Pennsylvania State University

**Sarah E. Hall**
Wheaton College, IL

**Stephen P. Hinshaw**
University of California, Berkeley

**Sara R. Jaffee**
Institute of Psychiatry, London

**Jerome Kagan**
Harvard University

**Erin A. Kaufman**
University of Utah

**Daniel N. Klein**
University at Stony Brook, NY

**Autumn J. Kujawa**
University at Stony Brook, NY

**Benjamin B. Lahey**
University of Chicago

**Mark F. Lenzenweger**
State University of New York at
Binghamton

**Andrea Kohn Maikovich-Fong**
Colorado Blood Cancer Institute at
Presbyterian/St. Luke's Hospital

**Sarah N. Mattson**
San Diego State University, CA

**Emily Neuhaus**
University of Colorado School of
Medicine

**Joel Nigg**
Oregon Health and Science University

**Alyssa L. Norris**
Washington State University

**Allison T. Pennock**
University at Stony Brook, NY

**Kristina Hiatt Racer**
University of Oregon

**Elizabeth A. Shirtcliff**
University of New Orleans, LA

**Wendy K. Silverman**
Florida International University

**Eric Stice**
Oregon Research Institute

**Kristin Tomlinson**
University of California, San Diego

**Irwin D. Waldman**
Emory University, GA

**Carl F. Weems**
University of New Orleans, LA

**Jennifer Winward**
University of California, San Diego

# PART I

## THE DEVELOPMENTAL PSYCHOPATHOLOGY APPROACH TO UNDERSTANDING MENTAL ILLNESS

# CHAPTER 1

# Developmental Psychopathology as a Scientific Discipline
## Rationale, Principles, and Advances

STEPHEN P. HINSHAW

FROM ITS "LAUNCH" BETWEEN three and four decades ago (see Achenbach, 1974; Cicchetti, 1984; Sroufe & Rutter, 1984), developmental psychopathology (DP) has become a force to be reckoned with. DP is at once a perspective on the origins of mental disorders that begin during childhood and adolescence, a multidisciplinary conceptual approach linking normative development to psychopathology, and a scientific discipline closely tied to clinical child/adolescent psychology and psychiatry but transcending the usual diagnosis-based emphasis of these fields (Cicchetti & Cohen, 2006; Cicchetti & Toth, 2009). Through its focus on the dynamic interplay of biology and context, genes and environments, and "inner" versus "outer" influences on the development of healthy and atypical functioning, it has come to dominate current thinking and research on psychopathology. Some of its core ideas are not new, having emerged in the context of embryology, systems theory, philosophy, and genetics long ago (see Cicchetti, 2006; Gottlieb & Willoughby, 2006, for elaboration). Yet the syntheses represented in this volume, reflecting DP's continuing growth, are truly cutting edge, given the relatively recent emergence of DP and given the knowledge explosion in recent years related to psychobiological influences as they transact with contextual forces. Today, scientists from diverse disciplines contribute to ever-expanding knowledge of this enterprise while clinicians benefit from and utilize its core principles. The underlying perspectives are no longer revolutionary; instead, they have come to comprise the dominant paradigm.

In this, our second edition of a graduate-level compendium on core aspects of this vast topic, we continue our tradition of providing current, conceptually based, clinically relevant, and developmentally informed information on causal mechanisms underlying child and adolescent psychopathology. Leading scientists across the entire field have contributed state-of-the-art summations of their particular areas of expertise; we owe them a great debt for their efforts toward translating the complex findings into each chapter synthesis. Indeed, every entry in this edition is brand new, which is entirely necessary given how much the science has advanced across the several years since the first edition (Beauchaine & Hinshaw, 2008).

## WHY DEVELOPMENTAL PSYCHOPATHOLOGY?

To contextualize and put into perspective why this entire area is so important, one must first consider the high levels of suffering involved in child and adolescent psychopathology, including the severe pain and restricted life opportunities experienced by not only affected children and adolescents but also by families, schools, and in some cases communities and society at large. Emotional and behavioral problems in youth are not only distressingly prevalent but also hugely impairing, leading to serious problems in such crucial domains as academic achievement, interpersonal competencies, and independent living skills. Distress is often intense; individuals may engage in behavior patterns that are highly destructive to their own development as well as the well-being of others.

For example, depression is associated with high degrees of hopelessness and despair, anxiety disorders with severe restrictions on exploration, bipolar disorder with disruption and chaos as well as high risk for suicidality, attention-deficit hyperactivity disorder with major deficits in academic and social arenas as well as risk for accidental injury, conduct problems with both violence and victimization, eating disorders with threats to physical well-being and healthy self-image, autism and other pervasive developmental disorders with severe isolation and major skill deficits, and substance use/abuse with squandered opportunities and major health risks. Child maltreatment is linked, in too many instances, to tragic developmental consequences, and the origins of personality disturbance are linked to major risk for self-harm and interpersonal disasters. Although lifelong pain and impairment are not inevitable, as we know from investigations of resilience (e.g., Luthar & Brown, 2007; Sapienza & Masten, 2011), mental disorders are quite likely to "up the ante" for devastation.

Second, the costs of mental disturbance are huge in other ways. Health care expenditures rise dramatically, educational and occupational milestones are likely to be hugely delayed or lost altogether, and deficits in later employability are often staggering, with major economic consequences (e.g., Murray & Lopez, 1996; Robb et al., 2011). Thus, beyond personal and family suffering, disabling skill deficits and harsh economic realities frequently accrue from mental disorder.

Third, not only do behavioral, emotional, and developmental disturbances in childhood and adolescence typically persist into adulthood, but what are often considered to be "adult" mental disorders often have precursors in the early years of development (Kessler et al., 2005). All too often, symptoms and impairments start early and remain problematic for years to come.

Given this set of deeply human, enormously costly, and persistent needs, why not rely on traditional clinical efforts in psychology and psychiatry, with their long, venerable histories? As detailed in earlier treatises, these efforts have too often yielded overly broad and static categories of mental disorders, with insufficient attention paid to biological vulnerabilities, contextual influences, multilevel chains of causation, dynamic and transactional influences, and divergent life-course pathways within a given diagnostic category (e.g., Cicchetti, 1990). The reciprocally deterministic nature of development, both typical and atypical, is not well captured in such diagnostic systems. As a function of the huge expansion of knowledge in a host of related fields and subfields, the complex yet compelling perspectives offered by DP have taken hold with increasing pace. Without them, traditional models seem sterile and impoverished.

Yet despite the utter scientific and clinical urgency surrounding this topic, important barriers stand in the way of increased scientific understanding and access to evidence-based treatment. Perhaps the primary reason is that mental disturbance at any age is still highly stigmatized (e.g., Hinshaw, 2007; Hinshaw & Stier, 2008). Intensive stigma and shame prevent help seeking and serve to render mental health a lower priority than physical health, despite the inextricable linkages between the two. Intriguingly, although we appear to be a far more open and accepting culture regarding mental health than half a century ago—and although public knowledge of mental illness has grown considerably since the 1950s—the U.S. public is *more* likely to link mental illness with dangerousness, and it wishes for *greater* social distance from those with mental disorders, than in the past (see Phelan, Link, Stueve, & Pescosolido, 2000). The reasons are complex but may relate to (a) increased numbers of seriously impaired individuals on the streets, without needed community services and resources; (b) enhanced public awareness that "dangerousness" is one of the few reasons that can still lead to involuntarily commitment; and (c) the tenuousness of the evidence that biogenetic ascriptions to mental illness (i.e., that it is a "brain disease" or a "disease like any other") can eliminate stigmatization (see Hinshaw, 2007; Jorm & Griffiths, 2008; Martinez, Piff, Mendoza-Denton, & Hinshaw, 2011; Pescosolido et al., 2010). DP perspectives promote complex as opposed to simplistic or reductionistic conceptions of mental disorder, leading to both enhanced scientific progress and, it is hoped, a more realistic view on the part of the general public, emphasizing multidetermined pathways but not personal weakness or blame.

In all, despite the major advances in basic science and clinical applications in recent years, which we highlight in the following pages, the field's knowledge of developing brains and minds in multiple, interacting contexts is still rudimentary. How could it be otherwise, given the sheer complexity of our topic matter? Still, for those who enjoy a challenge—and those who are excited by questions that will take many years and many great minds to answer, with the potential for a payoff of bettering the human condition—we sincerely hope that our chapters serve as a call to join the major scientific and clinical efforts needed in the decades ahead. Indeed, if the field is to continue to make headway toward understanding, treating, and preventing the serious clinical conditions that emerge during childhood and adolescence, the best minds of the current generation are required.

We admit that the multilayered nature of the topic at hand, paired with the huge numbers of risk factors (biological, experiential, and contextual) that promote disturbed functioning and the many protective factors that might mitigate such risk, can serve to delay needed translational efforts from DP-related insights to evidence-based treatment strategies (Cicchetti & Toth, 2009). Although this book is, by design, not a volume on intervention, our ultimate hope is that the intentional application of advances in basic science to clinical practice and prevention will occur at an ever-increasing pace.

## OVERVIEW OF APPROACH

In the chapters that follow, our core objective is to bring to life DP's core tenets and principles into a useful guide for students, clinicians, and scholars, in order to facilitate deepened understanding of the major forms of child and adolescent behavioral and emotional disturbance. To meet this aim, we have asked leaders in the field to present up-to-date material that is simultaneously developmentally based, clinically relevant, and directly inclusive of the types of psychobiological formulations that are gaining ascendancy in the entire mental health enterprise. In other words, we aim to supplement the kinds of developmental, process-oriented constructs typically linked to DP with appreciation of core findings in behavioral and molecular genetics, neural pathways, and brain plasticity that have risen to prominence in recent years.

Thus, in our instructions to the volume's contributors, we asked explicitly for coverage of historical context, epidemiologic factors, diagnostic issues, sex differences, cultural variables, developmental processes, and important psychobiological mechanisms that can illuminate the forms of pathology under discussion in their particular chapter. At the same time, we emphasized that neurobiological processes must not be represented in reductionistic fashion. Indeed, those contextual factors—familial, cultural, school-related—viewed as the predominant causal mechanisms throughout much of the last century are now known to interact and transact with biological vulnerabilities and risk variables to produce both maladaptation and healthy adaptation across development. Thus, we urged our authors to consider vulnerability and risk across multiple levels of analysis, emphasizing transaction across a range of individual and contextual factors in the genesis of (or desistance from) psychopathology. Indeed, modern views of behavioral and molecular genetics have placed into sharp relief the unique and interactive roles that environmental and cultural forces exert on development (e.g., Cicchetti & Curtis, 2006; Dodge & Rutter, 2011; Rutter, Moffitt, & Caspi, 2006).

Given page limitations and our desire for focused rather than exhaustive coverage, each chapter is relatively brief, with the goal of providing cogent, recent, and incisive commentary on conceptual issues, clinically relevant material, neuro-scientific advances, and interactive models. We strongly hope that readers use these contributions as a springboard for further exploration of conceptual frameworks, empirical research on etiology and mechanisms, and bases for prevention and treatment.

As noted earlier, despite the considerable advances that have been made, the road ahead is long. One can only wonder at what scholars a century from now will make of our preliminary attempts to model the hugely complex developmental pathways, processes, and trajectories linked to psychopathology. After all, the human genome was decoded only a decade ago, and high-resolution brain scanning is still a relatively young field of endeavor. Still, throughout the following pages, I highlight key advances that have been made in recent years regarding DP processes, methods, and models, signifying that the enterprise has already yielded unprecedented insights and discoveries.

## DP CONCEPTS AND PRINCIPLES

What characterizes a truly developmental view of psychopathology, as opposed to the kinds of descriptive, symptom-focused presentations that still dominate most classification systems and that still permeate many ideas in the field? As discussed in key readings (e.g., Cicchetti & Cohen, 2006; Cicchetti & Toth, 2009; Mash & Dozois, 2003; Rutter & Sroufe, 2000; Sameroff, Lewis, & Miller, 2000), several core points are commonly viewed as central to the DP perspective. These include the necessity of (a) interweaving studies of normal development and pathological functioning into a true synthesis; (b) examining developmental continuities and discontinuities of traits, behavior patterns, emotional responses, and disorders; (c) evaluating evidence across multiple levels of analysis (from genes to cultures, including the intermediate levels of individuals, families, schools, and neighborhoods); (d) incorporating distinct perspectives, including clinical and developmental psychology, child and adolescent psychiatry, genetics, neurology, public health, philosophy of science, and many others, into a truly multidisciplinary effort; (e) exploring both risk and protective factors and their interplay, so that competence, strength, and resilience as well as pathology and impairment can be understood; (f) involving reciprocal, transactional models of influence in the field's causal models, through which linear patterns of association and causation are replaced by probabilistic, dynamic, nonlinear, and complex conceptual models; and (g) capturing the importance of social and cultural context both in understanding the function and meaning of behavioral and emotional patterns and in interacting with biological predisposition to yield disordered functioning.

Three related principles bear emphasis. The first is that multiple pathways to pathology exist. Indeed, disparate routes may lead to a common condition or outcome, exemplifying the construct of *equifinality*. For example, aggressive behavior (or, diagnostically speaking, "conduct disorder") can result from physical abuse (Chapter 5), from a heritable tendency toward disinhibition (Chapter 3), from injury to the frontal lobes (Chapter 10), from coercive parenting interchanges with the developing child (Chapter 14), from prenatal and perinatal risk factors acting in concert with early experiences of insecure attachment or parental rejection (Chapter 9), or from different combinations of these vulnerabilities and risk factors (e.g., Jaffee, Strait, & Odgers, 2012; Raine, Brennan, & Mednick, 1997; Tremblay, 2010). In other words, separate—and in many cases interacting—causal influences can yield similar clinical endstates. In addition, the concept of *multifinality* applies when a given risk factor or initial state yields disparate outcomes across development. For instance, abuse may or may not lead to severe malaptation, depending on a host of intervening factors; extremes of inhibited temperament may produce shyness and social withdrawal, but other, healthier outcomes are also possible, depending on the presence or absence of additional risk or protective factors (see Cicchetti & Rogosch, 1996). Both equifinality and multifinality imply that linear models of association and simplistic categorical conceptions of disorder are incapable of facilitating full understanding of child and adolescent psychopathology. Indeed, such simplistic models may actually be misleading.

Second, DP models place emphasis on person-centered research designs, in which the typical practice of examining global effects of one or more risk/protective variables across an entire sample or population is supplemented by consideration of unique subgroups—whether defined by genotypes, personality variables, socialization practices, neighborhoods, or other key factors—and their particular developmental journeys across the life span (Bergman, von Eye, & Magnusson, 2006). Framed from a slightly different perspective, developmental continuities and discontinuities may well differ across homogeneous subgroups of participants. Even in variable-centered research, key moderator variables and mediator processes must always be considered (e.g., Fairchild & MacKinnon, 2009; Hinshaw, 2002; Howe, Reiss, & Yuh, 2002; Kraemer, Stice, Kazdin, Offord, & Kupfer, 2001) to ensure that (a) results are applicable to subsets of participants grouped on the basis of the moderator variable of interest (e.g., male versus female participants, those from different ethnic groups, those with different patterns of comorbidity) and (b) underlying mechanisms of change are considered explicitly.

Third, given the rapid growth in recent years of genetic and genomic models and brain imaging methods, DP researchers in the 21st century must pay increasing attention to the role of the brain—and to neuroscientific principles in general—to account for the wide range of extant pathologies and their devastating effects (Cicchetti & Curtis, 2006). Clearly, we have come a long way from the mid-20th century, when biological and temperamental factors were virtually ignored in accounts of child development and psychopathology.

As noted in the introductory chapter to the first edition (Hinshaw, 2008), a basic mathematical calculation may help to elucidate the underlying complexities here: Adults have approximately 100 billion neurons in their brains; children are born with even higher numbers, perhaps double that figure. Indeed a major developmental "task" over the earliest years of postnatal development is the pruning and migration of such neurons into a working, functional brain. But what is the rate of neural development during the 40 weeks of human gestation? To figure this out, one must divide 200 billion (a fair estimate of the number of neurons with which an infant is born) by the number of seconds in 40 weeks. The result—of dividing the numerator of 2 times 10 to the 11th power (the number of neurons) by the denominator of 2.4192 times 10 to the 7th power (the number of seconds)—is the astonishing figure that, on average, the embryo and fetus are producing approximately 8,000 new neurons *every second* throughout the entire course of prenatal development. This average is not constant, of course, given that the neural tube and brain do not even form for some weeks. Thus, in some crucial periods, this figure is even higher (see Giedd, Shaw, Wallace, Gogtay, & Lenroot, 2006, for additional information on the precise timing of neural development across pregnancy and childhood). Rates of connectivity in the developing brain yield numbers that are exponentially higher. As the cortex matures, revealing characteristic patterns of thickening and thinning, and as cortical neurons form rich and lasting connections with other brain regions, the number of synaptic connections goes into the trillions and beyond.

Given such staggering statistics, a key question involves the joint influence of genes, hormones, nutrition, life experiences, and contextual influences on the plasticity of the brain's development across childhood and adolescence. Without consideration of transactional processes, multilevel models, computational frameworks, gene-environment interplay, and a host of technological and conceptual advances related to the overall field of developmental neuroscience, we will not be able to solve the problem of gaining deep understanding of relevant mechanisms (see also Blakemore, Burnett, & Dahl, 2010; Romer & Walker, 2007; and Steinberg, 2010, for considerations of adolescent brain and behavioral development).

Key concepts and principles related to DP have been stated and restated across a large number of articles, chapters, and books. Indeed, detailed discussion of any one of them could easily fill a volume unto itself. The challenge for the current chapter is to encapsulate these tenets, in the service of foreshadowing and illuminating content on specific risk factors and specific disorders that fill the rest of the book. Because explanations of these concepts too often remain at a rather global and abstract level, leaving unresolved precisely what they suggest for the investigation and treatment of behavioral and emotional disorders, I try, in the following section, to bring these percepts to life.

## NORMAL AND ATYPICAL DEVELOPMENT ARE MUTUALLY INFORMATIVE

As opposed to the study of discrete, mutually exclusive categories of "disorder," DP models emphasize that phenomena defined as abnormal represent aberrations in normal developmental pathways and processes. Hence, without a full understanding of typical development, the study of pathology will remain incomplete and decontextualized. Taking just one example, illuminating the nature of attention-deficit/hyperactivity disorder (ADHD) requires thorough understanding of the normative development of attention, impulse control, and self-regulation (Nigg, 2006; Nigg, Hinshaw, & Huang-Pollack, 2006; Chapter 12). Similarly, investigations of autism must be fully integrated with the development of interpersonal awareness and empathy, which typically takes place over the first several years of life. Without such developmental templates, understanding autism may become an empty exercise of counting symptoms (for a developmental approach, see Dawson & Toth, 2006; Chapter 20). Additional instances exist across all forms of disordered emotion and behavior. Currently, few doubt the wisdom of understanding developmental sequences and processes associated with healthy outcomes as extremely relevant to the elucidation and explication of pathology.

Yet the process is conceptualized as a two-way street, with the corresponding view that investigations of pathological conditions—sometimes referred to as *adaptational failures* in DP terms (see Sroufe, 1997)—can and should provide a unique perspective on normal developmental mechanisms. In other words, the study of disrupted developmental progressions illuminates our understanding of what is normative.

Overall, this core tenet of DP—of the mutual interplay between the study of normality and pathology, along with the perspective that progress in each domain is dependent on progress in the other—is now widely held. Neurology abounds with relevant examples. For example, there is a long tradition utilizing the study of disrupted neural systems to enhance understanding of healthy brain functioning and vice versa. "Split-brain" patients (those who have had their cerebral hemispheres separated to provide relief from specific neurological disorders) provide unprecedented insights into normative brain processes, such that separable functions and even "personalities" subserved by the right versus left hemispheres become evident as a function of the pathology and resultant surgery. In parallel, famous case studies such as HM, in which key brain structures/regions have been surgically removed (in his case the hippocampus), greatly facilitate knowledge about human memory systems (see Gazzaniga, Ivry, & Mangun, 2009). Cicchetti and Curtis (2006) provide lucid detail on neuroscience-related approaches. For a specific example, the study of phenylketonuria (PKU) has implications for elaborating the normative development of executive functions (Diamond, Prevor, Callender, & Druin, 1997).

How might this perspective inform our understanding of psychological or psychiatric disorders that are the core subject matter of DP? In other words, beyond neurological conditions and formulations per se, can investigations of pathology inform normal development? Once again, it is now commonly accepted that the more we know about basic emotion, cognition, attention, memory, social awareness, self-regulation, and the like, the more investigations of psychopathology can benefit. Almost no form of mental disorder constitutes a clearly demarcated, qualitatively distinct category or taxon, meaning that processes applying to individuals near the center of the bell curve are likely to apply to those further out on the continuum as well. Nearly all forms of mental pathology appear consistent with a quantitative, dimensional perspective (Beauchaine, 2003), emphasizing the need for flow of information from normal developmental pathways to pathological functioning.

But what about the other direction? Specifically, what has been learned about normal developmental processes from studies of child and adolescent psychopathology? At first glance, the situation doesn't seem to be as heuristic as that in neurology; it may be that we have *not* gained the kinds of dramatic insights about typical psychological development from studies of child and adolescent psychopathology that have been realized in "harder" scientific endeavors. In other words, the complexity of mental disorders may limit parallels to more simply caused neurological conditions. In short, there are few behavioral and emotional equivalents to the surgical procedures of creating lesions in certain brain tracts or single-gene forms of pathology such as PKU.

Yet consider the work on autism by Baron-Cohen (2000). Relevant findings suggest that the lack of social connectedness experienced by individuals with autism may relate to a failure in attainment of a basic "theory of mind," which deals with the developing realization that other humans have mental states that differ from one's own. Most normal 4-year-olds can master theory-of-mind tests, suggesting that basic social understanding is predicated on a domain-specific cognitive module that, once operative, occurs almost automatically. On the other hand, a high percentage of youth with autistic disorder, even those with high levels of intellectual functioning, do not "pass" such psychological tests, suggesting that they have not come to the core realization that fellow humans have different minds and different psychological perspectives from their own.

I note that a number of individuals with high-functioning autism can eventually learn to pass the kinds of experimental tests used to test for theory of mind. Through effortful processing, they come to deduce that other children and adults have a different understanding of events in the world than they do. Yet this effortful skill does not mean that their social interactions become smooth, effortless, and "automatic." Indeed, the laborious kinds of calculations and inferences made by people with high-functioning autism to understand interpersonal dynamics are not usually accompanied by perfectly functional social interactions (Grandin, 2006). A key implication is that "normal" social-cognitive and social functioning is highly automatic and qualitatively distinct from the ability to deduce social situations analytically more typical in autism—which is time consuming and not perceived as skillful by peers. Thus, disruptions in social cognition and social performance in persons with autism may help to clarify the automatic and highly developed nature of the social cognitions and processes that underlie skilled interpersonal performance in normal development. Parenthetically, I note that current views of theory of mind posit that at least some aspects of understanding false beliefs appear far earlier in life, even toddlerhood and infancy, further challenging developmental models of both normative and atypical development (see, for example, Sodian, 2011).

Another example pertains to work on the reward sensitivity of individuals with ADHD (e.g., Sagvolden, Johansen, Aase, & Russell, 2005). Here, considerable evidence reveals that in people with this condition, large performance decrements occur when rewards are suddenly stopped, presumably related to a dopaminergically mediated problem with responding during extinction. More recent research (Volkow et al., 2009) reveals, in fact, that never-medicated adults with ADHD have markedly deficient numbers of dopamine receptors and transporters in reward and motivational brain pathways than do non-ADHD comparison subjects. This finding has served to revive "motivational" theories regarding the origins of ADHD, revealing a biologically driven undersensitivity to reward. Not only is extrinsic reward necessary to enhance task performance of affected individuals, but reward cessation would be expected to lead to larger-than-normal drop-off of task performance. In all, these insights foster understanding of basic developmental processes and mechanisms underlying dysregulated attention and impulse control, such that ADHD-related reward processes may well elucidate normative patterns of motivation, persistence, and effort.

A third instance, noted briefly, pertains to the horrific "experiments of nature" that occur when infants and toddlers are subjected to brutal institutionalization and lack of human contact during the earliest years of development (for review, see O'Connor, 2006). The development of specific symptom patterns (e.g., inattention and overactivity, as opposed to aggression; see Kreppner, O'Connor, Rutter, & the English and Romanian Adoptees Study Team, 2001), and the extent of social and cognitive "catch-up" following removal from the institutions, are extremely informative about normal-range development of secure relationships and cognitive performance. Such work has even incorporated experimental methods to understand whether in-home foster placements can mitigate the effects of early deprivation in terms of cognitive growth (Nelson et al., 2007). Indeed, for the previously institutionalized girls in this randomized trial, foster care placement led to improvements in girls' internalizing behavior patterns, mediated by the gaining of attachment security via the change from institutional care to family placements (McLaughlin, Zeanah, Fox, & Nelson, 2012). Thus, even in a harshly abandoned and deprived sample, attachment processes are implicated in reductions of anxiety and depression. Mediators of competence in more normative samples are still open to exploration.

## DEVELOPMENTAL CONTINUITIES AND DISCONTINUITIES

With this principle, it is commonly asserted that DP models must emphasize both continuous and discontinuous processes at work in the development of pathology. What precisely does this mean? Taking the example of externalizing and antisocial behavior, it is well known that antisocial behaviors show strong stability across time—meaning that correlations are substantial between early measures of aggressive and antisocial tendencies and those made at later times. In other words, the rank order remains relatively preserved, such that the most aggressive individuals at early points in development remain high in such behavior patterns across development. But does this mean that the precise forms of externalizing antisocial behavior remain constant? Clearly not, given that those children with extremes of temper tantrums and defiance during the toddler and preschool years are not especially likely to exhibit high rates of tantrums during adolescence. Rather, they have a high likelihood of displaying physical aggression in grade school, covert antisocial behaviors in preadolescence, and various forms of delinquency by their teen years (e.g., sexual assault, property crime, violence), followed by adult manifestations of antisocial behavior after adolescence (e.g., Moffitt, 1993, 2006). In short, continuities exist, but these are *heterotypic* in nature, as the actual form of the underlying antisocial trait changes form with development.

Another important consideration is that patterns of continuity may differ considerably across separable subgroups that display different developmental patterns or trajectories. Not all highly aggressive or antisocial children remain so, as some are prone to desist with the transition to adolescence. Others, however—the so-called early starter or life-course-persistent subgroup—maintain high rates through at least early adulthood (although, as just noted, the specific forms of the antisocial actions may well change with development). In addition, a large subset does not display major externalizing problems in childhood but instead shows a sharp increase with adolescence (for a review, see Moffitt, 2006). Understanding such continuities and discontinuities via homogeneous subgroups is likely to yield greater understanding than basic plots of overall curves of "growth" across the population. Sophisticated statistical strategies (e.g., growth mixture modeling; group-based trajectory modeling) are increasingly used to facilitate the search for separable trajectories or classes defined on patterns of change of the relevant dependent variable, leading to major insights about predictors, moderators, and mediators and emphasizing the major heterogeneity in multiple aspects of psychopathological functioning (see Muthén & Muthén, 2000; Nagin & Odgers, 2010a, 2010b).

## Multiple Levels of Analysis

The greatest potential for progress (and complexity) in the DP field is made when investigators travel back and forth between "micro" and "macro" levels, including intermediate steps or pathways, to understand mechanisms underlying the development of adjustment and maladjustment. The essential task for the next generations of DP investigators is to link events at the level of the gene (e.g., genetic polymorphisms; transcription and translation; epigenetic influences) to neurotransmission and neuroanatomical development, and subsequently into individual differences in temperament, social cognition, and emotional response patterns (for detailed discussion, see Cicchetti, 2008). At the same time, such bottom-up conceptions must be supplemented by top-down understanding of the ways in which family interaction patterns, peer relations, school factors, and neighborhood/community variables influence the developing, plastic brain, even at the level of gene expression, invoking the concept of epigenetic influences. Overall, progress in understanding pathological behavior will require multidisciplinary efforts in which investigators ranging from geneticists and biochemists, clinicians focusing on individual pathology, experts on family and neighborhood processes, investigators of clinical service systems, and public health officials must work collaboratively and in increasingly diversified ways. The phenomena under consideration are too complex, too dynamic, and too multifaceted to be understood by focusing exclusively on psychobiological processes, family factors, peer processes, or cultural factors in isolation. Performing the necessary kinds of investigations often mandates large scale, complex, and interdisciplinary/multidisciplinary work, necessitating collaborations across traditional academic boundaries. Although such collaboration is not simple, these kinds of efforts are undoubtedly where the payoffs will lie (for a key example, see Caspi, Hariri, Holmes, Uher, & Moffitt, 2010).

## Risk and Protective Factors

The key focus of a discipline such as DP—with the term *psychopathology* embedded in its title—is to discover the nature of behavioral and emotional problems, syndromes, and disorders. Many different definitional schemes have been invoked to define and explain psychopathological functioning, with none able to provide a complete picture (see Hinshaw, 2007, Chapter 1). Indeed, it is clear that biological vulnerabilities, psychological handicaps, environmental potentiators, and cultural-level norms all play a major role in defining and understanding behavioral manifestations that are considered abnormal and/or pathological in a particular social context. Risk factors (and constitutional vulnerabilities) are those antecedent variables that predict such dysfunction, and the ultimate goal is to discover those variables that are both malleable and potentially causal of the disorder in question (Kraemer et al., 1997).

Yet disordered behavior is not uniform, and risk factors are not inevitable predictors. Being female is a protective factor against most forms of psychopathology in the first decade of life but serves as a risk factor for internalizing conditions during adolescence (e.g., Hinshaw, 2009). As noted earlier, maltreatment is sometimes but not always a risk factor for later pathology. Furthermore, for most individuals with diagnosable forms of mental disorder, symptoms and impairments tend to wax and wane over time. It is often difficult to know when dysfunction precisely begins; it is also quite normative for periods of serious problems to be followed by healthier adjustment. In fact, the myth that mental disturbance is uniformly debilitating, handicapping, and permanent is a key reason for the continuing stigmatization of mental illness (Hinshaw, 2006, 2007).

*Resilience* is the term often used to define unexpectedly good outcomes, or competence, despite the presence of adversity or risk (Luthar, 2006; Sapienza & Masten, 2011). Indeed, the concept of multifinality, noted earlier, directly implies that, depending on a host of biological, environmental, and contextual factors, variegated outcomes will emanate from common risk factors, with the distinct possibility of positive adaptation in some cases.

DP is therefore centrally involved in the search for what have been called *protective factors*—those variables and processes that mitigate risk and promote more successful outcomes than would be expected. Yet controversy surrounds the construct of resilience, the nature of protective factors, and the nature of competent functioning (see Luthar & Brown, 2007; Masten, Burt, & Coatsworth, 2006). In fact, some have claimed that there is no need to invoke a set of special processes that are involved, given that a certain percentage of any sample exposed to a risk factor will show better-than-expected outcomes and that protective factors are all too often simply the opposite poles of what we typically think of as risk variables or vulnerabilities (e.g., higher rather than lower IQ; easier rather than more difficult temperament; warm and structured rather than cold and lax parenting). Even so, it is crucial to examine processes that may be involved in promoting competence and strength rather than disability and despair, given that such processes may be harnessed for prevention efforts and may provide key conceptual leads toward the understanding of both pathology and competence.

Indeed, recent advances in the study of resilience show that some aspects of resilient functioning have psychobiological and even genetic underpinnings and that a systemic, transactional, and even epigenetic model is needed to understand the multipronged nature of resilience-enhancing processes (see review in Sapienza & Masten, 2011). Furthermore, Luthar and Brown (2007) remind us that relationships are central to any conception of resilience, despite current work in psychobiological undercurrents. In short, gaining understanding of why some children born into poverty fare well in adolescence and adulthood, why some individuals with alleles that tend to confer risk for pathological outcomes do not evidence psychopathology, why some youth with difficult temperamental features develop into highly competent adults, and why some people who lack secure attachments or enriching environments during their early years nonetheless show academic and social competence, is essential for knowledge of both health and maladjustment. It is not just a luxury but a necessity to investigate positive developmental outcomes. Competence can shed light on the pathways that deflect away from pathology and, in so doing, may provide otherwise hidden insights into the necessary developmental components of adjustment versus maladjustment.

## Reciprocal, Transactional Models

Linear models of causation, in which static psychological variables are assumed to respond in invariant ways to the influence of risk or protective factors, are not adequate to the task of explaining psychopathology and its development (see Richters, 1997, who highlights that quite different explanatory systems are needed to deal with open systems such as individual people). Pathways from childhood to adolescent and adult functioning are marked by reciprocal patterns or chains, in which children influence parents, teachers, and peers, who shape the further individual development of the child. Such mutually interactive processes can themselves escalate over time, leading to what are termed *transactional models*. Furthermore, some developmental processes appear to operate via cascading, escalating chains (Masten et al., 2006; Masten & Cicchetti, 2010), whereas others may, as just noted, be dampened or altered by mediating, protective factors. Given the strong potential for nonlinear change in all of the above processes, dynamic systems models are needed to help explicate core developmental phenomena (see Granic & Hollenstein, 2006).

To be specific, it is now well known that a great many cognitive and personality outcomes are at least moderately heritable, meaning that genetic factors explain a sizable proportion of individual differences in the trait, attribute, or disorder in question. But via gene-environment correlations, environments (genetically associated with the trait in question) may amplify the expression of the trait, and individuals may seek or evoke environmental responses that further promote the trait's unfolding. Furthermore, as noted explicitly in Chapter 3, early-maturing brain regions that give rise to expression of key emotional and behavioral characteristics may influence the developmental maturation of other, later-maturing regions; environmental events and factors may actually aid in the "turning on" of genes that further reinforce similar neural and behavioral actions, through epigenetic processes. In addition, certain genotypes may become expressed only in the context of certain environmental factors, signifying the operation of gene-environment interactions (Rutter et al., 2006). Finally, as just noted, processes of development may operate in highly nonlinear ways, requiring a new set of tools and conceptual models for understanding change processes (Granic & Hollenstein, 2006). Sensitive data analytic strategies and innovative research designs are crucial tools for fostering greater understanding of such nonlinear phenomena.

## THE IMPORTANCE OF CONTEXT

A key tenet of DP, directly related to the above points, is that family, school-related, neighborhood, and wider cultural contexts are central for the unfolding of aberrant as well as adaptive behavior. This point cannot be overemphasized: What may have been adaptive behaviors at one point in human evolutionary history may be maladaptive in current times, given the major environmental and cultural changes that render certain genetically mediated traits far less advantageous than previously. As just two examples, consider [1] the storage of fat in times of uncertain meals and sudden need for survival-related activity, and [2] the presence of undue anxiety in relation to certain feared stimuli when conditions have markedly changed with respect to indoor, sedentary lifestyles. There are few absolutes in terms of either behavior patterns that are inherently maladaptive or risk factors that inevitably yield dysfunction. Cultural settings and context are all-important for shaping and even defining healthy versus unhealthy adaptation.

Similarly, key environmental factors (such as parenting styles) are not always uniformly positive or uniformly negative in terms of their developmental effects. Deater-Deckard and Dodge (1997) have shown, for example, that harsh, author-itarian parenting predicts antisocial behavior in white, middle-class children but not necessarily in African-American families. (On the other hand, parenting that crosses the line into abuse is uniformly harmful.) Many forms of mental disorder are present at roughly equivalent rates across multiple cultures, revealing key evidence for universality; but the effects of risk or protective factors may differ markedly depending on their developmental timing, the family and social context in which they are experienced by the developing child, and the niche or *space* that exists in a given culture for their expression and resolution (see, for example, Serafica & Vargas, 2006). In short, the DP perspective tells us clearly that setting and context are all-important (Cicchetti, 2006).

This discussion throws into sharp relief the surge of interest, in recent years, regarding the specific effects environments play, once biological vulnerabilities are taken into account. Rutter, Pickles, Murray, and Eaves (2001) provide a masterful account of how to understand specific, causal environmental forces and factors; Jaffee et al. (2012) provide an extremely useful guide to how nonexperimental designs and recent statistical advances can help facilitate just such understanding. As noted by Caspi et al. (2010), the leap in knowledge between environmental correlates and environmental "pathogens" (i.e., environmental factors that are causal) is a large one.

Along these lines, the process known as gene-environment interaction, discussed in more detail in Chapter 3 (and in the comprehensive volume of Dodge & Rutter, 2011), remains a hot topic. After groundbreaking research a decade ago on this topic (e.g., Caspi et al., 2003) revealing that genotypes may yield pathological outcomes only in certain environmental contexts, meta-analyses have challenged the size and strength of such findings (e.g., Risch et al., 2009). However, in an incisive rejoinder, Caspi et al. (2010) examine animal as well as human models of gene products and genetically mediated vulnerabilities, laying the groundwork for much-needed psychobiological pathways through which such moderated effects may occur. They also make the key point that many large-sample investigations—which receive the most "weight" in meta-analytic efforts—tend to utilize inferior assessments of environmental influences, such as those that are self-reported and retrospective. More precise environmental measures, in smaller studies, are thus discounted. Finally, Caspi et al. (2010) highlight that the serotonin transporter gene, implicated in a host of gene-environment interaction findings, exerts its effects not by conferring risk for any particular form of psychopathology but by enhancing sensitivity to key aspects of the environment—revealing the core DP principle that "nature" and "nurture" cannot fundamentally be separated.

Importantly, current models are moving away from the idea that certain genetic configurations are inevitably "risk" factors for psychopathology. Some, in fact, may yield better-than-expected outcomes in optimal contexts. In other words, they may serve as *plasticity* factors as opposed to risk factors per se, yielding differential susceptibility to both positive and negative environmental settings (e.g., Belsky & Pluess, 2009).

## Equifinality and Multifinality

As suggested earlier, there is overwhelming evidence that multiple pathways exist to both health and illness. It is a myth to think that all individuals displaying symptoms of a given mental disorder "got there" through similar mechanisms and processes. We know, for instance, that the broad syndrome of depression may emanate from heritable risks in some cases, from severe life losses and stressors in others, from the interaction of the two in a great many more, and from other early or contemporaneous risk factors in still others. ADHD, for example, is substantially heritable but the constituent symptomatology may also emerge from low birthweight, severe early deprivation, effects of teratogens like nicotine or tobacco in utero, or even from what were formerly thought to be low levels of environmental lead (Barkley, 2006; Nigg, 2006). In short, *equifinality*—the presence of multiple pathways leading to apparently similar outcome states—clearly operates with regard to the major entities of mental disturbance that we now recognize (Cicchetti & Rogosch, 1996).

In parallel, although inhibited temperament in infancy and toddlerhood is clearly predictive of risk for subsequent social anxiety, there is far from a 1:1 correspondence. Other risk and protective factors, including the presence of childrearing environments that gently but firmly "push" the child out of inhibited, withdrawn behavior patterns, may deflect any inevitable association between early inhibition and later internalizing conditions (see Kagan, 1997, and Chapter 7). Similarly, child maltreatment does not lead to a uniform set of outcomes but may instead yield a range of subsequent behavioral and emotional patterns even when the type or severity of abuse is held constant (Cicchetti & Valentino, 2006). Hence, through processes of *multifinality*, complex causal chains of influence render the operation of early risk factors as probabilistic rather than deterministic. In cases of pathology, the chain tends to intensify and widen, in a process termed *developmental cascades* (Masten & Cicchetti, 2010).

Thus, the DP model emphasizes malleability, flexibility, and plasticity in development, although the presence of multiple risk factors is clearly linked to lowered chances of recovery. Core issues in this regard involve, first, the attempt to disentangle the many potential developmental influences that may tip the individual toward health and competence versus disorder and failure; and second, the necessity of incorporating what is termed *probabilistic epigenesis* (Gottlieb & Willoughby, 2006) into causal models. This term means that genes do not provide a one-way causal influence on neural structures and behavior, because of highly interactive, reciprocal, and bidirectional influences with epigenetic factors (e.g., other brain structures and products, behavioral patterns, and environmental influences). Here we see that several DP principles—for example, nonlinear causal patterns, reciprocal/transactional models, and the importance of context—are closely linked. In an elegant musical metaphor, Boyce (2006) presents the notion of "symphonic causation" to illustrate the confluence of biological and contextual influences on development.

## PSYCHOBIOLOGICAL PRINCIPLES AND DISCOVERIES

The genomic era is upon us, and advances in brain imaging research and clinical techniques have made the developing brain far more accessible to scientific view than ever before (e.g., Giedd et al., 2006; Rende & Waldman, 2006). Although it is mistaken, as noted earlier, to give primacy to any given level of analysis in a DP perspective—brain, contextual, or other (Cicchetti & Toth, 2009)—we have asked contributors to pay particular attention to psychobiological factors and processes in their coverage.

Part of the reason is historical: Family systemic and environmental views dominated the field for much of the 20th century, and recent work on a range of psychobiological processes is not always featured in reviews and texts (Boyce, 2006). Another issue pertains to explanatory power: We now know that without understanding the potential effects of genes, physiological processes, and biological risk factors on psychopathology, we have little hope of understanding the most severe forms of disorder. Because the brain is remarkably plastic and because context influences biological unfolding, we have—as noted throughout this chapter—asked authors to emphasize contextualization of the psychobiological perspectives they present. In fact, reductionistic accounts of the primacy of single genes, the inevitable predictability of later functioning from early temperament, or the "placement" of psychopathology completely inside brightly colored brain images on journal or chapter pages are as short-sighted as the exclusively environmental accounts of psychopathology that dominated a half-century ago, such as the blaming of autism on emotional refrigeration by parents or schizophrenia by schizophregenic mothers.

## SUMMARY

Clearly, the development of psychopathological functioning is multidetermined, complex, interactive, transactional, and in many if not most instances nonlinear. It is nearly impossible to imagine otherwise, given the staggering complexity of the brain and the myriad influences, ranging from the microsocial to the macrosocial, that impinge on the developing infant, toddler, and child. For those who like problems and solutions wrapped in neat packages, the study of DP will undoubtedly be a frustrating endeavor, perhaps even unfathomable. On the other hand, for those who are intrigued by the diverse clinical presentations of various pathological conditions in childhood and adolescence; who are fascinated with how much remains to be learned about antecedent conditions and maintaining factors; who are possessed by an intense "need to know" about the underlying mechanisms of the conditions discussed in this volume; and who realize the need to consider healthy outcomes and competence as well as maladaptation, the DP perspective is a vital framework for the rapidly growing scientific enterprise linking normal and atypical development. Longitudinal, multilevel investigations are often required to gain the types of knowledge needed to understand psychopathology and competence from a developmental perspective, with the potential of high yield for developmental science and for informing prevention and intervention efforts. The study of DP is ever expanding, engaging scientists from large numbers of disciplines and perspectives. Progress is emerging quickly, but the territory to explore is vast and the road ahead is long.

## A GUIDE TO THE BOOK'S CONTENTS

Immediately following this chapter, Theodore P. Beauchaine, Daniel N. Klein, Nora L. Erickson, and Alyssa L. Norris (Chapter 2) provide a history of attempts to classify the vast domain of child and adolescent psychopathology, culminating in the newest editions of the *Diagnostic and Statistical Manual of Mental Disorders* and the *International Classification of Diseases*. This historical perspective throws into sharp relief the tensions between categorical versus continuous conceptions of psychopathological behavior and the still-vast territories to be investigated in order to reconcile basic science and current classifications. In Chapter 3, Theodore P. Beauchaine and Lisa M. Gatzke-Kopp provide rich detail on gene-environment interplay and on psychobiological forces more generally, given their strong implications in the genesis of child and adolescent psychopathology. This material is essential background for many of the disorder-specific chapters that follow later in the volume.

In the next section (Part II), Bruce E. Compas and Charissa Andreotti (Chapter 4) lead off by writing about cultural and contextual factors linked to the developmental of psychopathology. As discussed in the present chapter, such influences deserve equal billing with psychobiological factors and forces in current DP conceptualizations. In Chapter 5, Sara R. Jaffee and Andrea Kohn Maikovich-Fong cover maltreatment, which is known to be a clearly "environmental" contributor to psychopathology but one that (a) correlates and interacts with biological vulnerabilities and (b) may well produce biological as well as psychological consequences. Then, in Chapter 6, Emily Neuhaus and Theodore P. Beauchaine discuss the role of impulsivity as a risk factor for diverse forms of externalizing psychopathology. Providing rich historical coverage, they debunk earlier myths about the neural underpinnings of impulsivity and bring to life a host of core DP constructs. Chapter 7, by Jerome Kagan, is a witty and engaging account of behavioral inhibition and its consequences for a range of internalizing behavior patterns. This work also highlights many core DP principles, serving as a needed antidote to reductionism, either environmental or biological. In Chapter 8 Bruce J. Ellis, Marco Del Giudice, and Elizabeth A. Shirtcliff detail how exquisitely adaptive the human stress response system is, and the implications of this adaptability for both vulnerability to and protection from psychopathology. In Chapter 9, Nicole A. Crocker, Susanna L. Fryer, and Sarah N. Mattson discuss teratogens—substances either (a) transmitted from a pregnant mother to her embryo or fetus, or (b) encountered in the postnatal environment—that promote dysfunction in the developing organism. This work emphasizes the probabilistic rather than the deterministic nature of this pernicious risk factor. In Chapter 10, Katherine Shannon Bowen and Lisa M. Gatzke-Kopp cover various forms of brain injury, with emphasis on risk for dysfunction and potential recovery. This chapter deals with the specific "pathogens" of physical trauma and hypoxia, the construct of neural plasticity, and the potential for genetic factors to interact with trauma in the development of maladaptation. In Chapter 11, Pamela M. Cole, Sarah E. Hall, and Nastassia J. Hajal write a theoretically rich account of emotion dysregulation and its implications for psychopathological outcomes. In their view, emotions are inherently activating and organizing, but if attempts at their regulation are insufficient, if emotions are displayed in context-inappropriate fashion, or if emotions change either too quickly or too slowly, implications for dysfunction become apparent.

Part III covers disruptive or externalizing conditions. In Chapter 12, Joel Nigg provides rich coverage on the core processes of inattention, impulsivity, and hyperactivity that characterize ADHD, with an integration of psychological and psychobiological processes—and of both genetic and often-neglected environmental risk factors for this condition. Explicitly embracing the core tenets of DP, this chapter emphasizes the great need for integrated theoretical models in future work on this prevalent and distressing disorder. Chapter 13, by Irwin D. Waldman and Benjamin B. Lahey, presents a comprehensive, multilevel, integrative view of the development of aggressive and antisocial behavior, with specific reference to the diagnostic categories of oppositional defiant disorder and conduct disorder. A key issue for this domain of inquiry is the sheer number of pertinent risk factors, spanning intra-individual, familial, and wider contextual variables; Waldman and Lahey's integrative account is a welcome antidote to the often-chaotic feel of literature in this area. Thomas J. Dishion and Kristina Hiatt Racer, in Chapter 14, discuss principles and concepts underlying the development of antisocial personality, taking a life-span perspective as they do so, and featuring interplay among the myriad risk factors (individual, parental, peer-related, neighborhood level) that together yield adult antisocial outcomes and in some cases psychopathy. Chapter 15, by Sandra A. Brown, Kristin Tomlinson, and Jennifer Winward, discusses developmental trajectories of alcohol and substance problems, an area ripe for all of the DP principles discussed in this chapter, with major public health implications given the scope and consequences of early drug use and abuse.

Next, Part IV features internalizing conditions. Chapter 16, by Carl F. Weems and Wendy K. Silverman, covers the range of anxiety disorders, providing an integrative perspective on their origins and maintenance. Building from dimensional conceptions of anxiety and fear, they emphasize genetic and psychophysiological factors, social learning and cognitive processes, social and interpersonal variables, and interactions across these levels. Daniel N. Klein, Autumn J. Kujawa, Sarah R. Black, and Allison T. Pennock comprehensively review, in Chapter 17, known risk factors for and developmental issues related to child and adolescent depression. Covering the wide-ranging precursors to depressive outcomes (e.g., maladaptive cognitive patterns, stress reactivity, genetic vulnerability, disrupted parent–child relationships, to name some of the more salient), they provide an integrative developmental model. In Chapter 18, Sheila E. Crowell, Erin A. Kaufman, and Mark F. Lenzenweger provide essential commentary on borderline personality, self-injurious behavior, and their developmental antecedents. They emphasize genetic and neural risk factors, the clear role of parenting disruptions, and interactions among them, concluding that borderline personality and intentional self-injury constitute extremes of impulse control problems, particularly in relation to severe stressors. Note that the placement of this chapter in Part IV is somewhat arbitrary, given the admixture of dysphoric, internalizing features, and disinhibited, externalizing symptoms involved in these behavior patterns.

Finally, the coverage in Part V focuses on several additional, extremely important disorders. Bipolar disorder—also representing an extreme blend of externalizing and internalizing features—is the topic of Chapter 19, written by Joseph C. Blader and Gabrielle A. Carlson. This detailed chapter lays out the complex interactions and transactions (and strong heritability) of bipolar disorder, dealing directly with core developmental issues related to assessment, diagnosis, and symptom presentation. Chapter 20, written by Susan Faja and Geraldine Dawson, features autism spectrum disorder, an extremely "hot" area of both basic and applied research. This chapter presents a balanced and detailed perspective on the most promising of recent conceptual models, along with the promise of early intervention. Schizophrenia can and does exist in children, with major increases in prevalence throughout adolescence. In Chapter 21, Robert F. Asarnow tackles the important developmental issues related to, and the strong psychobiologic roots of, schizophrenia-spectrum conditions. Finally, Chapter 22, authored by Eric Stice and Cara Bohon, covers anorexia nervosa, bulimia nervosa, and binge eating disorder, once again featuring processes spanning psychobiological and psychosocial factors in such conditions while providing strong emphasis on a developmental neuroscience perspective.

As readers begin the rest of this volume, we highlight that smooth, packaged, easily digestible accounts are not found within these pages, as the kinds of reciprocal, interactive, cascading, and integrative models needed to facilitate further understanding are far from simple or linear. Yet for the next generation of investigators, clinicians, and policy makers—who, we hope will carry with them an appreciation of the systemic models and transactional processes embedded in DP conceptualizations—there can be no more fascinating venture. The study of atypical development is complex and clinically relevant, with the potential for elucidating the processes by which normal development occurs and for informing sorely needed intervention and prevention strategies. The questions herein are among the most important issues in all of science. Welcome to the journey ahead!

## REFERENCES

Achenbach, T. M. (1974). *Developmental psychopathology*. New York, NY: Ronald Press.

Barkley, R. A. (2006). *Attention deficit hyperactivity disorder: A handbook for diagnosis and treatment* (3rd ed.). New York, NY: Guilford Press.

Baron-Cohen, S. (2000). Theory of mind and autism: A fifteen-year review. In S. Baron-Cohen, H. Tager-Flusberg, & D. Cohen (Eds.), *Understanding other minds: Perspectives from developmental cognitive neuroscience* (pp. 3–20). Oxford, UK: Oxford University Press.

Beauchaine, T. P. (2003). Taxonometrics and developmental psychopathology. *Development and Psychopathology, 15*, 501–527.

Beauchaine, T. P., & Hinshaw, S. P. (Eds.). (2008). *Child and adolescent psychopathology*. Hoboken, NJ: Wiley.

Belsky, J., & Pluess, M. (2009). Beyond diathesis stress: Differential susceptibility to environmental influences. *Psychological Bulletin, 135*, 885–908.

Bergman, L. R., von Eye, A., & Magnusson, D. (2006). Person-oriented research strategies in developmental psychopathology. In D. Cicchetti & D. J. Cohen (Eds.), *Developmental psychopathology: Theory and method* (2nd ed., Vol. 1, pp. 850–888). Hoboken, NJ: Wiley.

Blakemore, S., Burnett, S., & Dahl, R. E. (2010). The role of puberty in the developing adolescent brain. *Human Brain Mapping, 31*, 926–933.

Boyce, T. (2006). Symphonic causation and the origins of childhood psychopathology. In D. Cicchetti & D. J. Cohen (Eds.), *Developmental psychopathology: Developmental neuroscience* (2nd ed., Vol. 2, pp. 797–817). Hoboken, NJ: Wiley.

Caspi, A., Hariri, A. R., Holmes, A., Uher, R., & Moffitt, T. E. (2010). Genetic sensitivity to the environment: The case of the serotonin transporter gene and its implications for studying complex diseases and traits. *American Journal of Psychiatry, 167*, 509–527.

Caspi, A., Sugden, K., Moffitt, T. E., Taylor, A., Craig, I. W., Harrington, H.... Poulton, R. (2003). Influence of life stress on depression: Moderation by a polymorphism in the 5-HTT gene. *Science, 301*, 386–389.

Cicchetti, D. (1984). The emergence of developmental psychopathology. *Child Development, 55*, 1–7.

Cicchetti, D. (1990). A historical perspective on the discipline of developmental psychopathology. In J. Rolf, A. Masten, D. Cicchetti, K. Nuechterlein, & S. Weintraub (Eds.), *Risk and protective factors in the development of psychopathology* (pp. 2–28). New York, NY: Cambridge University Press.

Cicchetti, D. (2006). Developmental psychopathology. In D. Cicchetti & D. J. Cohen (Eds.), *Developmental psychopathology: Theory and method* (2nd ed., Vol. 1, pp. 1–23). Hoboken, NJ: Wiley.

Cicchetti, D. (2008). A multiple-levels-of-analysis perspective on research in development and psychopathology. In T. P. Beauchaine & S. P. Hinshaw (Eds.), *Child and adolescent psychopathology* (pp. 27–57). Hoboken, NJ: Wiley.

Cicchetti, D., & Cohen, D. J. (Eds.). (2006). *Developmental psychopathology*. Hoboken, NJ: Wiley.

Cicchetti, D., & Curtis, W. J. (2006). The developing brain and neural plasticity: Implications for normality, psychopathology, and resilience. In D. Cicchetti & D. J. Cohen (Eds.), *Developmental psychopathology: Developmental neuroscience* (2nd ed., Vol. 2, pp. 1–64). Hoboken, NJ: Wiley.

Cicchetti, D., & Rogosch, F. (1996). Equifinality and multifinality in developmental psychopathology. *Development and Psychopathology, 8,* 597–600.

Cicchetti, D., & Toth, S. L. (2009). The past achievements and future promises of developmental psychopathology: The coming of age of a discipline. *Journal of Child Psychology and Psychiatry, 50,* 16–25.

Cicchetti, D., & Valentino, K. (2006). An ecological-transactional perspective on child maltreatment: Failure of the average expectable environment and its influence on child development. In D. Cicchetti & D. J. Cohen (Eds.), *Developmental psychopathology: Risk, disorder, and adaptation* (2nd ed., Vol. 3, pp. 317–357). Hoboken, NJ: Wiley.

Dawson, G., & Toth, K. (2006). Autism spectrum disorders. In D. Cicchetti & D. J. Cohen (Eds.), *Developmental psychopathology: Risk, disorder, and adaptation* (2nd ed., Vol. 3, pp. 317–357). Hoboken, NJ: Wiley.

Deater-Deckard, K., & Dodge, K. A. (1997). Externalizing behavior problems and discipline revisited: Nonlinear effects and variation by culture, context, and gender. *Psychological Inquiry, 8,* 161–175.

Diamond, A., Prevor, M. B., Callender, G., & Druin, D. P. (1997). Prefrontal cortex cognitive deficits in children treated early and continuously for PKU. *Monographs of the Society for Research in Child Development, 62* (Serial No. 4).

Dodge, K. A., & Rutter, M. (Eds.). (2011). *Gene-environment interactions in developmental psychopathology*. New York, NY: Guilford Press.

Fairchild, A. J., & MacKinnon, D. P. (2009). A general model for testing mediation and moderation effects. *Prevention Science, 10,* 87–99.

Gazzaniga, M. S., Ivry, R. B., & Mangun, G. R. (2009). *Cognitive neuroscience: The biology of the mind* (3rd ed.). New York, NY: Norton.

Giedd, J. N., Shaw, P., Wallace, G., Gogtay, N., & Lenroot, R. K. (2006). Anatomic brain imaging studies of normal and abnormal brain development in children and adolescents. In D. Cicchetti & D. J. Cohen (Eds.), *Developmental psychopathology: Developmental neuroscience* (2nd ed., Vol. 2, pp. 127–196). Hoboken, NJ: Wiley.

Gottlieb, G., & Willoughby, M. T. (2006). Probabalistic epigenesis of psychopathology. In D. Cicchetti & D. J. Cohen (Eds.), *Developmental psychopathology: Theory and method* (2nd ed., Vol. 1, pp. 673–700). Hoboken, NJ: Wiley.

Grandin, T. (2006). *Thinking in pictures: And other reports from my life with autism* (2nd ed.). New York, NY: Vintage.

Granic, I., & Hollenstein, T. (2006). A survey of dynamic systems methods for developmental psychopathology. In D. Cicchetti & D. J. Cohen (Eds.), *Developmental psychopathology: Theory and method* (2nd ed., Vol. 1, pp. 889–930). Hoboken, NJ: Wiley.

Hinshaw, S. P. (2002). Intervention research, theoretical mechanisms, and causal processes related to externalizing behavior patterns. *Development and Psychopathology, 14,* 789–818.

Hinshaw, S. P. (2006). Stigma and mental illness: Developmental issues and future prospects. In D. Cicchetti & D. J. Cohen (Eds.), *Developmental psychopathology: Risk, disorder, and adaptation* (2nd ed., Vol. 3, pp. 317–357). Hoboken, NJ: Wiley.

Hinshaw, S. P. (2007). *The mark of shame: Stigma of mental illness and an agenda for change.* New York, NY: Oxford University Press.

Hinshaw, S. P. (2008). Developmental psychopathology as a scientific discipline: Relevance to behavioral and emotional disorders of childhood and adolescence. In T. P. Beauchaine & S. P. Hinshaw (Eds.), *Child and adolescent psychopathology* (pp. 3–26). Hoboken, NJ: Wiley.

Hinshaw, S. P. (2009). *The triple bind: Saving our teenage girls from today's pressures.* New York, NY: Ballantine.

Hinshaw, S. P., & Stier, A. (2008). Stigma in relation to mental disorders. *Annual Review of Clinical Psychology, 4,* 269–293.

Howe, G. W., Reiss, D., & Yuh, J. (2002). Can prevention trials test theories of etiology? *Development and Psychopathology, 14,* 673–694.

Jaffee, S. R., Strait, L. B., & Odgers, C. L. (2012). From correlates to causes: Can quasi-experimental studies and statistical innovations bring us closer to understanding the causes of antisocial behavior? *Psychological Bulletin, 138,* 272–295.

Jorm, A. F., & Griffiths, K. M. (2008). The public's stigmatizing attitudes towards people with mental disorders: How important are biomedical conceptualizations? *Acta Psychiatrica Scandinavica, 118,* 315–321.

Kagan, J. (1997). Temperament and the reactions to unfamiliarity. *Child Development, 68,* 139–143.

Kessler, R. C., Berglund, P., Demler, O., Jin, R., Merikangas, K. R., & Walters, E. E. (2005). Lifetime prevalence and age-of-onset distributions of DSM-IV disorders in the national comorbidity survey replication. *Archives of General Psychiatry, 62,* 593–602.

Kraemer, H. C., Kazdin, A. E., Offord, D. R., Kessler, R. C., Jensen, P. S., & Kupfer, D. J. (1997). Coming to terms with the terms of risk. *Archives of General Psychiatry, 54,* 337–343.

Kraemer, H. C., Stice, E., Kazdin, A., Offord, D., & Kupfer, D. (2001). How do risk factors work together? Mediators, moderators, and independent, overlapping, and proxy risk factors. *American Journal of Psychiatry, 158,* 848–856.

Kreppner, J. M., O'Connor, T. G., Rutter, M., & the English and Romanian Adoptees Study Team. (2001). Can inattention/overactivity be a deprivation disorder? *Journal of Abnormal Child Psychology, 29,* 513–528.

Luthar, S. S. (2006). Resilience in development: A synthesis of research across five decades. In D. Cicchetti & D. J. Cohen (Eds.), *Developmental psychopathology: Risk, disorder, and adaptation* (2nd ed., Vol. 3, pp. 739–795). Hoboken, NJ: Wiley.

Luthar, S. S., & Brown, P. J. (2007). Maximizing resilience through diverse levels of inquiry: Prevailing paradigms, possibilities, and priorities for the future. *Development and Psychopathology, 19,* 931–955.

Martinez, A. G., Piff, P. K., Mendoza-Denton, R., & Hinshaw, S. P. (2011). The power of a label: Mental illness diagnoses, ascribed humanity, and social rejection. *Journal of Social and Clinical Psychology, 30*, 1–23.

Mash, E. J., & Dozois, D. J. A. (2003). Child psychopathology: A developmental-systems perspective. In E. J. Mash & R. A. Barkley (Eds.), *Child psychopathology* (2nd ed., pp. 3–71). New York, NY: Guilford Press.

Masten, A. S., Burt, K. B., & Coatsworth, J. D. (2006). Competence and psychopathology in development. In D. Cicchetti & D. J. Cohen (Eds.), *Developmental psychopathology: Risk, disorder, and adaptation* (2nd ed., Vol. 3, pp. 696–738). Hoboken, NJ: Wiley.

Masten, A. S., & Cicchetti, D. (2010). Developmental cascades. *Development and Psychopathology, 22*, 491–495.

McLaughlin, K. A., Zeanah, C. H., Fox, N. A., & Nelson, C. A. (2012). Attachment security as a mechanism linking foster care placement to improved mental health outcomes in previously institutionalized children. *Journal of Child Psychology and Psychiatry, 53*, 46–55.

Moffitt, T. E. (1993). "Life-course-persistent" and "adolescence-limited" antisocial behavior: A developmental taxonomy. *Psychological Review, 100*, 674–701.

Moffitt, T. E. (2006). Life course persistent versus adolescence limited antisocial behavior. In D. Cicchetti & D. J. Cohen (Eds.), *Developmental psychopathology: Risk, disorder, and adaptation* (2nd ed., Vol. 3, pp. 570–598). Hoboken, NJ: Wiley.

Murray, C. J., & Lopez, A. D. (Eds.). (1996). *The global burden of disease and injury series, Vol. 1. A comprehensive assessment of morbidity and disability from diseases, and risk factors in 1990 and projected to 2020.* Cambridge, MA: Harvard University Press.

Muthén, B. O., & Muthén, L. K. (2000). Integrating person centered and variable centered analyses: Growth mixture modeling with latent trajectory classes. *Alcoholism: Clinical and Experimental Research, 24*, 882–891.

Nagin, D. S., & Odgers, C. L. (2010a). Group-based trajectory modeling in clinical research. *Annual Review of Clinical Psychology, 6*, 109–138.

Nagin, D. S., & Odgers, C. L. (2010b). Group-based trajectory modeling (nearly) two decades later. *Journal of Quantitative Criminology, 26*, 445–453.

Nelson, C. A., Zeanah, C. H., Fox, N. A., Marshall, P. J., Smyke, A. T., & Guthrie, D. (2007). Cognitive recovery in socially deprived young children: The Bucharest early intervention project. *Science, 318*, 1937–1940.

Nigg, J. T. (2006). *What causes ADHD? Understanding what goes wrong and why.* New York, NY: Guilford Press.

Nigg, J. T., Hinshaw, S. P., & Huang-Pollack, C. (2006). Disorders of attention and impulse regulation. In D. Cicchetti & D. J. Cohen (Eds.), *Developmental psychopathology: Risk, disorder, and adaptation* (2nd ed., Vol. 3, pp. 358–403). Hoboken, NJ: Wiley.

O'Connor, T. G. (2006). The persisting effects of early experiences on psychological development. In D. Cicchetti & D. J. Cohen (Eds.), *Developmental psychopathology: Risk, disorder, and adaptation* (2nd ed., Vol. 3, pp. 202–234). Hoboken, NJ: Wiley.

Pescosolido, B. A., Martin, J. K., Long, J. S., Medina, T. R., Phelan, J. C., & Link, B. G. (2010). "A disease like any other?" A decade of change in public reactions to schizophrenia, depression, and alcohol dependence. *American Journal of Psychiatry*, *167*, 1321–1330.

Phelan, J. C., Link, B. G., Stueve, A., & Pescosolido, B. A., (2000). Public conceptions of mental illness in 1950 and 1996: What is mental illness and is it to be feared? *Journal of Health and Social Behavior*, *41*, 188–207.

Raine, A., Brennan, P., & Mednick, S. A. (1997). Interaction between birth complications and early maternal rejection in predisposing individuals to adult violence: Specificity to serious, early-onset violence. *American Journal of Psychiatry*, *154*, 1265–1271.

Rende, R., & Waldman, I. (2006). Behavioral and molecular genetics and developmental psychopathology. In D. Cicchetti & D. J. Cohen (Eds.), *Developmental psychopathology: Developmental neuroscience* (2nd ed., Vol. 2, pp. 427–464). Hoboken, NJ: Wiley.

Richters, J. E. (1997). The Hubble hypothesis and the developmentalist's dilemma. *Development and Psychopathology*, *9*, 193–229.

Risch, N., Herrell, R., Lehner, T., Liang, R. Y., Eaves, L., Hoh, J. . . . Merikangas, K. R. (2009). Interaction between the serotonin transporter gene (5-HTTLPR), stressful life events, and risk of depression: A meta-analysis. *Journal of the American Medical Association*, *301*, 2462–2471.

Robb, J. A., Sibley, M. H., Pelham, W. E., Foster, E. M., Molina, B. S. G., Gnagy, E. M., & Kuriyan, A. B. (2011). The estimated annual cost of ADHD to the US education system. *School Mental Health*, *3*, 169–177.

Romer, D., & Walker, E. F. (Eds.). (2007). *Adolescent psychopathology and the developing brain*. New York, NY: Oxford University Press.

Rutter, M., Moffitt, T. E., & Caspi, A. (2006). Gene-environment interplay and psychopathology: Multiple varieties but real effects. *Journal of Child Psychology and Psychiatry*, *47*, 226–261.

Rutter, M., Pickles, A., Murray, R., & Eaves, L. (2001). Testing hypotheses on specific environmental causal effects on behavior. *Psychological Bulletin*, *127*, 291–324.

Rutter, M., & Sroufe, L. A. (2000). Developmental psychopathology: Concepts and challenges. *Development and Psychopathology*, *12*, 265–296.

Sagvolden, T., Johansen, E. B., Aase, H., & Russell, V. A. (2005). A dynamic developmental theory of attention-deficit/hyperactivity disorder (ADHD) predominantly hyperactive/impulsive and combined types. *Behavioral and Brain Sciences*, *28*, 397–419.

Sameroff, A. J., Lewis, M., & Miller, S. M. (Eds.). (2000). *Handbook of developmental psychopathology* (2nd ed.). New York, NY: Kluwer Academic/Plenum.

Sapienza, J. K., & Masten, A. S. (2011). Understanding and promoting resilience in children and youth. *Current Opinion in Psychiatry*, *24*, 267–273.

Serafica, F. C., & Vargas, L. A. (2006). Cultural diversity in the development of child psychopathology. In D. Cicchetti & D. J. Cohen (Eds.), *Developmental psychopathology: Theory and method* (2nd ed., Vol. 1, pp. 588–626). Hoboken, NJ: Wiley.

Sodian, B. (2011). Theory of mind in infancy. *Child Development Perspectives, 5,* 39–43.

Sroufe, L. A. (1997). Psychopathology as an outcome of development. *Development and Psychopathology, 9,* 251–268.

Sroufe, L. A., & Rutter, M. (1984). The domain of developmental psychopathology. *Child Development, 55,* 17–29.

Steinberg, L. (2010). A dual systems model of adolescent risk-taking. *Developmental Psychobiology, 52,* 316–224.

Tremblay, R. E. (2010). Developmental origins of disruptive behavior problems: The "original sin" hypothesis, epigenetics, and their consequences for prevention. *Journal of Child Psychology and Psychiatry, 51,* 341–367.

Volkow, N. D., Wang, G-J., Kollins, S. H., Wigal, T. L., Newcorn, J. H., Telang, F. . . . Swanson, J. M. (2009). Evaluating dopamine reward pathway in ADHD: Clinical implications. *Journal of the American Medical Association, 302,* 1084–1091.

# CHAPTER 2

# Developmental Psychopathology and the Diagnostic and Statistical Manual of Mental Disorders

THEODORE P. BEAUCHAINE, DANIEL N. KLEIN,
NORA L. ERICKSON, AND ALYSSA L. NORRIS

A LL SCIENTIFIC DISCIPLINES HAVE rules for classifying phenomena and events that fall within their purview. Chemistry, for example, among the more advanced physical sciences, has fundamental laws describing what constitutes an element (i.e., the number of protons in an atomic nucleus), what gives rise to similarities among elements (e.g., common bonding properties), how elements differ (e.g., solubility versus inertness), and how elements interact across levels of analysis to create what might otherwise be inexplicable phenomena (e.g., the high boiling point of water conferred by hydrogen bonds). For chemistry, these and other properties are summarized in the periodic table, which represents an abbreviated *taxonomy* of elements. Although issues of taxonomy in chemistry are far more complex than this paragraph implies, the example illustrates how important precise classification is in any discipline. Indeed, accurate classification ultimately leads to better prediction and control of external events—the fundamental objectives of science (Braithwaite, 1953; see also Beauchaine, Gatzke-Kopp, & Mead, 2007). In chemistry, control of chemical reactions and molecular compounds has led to astounding advances in processes such as water purification, affecting the lives of millions. As outlined in Chapter 1, a major goal of developmental psychopathology research is to improve prediction and control of mental illness, which should ultimately lead to more effective prevention and intervention programs, alleviating considerable human suffering (see also Beauchaine, Neuhaus, Brenner, & Gatzke-Kopp, 2008).

Following from this brief discussion, in this chapter we describe the predominant classification system of psychopathology in the United States—the *Diagnostic and Statistical Manual of Mental Disorders* (*DSM*, American Psychiatric Association [APA], 2000). In doing so we (1) outline the history of the *DSM*; (2) highlight important issues and difficulties that emerge when diagnosing psychopathology; (3) juxtapose the *DSM-IV-TR* and its limitations with alternative perspectives and theoretical orientations, and (4) describe likely changes to appear in the forthcoming *DSM-5*, scheduled for publication in 2013.

## HISTORICAL CONTEXT

Unlike the physical sciences, psychology and psychiatry are relatively new. In fact, the first well-organized attempt in the United States at devising a classification system of psychopathology occurred only 60 years ago with publication of the first edition of the *DSM* (APA, 1952). As a result, psychology and psychiatry are replete with unresolved taxonomic issues,[1] some of which are specific to children and adolescents (see Achenbach & Rescorla, 2006; Beauchaine, Klein, Crowell, Derbidge, & Gatzke-Kopp, 2009; Beauchaine & Marsh, 2006; Eaton, Krueger, South, Simms, & Clark, 2011; Jensen, Knapp, & Mrazek, 2006; Krueger et al., 2011; World Health Organization [WHO], 1996). Many of these issues are described in sections to follow.

### EARLY VERSIONS OF THE *DSM*

The current version of the *DSM* is the *DSM-IV-TR* (APA, 2000). This is actually the seventh in a series of *DSMs* (including both major and minor revisions) dating to 1952 (*DSM-I*, 1952; *DSM-II*, 1968; *DSM-II*, seventh printing, 1974; *DSM-III*, 1980; *DSM-III-R*, 1987; *DSM-IV*, 1994; *DSM-IV-TR*, 2000).

*DSM-I.* The *DSM-I* (APA, 1952) was an effort by the APA to produce a single nomenclature for psychopathology. Prior to the *DSM-I*, there were several different classification systems, none of which were used consistently across the U.S. (see Blashfield, 1998). The *DSM-I* was influenced strongly by Adolph Meyer's psychobiology, which viewed psychopathology as a reaction to stress (e.g., Meyer, Bentley, & Cowdry, 1934). Hence, all disorders included "reaction" in their titles (e.g., depressive reaction). In formulating the *DSM-I*, the APA relied on the broad opinion of its membership. To do so, it sent detailed questionnaires to 10% of its members, from which proposed categories of psychopathology were derived. Three broad classes of psychopathology emerged from this process, including organic brain syndromes, functional disorders, and mental deficiency. Within these broad classes, 108 specific diagnoses were created (depending on the method of counting), only one of which could be applied to children (adjustment reaction of childhood/adolescence). Final approval of psychiatric classes and specific diagnoses was obtained through a vote of the APA membership. As this description implies, the *DSM-I* had little if any basis in empirical research.

*DSM-II.* The *DSM-II* (APA, 1968), which contained about 182 diagnoses (again, depending on the method of counting), was published with few changes in process or philosophy. A major goal in formulating the *DSM-II* was to improve communication

---

1. We do not mean to imply that taxonomic questions have been resolved in other sciences. Issues of classification continue to be debated in diverse fields including evolutionary biology (see, e.g., Laurin, 2010) and paleontology (see Beauchaine, 2003).

among mental health professionals—especially psychiatrists (e.g., Scotti & Morris, 2000). The *DSM-II* had strong psychoanalytic overtones, reflecting the training of most psychiatrists at the time. Major diagnostic classes of psychopathology were expanded from 3 to 11, and a number of childhood and adolescent disorders were added, including group delinquent reaction, hyperkinetic reaction, overanxious reaction, runaway reaction, unsocialized aggressive reaction, and withdrawing reaction.

Beginning with publication of the *DSM-II*, international treaty has dictated that the *DSM* and International Classification of Diseases (ICD) be compatible. The ICD, published by the World Health Organization, is the classification system used in most other countries to diagnose mental illness. Some changes made to the *DSM-II* were needed to render it more similar to the ICD-8 (WHO, 1966). Currently, the ICD is in its 10th edition—revised (ICD-10), which was published in 2008. The ICD-11 is expected in 2014.

*DSM-II, seventh printing.* In the seventh printing of the *DSM-II* (APA, 1974), homosexuality was removed as a mental disorder, following protests by gay rights activists at the 1970 annual convention of the APA in San Francisco. This landmark event illustrates several inter-related points about diagnosis of mental illness. First, diagnostic systems such as the *DSM*, which are constructed by social institutions, often reflect social values (see, e.g., McCarthy & Gerring, 1994). Second, psychiatry and related disciplines at times reinforce prevailing social value systems, which may lead to stigmatization of certain members of society, with considerable potential for negative effects on mental health (see, e.g., Prilleltensky, 1989). Finally, as a social institution, the APA is not indifferent to sociopolitical influence. Removing homosexuality from the *DSM-II* also foreshadowed struggles to deal with validity of psychiatric diagnosis more broadly, a major issue confronted in later revisions of the *DSM*.

## RELIABILITY, VALIDITY, AND SUBSEQUENT VERSIONS OF THE *DSM*

In contrast to the *DSM-I* (APA, 1952) and *DSM-II* (APA, 1968), the *DSM-III* (APA, 1980) was designed to be descriptive and largely atheoretical, so it would appeal to and be useful to professionals from a variety of disciplines and conceptual orientations in addition to psychiatry. Research on the clinical features and etiology of major forms of psychopathology was also weighted heavily in formulating the *DSM-III*—a major shift from the consensus opinion approach to constructing earlier versions (see above). Thus, introduction of the *DSM-III* in 1980 was a watershed event in modern classification of psychopathology. Prior to 1970, most mental health professionals in the United States were not especially concerned with psychiatric diagnosis. The dominant paradigm was psychoanalysis, which did not place much stock in diagnosis. However, in the 1960s a new paradigm, often referred to as biological psychiatry, challenged and ultimately supplanted psychoanalysis as the dominant perspective in the United States. One agenda of biological psychiatry proponents was to make the discipline more scientific by increasing its emphasis on empirical research, particularly on the biological bases and treatment of psychopathology, thereby bringing psychiatry into the mainstream of modern medicine.

Diagnosis played a central role in this agenda, as a reliable and valid classification system was necessary for the enterprise. Indeed, how successful could research on biological causes/correlates of psychopathology be if the major independent variable, diagnosis, was unreliable or invalid? Since diagnosis was a cornerstone of well-developed specialties in mainstream medicine (e.g., Engel, 1977), emphasis on reliable diagnosis was paramount. However, there was a major obstacle: Limited evidence of inter-rater reliability of psychiatric diagnosis (e.g., Spitzer & Fleiss, 1974).

Problems with reliability were hard to ignore. First, rates of various diagnoses differed dramatically between the United States and most European countries. For example, the rate of schizophrenia was many times higher in the United States than in the United Kingdom. To address this issue, a team of researchers in the United States and United Kingdom launched the Cross-National Diagnostic Project (for a description see Gurland, 1976). Using the same diagnostic criteria and assessment procedures, they found that differences in clinical diagnoses between hospitals in New York and London were attributable entirely to different diagnostic practice; patients' symptoms were virtually identical in both cities. Furthermore, clinical diagnoses of British psychiatrists corresponded more closely to patients' actual clinical presentations than those of U.S. psychiatrists, who greatly overdiagnosed schizophrenia and underdiagnosed mood disorders.

Second, almost all studies addressing diagnostic reliability conducted to that time indicated very low inter-rater agreement. Spitzer and Fleiss (1974) aggregated data from these studies, and calculated inter-rater reliability using the kappa ($\kappa$) statistic, which measures the degree of association between categorical constructs such as presence versus absence of a diagnosis, correcting for chance levels of agreement. In general, $\kappa$s ranging from 0 to .20 indicate slight agreement, .21 to .40 fair agreement, .41 to .60 moderate agreement, .61 to .80 substantial agreement, and .81 to 1.0 excellent agreement (Landis & Koch, 1977). Spitzer and Fleiss reported that $\kappa$s from previous inter-rater reliability studies were .41 for depression; .33 for mania; .45 for anxiety neurosis; .57 for schizophrenia; and .71 for alcoholism. Only the latter could be considered adequate.

Spitzer and Fleiss (1974) attributed the low inter-rater reliability to two sources: criterion variance and information variance. Criterion variance refers to diagnosticians relying on different criteria when making a diagnosis. Thus, if one clinician diagnoses schizophrenia on the basis of even mild indications of cognitive slippage (a form of thought disorder), whereas another reserves the diagnosis only for patients who exhibit severe delusions or hallucinations, agreement will be low. In this regard, the DSM-I (APA, 1952) and DSM-II (APA, 1968) were not helpful because their diagnostic criteria were extremely vague. Each diagnosis was described in several sentences listing characteristic signs and symptoms, yet there was no specification of how many symptoms were required, how long a symptom had to be present, or whether other symptoms might rule out a diagnosis (e.g., in a patient with visual hallucinations, could schizophrenia be diagnosed in the context of acute alcohol withdrawal?).

## OPERATIONALIZING DIAGNOSTIC CRITERIA: REDUCING CRITERION VARIANCE

The criterion variance problem was addressed initially by Mandel Cohen, who was interested in developing a more empirical approach to studying psychopathology. Cohen conducted several pioneering studies of mood, anxiety, and somatoform disorders. These involved formulating careful criteria for diagnosis, applying them to what at the time were large samples of patients, and examining patients' clinical presentations, family histories, and clinical course (see Healy, 2002). Psychiatric journals were not particularly interested in this work, and most of Cohen's papers were published in general medical journals (e.g., Cohen, Cassidy, Flanagan, & Spellman, 1937; Cohen, Robins, & Purtell, 1952), with little effect on psychiatry or psychology.

One of Cohen's students was Eli Robins, who moved to St. Louis to become chair of the Department of Psychiatry at Washington University. Throughout the 1960s, Robins and several colleagues, including Guze and Winokur, applied Cohen's approach in a series of landmark studies of psychopathology (e.g., Arkonac & Guze, 1963; Reich, Clayton, & Winokur, 1969). One of the hallmarks of the Washington University approach was the development of systematic operational (i.e., explicit) diagnostic criteria for a selected group of diagnoses. This systematic approach was explicated by E. Robins and Guze (1970), who published a brief yet highly influential paper in which they advanced a five-step process toward ensuring that psychiatric classes were specific, objective, and nonarbitrary. Using the example of schizophrenia, Robins and Guze suggested that diagnostic validity can be established only when a clinical syndrome is characterized by (a) a cluster of covarying symptoms and etiological precursors (obtained from clinical description); (b) reliable physiological, biological, and/or psychological markers (obtained from laboratory studies); (c) readily definable exclusionary criteria; (d) a predictable course (assessed through follow-up studies), and (e) increased rates of the same disorder among first-degree relatives (assessed through family studies). The Robins and Guze method was soon used by Feighner et al. (1972) to develop the first set of psychiatric disorders that were validated systematically. The associated symptom lists are now referred to as the *Feighner Criteria*. Although the primary motivation in formulating the Feighner Criteria was to validate psychiatric disorders (see Kendler, Munoz, & Murphy, 2009), doing so required specification of explicit operational criteria.

Not long after the Feighner Criteria (1972) were published, the National Institute of Mental Health (NIMH) sponsored the Collaborative Study of the Psychobiology of Depression Study, a multisite investigation of the clinical features, family history, biological correlates, and course of depression (see Katz, Secunda, Hirschfeld, & Koslow, 1979). As part of this study, NIMH contracted with Spitzer and Endicott to develop a revised version of the Feighner criteria, which came to be known as the Research Diagnostic Criteria (RDC; Spitzer, Endicott, & Robins, 1978). Thus, by the late 1970s, the importance of specifying operational criteria for psychiatric disorders was widely recognized among the psychopathology research community, which strongly influenced development of the *DSM-III* (APA, 1980) and all subsequent versions of the *DSM* (see e.g., Cloninger, 1989; Kendler et al., 2009).

## Structured Interviews: Reducing Information Variance

A major task of the U.S.–U.K. Cross-National Project was to standardize collection of data on symptoms by British and American clinicians. Accordingly, Wing, Cooper, and Sartorius (1974) developed a standardized clinical interview, which provided (1) specific questions to be asked by the interviewer, (2) specific rating scales for each symptom, (3) conventions for making ratings, and (4) a detailed glossary defining each symptom. This instrument was called the present state examination (PSE), designed to allow experienced clinicians to obtain a systematic assessment of patients' current symptoms. It did not collect information on previous course or history, and therefore could not be used to make diagnoses. However, it was an important advance in standardizing collection of information across clinicians and sites.

At the same time, psychiatrists at Washington University had developed a semi-structured diagnostic interview for use in various research projects being conducted in their department. Like the PSE, it included standardized questions and rating scales. However, it also provided a systematic assessment of the development and course of psychopathology, rather than focusing only on the patient's current state (Woodruff, Goodwin, & Guze, 1974). Thus, it included all information necessary to make diagnoses according to criteria established at the time (see above).

Soon afterward, as part of their role in the NIMH Collaborative Study of the Psychobiology of Depression Study, Endicott and Spitzer (1978) developed a semi-structured diagnostic interview called the Schedule for the Affective Disorders and Schizophrenia (SADS). This interview allowed trained clinicians to collect systematic and reliable data on both current symptoms and history of most major psychiatric disorders. Thus, use of the SADS also allowed clinicians to make specific diagnoses.

By the time *DSM-III* was published in 1980, structured diagnostic interviews had been accepted as the state-of-the-art in psychiatric assessment. However, both the PSE and SADS were quite time-consuming, and neither was matched to the *DSM-III*. Hence, Spitzer and Williams (1983) developed a new instrument, the Structured Clinical Interview for *DSM-III* (SCID), which eventually assessed all major disorders in the *DSM-III*, and later the *DSM-III-R* (e.g., Spitzer, Williams, Gibbon, & First, 1990) and the *DSM-IV* (e.g., First, Spitzer, Gibbon, & Williams, 2002). One objective was that the SCID be user-friendly enough to be adopted in routine clinical practice in addition to research, although this has not occurred.

Another major development in structured interviewing was construction of the Diagnostic Interview Schedule (DIS; Robins, Helzer, Croughan, & Ratcliff, 1981), by Lee Robins (not to be confused with E. Robins, her spouse), a sociologist at Washington University who pioneered research on antisocial personality disorder (Chapter 14). The impetus for the development of the DIS was a report by the Carter

Administration's Presidential Commission on Mental Health, which stressed the need to collect better data on the prevalence of mental disorders in the United States. This report led to the NIMH Epidemiological Catchment Area (ECA) survey, the largest epidemiological study of mental disorders ever conducted (see Regier et al., 1984). A problem in designing this study, however, was that it was prohibitively expensive to hire trained clinicians to conduct diagnostic interviews with more than 18,000 participants. Accordingly, L. Robins and colleagues developed the DIS so it could be used by lay interviewers with no previous training in psychopathology. Because it was designed for use by nonclinicians, the DIS is much more structured than other diagnostic interviews, and, unlike the PSE, SADS, and SCID, leaves no room for interviewer judgment in formulating questions and rating symptoms. With these other interviews, the interviewer is expected to probe respondents' answers until confident they understand the question and are reporting a clinically significant experience that is relevant to the construct being assessed. In contrast, with the DIS, interviewers take the respondents' report at face value. Thus, it is a respondent-based, as opposed to an interviewer-based interview (Angold & Fisher, 1999). Diagnoses are derived by computer using *DSM* criteria.

Finally, to assess rates of psychopathology in large epidemiological samples of children and adolescents, NIMH later undertook development of the Diagnostic Interview Schedule for Children (DISC; Costello, Edelbrock, Dulcan, Kalas, & Klaric, 1984). The current version of the DISC assesses 30 *DSM-IV-TR* (APA, 2000) psychiatric disorders, designed for use with parents of children ages 6 to 17 and with children and adolescents ages 9 to 17. Like the DIS, it is administered by lay interviewers (Shaffer, Fischer, Lucas, Dulcan, & Schwab-Stone, 2000). Both the DIS and DISC have been controversial, with some questioning the validity of diagnoses so completely based on self-report—especially among children (see, e.g., Renou, Hergueta, Flament, Mouren-Simeoni, & Lecrubier, 2004). Indeed, adolescents who suffer from disruptive behavior disorders such as ADHD and conduct disorder often underreport symptoms (e.g., Sibley et al., 2010). Nevertheless, considerable evidence points toward reliability of the DISC (see Shaffer et al., 2000), and its use in research settings is now commonplace.

## The *DSM-III, DSM-III-R,* and *DSM-IV*

*DSM-III.* Following from his extensive work on psychiatric diagnosis outlined above, Spitzer was chosen to lead revisions to the *DSM III*. Rather than continuing with tradition, he looked toward the Feighner et al. (1972) criteria and the RDC (Spitzer et al., 1978) as a means of solving the problem of criterion variance. The *DSM-III* therefore became the first official classification system in psychopathology that used specific symptoms, including inclusion, exclusion, and duration criteria for each diagnosis. This required a major expansion of the Feighner Criteria and RDC, which covered no more than 15 or so disorders.

The *DSM-III* (APA, 1980) also introduced multiaxial classification. Thus, in addition to classifying major psychiatric syndromes (Axis I), separate axes were created for personality disorders (Axis II); physical conditions that are relevant to understanding a person's presenting problem (Axis III), psychosocial and environ-mental stressors and problems (Axis IV), and overall severity, or global assessment of functioning (GAF; Axis V). Use of multiple axes is a means of addressing patients' uniqueness in making a diagnosis: Not every patient with the same diagnosis is the same in all respects. This is a particularly important consideration in developmental psychopathology research (see Chapter 1), which emphasizes contextual influences on the development of mental illness (Chapter 4).

*DSM-III-R.* A revised version of the *DSM-III* (APA, 1987) was published only seven years later. In large part because so little new research was available, changes were minimal, and the revision was not felt to be extensive enough to warrant being called a fourth edition. The rationale for the revision was that some diag-nostic criteria were inconsistent, unclear, or contradicted by subsequent research (APA, 1987).

Nevertheless, one set of changes had major consequences. Following publication of the *DSM-III* (APA, 1980), several studies were published questioning the widespread use of exclusion criteria. Exclusion criteria are a means of implementing diagnostic hierarchies, which serve to simplify diagnosis. Patients typically present with a wide array of symptoms. Traditionally, a major task of diagnosing has been differential diagnosis—deciding what the most appropriate diagnosis is among the many possibilities suggested by the patient's clinical presentation. Diagnostic hierarchies are useful in differential diagnosis because they indicate which symptoms should receive priority. Prior to the *DSM-III-R*, *organic* mental disorders (syndromes attributable to central nervous system disease, brain trauma, or significant substance abuse) were at the top of the diagnostic hierarchy. Next came schizophrenia. Then came major mood disorders, with neurotic and personality disorders at the bottom. Thus, in the absence of organic factors, schizophrenia symptoms were accorded priority in diagnosis, regardless of the presence of major mood, neurotic, and/or personality disorder features. In the absence of both organic factors and schizophrenia symptoms, mood disorder symptoms took precedence regardless of neurotic and personality disorder features. Finally, neurotic and personality disorder diagnoses were only considered if organic, schizophrenia, and mood disorder features were absent.

Several studies in the early 1980s demonstrated that exclusion criteria in the *DSM-III* (APA, 1980) were often arbitrary and lost significant information. For example, family histories of patients with major depression and panic disorder differed from those of patients with major depression alone (Leckman, Weissman, Merikangas, Pauls, & Prusoff, 1983). Hence, comorbid panic disorder appeared to be important, and excluding the diagnosis in patients with major depression represented a loss of potentially important information. In light of these data, many exclusion criteria were eliminated from the *DSM-III-R* (APA, 1987), except those used to rule out organic (general medical or substance-induced) causes of disorder.

As might be expected, eliminating exclusion criteria led to a significant increase in rates of comorbidity, or the co-occurrence of two or more disorders (see Klein & Riso, 1993). As a consequence, understanding comorbidity has been a top agenda item in psychopathology research ever since (see, e.g., Angold, Costello, & Erkanli, 1999;

Beauchaine, Hinshaw, & Pang, 2010). At the same time, the reduction of hierarchical exclusion criteria has resulted in a diminished role for differential diagnosis in the diagnostic process.

*DSM-IV.* In 1994 the *DSM-IV* (APA, 1994) was published. One motivation for publishing a new version so soon was the international treaty requirement that it be consistent with the ICD (see earlier), which was undergoing revision. Although content changes were relatively minor, the process through which *DSM-IV* revisions were derived witnessed a marked change. Specifically, revisions were driven much more by data than in previous versions, and the process was more systematic and better documented. As outlined in the *DSM-IV* itself: (1) review papers were commissioned by the APA addressing relevant literature for almost all existing and proposed categories; (2) NIMH funded 12 multisite field trials to collect data to inform decisions about revisions to criteria; (3) the McArthur Foundation provided funding for several investigators to reanalyze existing data sets, thereby providing additional data relevant to proposed revisions; and, (4) the literature reviews, results of field trials, reanalyses, and rationales for all revisions were published in a multivolume *DSM-IV* Sourcebook (e.g., APA, 1996). A similar process has been carried forward in the forthcoming *DSM 5*, described in later sections.

*DSM-IV-TR.* In the text revision to the *DSM-IV*, published in 2000 (APA, 2000), diagnostic categories and their criteria were left almost completely unchanged. Rather, factual errors were corrected; sections of text describing each diagnostic category, associated features, advances in laboratory and clinical research, and so on, were revised based on new research; and diagnostic codes that had changed in the latest edition of the ICD were updated.

## THE *DSM* AND DEVELOPMENTAL PSYCHOPATHOLOGY

Although it is important for any student of psychopathology to understand the history behind, rationale for, and use of the predominant classification system of mental disorders in the United States, it is equally important to understand limitations of that system. Indeed, certain departures in philosophy underlying the *DSM* and developmental psychopathology approaches are clearly apparent. Historically, criticisms of the *DSM* have come from both within and outside psychiatry (see, e.g., McCarthy & Gerring, 1994), with developmental psychopathologists providing some of the most incisive critiques (e.g., Richters & Cicchetti, 1993). We and others have summarized these critiques and provided a few of our own elsewhere (e.g., Beauchaine, 2003; Beauchaine et al., 2009; Cummings, Davies, & Campbell, 2000; Hinshaw & Park, 1999; Hudziak, Achenbach, Altoff, & Pine, 2007). Here we include a brief overview.

### CRITICISMS OF THE *DSM* APPROACH

*Problems with construct validity.* Although application of the Feighner Criteria and the RDC to some (though not nearly all) disorders represents an attempt to ensure diagnostic validity, reliability has been of far greater concern from the *DSM-III* onward (APA, 1980; see e.g., Kraemer, Kupfer, Narrow, Clarke, & Regier, 2010). Yet reliability does not ensure validity. To use a somewhat hyperbolic example, separate raters can agree with very high precision that a person is over 6′ 5′, but such agreement says nothing about height being a symptom of mental illness. Indeed, any such assertion would be arbitrary at best—a situation that applied to sexual orientation before the seventh printing of the *DSM-II* (APA, 1974), when homosexuality was considered a mental disorder (see earlier).

In developmental psychopathology research, *construct validity* refers to the extent to which symptoms of a diagnosis mark an objective, nonarbitrary entity that relates to mental health outcomes. Construct validity should be considered whenever the cause of a trait cannot be observed directly (Cronbach & Meehl, 1955), which is usually the case for psychopathology. To borrow an example we have used elsewhere (Beauchaine & Marsh, 2006), consider the difference between a medical syndrome such as pancreatic cancer, and a common psychiatric condition such as major depressive disorder. In the former case, a patient presents at his or her physician's office with a collection of symptoms, which might include weight loss, dark urine, nausea, and abdominal pain. This collection of symptoms, or *manifest indicators*, leads to a hypothesis on the part of the physician regarding its unobserved, or *latent* cause. Importantly, for a medical condition such as pancreatic cancer, the hypothesis is either confirmed or disconfirmed by a biopsy or other diagnostic test. If the biopsy is positive, the cause of the disorder becomes known. If the biopsy is negative, a new hypothesis is generated and tested.

Compare this with a depressed individual, who also presents with a collection of symptoms, including depressed mood, anhedonia, fatigue, weight loss, and insomnia. In contrast to the case of pancreatic cancer, there are no diagnostic tests that can identify the cause of depression (although certain medical conditions such as hypothyroidism should be ruled out). Thus, we are left with a somewhat tautological definition of depression: The patient is depressed because she or he presents with a collection of symptoms, and the patient presents with a collection of symptoms because she or he is depressed. We are therefore forced to infer psychopathology with no gold standard or pathognomonic sign of disease state.

Under such conditions, difficulties posed for construct validation of psychiatric disorders are often formidable. Prior to publication of the *DSM-III* (APA, 1980), almost no evidence existed for the construct validity of any diagnostic category (Kendell, 1989), because all were derived clinically rather than through systematic research (see above). At present, even after decades of relevant research, unanswered questions about the construct validity of many psychiatric disorders abound. For example, in research on pediatric bipolar disorder, issues regarding proper diagnostic cutoffs and delimitation from other disorders including ADHD have not been addressed fully (see Chapter 19).

*Heterogeneity within diagnostic classes.* A related issue follows from the observation that diverse etiologies often result in what appears to be a single disorder, a phenomenon known as *equifinality* (see Chapter 1). For example, impulsivity may arise from one of several sources, each of which is expressed behaviorally as ADHD (Chapter 12). However, since *DSM* diagnoses are all derived syndromally (i.e., from symptoms with little if any regard to etiology), different underlying causes of a disorder may never be ascertained, even when it is possible to do so.

Both treatment and prevention are often improved when pathophysiological and etiological diagnoses are used rather than syndromal diagnosis (Preskorn & Baker, 2002). For example, if hypothyroidism is identified in the pathophysiology of depression, treatment follows a different course (synthetic thyroxine treatment) than antidepressant use and/or psychotherapy. Furthermore, if the specific etiology of hypothyroidism is identified as radiation-induced (as opposed to one of several heritable variants), identification of the radiation source might be facilitated, thereby preventing others from incurring similar exposure. Although this example may seem extreme, potentially meaningful distinctions among depression subtypes are underemphasized in the *DSM-IV-TR* (APA, 2000). For example, melancholia—a subtype of depression that appears to arise from different etiological mechanisms than nonmelancholic depression (see Leventhal & Rehm, 2005)—may confer increased risk of adverse long-term functional outcomes including suicide (e.g., Carroll, Greden, & Feinberg, 1980; Coryell & Schlesser, 2001). Yet it is not currently classified as a separate mood disorder (although some have argued ardently for doing so in the *DSM-5*; see, e.g., Parker et al., 2010).

*Categorical versus dimensional measurement.* One of the most persistent criticisms of the *DSM* is that all psychiatric disorders are diagnosed categorically (i.e., present versus absent), even though overwhelming research evidence indicates that most forms of psychopathology reflect extreme expressions of continuously distributed traits (see, e.g., Beauchaine, 2007; Haslam, Holland, & Kuppens, 2012; Hudziak et al., 2007; Krueger, Watson, & Barlow, 2005; Trull & Durrett, 2005). Furthermore, even in rare exceptions when psychiatric vulnerability is distributed categorically (e.g., schizotypy; see Lenzenweger, McLachlan, & Rubin, 2007), individual differences in symptom expression are nevertheless observed (Beauchaine, Lenzenweger, & Waller, 2008), and may provide key information about current functioning and long-term prognosis that is lost by categorizing.

Other adverse consequences of categorizing dimensions include difficulty ascertaining optimal diagnostic cutoffs (e.g., 95th percentile? 98th percentile? see Meehl, 1995), and loss of statistical information (see MacCallum, Zhang, Preacher, & Rucker, 2002). Individuals in need of intervention may also be turned away because they fail to meet diagnostic criteria even though they suffer considerable impairment. To address such problems, hybrid classification systems have been proposed in which both presence vs. absence and severity of psychopathology are assessed (e.g., Hudziak et al., 2007). This approach is likely to be implemented in certain parts of the *DSM-5* (see below). Notably, dimensional assessment has long been used in child psychopathology research, even when using *DSM* criterion sets, given limitations of categorical classification (e.g., Achenbach & Edelbrock, 1991; Conners, Sitarenios, Parker, & Epstein, 1998; Gadow & Sprafkin,1997; Robinson, Eyberg, & Ross, 1980).

*Failure to consider development.* Developmental psychopathologists have been especially critical of the *DSM* because it fails to consider issues of development in diagnosis (e.g., Richters & Cicchetti, 1993; Sroufe, 1997). With few exceptions (e.g., early-onset conduct disorder; see Chapter 13), child and adolescent psychopathology are assessed and diagnosed without careful consideration of normative developmental trends in behavior, and without acknowledgement that single behavioral traits—including those that confer vulnerability to psychopathology—may be expressed differently at different ages. *Heterotypic continuity* refers to such changes in the behavioral expression of psychopathology across development. For example, we have known for about 50 years that delinquent adult males almost invariably follow a developmental pathway that begins with severe hyperactivity impulsivity as early as toddlerhood, followed in rough temporal sequence by oppositional/defiant disorder (ODD; Chapter 13) in preschool, early-onset conduct disorder (CD; Chapter 13) in elementary school, substance use disorders (SUDs; Chapter 15) in adolescence, and antisocial personality disorder (ASPD; Chapter 14) in adulthood (see, e.g., Loeber & Hay, 1997; Lynam, 1998; Robins, 1966). Thus, even though continuity in externalizing conduct is common among those on this trajectory, specific behaviors vary considerably across development (Hinshaw, Lahey, & Hart, 1993). Among other consequences, failure to consider such heterotypic continuity results in (a) a research literature that is often fractionated based on topographies of behavior (e.g., tantrums in toddlerhood, truancy in elementary school, substance use in adulthood) rather than etiology, (b) alternative treatment strategies for conditions such as CD and SUDs that are not informed by one another when they would benefit from being so (see Beauchaine et al., 2008), and (c) faulty conclusions about etiology and comorbidity of externalizing disorders (see Beauchaine et al., 2010).

*The Axis I–Axis II distinction.* Several criticisms have also arisen around the *DSM* distinction between major psychiatric syndromes (Axis I) and personality disorders (Axis II), and around the assumption that personality disorders can only be diagnosed among adults. As defined in the *DSM-IV-TR* (APA, 2000), Axis II disorders should be characterized by (a) an enduring pattern of experience and behavior that deviates markedly from societal expectations, manifested in two or more of the following: cognition, affect, interpersonal functioning, and impulse control; (b) the pattern is inflexible and pervasive across many situations; (c) clinically significant distress or impairment; and (d) stability and of long duration, with an onset age that can be traced back to at least adolescence or early adulthood.

As we have summarized elsewhere (Beauchaine et al., 2009), however, the basis for the distinction between Axis I and Axis II is often arbitrary. Indeed, many if not most Axis I disorders (e.g., schizophrenia, dysthymia, obsessive-compulsive disorder, anorexia nervosa) meet the conceptual requirements for personality disorders outlined above, with adolescent or early adult onset, chronic course, and pervasive effects on psychological and social functioning.

Furthermore, several personality disorders share etiological influences with Axis I disorders, including schizotypal personality disorder and schizophrenia, as well as avoidant personality disorder and generalized social phobia, among others.

*Failure to consider culture and other contextual issues.* In general, the *DSM* is indifferent to both (a) culturally induced individual differences in behavior that might be mistaken for psychopathology (see, e.g., Marsella & Yamada, 2010), and (b) cultural, socioeconomic, and other contextually driven individual differences in the expression of psychopathology (see, e.g., Gone & Kirmayer, 2010; Lewis-Fernández et al., 2010). As a result, strict adherence to *DSM* criterion sets without consideration of race, ethnicity, and class can lead to both false positive and false negative conclusions regarding the presence versus absence of psychopathology. One objective of the developmental psychopathology approach is to construct a discipline that acknowledges the role of context in shaping behavior, and that does not assume (even implicitly) that group differences in behavior between members of the dominant social class and other cultural subgroups always imply deficits in functioning among the latter (e.g., Cicchetti & Toth, 2009; Garcia-Coll, Akerman, & Cicchetti, 2000; see Chapter 4).

## CHANGES TO THE UPCOMING *DSM-5*

The task force charged with formulating the *DSM-5* appears responsive to some, though not all, of these criticisms. For example, although personality disorders will now be assessed dimensionally, externalizing disorders including ADHD, ODD, CD, and so on, will remain distinct, with limited if any consideration of heterotypic comorbidity. In this section, we briefly (1) describe anticipated changes to the upcoming *DSM-5*, which is expected to be published in May 2013, and (2) consider how these changes offer improvements over past versions of the *DSM*, with some of the specific criticisms outlined above in mind.

Procedurally, revising the *DSM-IV-TR* (APA, 2000) began in 1999 with an informal discussion about the need to improve validity of psychiatric diagnosis between Steven Hyman, director of NIMH, Steven Mirin, medical director of the APA, and David Kupfer, chair of the APA Committee on Psychiatric Diagnosis and Assessment at NIMH (APA, 2012a). This discussion spawned the initial *DSM-5* Research Planning Conference in 1999, sponsored by both the APA and NIMH. Participants invited to this conference included experts in behavioral genetics, molecular genetics, neuroscience, life-span development, cognition, and behavior. Notably, many of those involved in the *DSM-IV* revision were not invited, with the explicit purpose of encouraging new thinking. The committee commissioned a series of white papers to identify (1) areas of needed research, (2) cross-cutting unresolved issues in psychiatric diagnosis, (3) ways in which the burgeoning research base in neuroscience could inform psychiatric diagnosis, and (4) issues of culture in psychopathology, among others. Soon after the conference, Darrel Regier was recruited to coordinate development of the *DSM-5*. Regier became vice chair of the *DSM-5* Task Force, which was chaired by David Kupfer. A first set of white papers appeared in 2002 (Kupfer, First, & Regier, 2002), and a second set appeared in 2007 (Narrow, First, Sirovatka, & Regier, 2007). These edited volumes identified specific areas in which new research was needed.

Between 2004 and 2008, 13 conferences were held among experts from NIMH, the APA, the WHO, the American Psychiatric Institute for Research and Education (APIRE), the National Institute on Drug Abuse (NIDA), and the National Institute on Alcoholism and Alcohol Abuse (NIAAA). Participants from both the United States and other nations wrote a series of review papers, from which more specific research agendas were developed (APA, 2012b).

In 2006, Kupfer and Regier nominated chairs of the diagnostic work groups for the *DSM-5* Task Force, who were approved by the APA Board of Trustees in 2007. These chairs then recruited leading experts in their fields to populate the individual work groups, which were approved by the APA in 2008, after they had already begun meeting. Thirteen work groups were formed, representing diagnostic categories in the *DSM-IV-TR* (APA, 2000).

As with previous revisions (see earlier), the *DSM-5* Task Force implemented a series of field trials, this time to ascertain the validity, reliability, feasibility, and clinical utility of proposed criteria, including new dimensional indices—an approach never used in previous versions of the *DSM*. Based primarily on results of the field trials, revised criteria were drafted and are now being finalized (APA, 2012c). One goal of the field trials is to develop diagnostic criteria that are useful in both research and clinical settings. Since this text is organized around the developmental psychopathology perspective, we do not provide a complete list of likely changes to diagnostic criteria. Nevertheless, we summarize changes to selected common disorders of childhood and adolescence in Table 2.1. Readers will find more detailed coverage of changes to the *DSM-5* in disorder-specific chapters to follow.

Structurally, the *DSM-5* will be considerably different than its predecessors, even though most diagnostic categories will be retained. To make the *DSM-5* more user-friendly for clinicians, the 20 chapters are sequenced developmentally, with disorders usually diagnosed in infancy listed first, followed by disorders of childhood, adolescence, and so on.

Among the biggest changes to the *DSM-5* are revisions to personality disorder criteria and diagnosis. These changes follow from long-standing concerns about reliability, validity, and arbitrarily categorizing dimensional personality traits (see above). Among other changes, the number of personality disorders will be reduced from 10 to 6, and ratings in three different areas will be used to diagnose personality pathology. These include (1) a general definition of personality disorder requiring at least mild impairment in personality functioning (defined as disturbances in how patients view themselves and how well they function in interpersonal relationships); (2) six specific personality disorder diagnoses, defined using up to six personality traits (negative affectivity, detachment, antagonism, disinhibition, psychoticism) and their facets, selected largely on the basis of the *DSM-IV* diagnostic criteria for these six disorders; and (3) ratings of pathological personality traits using the trait domains and their facets. Finally, the behavior pattern must be stable across time and situations.

The multiaxial system of diagnosis is also likely to change. Whereas the *DSM-IV-TR* (APA, 2000) uses a five axis system (see above), the *DSM-5* will include three axes. This will be accomplished by subsuming *DSM-IV-TR* Axes I (clinical disorders), II (developmental and personality disorders), and III (general medical conditions) into Axis I of the *DSM-5* (psychiatric and medical diagnoses). Axis IV of the *DSM-IV-TR* (psychosocial and environmental problems) will become Axis II in the *DSM-5*, and Axis V of the *DSM-IV-TR* (global assessment of functioning) will be replaced by Axis III of the *DSM-5* (specific rating scale of severity for each disorder).

**Table 2.1**

Upcoming Changes to Selected *DSM-IV* Disorders of Childhood/Adolescence and Their Criterion Sets for the *DSM-5*

| Current diagnostic class | Specific disorder (relevant chptr) | *DSM-IV* criterion or criteria being changed | Description of key changes for *DSM-5* and abbreviated rationale |
|---|---|---|---|
| Disruptive, impulse control, and conduct disorders | Attention deficit/ hyperactivity disorder (12) | A. Either (1) or (2): <br> 1. Six (or more) of the following symptoms of inattention have persisted for at least 6 months to a degree that is maladaptive and inconsistent with developmental level: Inattention <br> (a) Often fails to give close attention to details or makes careless mistakes in schoolwork, work, or other activities <br> (b) Often has difficulty sustaining attention in tasks or play activities <br> (c) Often does not seem to listen when spoken to directly <br> (d) Often does not follow through on instructions and fails to finish schoolwork, chores, or duties in the workplace (not due to oppositional behavior or failure to understand instructions) <br> (e) Often has difficulty organizing tasks and activities | A. Either (1) and/or (2). <br> 1. Inattention: Six (or more) of the following symptoms have persisted for at least 6 months to a degree that is inconsistent with developmental level and that impact directly on social and academic/occupational activities. Note: for older adolescents and adults (ages 17 and older), only 4 symptoms are required. The symptoms are not due to oppositional behavior, defiance, hostility, or a failure to understand tasks or instructions. <br> (a) Often fails to give close attention to details or makes careless mistakes in schoolwork, at work, or during other activities (for example, overlooks or misses details, work is inaccurate) <br> (b) Often has difficulty sustaining attention in tasks or play activities (for example, has difficulty remaining focused during lectures, |

*(continued overleaf)*

**Table 2.1** (*continued*)

| Current diagnostic class | Specific disorder (relevant chptr) | DSM-IV criterion or criteria being changed | Description of key changes for DSM-5 and abbreviated rationale |
|---|---|---|---|
| | | (f) Often avoids, dislikes, or is reluctant to engage in tasks that require sustained mental effort (such as schoolwork or homework) | conversations, or reading lengthy writings) |
| | | | (c) Often does not seem to listen when spoken to directly (mind seems elsewhere, even in the absence of any obvious distraction) |
| | | (g) Often loses things necessary for tasks or activities (e.g., toys, school assignments, pencils, books, or tools) | (d) Frequently does not follow through on instructions (starts tasks but quickly loses focus and is easily sidetracked, fails to finish |
| | | (h) Is often easily distracted by extraneous stimuli | schoolwork, household chores, or tasks in the workplace) |
| | | (i) Is often forgetful in daily activities | (e) Often has difficulty organizing tasks and activities. (Has difficulty managing sequential tasks and keeping materials and belongings in order. Work is messy and disorganized. Has poor time management and tends to fail to meet deadlines.) |

(f) Characteristically avoids, seems to dislike, and is reluctant to engage in tasks that require sustained mental effort (such as schoolwork or homework or, for older adolescents and adults, preparing reports, completing forms, or reviewing lengthy papers)

(g) Frequently loses objects necessary for tasks or activities (e.g., school assignments, pencils, books, tools, wallets, keys, paperwork, eyeglasses, or mobile telephones)

(h) Is often easily distracted by extraneous stimuli (for older adolescents and adults may include unrelated thoughts)

(i) Is often forgetful in daily activities, chores, and running errands (for older adolescents and adults, returning calls, paying bills, and keeping appointments)

*A number of criticisms have been levied against DSM-IV criteria, including the instability of inattention (I) and hyperactivity-impulsivity (HI) subtypes, categorical/dimensional*

*(continued overleaf)*

**Table 2.1** (continued)

| Current diagnostic class | Specific disorder (relevant chptr) | DSM-IV criterion or criteria being changed | Description of key changes for DSM-5 and abbreviated rationale |
|---|---|---|---|
| | | | *debate over subtypes, lack of substantial evidence for subtype entities, threshold artifacts due to subtype delineation (i.e., child may present with 10 criteria, but if only 5 in each subtype would not receive a diagnosis), arbitrary age of onset, and a lack of representation of adult ADHD manifestations in the criteria.* |
| | | | *At this time, the task force has proposed numerous options for revisions to existing criteria. Perhaps most importantly regarding symptoms required in Criterion A, the proposed changes include examples for each symptom. Although the examples are not meant to be exhaustive, they are intended to make the particular symptoms easier to recognize and the criteria easier to implement in clinical settings.* |
| | | | *e.g., American Psychiatric Association, 2010e* |

2. Six (or more) of the following symptoms of hyperactivity/impulsivity have persisted for at least 6 months to a degree that is maladaptive and inconsistent with developmental level:Hyperactivity

a. Often fidgets with hands or feet or squirms in seat

b. Often leaves seat in classroom or in other situations in which remaining seated is expected

c. Often runs about or climbs excessively in situations in which it is inappropriate (in adolescents or adults, may be limited to subjective feelings of restlessness)

d. Often has difficulty playing or engaging in leisure activities quietly

e. Is often "on the go" or often acts as if "driven by a motor"

f. Often talks excessively/impulsively

g. Often blurts out answers before questions have been completed

h. Often has difficulty awaiting turn

i. Often interrupts or intrudes on others (e.g., butts into conversations or games)

2. Hyperactivity and Impulsivity: Six (or more) of the following symptoms have persisted for at least 6 months to a degree that is inconsistent with developmental level and that impact directly on social and academic/occupational activities.
Note: For older adolescents and adults (ages 17 and older), only 4 symptoms are required. The symptoms are not due to oppositional behavior, defiance, hostility, or a failure to understand tasks or instructions.

a. Often fidgets or taps hands or feet or squirms in seat

b. Is often restless during activities when others are seated (may leave his or her place in the classroom, office or other workplace, or in other situations that require remaining seated)

c. Often runs about or climbs on furniture and moves excessively in inappropriate situations. In adolescents or adults, may be limited to feeling restless or confined

d. Is often excessively loud or noisy during play, leisure, or social activities

(continued overleaf)

**Table 2.1** *(continued)*

| Current diagnostic class | Specific disorder (relevant chptr) | *DSM-IV* criterion or criteria being changed | Description of key changes for *DSM-5* and abbreviated rationale |
|---|---|---|---|
| | | | e. Is often "on the go," acting as if "driven by a motor." Is uncomfortable being still for an extended time, as in restaurants, meetings, etc. Seen by others as being restless and difficult to keep up with |
| | | | f. Often talks excessively |
| | | | g. Often blurts out an answer before a question has been completed. Older adolescents or adults may complete people's sentences and "jump the gun" in conversations |
| | | | h. Has difficulty waiting his or her turn or waiting in line |
| | | | i. Often interrupts or intrudes on others (frequently butts into conversations, games, or activities; may start using other people's things without asking or receiving permission; adolescents or adults may intrude into or take over what others are doing) |
| | | | j. Tends to act without thinking, such as starting tasks without adequate preparation or avoiding reading or listening to instructions. May speak |

out without considering consequences or make important decisions on the spur of the moment, such as impulsively buying items, suddenly quitting a job, or breaking up with a friend

k. Is often impatient, as shown by feeling restless when waiting for others and wanting to move faster than others, wanting people to get to the point, speeding while driving, and cutting into traffic to go faster than others

l. Is uncomfortable doing things slowly and systematically and often rushes through activities or tasks

m. Finds it difficult to resist temptations or opportunities, even if it means taking risks (A child may grab toys off a store shelf or play with dangerous objects; adults may commit to a relationship after only a brief acquaintance or take a job or enter into a business arrangement without doing due diligence)

*(continued overleaf)*

49

**Table 2.1** *(continued)*

| Current diagnostic class | Specific disorder (relevant chptr) | DSM-IV criterion or criteria being changed | Description of key changes for DSM-5 and abbreviated rationale |
|---|---|---|---|
| | | | *Structure:* |
| | | | *Option 1: Existing structure with three subtypes-predominantly inattentive (PI), predominantly hyperactive (PH), combined (C).* |
| | | | *Option 2: Existing structure without subtypes using HI and I criteria as behavior-specific dimension scores.* |
| | | | *Option 3: Replace existing structure with "Combined ADHD" alone.* |
| | | | *Dealing with AD without Hyperactivity:* |
| | | | *Option 1: No change/PI has separate code. Including HA items may distinguish the disorder from general inattention, but might not be validated empirically.* |
| | | | *Option 2: Redefine "Restrictive PI" with limited presence of HI as fourth subtype requiring no more than 2 current and no past history of HI criteria. Would add descriptive and heuristic value, but sharing the same code would make it hard to determine its clinical usage.* |

*Option 3: New diagnosis of "Attention-Deficit Disorder" with its own code.*

*Criteria Distribution and Content*
*Add four new impulsivity criteria to counter the under-representation of impulsivity criteria: acts without thinking, impatient, rushes through tasks, and difficulty resisting immediate temptations. Counters the relative under-representation of impulsivity criteria, but increases the number of criteria that must be remembered, potentially leading to false negatives/positives, and it is not known whether new criteria would overlap with HI items.*

*Adult ADHD*
*Lower threshold for ADHD-C from 6 to 3 criteria from either I or HI. Research shows symptoms decrease over time, but impairment persists into adulthood.*

*e.g., Barkley, Murphy, & Fischer, 2008; Kieling et al., 2010; Mannuzza, 2008; Polanczyk, Caspi, Houts, Kollins, Rohde, & Moffitt, 2010.*

*(continued overleaf)*

**Table 2.1** (continued)

| Current diagnostic class | Specific disorder (relevant chptr) | DSM-IV criterion or criteria being changed | Description of key changes for DSM-5 and abbreviated rationale |
|---|---|---|---|
| | | B. Some hyperactive-impulsive or inattentive symptoms that caused impairment were present before age 7 years. | B. Several noticeable inattentive or hyperactive-impulsive symptoms were present by age 12. *Instead of focusing on impairment before a certain age, individuals now fulfill this criteria through the presence of symptoms. Increase age of onset of symptoms to be present on or before age 12. Although it is not known whether raising the age of onset would increase false positives by increasing the prevalence of diagnoses, children with later onset appear to have the same disorder course as those with earlier onset. In addition, identifying symptoms rather than impairment avoids disentangling comorbidity issues.* |
| | Conduct disorder (13) | | No proposed revision to main criteria, but proposed additional specifier: "Callous and Unemotional Traits in Conduct Disorder." 1. Meets full criteria for Conduct Disorder. |

2. Shows 2 or more of the following characteristics persistently over at least 12 months and in more than one relationship or setting. The clinician should consider multiple sources of information to determine the presence of these traits, such as whether the person self-reports them as being characteristic of him or herself and if they are reported by others (e.g., parents, other family members, teachers, peers) who have known the person for significant periods of time.

   (a) Lack of Remorse or Guilt: Does not feel bad or guilty when he/she does something wrong (except if expressing remorse when caught and/or facing punishment).

   (b) Callous-Lack of Empathy: Disregards and is unconcerned about the feelings of others.

   (c) Unconcerned about Performance: Does not show concern about poor/problematic performance at school, work, or in other important activities.

*(continued overleaf)*

**Table 2.1** *(continued)*

| Current diagnostic class | Specific disorder (relevant chptr) | *DSM-IV* criterion or criteria being changed | Description of key changes for *DSM-5* and abbreviated rationale |
|---|---|---|---|
| | | | (d) Shallow or Deficient Affect: Does not express feelings or show emotions to others, except in ways that seem shallow or superficial (e.g., emotions are not consistent with actions; can turn emotions "on" or "off" quickly) or when they are used for gain (e.g., to manipulate or intimidate others).<br><br>*Current diagnostic criteria for CD has resulted in a heterogeneous group of individuals, and adding this specifier could provide greater delineation among those meeting criteria based on severity, life course, and etiology. Recent advances in research on the manifestation of psychopathic traits in children and adolescents have demonstrated important etiological and clinical distinctions based on the* |

*presence of these symptoms. By including this specifier, clinicians and researchers could begin to harness these distinctions in their work on conduct disorder.*

*e.g., Frick & Moffitt (2010)*

Oppositional defiant disorder (13)

A. A pattern of negativistic, hostile, and defiant behavior lasting at least 6 months, during which four (or more) of the following are present:
1. Often loses temper
2. Often argues with adults
3. Often actively defies or refuses to comply with adults' requests or rules
4. Often deliberately annoys people
5. Often blames others for his or her mistakes or misbehavior
6. Is often touchy or easily annoyed by others
7. Is often angry and resentful
8. Is often spiteful or vindictive
Note: Consider a criterion met only if the behavior occurs more frequently than is typically observed in individuals of comparable age and developmental level.

A. A persistent pattern of angry and irritable mood along with defiant and vindictive behavior as evidenced by four (or more) of the following symptoms being displayed with one or more persons other than siblings.
Angry/Irritable Mood
1. Loses temper
2. Is touchy or easily annoyed by others
3. Is angry and resentful
Defiant/Headstrong Behavior
4. Argues with adults
5. Actively defies or refuses to comply with adults' request or rules
6. Deliberately annoys people
7. Blames others for his or her mistakes or misbehavior
8. Vindictiveness: Has been spiteful or vindictive at least twice within the past six months

*Although there are no proposed changes to the symptoms or structure of the ODD criteria, there has been a shift to move beyond subjective*

*(continued overleaf)*

**Table 2.1** *(continued)*

| Current diagnostic class | Specific disorder (relevant chptr) | *DSM-IV* criterion or criteria being changed | Description of key changes for *DSM-5* and abbreviated rationale |
|---|---|---|---|
| | | | *frequency criteria (i.e., "often") to objective definitions. The work group recognizes, however, that ongoing research is needed to determine appropriate criteria and cut points.* |
| | | | *Recommendation 3: Organize symptoms in the criteria for ODD by emotional and behavioral symptoms. Although all symptoms are correlated, emotional symptoms do uniquely predict emotional disorders.* |
| | | | *e.g., Stringaris & Goodman, 2009* |
| | | B. The disturbance in behavior causes clinically significant impairment in social, academic, or occupational functioning. | B. (NOTE: UNDER CONSIDERATION) The persistence and frequency of these behaviors should be used to distinguish a behavior that is within normal limits from a behavior that is symptomatic to determine if they should be considered a symptom of the disorder. For children under 5 years of age, the behavior must occur on most days for a period of at least six months unless otherwise noted (see Symptom #8). For individuals 5 years or older, the behavior must occur at least |

once per week for at least six months, unless otherwise noted (see Symptom #8). While these frequency criteria provide a minimal level of frequency to define symptoms, other factors should also be considered such as whether the frequency and intensity of the behaviors are non-normative given the person's developmental level, gender, and culture.

D. Criteria are not met for conduct disorder, and, if the individual is age 18 years or older, criteria are not met for antisocial personality disorder.

D. *The behaviors may be confined to only one setting or, in more severe cases, present in multiple settings.*

*Recommendation 2: Remove exclusionary criteria for CD.*

*Develop a severity index based on the presence of symptoms across contexts. Children meeting ODD criteria through both teacher and parent reports may demonstrate greater impairment than those meeting criteria via parent report alone.*

*e.g., Munkvold, Lundervold, Lie, & Manger, 2009*

Intermittent explosive disorder† | *New addition to the DSM-5.* | Proposals being finalized; not yet published.

*(continued overleaf)*

57

**Table 2.1** (continued)

| Current diagnostic class | Specific disorder (relevant chptr) | DSM-IV criterion or criteria being changed | Description of key changes for DSM-5 and abbreviated rationale |
|---|---|---|---|
| | Dyssocial personality disorder* (14) | *Formerly antisocial personality disorder*<br><br>However, the new proposed structure of personality disorders represents a radical departure from previous iterations of the DSM. The new general criteria can be seen at right: | A. Significant impairments in self (identity or self-direction) and interpersonal (empathy or intimacy) functioning.<br>B. One or more pathological personality trait domains or trait facets.<br>C. The impairments in personality functioning and the individual's personality trait expression are relatively stable across time and consistent across situations.<br>D. The impairments in personality functioning and the individual's personality trait expression are not better understood as normative for the individual's developmental stage or socio-cultural environment.<br>E. The impairments in personality functioning and the individual's personality trait expression are not solely due to the direct physiological effects of a substance (e.g., a drug of abuse, medication) or a general medical condition (e.g., severe head trauma).<br><br>*The proposed new hybrid dimensional-categorical model of personality disorders (see text).*<br><br>*American Psychiatric Association (2010b, 2010c)* |

A. Significant impairments in personality functioning manifest by:

1. Impairments in self-functioning (a or b):

   (a) Identity: Ego-centrism; self-esteem derived from personal gain, power, or pleasure.

   (b) Self-direction: Goal-setting based on personal gratification; absence of prosocial internal standards associated with failure to conform to lawful or culturally normative ethical behavior.

   *and*

2. Impairments in interpersonal functioning (a or b):

   (a) Empathy: Lack of concern for feelings, needs, or suffering of others; lack of remorse after hurting or mistreating another.

   (b) Intimacy: Incapacity for mutually intimate relationships, as exploitation is a primary means of relating to others, including by deceit and coercion; use of dominance or intimidation to control others.

*For now, the rationale for the proposed changes reflect the shift to the new model of PDs more so than specific changes to the criteria for this disorder in particular. Information specific to changes to criteria for this disorder have yet to be supplied.*

*(continued overleaf)*

**Table 2.1** (*continued*)

| Current diagnostic class | Specific disorder (relevant chptr) | DSM-IV criterion or criteria being changed | Description of key changes for DSM-5 and abbreviated rationale |
|---|---|---|---|
| | | A. There is a pervasive pattern of disregard for and violation of the rights of others occurring since age 15 years, as indicated by three (or more) of the following: <br><br> 1. Failure to conform to social norms with respect to lawful behaviors as indicated by repeatedly performing acts that are grounds for arrest <br><br> 2. Deceitfulness, as indicated by repeated lying, use of aliases, or conning others for personal profit or pleasure <br><br> 3. Impulsivity or failure to plan ahead <br><br> 4. Irritability and aggressiveness, as indicated by repeated physical fights or assaults <br><br> 5. Reckless disregard for safety of self or others <br><br> 6. Consistent irresponsibility, as indicated by repeated failure to sustain consistent work behavior or honor financial obligations <br><br> 7. Lack of remorse, as indicated by being indifferent to or rationalizing having hurt, mistreated, or stolen from another | B. Pathological personality traits in the following domains: <br><br> 1. Antagonism, characterized by: <br><br> (a) Manipulativeness: Frequent use of subterfuge to influence or control others; use of seduction, charm, glibness, or ingratiation to achieve one's ends <br><br> (b) Deceitfulness: Dishonesty and fraudulence; misrepresentation of self; embellishment or fabrication when relating events <br><br> (c) Callousness: Lack of concern for feelings or problems of others; lack of guilt or remorse about the negative or harmful effects of one's actions on others; aggression; sadism <br><br> (d) Hostility: Persistent or frequent angry feelings; anger or irritability in response to minor slights and insults; mean, nasty, or vengeful behavior <br><br> 2. Disinhibition, characterized by: <br><br> (a) Irresponsibility: Disregard for—and failure to honor—financial and other |

obligations or commitments; lack of respect for—and lack of follow through on—agreements and promises.

(b) Impulsivity: Acting on the spur of the moment in response to immediate stimuli; acting on a momentary basis without a plan or consideration of outcomes; difficulty establishing and following plans.

(c) Risk taking: Engagement in dangerous, risky, and potentially self-damaging activities, unnecessarily and without regard for consequences; boredom proneness and thoughtless initiation of activities to counter boredom; lack of concern for one's limitations and denial of the reality of personal danger.

C. The impairments in personality functioning and the individual's personality trait expression are relatively stable across time and consistent across situations.

D. The impairments in personality functioning and the individual's personality trait expression are not better understood as normative for the individual's developmental stage or sociocultural environment.

B. The individual is at least age 18 years.

C. There is evidence of conduct disorder with onset before age 15 years.

*(continued overleaf)*

61

**Table 2.1** (continued)

| Current diagnostic class | Specific disorder (relevant chptr) | DSM-IV criterion or criteria being changed | Description of key changes for DSM-5 and abbreviated rationale |
|---|---|---|---|
| Addiction and related disorders* | Substance use disorder†† (15) | New disorder that subsumes what were substance abuse and substance dependence in the DSM-IV. | A. A maladaptive pattern of substance use leading to clinically significant impairment or distress, as manifested by 2 (or more) of the following, occurring within a 12-month period: |
| | | | 1. Recurrent substance use resulting in a failure to fulfill major role obligations at work, school, or home (e.g., repeated absences or poor work performance related to substance use; substance-related absences, suspensions, or expulsions from school; neglect of children or household) |
| | | | 2. Recurrent substance use in situations in which it is physically hazardous (e.g., driving an automobile or operating a machine when impaired by substance use) |
| | | | 3. Continued substance use despite having persistent or recurrent social or interpersonal problems caused or exacerbated by the effects of the substance (e.g., arguments with spouse about consequences of intoxication, physical fights) |

4. Tolerance, as defined by either of the following:
   a. A need for markedly increased amounts of the substance to achieve intoxication or desired effect
   b. Markedly diminished effect with continued use of the same amount of the substance
      (Note: Tolerance is not counted for those taking medications under medical supervision such as analgesics, antidepressants, anti-anxiety medications or beta-blockers.)

5. Withdrawal, as manifested by either of the following:
   a. The characteristic withdrawal syndrome for the substance (refer to Criteria A and B of the criteria sets for withdrawal from the specific substances)
   b. The same (or a closely related) substance is taken to relieve or avoid withdrawal symptoms
      (Note: Withdrawal is not counted for those taking medications under medical supervision such as analgesics, antidepressants, anti-anxiety medications, or beta-blockers.)

*(continued overleaf)*

**Table 2.1** (*continued*)

| Current diagnostic class | Specific disorder (relevant chptr) | *DSM-IV* criterion or criteria being changed | Description of key changes for *DSM-5* and abbreviated rationale |
|---|---|---|---|
| | | | 6. The substance is often taken in larger amounts or over a longer period than was intended. |
| | | | 7. There is a persistent desire or unsuccessful efforts to cut down or control substance use. |
| | | | 8. A great deal of time is spent in activities necessary to obtain the substance, use the substance, or recover from its effects. |
| | | | 9. Important social, occupational, or recreational activities are given up or reduced because of substance use. |
| | | | 10. The substance use is continued despite knowledge of having a persistent or recurrent physical or psychological problem that is likely to have been caused or exacerbated by the substance. |
| | | | 11. Craving or a strong desire or urge to use a specific substance. |

*Broadly referring to substance-related disorders, the task force has proposed combining substance abuse and substance dependence into one disorder. Factor analyses and latent class analyses support the dimensional nature of substance use disorders through support for one-factor models, high correlations among two factors (if present), or classes based on severity rather than separate classes for abuse and dependence. For example, using quantity and frequency of drinking and drunkenness to assess alcohol use, Borges et al. (2010) revealed no distinction between abuse and dependence. However, current criteria did identify those in the middle-upper end of the alcohol use continuum, indicating criteria could be expanded to fully capture the continuum using consumption variables in addition to DSM-IV diagnostic criteria.*

*e.g., Borges et al., 2010*

*(continued overleaf)*

**Table 2.1** (continued)

| Current diagnostic class | Specific disorder (relevant chptr) | DSM-IV criterion or criteria being changed | Description of key changes for DSM-5 and abbreviated rationale |
|---|---|---|---|
| Anxiety disorders Proposed changes to provide greater consistency across anxiety disorders as a whole (e.g., "marked fear" rather than "intense" fear or anxiety). In addition, scales are proposed to serve as measures of severity across the cluster of anxiety disorders (Craske, Rauch, Ursano, Prenoveau, Pine, & Zinbarg, 2009). | Separation anxiety disorder (16) | A. Developmentally inappropriate and excessive anxiety concerning separation from home or from those to whom the individual is attached, as evidenced by three (or more) of the following:<br><br>1. Recurrent excessive distress when separation from home or major attachment figures occurs or is anticipated<br><br>2. Persistent and excessive worry about losing, or about possible harm befalling, major attachment figures<br><br>3. Persistent and excessive worry that an untoward event will lead to separation from a major attachment figure (e.g., getting lost or being kidnapped)<br><br>4. Persistent reluctance or refusal to go to school or elsewhere because of fear of separation<br><br>5. Persistently and excessively fearful or reluctant to be alone or without major attachment figures at home or without significant adults in other settings | A. Developmentally inappropriate and excessive anxiety concerning separation from home or from those to whom the individual is attached, as evidenced by three (or more) of the following:<br><br>1. Recurrent excessive distress when separation from home or major attachment figures occurs or is anticipated<br><br>2. Persistent and excessive worry about losing, or about possible harm befalling, major attachment figures (e.g., health, accidents, death)<br><br>3. Persistent and excessive worry that an untoward event will lead to separation from a major attachment figure (e.g., getting lost or being kidnapped)<br><br>4. Persistent reluctance or refusal to go to school, work, or elsewhere because of fear of separation<br><br>5. Persistent and excessive fear about or reluctance to be alone or without major attachment figures |

6. Persistent reluctance or refusal to go to sleep without being near a major attachment figure or to sleep away from home
7. Repeated nightmares involving the theme of separation
8. Repeated complaints of physical symptoms (such as headaches, stomachaches, nausea, or vomiting) when separation from major attachment figures occurs or is anticipated

*Proposed changes have aimed to create more valid evaluations of worries through the inclusion of examples. Criteria have also been expanded to include worries about events that could befall attachment figures, not just the child him/herself. In addition, criteria was expanded to address separation anxiety disorder in adult populations [i.e., "work" under (4) and removal of "without significant adults" in (5)].*

*e.g., Bögels et al. (2010)*

6. Persistent reluctance or refusal to go to sleep without being near a major attachment figure or to sleep away from home
7. Repeated nightmares involving the theme of separation
8. Repeated complaints of physical symptoms (such as headaches, stomachaches, nausea, or vomiting) when separation from major attachment figures occurs or is anticipated

*(continued overleaf)*

**Table 2.1** (continued)

| Current diagnostic class | Specific disorder (relevant chptr) | *DSM-IV* criterion or criteria being changed | Description of key changes for *DSM-5* and abbreviated rationale |
| --- | --- | --- | --- |
| | | B. The disturbance causes clinically significant distress or impairment in social, academic (occupational), or other important areas of functioning. | B. The disturbance causes clinically significant distress or impairment in social, academic (occupational), or other important areas of functioning. *Utilize the Spence Children's Anxiety Scale-Separation Anxiety Disorder Subscale to specifically assess diagnostic criteria.* |
| | Agoraphobia† (16) | Note: Agoraphobia is not a codable disorder. Code the specific disorder in which the Agoraphobia occurs (e.g., 300.21 Panic Disorder With Agoraphobia or 300.22 Agoraphobia Without History of Panic Disorder). | *Agoraphobia will now be established as its own codable disorder separate from panic disorder based on genetic data, prior psychiatric history, comorbidity, course of illness, response to treatment, and reliability.* e.g., *Wittchen, Gloster, Beesdo-Baum, Fava, & Craske, 2010* |
| | | A. Anxiety about being in places or situations from which escape might be difficult (or embarrassing) or in which help may not be available in the event of having an unexpected or situationally predisposed Panic Attack or panic-like symptoms. Agoraphobic fears typically | A. Marked fear or anxiety about at least two agoraphobic situations, such as the following (see text for more examples): 1. being outside of the home alone; 2. public transportation (for example, traveling in buses, trains, ships, planes); |

A. Involve characteristic clusters of situations that include being outside the home alone; being in a crowd or standing in a line; being on a bridge; and traveling in a bus, train, or automobile.

3. open spaces (for example, parking lots, marketplace);
4. being in shops, theaters, or cinemas; or
5. standing in line or being in a crowd.

Fear or anxiety is related exclusively to specific listed situations in an effort to operationalize Agoraphobia as distinct from panic disorder.

Specific phobia (16)

A. Marked and persistent fear that is excessive or unreasonable, cued by the presence or anticipation of a specific object or situation (e.g., flying, heights, animals, receiving an injection, seeing blood).

A. Marked fear or anxiety about a specific object or situation (e.g., flying, heights, animals, receiving an injection, seeing blood).

*Broadly, changes to the criteria for specific phobias involve word changes to reflect consistency across anxiety disorders (e.g., "marked" in place of "intense"; "fear or anxiety"), the diagnostic threshold based on symptom severity, and the operationalization of vague terms, such as "excessive or unreasonable." In general, however, the work group argued that further data analysis is needed on the duration cutoff of 6 months as well as whether a separate criteria is needed any longer for significant distress considering the changes made in Criterion A, C, and E.*

*e.g., Craske et al., 2009; LeBeau et al., 2010*

*(continued overleaf)*

**Table 2.1** *(continued)*

| Current diagnostic class | Specific disorder (relevant chptr) | *DSM-IV* criterion or criteria being changed | Description of key changes for *DSM-5* and abbreviated rationale |
|---|---|---|---|
| | | B. Exposure to the phobic stimulus almost invariably provokes an immediate anxiety response, which may take the form of a situationally bound or situationally predisposed panic attack. Note: In children, the anxiety may be expressed by crying, tantrums, freezing, or clinging. | B. The phobic object or situation consistently provokes fear or anxiety. Note: In children, the fear or anxiety may be expressed by crying, tantrums, freezing, or clinging. |
| | Social anxiety disorder* (16) | *Formerly Social Phobia* <br><br> A. A marked and persistent fear of one or more social or performance situations in which the person is exposed to unfamiliar people or to possible scrutiny by others. The individual fears that he or she will act in a way (or show anxiety symptoms) that will be humiliating or embarrassing. Note: In children, there must be evidence of the capacity for age-appropriate social relationships with familiar people and the anxiety must occur in peer settings, not just in interactions with adults. | A. Marked fear or anxiety about one or more social situations in which the person is exposed to possible scrutiny by others. Examples include social interactions (e.g., having a conversation), being observed (e.g., eating or drinking), or performing in front of others (e.g., giving a speech). <br><br> *Broadly, the work group has proposed wording changes to reflect consistency across anxiety disorders (e.g., "marked" in place of "intense").* <br><br> e.g., Bögels et al., 2010; Lewis-Fernández et al., 2010 |

C. The social situations consistently provoke fear or anxiety. Note: In children, the fear or anxiety may be expressed by crying, tantrums, freezing, clinging, shrinking, or refusal to speak in social situations.

*Emphasis shifted from an individual's identification of fear as "excessive or unreasonable" to an emphasis on the manifestation of fear or anxiety.*

C. The person recognizes that the fear is excessive or unreasonable. Note: In children, this feature may be absent.

G. The fear, anxiety, and avoidance cause clinically significant distress or impairment in social, occupational, or other important areas of functioning.

*Severity Measures:*
*Social phobia inventory or mini-social phobia inventory*

E. The avoidance, anxious anticipation, or distress in the feared social or performance situation(s) interferes significantly with the person's normal routine, occupational (academic) functioning, or social activities or relationships, or there is marked distress about having the phobia.

Generalized anxiety disorder (16)

A. Excessive anxiety and worry (apprehensive expectation) about two (or more) domains of activities or events (for example, domains like family, health, finances, and school/work difficulties)

A. Excessive anxiety and worry (apprehensive expectation), occurring more days than not for at least 6 months, about a number of events or activities (such as work or school performance).

*It is possible there will be a name change in either DSM-V or future classifications of this disorder to better reflect worry, argued to be the primary component of GAD. In addition to this proposed change, the work group has suggested lowering diagnostic thresholds (time, symptoms) to better capture a greater number of clinically significant cases.*

*e.g., Andrews et al., 2010*

*(continued overleaf)*

**Table 2.1** *(continued)*

| Current diagnostic class | Specific disorder (relevant chptr) | *DSM-IV* criterion or criteria being changed | Description of key changes for *DSM-5* and abbreviated rationale |
|---|---|---|---|
| | | C. The anxiety and worry are associated with three (or more) of the following six symptoms (with at least some symptoms present for more days than not for the past 6 months). Note: Only one item is required in children.<br>1. Restlessness or feeling keyed up or on edge<br>2. Being easily fatigued<br>3. Difficulty concentrating or mind going blank<br>4. Irritability<br>5. Muscle tension<br>6. Sleep disturbance (difficulty falling or staying asleep, or restless unsatisfying sleep) | C. The anxiety and worry are associated with one or more of the following symptoms:<br>1. Restlessness or feeling keyed up or on edge<br>2. Being easily fatigued<br>3. Difficulty concentrating or mind going blank<br>4. Irritability<br>5. Muscle tension<br>6. Sleep disturbance (difficulty falling or staying asleep, or restless unsatisfying sleep)<br><br>*Suggest reducing the number of symptoms from three to one or more due to lack of evidence for the clinical significance of DSM-IV threshold. Thus, this would also allow for the identification of a greater number of meaningful cases.* |
| | | E. The anxiety, worry, or physical symptoms cause clinically significant distress or impairment in social, occupational, or other important areas of functioning. | F. The anxiety, worry, or physical symptoms cause clinically significant distress or impairment in social, occupational, or other important areas of functioning.<br><br>*Considering removal of this criterion.* |

| Obsessive-compulsive and related disorders | Obsessive-compulsive disorder (16) | A. Either obsessions or compulsions: Obsessions as defined by (1), (2), (3), and (4): 1. Recurrent and persistent thoughts, impulses, or images that are experienced, at some time during the disturbance, as intrusive and inappropriate and that cause marked anxiety or distress. 2. The thoughts, impulses, or images are not simply excessive worries about real-life problems. 3. The person attempts to ignore or suppress such thoughts, impulses, or images, or to neutralize them with some other thought or action. 4. The person recognizes that the obsessional thoughts, impulses, or images are a product of his or her own mind (not imposed from without as in thought insertion). Compulsions as defined by (1) and (2): 1. Repetitive behaviors (e.g., hand washing, ordering, checking) or mental acts (e.g., praying, counting, repeating words silently) that the person feels driven to perform in response to an obsession, or according to rules that must be applied rigidly. 2. The behaviors or mental acts are aimed at preventing or reducing | A. Either obsessions or compulsions: Obsessions as defined by (1) and (2): 1. Recurrent and persistent thoughts, urges, or images that are experienced, at some time during the disturbance, as intrusive and unwanted and that in most individuals cause marked anxiety or distress. 2. The person attempts to ignore or suppress such thoughts, urges, or images, or to neutralize them with some other thought or action (i.e., by performing a compulsion). Compulsions as defined by (1) and (2): 1. Repetitive behaviors (e.g., hand washing, ordering, checking) or mental acts (e.g., praying, counting, repeating words silently) that the person feels driven to perform in response to an obsession, or according to rules that must be applied rigidly. 2. The behaviors or mental acts are aimed at preventing or reducing anxiety or distress, or preventing some dreaded event or situation; however, these behaviors or mental acts either are not connected in a realistic way with what they are designed to neutralize or prevent, or are clearly excessive. |
| --- | --- | --- | --- |

*(continued overleaf)*

Table 2.1 *(continued)*

| Current diagnostic class | Specific disorder (relevant chptr) | DSM-IV criterion or criteria being changed | Description of key changes for DSM-5 and abbreviated rationale |
|---|---|---|---|
| | | distress or preventing some dreaded event or situation; however, these behaviors or mental acts either are not connected in a realistic way with what they are designed to neutralize or prevent or are clearly excessive. | *A number of wording changes are proposed for the definitions of obsessions and compulsions, including replacing "impulse" with "urge" as well as "inappropriate" with "unwanted" to reflect the ego-dystonic nature of obsessions.* |
| | | | *The work group is also considering adding avoidance to the definition of obsessions.* |
| | | | *e.g., Leckman et al., 2010* |
| Trauma- and stressor-related disorders | Posttraumatic stress disorder (16) | A. The person has been exposed to a traumatic event in which both of the following were present: <br> 1. The person experienced, witnessed, or was confronted with an event or events that involved actual or threatened death or serious injury, or a threat to the physical integrity of self or others. <br> 2. The person's response involved intense fear, helplessness, or horror. Note: In children, this may be expressed instead by disorganized or agitated behavior. | A. The person was exposed to one or more of the following event(s): death or threatened death, actual or threatened serious injury, or actual or threatened sexual violation, in one or more of the following ways: <br> 1. Experiencing the event(s) him- or herself <br> 2. Witnessing, in person, the event(s) as they occurred to others <br> 3. Learning that the event(s) occurred to a close relative or close friend; in such cases, the actual or threatened death must have been violent or accidental |

74

4. Experiencing repeated or extreme exposure to aversive details of the event(s) (e.g., first responders collecting body parts; police officers repeatedly exposed to details of child abuse); this does not apply to exposure through electronic media, television, movies, or pictures, unless this exposure is work related.

*Criterion A has been altered to create a better distinction between "traumatic" events and distressing events that do not meet this threshold. Criterion A2 has been removed.*

*e.g., Hinton & Lewis-Fernandez, 2011*

D. Negative alterations in cognitions and mood that are associated with the traumatic event(s) (that began or worsened after the traumatic event[s]), as evidenced by 3 or more of the following: Note: In children, as evidenced by 2 or more of the following:

Inability to remember an important aspect of the traumatic event(s) (typically dissociative amnesia; not due to head injury, alcohol, or drugs)

Persistent and exaggerated negative expectations about one's self, others, or the world (e.g., "I am bad," "no one can be trusted," "I've lost my soul forever,"

*(continued overleaf)*

**Table 2.1** (continued)

| Current diagnostic class | Specific disorder (relevant chptr) | DSM-IV criterion or criteria being changed | Description of key changes for DSM-5 and abbreviated rationale |
|---|---|---|---|
| | | | "my whole nervous system is permanently ruined," "the world is completely dangerous") |
| | | | Persistent distorted blame of self or others about the cause or consequences of the traumatic event(s) |
| | | | Pervasive negative emotional state—for example: fear, horror, anger, guilt, or shame |
| | | | Markedly diminished interest or participation in significant activities |
| | | | Feeling of detachment or estrangement from others |
| | | | Persistent inability to experience positive emotions (e.g., unable to have loving feelings, psychic numbing). |
| | | | *New diagnostic cluster representing a division of formerly Cluster C criterion in line with supporting evidence from confirmatory factor analyses.* |
| | Posttraumatic stress disorder in preschool children† (16) | *New addition to the DSM-5.* | A. The child (less than 6 years old) was exposed to the following event(s): death or threatened death, actual or threatened |

serious injury, or actual or threatened sexual violation, in one or more of the following ways:

1. Experiencing the event(s) him- or herself
2. Witnessing the event(s) as it (they) occurred to others, especially primary caregivers
3. Learning that the event(s) occurred to a close relative or close friend

Note: Witnessing does not include events that are witnessed only in electronic media, television, movies or pictures.

*Since the publication of DSM-IV, studies have examined the symptoms and signs of PTSD in samples of children and adolescents under the age of 15, which had not previously been done. With this new information, the work group has proposed a specified diagnosis of PTSD in preschool children to highlight a more behavioral focus of symptoms and signs (e.g., "constriction in play" in C4) in place of measures of subjective experience.*

*e.g., Zeanah, 2010*

B. Intrusion symptoms that are associated with the traumatic event (that began after

*(continued overleaf)*

**Table 2.1** *(continued)*

| Current diagnostic class | Specific disorder (relevant chptr) | DSM-IV criterion or criteria being changed | Description of key changes for DSM-5 and abbreviated rationale |
| --- | --- | --- | --- |
| | | | the traumatic event), as evidenced by 1 or more of the following: |
| | | | 1. Spontaneous or cued recurrent, involuntary, and intrusive distressing memories of the traumatic event. Note: Spontaneous and intrusive memories may not necessarily appear distressing and may be expressed as play reenactment. |
| | | | 2. Recurrent distressing dreams related to the traumatic event (Note: It may not be possible to ascertain that the content is related to the traumatic event) |
| | | | 3. Dissociative reactions in which the individual feels or acts as if the traumatic event(s) were recurring (such reactions may occur on a continuum with the most extreme expression being a complete loss of awareness of present surroundings) |
| | | | 4. Intense or prolonged psychological distress at exposure to internal or external cues that symbolize or resemble an aspect of the traumatic event(s) |
| | | | 5. Marked physiological reactions to reminders of the traumatic event(s) |
| | | | *Compared to the criteria for adults, the work group has recommended* |

| | | | |
|---|---|---|---|
| | | *(but currently still retained) the qualifier of intrusions as distressing. This change will likely be emphasized in a note.* | |
| Acute stress disorder | A. The person has been exposed to a traumatic event in which both of the following were present:<br><br>1. The person experienced, witnessed, or was confronted with an event or events that involved actual or threatened death or serious injury, or a threat to the physical integrity of self or others.<br>2. The person's response involved intense fear, helplessness, or horror. | A. The person was exposed to one or more of the following event(s): death or threatened death, actual or threatened serious injury, or actual or threatened sexual violation, in one or more of the following ways:<br><br>1. Experiencing the event(s) him- or herself<br>2. Witnessing, in person, the event(s) as they occurred to others<br>3. Learning that the event(s) occurred to a close relative or close friend; in such cases, the actual or threatened death must have been violent or accidental<br>4. Experiencing repeated or extreme exposure to aversive details of the event(s) (e.g., first responders collecting body parts; police officers repeatedly exposed to details of child abuse); this does not apply to exposure through electronic media, television, movies or pictures, unless this exposure is work related. | *The work group has removed some of the DSM-IV acute stress disorder criteria (criterion A2; dissociative symptoms B3–5) due to a lack of clinical utility.*<br><br>*e.g., Bryant, Friedman, Spiegel, Ursano, & Strain, 2011; Hinton & Lewis-Fernandez, 2011* |

*(continued overleaf)*

**Table 2.1** (continued)

| Current diagnostic class | Specific disorder (relevant chptr) | DSM-IV criterion or criteria being changed | Description of key changes for DSM-5 and abbreviated rationale |
|---|---|---|---|
| | | B. Either while experiencing or after experiencing the distressing event, the individual has three (or more) of the following dissociative symptoms:<br><br>1. Subjective sense of numbing, detachment, or absence of emotional responsiveness<br>2. A reduction in awareness of his or her surroundings (e.g., "being in a daze")<br>3. Derealization<br>4. Depersonalization<br>5. Dissociative amnesia (i.e., inability to recall an important aspect of the trauma) | B. Eight (or more) of the following symptoms are present that were not present prior to the traumatic event or have worsened since: Intrusion Symptoms<br><br>1. Spontaneous or cued recurrent, involuntary, and intrusive distressing memories of the traumatic event<br>2. Recurrent distressing dreams in which the content and/or affect of the dream is related to the traumatic event<br>3. Dissociative reactions (e.g., flashbacks) in which the individual feels or acts as if the traumatic event were recurring<br>4. Intense or prolonged psychological distress or physiological reactivity at exposure to internal or external cues that symbolize or resemble an aspect of the traumatic event<br>5. Dissociative Symptoms: A subjective sense of numbing, detachment from others, or reduced responsiveness to events that would normally elicit an emotional response |

1. An altered sense of the reality of one's surroundings or oneself (e.g., seeing oneself from another's perspective, being in a daze, time slowing)
2. Inability to remember at least one important aspect of the traumatic event (typically dissociative amnesia; not due to head injury, alcohol, drugs)
3. Avoidance Symptoms: Persistent and effortful avoidance of thoughts, conversations, or feelings that arouse recollections of the traumatic event
4. Persistent and effortful avoidance of activities, places, or physical reminders that arouse recollections of the traumatic event
5. Sleep disturbance (for example, difficulty falling or staying asleep, or restless sleep)
6. Hypervigilance
7. Irritable or aggressive behavior
8. Exaggerated startle response
9. Agitation or restlessness

*All symptoms have been collapsed into a single cluster, while also providing greater specification rather than general cluster descriptions. They have done so because research has demonstrated that reactions do not necessarily include dissociative or other symptom clusters specified in DSM-IV.*

(continued overleaf)

**Table 2.1** *(continued)*

| Current diagnostic class | Specific disorder (relevant chptr) | *DSM-IV* criterion or criteria being changed | Description of key changes for *DSM-5* and abbreviated rationale |
|---|---|---|---|
| Depressive disorders | Disruptive mood dysregulation disorder† (17) | New addition to the DSM-5. | A. The disorder is characterized by severe recurrent temper outbursts in response to common stressors.<br>1. The temper outbursts are manifest verbally and/or behaviorally, such as in the form of verbal rages, or physical aggression towards people or property.<br>2. The reaction is grossly out of proportion in intensity or duration to the situation or provocation.<br>3. The responses are inconsistent with developmental level.<br><br>*A dramatic increase in the diagnostic rates of pediatric bipolar disorder supports the need for a syndrome that describes severe, nonepisodic irritability in children. These children have psychiatric impairment, but have not previously fit well within any existing category in the DSM.*<br><br>*American Psychiatric Association, Task Force on DSM-5 childhood and adolescent disorders, 2010* |

B. Frequency: The temper outbursts occur, on average, three or more times per week.

C. Mood between temper outbursts:

1. Nearly every day, the mood between temper outbursts is persistently negative (irritable, angry, and/or sad).

2. The negative mood is observable by others (e.g., parents, teachers, peers).

Major depressive episode (17)

A. Five (or more) of the following symptoms have been present during the same 2-week period and represent a change from previous functioning; at least one of the symptoms is either (1) depressed mood or (2) loss of interest or pleasure. Note: Do not include symptoms that are clearly due to a general medical condition, or mood-incongruent delusions or hallucinations.

1. Depressed mood most of the day, nearly every day, as indicated by either subjective report (e.g., feels sad or empty) or observation made by others (e.g., appears tearful). Note: In children and adolescents, can be irritable mood.

2. Markedly diminished interest or pleasure in all, or almost all, activities most of the day, nearly every day (as indicated by either subjective account or observation made by others)

A. Five (or more) of the following criteria have been present during the same 2-week period and represent a change from previous functioning; at least one of the symptoms is either (1) depressed mood or (2) loss of interest or pleasure. Note: Do not include symptoms that are clearly due to a medical condition.

1. Depressed mood most of the day, nearly every day, as indicated by either subjective report (e.g., feels sad or empty) or observation made by others (e.g., appears tearful). Note: In children and adolescents, can be irritable mood.

2. Markedly diminished interest or pleasure in all, or almost all, activities most of the day, nearly every day (as indicated by either subjective account or observation made by others)

3. Significant weight loss when not dieting or weight gain (e.g., a change

(continued overleaf)

**Table 2.1** (*continued*)

| Current diagnostic class | Specific disorder (relevant chptr) | *DSM-IV* criterion or criteria being changed | Description of key changes for *DSM-5* and abbreviated rationale |
|---|---|---|---|
| | | 3. Significant weight loss when not dieting or weight gain (e.g., a change of more than 5% of body weight in a month), or decrease or increase in appetite nearly every day. Note: In children, consider failure to make expected weight gains.<br><br>4. Insomnia or hypersomnia nearly every day<br><br>5. Psychomotor agitation or retardation nearly every day (observable by others, not merely subjective feelings of restlessness or being slowed down)<br><br>6. Fatigue or loss of energy nearly every day<br><br>7. Feelings of worthlessness or excessive or inappropriate guilt (which may be delusional) nearly every day (not merely self-reproach or guilt about being sick)<br><br>8. Diminished ability to think or concentrate, or indecisiveness, nearly every day (either by subjective account or as observed by others)<br><br>9. Recurrent thoughts of death (not just fear of dying), recurrent suicidal ideation without a specific plan, or a | of more than 5% of body weight in a month), or decrease or increase in appetite nearly every day. Note: In children, consider failure to make expected weight gain<br><br>4. Insomnia or hypersomnia nearly every day<br><br>5. Psychomotor agitation or retardation nearly every day (observable by others, not merely subjective feelings of restlessness or being slowed down)<br><br>6. Fatigue or loss of energy nearly every day<br><br>7. Feelings of worthlessness or excessive or inappropriate guilt (which may be delusional) nearly every day (not merely self-reproach or guilt about being sick)<br><br>8. Diminished ability to think or concentrate, or indecisiveness, nearly every day (either by subjective account or as observed by others)<br><br>9. Recurrent thoughts of death (not just fear of dying), recurrent suicidal ideation without a specific plan, or a suicide attempt or a specific plan for committing suicide |

suicide attempt or a specific plan for committing suicide

*The term "criteria" replaces "symptoms" with the hope of preventing confusion between number of symptoms and number of criteria necessary for diagnosis.*

*In the first note, "Do not include symptoms due to ...mood-incongruent delusions or hallucinations" is eliminated as the meaning and purpose were deemed unclear.*

B. The symptoms do not meet criteria for a mixed episode.

*This criterion is being removed and replaced by a mixed features specifier.*

D. The symptoms are not due to the direct physiological effects of a substance (e.g., a drug of abuse, a medication) or a general medical condition (e.g., hypothyroidism).

C. The episode is not due to the direct physiological effects of a substance or antidepressant intervention (e.g., a drug of abuse, a medication, or other treatment). Note: A full hypomanic or manic episode emerging during antidepressant treatment (medication, ECT, etc.) and persisting beyond the physiological effect of that treatment is sufficient evidence for a hypomanic or manic episode diagnosis. However, caution is indicated so that one or two symptoms (particularly increased irritability, edginess or agitation following antidepressant use) are not taken as sufficient for diagnosis of a hypomanic or manic episode.

*e.g, Ziscook & Kendler, 2007*

*(continued overleaf)*

**Table 2.1** *(continued)*

| Current diagnostic class | Specific disorder (relevant chptr) | *DSM-IV* criterion or criteria being changed | Description of key changes for *DSM-5* and abbreviated rationale |
|---|---|---|---|
| | | E. The symptoms are not better accounted for by bereavement, i.e., after the loss of a loved one, the symptoms persist for longer than 2 months or are characterized by marked functional impairment, morbid preoccupation with worthlessness, suicidal ideation, psychotic symptoms, or psychomotor retardation. | This criterion is being removed. *The exclusion of symptoms "not better accounted for by bereavement" is removed; separating loss of a loved one from other stressors is not supported by evidence.* |
| | Chronic depressive disorder* (17) | *Formerly dysthymic disorder.* This category will replace the previous criteria for dysthymic disorder. | The proposed criteria for chronic depressive disorder have been gleaned from the definition of dysthymia after the elimination of Criterion D (excluding those with major depressive episodes in the first two years of illness) and of Criterion E (a history of mania or hypomania). *Studies comparing chronic nonbipolar major depression to dysthymia (with or without superimposed major depression) have found no significant differences in demographic variables, pattern of symptoms, response to treatment, or family history. It is therefore proposed that the category of major depression with chronic specifier be combined with* |

*dysthymic disorder under the term "chronic depressive disorder."*

*e.g., McCullough et al., 2000; Yang & Dunner, 2001*

This criterion is being removed.

This criterion is being removed.

The patient has three or four of the symptoms of major depression (which must include depressed mood and/or anhedonia), and they are accompanied by anxious distress. The symptoms must have lasted at least 2 weeks, and no other DSM diagnosis of anxiety or depression must be present, and they are both occurring at the same time.

Anxious distress is defined as having two or more of the following symptoms: irrational worry, preoccupation with unpleasant worries, having trouble relaxing, motor tension, fear that something awful may happen.

D. No major depressive episode has been present during the first 2 years of the disturbance (1 year for children and adolescents); i.e., the disturbance is not better accounted for by chronic major depressive disorder, or major depressive disorder; in partial remission.

E. There has never been a manic episode, a mixed episode, or a hypomanic episode, and criteria have never been met for cyclothymic disorder.

Mixed anxiety/depression

A. Persistent or recurrent dysphoric mood lasting at least 1 month.

B. The dysphoric mood is accompanied by at least 1 month of four (or more) of the following symptoms:

1. Difficulty concentrating or mind going blank
2. Sleep disturbance (difficulty falling or staying asleep, or restless, unsatisfying sleep)
3. Fatigue or low energy
4. Irritability
5. Worry
6. Being easily moved to tears
7. Hypervigilance

*(continued overleaf)*

**Table 2.1** (*continued*)

| Current diagnostic class | Specific disorder (relevant chptr) | *DSM-IV* criterion or criteria being changed | Description of key changes for *DSM-5* and abbreviated rationale |
|---|---|---|---|
| | | 8. Anticipating the worst<br>9. Hopelessness (pervasive pessimism about the future)<br>10. Low self-esteem or feelings of worthlessness<br>C. The symptoms cause clinically significant distress or impairment in social, occupational, or other important areas of functioning.<br>D. The symptoms are not due to the direct physiological effects of a substance (e.g., a drug of abuse, a medication) or a general medical condition.<br>E. All of the following:<br>  1. Criteria have never been met for major depressive disorder, dysthymic disorder, panic disorder, or generalized anxiety disorder.<br>  2. Criteria are not currently met for any other anxiety or mood disorder (including an anxiety or mood disorder, in partial remission).<br>  3. The symptoms are not better accounted for by any other mental disorder. | *Support for the inclusion of this disorder is based on research suggesting high comorbidity rates between anxiety and depression, as well as convergent evidence that anxious symptoms during a depressive episode are associated with greater symptom severity and episode duration.*<br><br>*e.g., Clayton, Grove, Coryell, & Keller, 1991* |

| Personality disorders | Borderline personality disorder (18) | A pervasive pattern of instability of interpersonal relationships, self-image, and affects, and marked impulsivity beginning by early adulthood and present in a variety of contexts, as indicated by five (or more) of the following: | A. Significant impairments in personality functioning manifest by: |
|---|---|---|---|

1. Frantic efforts to avoid real or imagined abandonment. Note: Do not include suicidal or self-mutilating behavior covered in Criterion 5.

2. A pattern of unstable and intense interpersonal relationships characterized by alternating between extremes of idealization and devaluation

3. Identity disturbance: markedly and persistently unstable self-image or sense of self

4. Impulsivity in at least two areas that are potentially self-damaging (e.g., spending, sex, substance abuse, reckless driving, binge eating). Note: Do not include suicidal or self-mutilating behavior covered in Criterion 5.

5. Recurrent suicidal behavior, gestures, threats, or self-mutilating behavior

6. Affective instability due to a marked reactivity of mood (e.g., intense episodic dysphoria, irritability, or anxiety usually lasting a few hours and only rarely more than a few days)

1. Impairments in self-functioning (a or b): a. Identity: Markedly impoverished, poorly developed, or unstable self-image, often associated with excessive self-criticism; chronic feelings of emptiness; dissociative states under stress; b. Self-direction: Instability in goals, aspirations, values, or career plans.

2. Impairments in interpersonal functioning (a or b): a. Empathy: Compromised ability to recognize the feelings and needs of others associated with interpersonal hypersensitivity (i.e., prone to feel slighted or insulted); perceptions of others selectively biased toward negative attributes or vulnerabilities; b. Intimacy: Intense, unstable, and conflicted close relationships, marked by mistrust, neediness, and anxious preoccupation with real or imagined abandonment; close relationships often viewed in extremes of idealization and devaluation and alternating between over involvement and withdrawal.

*See above section on general changes to personality disorders.*

*(continued overleaf)*

**Table 2.1** (continued)

| Current diagnostic class | Specific disorder (relevant chptr) | *DSM-IV* criterion or criteria being changed | Description of key changes for *DSM-5* and abbreviated rationale |
|---|---|---|---|
| | | 7. Chronic feelings of emptiness<br>8. Inappropriate, intense anger or difficulty controlling anger (e.g., frequent displays of temper, constant anger, recurrent physical fights)<br>9. Transient, stress-related paranoid ideation or severe dissociative symptoms | B. Pathological personality traits in the following domains:<br>1. Negative affectivity, characterized by:<br>(a) Emotional lability: Unstable emotional experiences and frequent mood changes; emotions that are easily aroused, intense, and/or out of proportion to events and circumstances.<br>(b) Anxiousness: Intense feelings of nervousness, tenseness, or panic, often in reaction to interpersonal stresses; worry about the negative effects of past unpleasant experiences and future negative possibilities; feeling fearful, apprehensive, or threatened by uncertainty; fears of falling apart or losing control. |

(c) Separation insecurity: Fears of rejection by—and/or separation from—significant others, associated with fears of excessive dependency and complete loss of autonomy.

(d) Depressivity: Frequent feelings of being down, miserable, and/or hopeless; difficulty recovering from such moods; pessimism about the future; pervasive shame; feeling of inferior self-worth; thoughts of suicide and suicidal behavior.

2. Disinhibition, characterized by:

(a) Impulsivity: Acting on the spur of the moment in response to immediate stimuli; acting on a momentary basis without a plan or consideration of outcomes; difficulty establishing or following plans; a sense of urgency and self-harming behavior under emotional distress.

(b) Risk taking: Engagement in dangerous, risky, and potentially self-damaging activities, unnecessarily and without regard to consequences; lack of concern for one's limitations and denial of the reality of personal danger.

*(continued overleaf)*

**Table 2.1** (continued)

| Current diagnostic class | Specific disorder (relevant chptr) | DSM-IV criterion or criteria being changed | Description of key changes for DSM-5 and abbreviated rationale |
|---|---|---|---|
| | Nonsuicidal self-injury† (18) | New addition to the DSM-5. | 3. Antagonism, characterized by: (a) Hostility: Persistent or frequent angry feelings; anger or irritability in response to minor slights and insults. A new disorder should be unrepresented or inappropriately represented in DSM-IV; have clinical value, improving accurate identification and/or treatment; and be prevalent, impairing, and distinctive. *Studies conducted among both adult and adolescent inpatients and outpatients have demonstrated that repeated self-injury co-occurs in conjunction with a variety of diagnoses (i.e., self-injury is not specific to borderline personality disorder).* *e.g., Herpertz, 1995; Jacobson, Muehlenkamp, Miller, & Turner, 2008* |

A. In the last year, the individual has, on 5 or more days, engaged in intentional self-inflicted damage to the surface of his or her body, of a sort likely to induce bleeding or bruising or pain (e.g., cutting, burning, stabbing, hitting, excessive rubbing), for purposes not socially sanctioned (e.g., body piercing, tattooing), but performed with the expectation that the injury will lead to only minor or moderate physical harm. The absence of suicidal intent is either reported by the patient or can be inferred by frequent use of methods that the patient knows, by experience, not to have lethal potential. (When uncertain, code with NOS 2.) The behavior is not of a common and trivial nature, such as picking at a wound or nail biting.

*Research indicates that among a large group of consecutive patients with borderline personality disorder who were engaging in self-injurious behavior, those who had self-injured more than 5 times were more likely to be in treatment and to meet criteria for an additional psychiatric diagnosis. In addition, a deliberate move away from general terms such as "self-harm" is based in its previously broad application to include both suicide attempts and nonsuicidal injuries, as well as behaviors or attitudes conveying a degree risk of harmful consequences (e.g., substance abuse).*

e.g., Brausch & Gutierrez, 2010; Dulit, Fyer, Leon, Brodsky, & Frances, 1994

(continued overleaf)

**Table 2.1** (continued)

| Current diagnostic class | Specific disorder (relevant chptr) | DSM-IV criterion or criteria being changed | Description of key changes for DSM-5 and abbreviated rationale |
|---|---|---|---|
| | | | B. The intentional injury is associated with at least 2 of the following: <br> 1. Negative feelings or thoughts, such as depression, anxiety, tension, anger, generalized distress, or self-criticism, occurring in the period immediately prior to the self-injurious act <br> 2. Prior to engaging in the act, a period of preoccupation with the intended behavior that is difficult to resist <br> 3. The urge to engage in self-injury occurs frequently, although it might not be acted on <br> 4. The activity is engaged in with a purpose; this might be relief from a negative feeling/cognitive state or interpersonal difficulty or induction of a positive feeling state. The patient anticipates these will occur either during or immediately following the self-injury. |
| Bipolar and related disorders | Bipolar I disorder (19) | A. There are six separate Criterion A sets: bipolar I disorder (most recent episode manic, hypomanic, mixed, or depressed). There are also several specifiers. | Addition of "and present most of the day, nearly every day" to the A criterion |

B. During the period of mood disturbance, three (or more) of the following symptoms have persisted (four if the mood is only irritable) and have been present to a significant degree.

Addition of "and represent a noticeable change from usual behavior" to the stem language for the B criteria

*To maintain consistency with major depressive disorder in terms of qualifiers and precision, parallel episode definitions in mania or hypomania are suggested.*

*American Psychiatric Association, Task Force on DSM-5 Mood Disorders (2010a)*

Bipolar II disorder (19)
Cyclothymic disorder (19)

A. For at least 2 years, the presence of numerous periods with hypomanic symptoms and numerous periods with depressive symptoms that do not meet criteria for a major depressive episode. Note: In children and adolescents, the duration must be at least 1 year.

B. During the above 2-year period (1 year in children and adolescents), the person has not been without the symptoms in Criterion A for more than 2 months at a time.

C. No major depressive episode, manic episode, or mixed episode has been present during the first 2 years of the disturbance.

See above under bipolar I disorder.
The only proposed change is the removal of "Mixed Episode" from Criterion C.

*(continued overleaf)*

**Table 2.1** *(continued)*

| Current diagnostic class | Specific disorder (relevant chptr) | *DSM-IV* criterion or criteria being changed | Description of key changes for *DSM-5* and abbreviated rationale |
|---|---|---|---|
| Neurodevelopmental disorders | Autism spectrum disorder†† (20) | This diagnostic category is new to the DSM-5 and subsumes what were previously autistic disorder (autism), Asperger's disorder, childhood disintegrative disorder, and pervasive developmental disorder not otherwise specified. | New diagnostic category that includes autistic disorder (autism), Asperger's disorder, childhood disintegrative disorder, and pervasive developmental disorder not otherwise specified. *General consensus that autism is defined by a common set of behaviors supports a single spectrum disorder and diagnostic category, adapted to the individual's clinical presentation by inclusion of clinical specifiers (e.g., severity, verbal abilities and others) and associated features (e.g., known genetic disorders, epilepsy, intellectual disability and others).* e.g., *Mandy, Charman, & Skuse, 2012; Wiggins, Robins, Adamson, Bakeman, & Henrich, 2011* |

| Schizophrenia spectrum disorders | Schizophrenia (21) | A. Characteristic symptoms: Two (or more) of the following, each present for a significant portion of time during a 1-month period (or less if successfully treated): <br> 1. Delusions <br> 2. Hallucinations <br> 3. Disorganized speech (e.g., frequent derailment or incoherence) <br> 4. Grossly disorganized or catatonic behavior <br> 5. Negative symptoms, i.e., affective flattening, alogia, or avolition <br><br> Note. Only one Criterion A symptom is required if delusions are bizarre or hallucinations consist of a voice keeping up a running commentary on the person's behavior or thoughts, or two or more voices conversing with each other. | A. Characteristic symptoms: Two (or more) of the following, each present for a significant portion of time during a 1-month period (or less if successfully treated). At least one of these should include 1 to 3. <br> 1. Delusions <br> 2. Hallucinations <br> 3. Disorganized speech <br> 4. Grossly abnormal psychomotor behavior, such as catatonia <br> 5. Negative symptoms, i.e., restricted affect or avolition/asociality | *By requiring that at least one of the characteristic symptoms be delusions, hallucinations, or disorganized speech, these criteria now fit the definition of schizophrenia as a "psychotic disorder and psychosis characterized by reality distortion and severe disorganization." Additionally, the criteria have been modified to clarify the negative symptoms, distinguish between disorganized behavior and catatonia, and remove the requirement that only one characteristic symptom need be present if it is a bizarre delusion or a Schneiderian first-rank symptom hallucination.* <br><br> *e.g., Fiedorowicz, Epping, & Flaum, 2008; Regier, 2007* |

*(continued overleaf)*

**Table 2.1** *(continued)*

| Current diagnostic class | Specific disorder (relevant chptr) | *DSM-IV* criterion or criteria being changed | Description of key changes for *DSM-5* and abbreviated rationale |
|---|---|---|---|
| | | Schizophrenia subtypes: paranoid, disorganized, catatonic, undifferentiated, residual | The work group is recommending that these subtypes not be included in DSM-5. |
| | | | These subgroups have had minimal clinical utility and diagnostic stability. |
| Feeding and eating disorders | Anorexia nervosa (22) | A. Refusal to maintain body weight at or above a minimally normal weight for age and height (e.g., weight loss leading to maintenance of body weight less than 85% of that expected; or failure to make expected weight gain during period of growth, leading to body weight less than 85% of that expected). | A. Restriction of energy intake relative to requirements leading to a significantly low body weight in the context of age, sex, developmental trajectory, and physical health. Significantly low weight is defined as a weight that is less than minimally normal, or, for children and adolescents, less than that minimally expected. |
| | | | *The word "refusal" has been removed as it implies intention and may contribute to difficulties with assessment. Instead, a focus on behavior has been suggested. e.g., Becker, Eddy, & Perloe, 2009* |
| | | B. Intense fear of gaining weight or becoming fat, even though underweight | B. Intense fear of gaining weight or becoming fat, or persistent behavior that interferes with weight gain, even though at a significantly low weight. |

98

D. In postmenarcheal females, amenorrhea, i.e., the absence of at least three consecutive menstrual cycles. (A woman is considered to have amenorrhea if her periods occur only following hormone, e.g., estrogen, administration.)

*The addition of a behavioral component contributes to a more inclusive criterion that now encompasses the small subset of individuals with the syndrome who explicitly deny a "fear of weight gain."*

D. Removal of amenorrhea criterion

*In DSM-IV, amenorrhea is required; however, this criterion excludes those individuals who exhibit all other symptoms of anorexia nervosa but maintain some menstrual activity. In addition, this criterion previously excluded pre-menarchal females, females taking oral contraceptives, post-menopausal females, or males from meeting diagnostic criteria.*

*e.g., Attia & Roberto, 2009*

Specify type:
Restricting Type: During the current episode of anorexia nervosa, the person has not regularly engaged in binge eating or purging behavior (i.e., self-induced vomiting or the misuse of laxatives, diuretics, or enemas).
Binge-Eating/Purging Type: During the current episode of anorexia nervosa, the person has regularly engaged in binge

Specifying current type: Restricting Type: during the past 3 months, the person has not engaged in recurrent episodes of binge eating or purging behavior (i.e., self-induced vomiting or the misuse of laxatives, diuretics, or enemas); binge-eating/purging type: during the past 3 months, the person has engaged in recurrent episodes of binge eating or purging behavior (i.e., self-induced vomiting or the misuse of laxatives, diuretics, or enemas)

*(continued overleaf)*

**Table 2.1** *(continued)*

| Current diagnostic class | Specific disorder (relevant chptr) | DSM-IV criterion or criteria being changed | Description of key changes for DSM-5 and abbreviated rationale |
|---|---|---|---|
| | | eating or purging behavior (i.e., self-induced vomiting or the misuse of laxatives, diuretics, or enemas). | *Although subtyping may hold certain utility for clinical and research purposes, data indicate significant cross-over between subtypes; as a result, it may be difficult to specify the subtype for the "current episode." It is suggested that the subtyping instead be specified for the past 3 months, consistent with the time frame used for bulimia nervosa and binge eating disorder.* |
| | | | *e.g., Peat, Mitchell, Hoek, & Wonderlich, 2009* |
| | Binge eating disorder° (22) | *Formerly in Appendix B.* | It is recommended that it be formally included as a disorder in DSM-5. |
| | | | *Across numerous studies, BED has distinguished itself from obesity and the other eating disorders across a wide range of validators.* |

Given the scope of these and other changes, it will take years of research to determine how effective the newest revision of the *DSM* will be in increasing the validity of psychiatric diagnosis—a major objective of the *DSM-5* Task Force, the APA, and other interested parties (see, e.g., Kraemer et al., 2010). Because most disorders will still be classified categorically, and because diagnoses will remain syndromal as opposed to pathophysiological or etiological, dissatisfaction among some is likely to persist. In research settings, for example, it is widely recognized that most forms of psychopathology are (1) distributed across dimensions—not categories (see above), and (2) rooted in specific neural systems subserving behavior. Weaknesses of the *DSM* approach in these areas comprise the impetus for an alternative classification system being developed by the NIMH.

## THE RESEARCH DOMAIN CRITERIA

Part of the NIMH Strategic Plan calls for a new, dimensional system of classifying psychopathology, based on identifiable neurobiological processes and observable behavior (NIMH, 2012). This system, known as the Research Domain Criteria (RDoC; e.g., Insel et al., 2010; Sanislow et al., 2010), is now under development. A major objective of the RDoC project is to identify dimensions of behavior, such as trait impulsivity, and map their underlying biobehavioral substrates, spanning genes to behavior. As outlined in Chapter 6, for example, several candidate genes, including the dopamine transporter (DAT), the monoamine oxidase-A (MAO-A) gene, and the catechol-*o*-methyltransferase (COMT) gene, have been implicated in trait impulsivity. Through their effects on neurotransmitter function and other central nervous system processes, these genes give rise to less reactive dopamine responses in neural structures (e.g., nucleus accumbens, anterior cingulate cortex) implicated in reward and associative learning. In turn, underreactive dopamine responding is expressed peripherally as cardiac insensitivity to incentives, and behaviorally as reward-seeking tendencies including delinquency (see Beauchaine et al., 2009; Beauchaine & Gatzke-Kopp, 2012; Chapter 6). Importantly, trait impulsivity underlies disorders across the externalizing spectrum (see, e.g., Krueger et al., 2002), yet is also observed in other forms of psychopathology not traditionally classified as externalizing, including borderline personality disorder (see Crowell, Beauchaine, & Linehan, 2009). Identifying traits that cut across traditional diagnostic boundaries and therefore "carve nature at its joints" is a primary objective of the RDoC project. Major assumptions of this approach are that it will (a) improve construct validity vis-à-vis the *DSM*; (b) identify more genetically homogenous populations for psychiatric genetics studies, an area of research that has been hampered by the current approach of mapping genes onto behavioral syndromes that arise from heterogeneous causes (i.e., equifinality; see Chapter 1); and (c) result in better treatments because our understanding of etiology will improve, allowing us to better match patients to specific interventions.

To advance the RDoC agenda, NIMH formed an internal work group in 2009, and has solicited input from researchers around the world. Several workshops have also been held, including those addressing cognitive systems, social process systems, arousal/regulatory systems, working memory systems, negative valence systems, and positive valence systems. In addition, NIMH released a request for grant applications in 2012 entitled, *Dimensional Approaches to Research Classification in Psychiatric Disorders*. Thus, the RDoC project remains in the development stage.

## CONCLUSIONS

In this chapter, we reviewed historical developments in psychiatric diagnosis—particularly emergence of the *DSM*—and identified core issues confronted by those who seek to classify psychopathology. As our review indicates, the history of the *DSM* and the complexities behind its development are far more intricate than might be surmised from thumbing through its pages. Although considerable efforts of many talented scientists have contributed to revising the *DSM*, long-standing issues of validity, and to a lesser extent reliability, remain to be addressed fully. Among the most important limitations of the *DSM* framework are its failures to (a) capture developmental processes underlying current and future risk for psychopathology, (b) specify pathophysiological and etiological mechanisms of psychopathology, (c) map broad biobehavoioral traits that predispose to psychopathology across traditional diagnostic boundaries, and (d) account fully for contextual influences such as ethnicity and culture on the development of psychopathology. As outlined in Chapter 1, these issues are central to the developmental psychopathology perspective, and are therefore addressed in chapters to follow.

## REFERENCES

Achenbach, T. M., & Edelbrock, C. S. (1991). *Manual for the child behavior checklist and revised child behavior profile*. Burlington, VT: University Associates in Psychiatry.

Achenbach, T. M., & Rescorla, L. A. (2006). Developmental issues in assessment, taxonomy, and diagnosis of psychopathology: Lifespan and multicultural perspectives. In D. Cicchetti & D. Cohen (Eds.), *Developmental psychopathology* (2nd ed., pp. 139–180). Hoboken, NJ: Wiley.

American Psychiatric Association. (1952). *Diagnostic and statistical manual of mental disorders*. Washington, DC: Author.

American Psychiatric Association. (1968). *Diagnostic and statistical manual of mental disorders* (2nd ed.). Washington, DC: Author.

American Psychiatric Association. (1974). *Diagnostic and statistical manual of mental disorders* (2nd ed., seventh printing). Washington, DC: Author.

American Psychiatric Association. (1980). *Diagnostic and statistical manual of mental disorders* (3rd ed.). Washington, DC: Author.

American Psychiatric Association. (1987). *Diagnostic and statistical manual of mental disorders* (3rd ed., revised). Washington, DC: Author.

American Psychiatric Association. (1994). *Diagnostic and statistical manual of mental disorders* (4th ed.). Washington, DC: Author.

American Psychiatric Association. (1996). *DSM-IV sourcebook* (Vol. 3). Washington, DC: Author.

American Psychiatric Association. (2000). *Diagnostic and statistical manual of mental disorders* (4th ed., text revision). Washington, DC: Author.

American Psychiatric Association. (2010a). *DSM-5: Options being considered for ADHD*. Retrieved from http://www.dsm5.org/Proposed%20Revision%20Attachments/APA%20Options%20for%20ADHD.pdf

American Psychiatric Association. (2010b). *Brief rationale and status of the development of a trait dimensional diagnostic system for personality disorder in DSM-5*. Retrieved from http://www.dsm5.org/Documents/APA%20Trait%20System%20Rationale.pdf

American Psychiatric Association. (2010c). *Rationale for a revised "A" criteria for personality disorders and the levels of personality functioning*. Retrieved from http://www.dsm5.org/Proposed%20Revision%20Attachments/APA%20Rationale%20for%20a%20Revised%20Criterion%20A%206-20-11.pdf

American Psychiatric Association. (2012a). *DSM-5: The future manual*. Retrieved from http://www.psych.org/mainmenu/research/dsmiv/dsmv.aspx

American Psychiatric Association. (2012b). *DSM-5: The future of psychiatric diagnosis*. Retrieved from http://www.dsm5.org/Pages/Default.aspx

American Psychiatric Association. (2012c). *DSM-5 field trials*. Retrieved from http://www.dsm5.org/Research/Pages/DSM-5FieldTrials.aspx

American Psychiatric Association, task force on DSM-5 childhood and adolescent disorders (2010d). *Justification for Temper Dysregulation Disorder with Dysphoria*. Retrieved from http://www.dsm5.org/ProposedRevision/Pages/proposedrevision.aspx?rid=397#

American Psychiatric Association, Task Force on DSM-5 Mood Disorders. (2010e). *Issues pertinent to a developmental approach to bipolar disorder in DSM-5*. Retrieved from http://www.dsm5.org/ProposedRevision/Pages/proposedrevision.aspx?rid=154#

Andrews, G., Hobbs, M. L., Borkovec, T. D., Beesdo, K., Craske, M. G., Heimberg, R. G., . . . Stanley, M.A. (2010). Generalized Worry Disorder: A review of DSM-IV Generalized Anxiety Disorder and options for DSM-V. *Depression and Anxiety, 27,* 134–147.

Angold, A., Costello, E. J., & Erkanli, A. (1999). Comorbidity. *Journal of Child Psychology and Psychiatry, 40,* 57–87.

Angold, A., & Fisher, P. W. (1999). Interviewer-based interviews. In D. Shaffer, C. P. Lucas, & J. E. Richters (Eds.), *Diagnostic assessment in child and adolescent psychopathology* (pp. 34–64). New York, NY: Guilford Press.

Arkonac, O., & Guze, S. B. (1963). A family study of hysteria. *New England Journal of Medicine, 268,* 239–242.

Attia, E., & Roberto, C. A. (2009). Should amenorrhea be a diagnostic criterion for anorexia nervosa? *International Journal of Eating Disorders, 42,* 581–589.

Barkley, R. A., Murphy, K. R., & Fischer, M. (2008). *ADHD in adults: What the science says*. New York, NY: Guilford Press.

Beauchaine, T. P. (2003). Taxometrics and developmental psychopathology. *Development and Psychopathology, 15,* 501–527.

Beauchaine, T. P. (2007). A brief taxometrics primer. *Journal of Clinical Child and Adolescent Psychology, 36,* 654–676.

Beauchaine, T. P., & Gatzke-Kopp, L. M. (2012). Instantiating the multiple levels of analysis perspective into a program of study on the development of antisocial behavior. *Development and Psychopathology, 24*, 1003–1018.

Beauchaine, T. P., Gatzke-Kopp, L., & Mead, H. K. (2007). Polyvagal theory and developmental psychopathology: Emotion dysregulation and conduct problems from preschool to adolescence. *Biological Psychology, 74*, 174–184.

Beauchaine, T. P., Hinshaw, S. P., & Pang, K. L. (2010). Comorbidity of attention-deficit/hyperactivity disorder and early-onset conduct disorder: Biological, environmental, and developmental mechanisms. *Clinical Psychology: Science and Practice, 17*, 327–336.

Beauchaine, T. P., Klein, D. N., Crowell, S. E., Derbidge, C., & Gatzke-Kopp, L. M. (2009). Multifinality in the development of personality disorders: A Biology × Sex × Environment interaction model of antisocial and borderline traits. *Development and Psychopathology, 21*, 735–770.

Beauchaine, T. P., Lenzenweger, M. F., & Waller, N. (2008). Schizotypy, taxometrics, and disconfirming theories in soft science. *Personality and Individual Differences, 44*, 1652–1662.

Beauchaine, T. P., & Marsh, P. (2006). Taxometric methods: Enhancing early detection and prevention of psychopathology by identifying latent vulnerability traits. In D. Cicchetti & D. Cohen (Eds.), *Developmental psychopathology* (2nd ed., pp. 931–967). Hoboken, NJ: Wiley.

Beauchaine, T. P., Neuhaus, E., Brenner, S. L., & Gatzke-Kopp, L. (2008). Ten good reasons to consider biological processes in prevention and intervention research. *Development and Psychopathology, 20*, 745–774.

Becker, A. E., Eddy, K. T., & Perloe, A. (2009). Clarifying criteria for cognitive signs and symptoms for eating disorders in DSM-V. *International Journal of Eating Disorders, 42*, 611–619.

Blashfield, R. K. (1998). Diagnostic models and systems (pp. 57–80). In A. S. Bellack & M. Hersen (Eds.), *Comprehensive clinical psychology*. New York, NY: Pergamon.

Bögels, S. M., Alden, L., Beidel, D. C., Clark, L. A., Pine, D. S., Stein, M. B., & Voncken, M. (2010). Social anxiety disorder: Questions and answers for the DSM-V. *Depression and Anxiety, 27*, 168–189.

Borges, G., Ye, Y., Bond, J., Cherpital, C. J., Cremonte, M., Moskalewicz, J., Swiatkiewicz, G., & Rubio-Stipec M. (2010). The dimensionality of alcohol use disorders and alcohol consumption in a cross-national perspective. *Addiction, 105*, 240–254.

Braithwaite, R. B. (1953). *Scientific explanation*. Cambridge, United Kingdom: Cambridge University Press.

Brausch, A. M., & Gutierrez, P. M. (2010). Differences in non-suicidal self-injury and suicide attempts in adolescents. *Journal of Youth and Adolescence, 39*, 233–242.

Bryant, R. A., Friedman, M. J., Spiegel, D., Ursano, R., & Strain, J. (2011). A review of acute stress disorder in DSM-5. *Depression and Anxiety, 28*, 802–817.

Carroll, B. J., Greden, J. R., & Feinberg, M. (1980). Suicide, neuroendocrine dysfunction and CSF 5-HIAA concentrations in depression. In B. Angrist (Ed.), *Proceedings of the 12th CINP congress* (pp. 307–313). Oxford, United Kingdom: Pergamon Press.

Cicchetti, D., & Toth, S. L. (2009). The past achievements and future promises of developmental psychopathology: The coming of age of a discipline. *Journal of Child Psychology and Psychiatry, 50*, 16–25.

Clayton, P. J., Grove, W. M., Coryell, W. H., & Keller, M. B. (1991). Follow-up and family study of anxious depression. *American Journal of Psychiatry, 148*, 1512–1517.

Cloninger, C. R. (1989). Establishment of diagnostic validity in psychiatric illness: Robins and Guze's method revisited. In L. N. Robins & J. E. Barrett (Eds.), *The validity of psychiatric diagnosis* (pp. 9–18). New York, NY: Raven.

Cohen, M. E., Cassidy, W. L., Flanagan, N. B., & Spellman, M. (1937). Clinical observations in manic-depressive disease—A quantitative study of 100 manic-depressive patients 50 medically sick controls. *Journal of the American Medical Association, 164*, 1535–1546.

Cohen, M. E., Robins, E., & Purtell, J. J. (1952). "Hysteria" in men. A study of 38 patients so diagnosed and 194 control subjects. *New England Journal of Medicine, 246*, 677–685.

Conners, C. K., Sitarenios, G., Parker, J. D. A., & Epstein, J. N. (1998). The revised Conners' parent rating scale (CPRS-R): Factor structure, reliability, and criterion validity. *Journal of Abnormal Child Psychology, 26*, 257–268.

Coryell, W., & Schlesser, M. (2001). The dexamethasone suppression test and suicide prediction. *American Journal of Psychiatry, 158*, 748–753.

Costello, A. J., Edelbrock, C. S., Dulcan, M. D., Kalas, R., & Klaric, S. H. (1984), *Report of the NIMH diagnostic interview schedule for children (DISC)*. Washington, DC: NIMH.

Craske, M. G., Rauch, S. L., Ursano, R., Prenoveau, J., Pine, D. S., & Zinbarg, R. E. (2009). What is an Anxiety Disorder? *Depression and Anxiety, 26*, 1066–1085.

Cronbach, L. J., & Meehl, P. E. (1955). Construct validity in psychological tests. *Psychological Bulletin, 52*, 281–302.

Crowell, S. E., Beauchaine, T. P., & Linehan, M. (2009). A biosocial developmental model of borderline personality: Elaborating and extending Linehan's theory. *Psychological Bulletin, 135*, 495–510.

Cummings, E. M., Davies, P. T., & Campbell, S. B. (2000). *Developmental psychopathology and family process*. New York, NY: Guilford Press.

Dulit, R. A., Fyer, M. R., Leon, A. C., Brodsky, B. S., & Frances, A. J. (1994). Clinical correlates of self-mutilation in borderline personality disorder. *American Journal of Psychiatry, 151*, 1305–1311.

Eaton, N. R., Krueger, R. F., South, S. C., Simms, L. J., & Clark, L. A. (2011). Contrasting prototypes and dimensions in the classification of personality pathology: Evidence that dimensions, but not prototypes, are robust. *Psychological Medicine, 41*, 1151–1163.

Endicott, J., & Spitzer, R. L. (1978). A diagnostic interview: The schedule for affective disorders and schizophrenia. *Archives of General Psychiatry, 35*, 837–844.

Engel, G. L. (1977). The need for a new medical model: A challenge for biomedicine. *Science, 196*, 129–136.

Feighner, J. P., Robins, E., Guze, S. B., Woodruff, R. A., Winokur, G., & Munoz, R. (1972). Diagnostic criteria for use in psychiatric research. *Archives of General Psychiatry, 26*, 57–63.

Fiedorowicz J. G., Epping E. A., & Flaum, M. (2008). Toward defining schizophrenia as a more useful clinical construct. *Current Psychiatry Reports, 10*, 344–351.

First, M. B., Spitzer, R. L., Gibbon, M., & Williams, J. B. W. (2002). *Structured clinical interview for DSM-IV-TR axis I disorders, research version, patient edition (SCID-IP).* New York, NY: Biometrics Research.

Frick, P. J., & Moffitt, T. E. (2010). *A proposal to the DSM-V childhood disorders and the ADHD and disruptive behavior disorders work group to include a specifier to the diagnosis of conduct disorder based on the presence of callous-unemotional traits.* Retrieved from http://www.dsm5.org/Proposed%20Revision%20Attachments/Proposal%20for%20Callous%20and%20Unemotional%20Specifier%20of%20Conduct%20Disorder.pdf

Gadow, K. D., & Sprafkin, J. (1997). *Child symptom inventories norms manual.* Stony Brook, NY: Checkmate Plus.

Garcia-Coll, C., Akerman, A., & Cicchetti, D. (2000). Cultural influences on developmental processes and outcomes: Implications for the study of development and psychopathology. *Development and Psychopathology, 12*, 333–356.

Gone, J. P., & Kirmayer, L. J. (2010). On the wisdom of considering culture and context in psychopathology. In T. Millon, R. F. Krueger, & E. Simonsen (Eds.), *Contemporary directions in psychopathology: Scientific foundations of the DSM-V and ICD-11* (pp. 72–96). New York, NY: Guilford Press.

Gurland, B. (1976). Aims, organization, and initial studies of the cross-national project. *International Journal of Aging and Human Development, 7*, 283–293.

Haslam, N., Holland, E., & Kuppens, P. (2012). Categories versus dimensions in personality and psychopathology: A quantitative review of taxometric research. *Psychological Medicine, 42*, 903–920.

Healy, D. (2002). Mandel Cohen and the origins of the diagnostic and statistical manual of mental disorders, third edition: DSM-III. *History of Psychiatry, 13*, 209–230.

Herpertz, S. (1995). Self-injurious behavior: Psychopathological and nosological characteristics in subtypes of self-injurers. *Acta Psychiatrica Scandanavia, 91*, 57–68.

Hinshaw, S. P., Lahey, B. B., & Hart, E. L. (1993). Issues of taxonomy and comorbidity in the development of conduct disorder. *Development and Psychopathology, 5*, 31–49.

Hinshaw, S. P., & Park, T. (1999). Research problems and issues: Toward a more definitive science of disruptive behavior disorders. In H. C. Quay & A. E. Hogan (Eds.), *Handbook of disruptive behavior disorders* (pp. 593–620). New York, NY: Plenum Press.

Hinton, D. E., & Lewis-Fernandez, R. (2011). The cross-cultural validity of post-traumatic stress disorder: Implications for DSM-5. *Depression and Anxiety, 28*, 783–801.

Hudziak, J. J., Achenbach, T. M., Altoff, R. R., & Pine, D. S. (2007). A dimensional approach to developmental psychopathology. *International Journal of Methods in Psychiatric Research, S1*, 16–23.

Insel, T. R., Cuthbert, B. N., Garvey, M. A., Heinssen, R. K., Pine, D. S., Quinn, K. J.,...Wang, P. S. (2010). Research domain criteria (RDoC): Toward a new classification framework for research on mental disorders. *American Journal of Psychiatry, 167*, 748–751.

Jacobson, C. M., Muehlenkamp, J. J., Miller, A. L., & Turner, E. B. (2008). Psychiatric impairment among adolescents engaging in different types of deliberate self-harm. *Journal of Clinical Child and Adolescent Psychology, 37*, 363–375.

Jensen, P. S., Knapp, P., & Mrazek, D. A. (2006). *Toward a new diagnostic system for child psychopathology: Moving beyond the DSM.* New York, NY: Guilford Press.

Katz, M. M., Secunda, S. K., Hirschfeld, R. M. A., & Koslow, S. H. (1979). NIMH—Clinical research branch collaborative program on the psychobiology of depression. *Archives of General Psychiatry, 36*, 765–771.

Kendell, R. E. (1989). Clinical validity. *Psychological Medicine, 19*, 45–55.

Kendler, K. S., Munoz, R. A., & Murphy, G. (2009). The development of the Feighner criteria: A historical perspective. *American Journal of Psychiatry, 167*, 134–142.

Kieling, C., Kieling, R., Rohde, L. A., Frick, P. J., Moffitt, T., Nigg, J., . . . Castellanos, F. X. (2010). The age-at-onset of ADHD. *American Journal of Psychiatry, 167*, 14–16.

Klein, D. N., & Riso, L. P. (1993). Psychiatric disorders: Problems of boundaries and comorbidity. In C. G. Costello (Ed.), *Basic issues in psychopathology* (pp. 19–66). New York, NY: Guilford Press.

Kraemer, H. C., Kupfer, D. J., Narrow, W. E., Clarke, D. E., & Regier, D. A. (2010). Moving toward DSM-5: The field trials. *American Journal of Psychiatry, 167*, 1158–1160.

Krueger, R. F., Eaton, N. R., Clark, L. A., Watson, D., Markon, K. E., Derringer, J., . . . Livesley, W. J. (2011). Deriving an empirical structure of personality pathology for DSM-5. *Journal of Personality Disorders, 25*, 170–191.

Krueger, R. F., Hicks, B. M., Patrick, C. J., Carlson, S. R., Iacono, W. G., & McGue, M. (2002). Etiologic connections among substance dependence, antisocial behavior, and personality: Modeling the externalizing spectrum. *Journal of Abnormal Psychology, 111*, 411–424

Krueger, R. F., Watson, D., & Barlow, D. H. (2005). Toward a dimensionally based taxonomy of psychopathology [Special section]. *Journal of Abnormal Psychology, 114*, 491–569.

Kupfer, D. J., First, M. B., & Regier, D. A. (2002). *A research agenda for DSM-V.* Washington, DC: American Psychiatric Association.

Landis, J. R., & Koch, G. G. (1977). The measurement of observer agreement for categorical data. *Biometrics, 33*, 159–174.

Laurin, M. (2010). The subjective nature of Linnaean categories and its impact in evolutionary biology and biodiversity studies. *Contributions to Zoology, 79*, 131–146.

LeBeau, R. T., Glenn, D., Liao, B., Wittchen, H.-U., Beesdo-Baum, K., Ollendick, T., & Craske, M. G. (2010). Specific phobia: A review of DSM-IV specific phobia and preliminary recommendations for DSM-V. *Depression and Anxiety, 27*, 148–167.

Leckman, J. F., Denys, D., Simpson, H. B., Mataix-Cols, D., Hollander, E., Saxena, S., . . . Stein, D. J. (2010). Obsessive-compulsive disorder: A review of the diagnostic criteria and possible subtype and dimensional specifiers for DSM-V. *Depression and Anxiety, 27*, 507–527.

Leckman, J. F., Weissman, M. M., Merikangas, K. R., Pauls, D. L., & Prusoff, B. A. (1983). Panic disorder and major depression: Increased risk of depression, alcoholism, panic, and phobic disorders in families of depressed probands with panic disorder. *Archives of General Psychiatry, 40*, 1055–1060.

Lenzenweger, M. F., McLachlan, G., & Rubin, D. B. (2007). Resolving the latent structure of schizophrenia endophenotypes using expectation-maximization-based finite mixture modeling. *Journal of Abnormal Psychology, 116*, 16–29.

Leventhal, A. M., & Rehm, L. P. (2005). The empirical status of melancholia: Implications for psychology. *Clinical Psychology Review, 25*, 25–44.

Lewis-Fernández, R., Hinton, D. E., Laria, A. J., Patterson, E. H., Hofmann, S. G., Craske, M. G., . . . Liao, B. (2010). Culture and the anxiety disorders: Recommendations for DSM-V. *Depression and Anxiety, 27*, 212–229.

Loeber, R., & Hay, D. (1997). Key issues in the development of aggression and violence from childhood to early adulthood. *Annual Review of Psychology, 48*, 371–410.

Lynam, D. R. (1998). Early identification of the fledgling psychopath: Locating the psychopathic child in the current nomenclature. *Journal of Abnormal Psychology, 107*, 566–575.

MacCallum, R. C., Zhang, S., Preacher, C. J., & Rucker, D. D. (2002). On the practice of dichotomization of quantitative variables. *Psychological Methods, 7*, 19–40.

Mandy, W. P. L., Charman, T., & Skuse, D. H. (2012). Testing the construct validity of the proposed criterion for DSM-5 autism spectrum disorder. *Journal of the American Academy of Child and Adolescent Psychiatry, 51*, 41–50.

Mannuzza, S. (2008). *Diagnosing ADHD in adults: DSM-IV controversies and DSM-V recommendations*. Review conducted for American Psychiatric Association, DSM-V Disruptive Behavior Disorders Workgroup.

Marsella, A. J., & Yamada, A. M. (2010). Culture and psychopathology: Foundations, issues, directions. *Journal of Pacific Rim Psychology, 4*, 103–115.

McCarthy, L. P., & Gerring, J. P. (1994). Revising psychiatry's charter document. *Written Communication, 11*, 147–192.

McCullough, J. P., Klein, D. N., Keller, M. B., Holzer, C. E., Davis, S. M., Kornstein, S. G., . . . Harrison, W. M. (2000). Comparison of DSM-III major depression and major depression superimposed on dysthymia (double depression): Validity of the distinction. *Journal of Abnormal Psychology, 109*, 419–427.

Meehl, P. E. (1995). Bootstraps taxometrics: Solving the classification problem in psychopathology. *American Psychologist, 50*, 266–275.

Meyer, A. Bentley, M., & Cowdry, E. V. (1934). *The problem of mental disorder: A study undertaken by the committee on psychiatric investigations, national research council* (pp. 51–70). New York, NY: McGraw-Hill.

Munkvold, L., Lundervold, A., Lie, S. A., & Manger, T. (2009). Should there be separate parent and teacher-based categories of ODD? Evidence from a general population. *Journal of Child Psychology and Psychiatry, 50*, 1264–1272.

Narrow, W. E., First, M. B., Sirovatka, P. J., & Regier, D. A. (2007). *Age and gender considerations in psychiatric diagnosis: A research agenda for DSM-V*. Washington, DC: American Psychiatric Association.

National Institute of Mental Health. (2012). *Research Domain Criteria (RDoC)*. Retrieved from http://www.nimh.nih.gov/research-funding/rdoc/index.shtml

Parker, G., Fink, M., Shorter, E., Taylor, M. A., Akiskal, H., Berrios, G., . . . Swartz, C. (2010). Whither melancholia? The case for its classification as a mood disorder. *American Journal of Psychiatry, 167*, 745–747.

Peat, C., Mitchell, J. E., Hoek, H. W., & Wonderlich, S. A. (2009). Validity and utility of subtyping anorexia nervosa. *International Journal of Eating Disorders, 42,* 590–594.

Polanczyk, G., Caspi, A., Houts, R., Kollins, S. H., Rohde, L. A., & Moffitt, T. (2010). Implications of extending the ADHD age-of-onset criterion to age 12: Results from a prospectively studied birth cohort. *Journal of the American Academy of Child and Adolescent Psychiatry, 49,* 210–216.

Preskorn, S. H., & Baker, B. (2002). The overlap of DSM-IV syndromes: Potential implications for the practice of polypsychopharmacology, psychiatric drug development, and the human genome project. *Journal of Psychiatric Practice, 8,* 170–177.

Prilleltensky, I. (1989). Psychology and the status quo. *American Psychologist, 44,* 795–802.

Regier, D. A. (2007). Time for a fresh start? Rethinking psychosis in DSM-V. *Schizophrenia Bulletin, 33,* 843–845.

Regier, D. A., Myers, J. K., Kramer, M., Robins, L. N., Blazer, D. G., Hough, R. L., . . . Locke, B. Z. (1984). The NIMH epidemiologic catchment area program. Historical context, major objectives, and study population characteristics. *Archives of General Psychiatry, 41,* 934–941.

Reich, T., Clayton, P. J., & Winokur, G. (1969). Family history studies: V. The genetics of mania. *American Journal of Psychiatry, 125,* 1358–1369.

Renou, S., Hergueta, T., Flament, M., Mouren-Simeoni, M. C., & Lecrubier, Y. (2004). Diagnostic structured interviews in child and adolescent psychiatry. *Encephale, 30,* 122–134.

Richters, J. E., & Cicchetti, D. (1993). Mark Twain meets DSM-III-R: Conduct disorder, development, and the concept of harmful dysfunction. *Development and Psychopathology, 5,* 5–29.

Robins, E., & Guze, S. B. (1970). Establishment of diagnostic validity in psychiatric illness: Its application to schizophrenia. *American Journal of Psychiatry, 126,* 983–987.

Robins, L. N. (1966). *Deviant children grown up.* Baltimore, MD: Williams and Wilkins.

Robins, L. N., Helzer, J. E., Croughan, J., & Ratcliff, K. S. (1981). NIMH diagnostic interview schedule. *Archives of General Psychiatry, 38,* 381–389.

Robinson, E. A., Eyberg, S. M., & Ross, A. W. (1980). The standardization of an inventory of child conduct problem behaviors. *Journal of Clinical Child Psychology, 9,* 22–28.

Sanislow, C. A., Pine, D. S., Quinn, K. J., Kozak, M. J., Garvey, M. A., Heinssen, R. K., . . . . Cuthbert, B. N. (2010). Developing constructs for psychopathology research: Research domain criteria. *Journal of Abnormal Psychology, 119,* 631–639.

Scotti, J. R., & Morris, T. L. (2000). Diagnosis and classification. In M. Hersen & R. T. Ammerman (Eds.), *Advanced abnormal child psychology* (pp.15–32). Mahwah, NJ: Erlbaum.

Shaffer, D., Fischer, P., Lucas, C. P., Dulcan, M. K., & Schwab-Stone, M. E. (2000). NIMH diagnostic interview schedule for children version IV (NIMH DISC-IV): Description, differences from previous versions, and reliability of some common diagnoses. *Journal of the American Academy of Child and Adolescent Psychiatry, 39,* 28–38.

Sibley, M. H., Pelham, W. E., Molina, B. S. G., Waschbusch, D. A., Gnagy, E. M., Babinski, D. E., & Biswas, A. (2010). Inconsistent self-report of delinquency by adolescents and young adults with ADHD. *Journal of Abnormal Child Psychology, 38,* 645–656.

Spitzer, R. L., Endicott, J., & Robins, E. (1978). Research diagnostic criteria. *Archives of General Psychiatry, 35,* 773–782.

Spitzer, R. L., & Fleiss, J. L. (1974). A re-analysis of the reliability of psychiatric diagnosis. *British Journal of Psychiatry, 125,* 341–347.

Spitzer, R. L., & Williams, J. B. W. (1983). The DSM-III classification of affective disorders. *Acta Psychiatrica Scandanavia, S310,* 106–116.

Spitzer, R. L., Williams, J. B. W., Gibbon, M., & First, M. B. (1990). Structured clinical interview for DSM-III-R, patient edition/non-patient edition *(SCID-P/SCID-NP).* Washington, DC: American Psychiatric Press.

Sroufe, L. A. (1997). Psychopathology as an outcome of development. *Development and Psychopathology, 9,* 17–29.

Stringaris, A., & Goodman, R. (2009). Longitudinal outcome of youth oppositionality: Irritable, headstrong, and hurtful behaviors have distinctive predictions. *Journal of the American Academy of Child and Adolescent Psychiatry, 48,* 404–412.

Trull, T. J., & Durrett, C. A. (2005). Categorical and dimensional models of personality disorder. *Annual Review of Clinical Psychology, 1,* 355–380.

Wiggins, L. D., Robins, D. L., Adamson, L. B., Bakeman, R., & Henrich, C. C. (2011). Support for a dimensional view of autism spectrum disorders in toddlers. *Journal of Autism and Developmental Disorders, 42,* 191–200.

Wing, J. K., Cooper, J. F., & Sartorius, N. (1974). *The measurement and classification of psychiatric symptoms.* London, United Kingdom: Cambridge University Press.

Wittchen, H.-U., Gloster, A. T., Beesdo-Baum, K., Fava, G. A., & Craske, M. G. (2010). Agoraphobia: A review of the diagnostic classificatory position and criteria. *Depression and Anxiety, 27,* 113–133.

Woodruff, R. A., Goodwin, D. W., & Guze, S. B. (1974). *Psychiatric diagnosis.* New York, NY: Oxford University Press.

World Health Organization. (1966). ICD-8: International statistical classification of diseases and related health problems *(10th* Rev. ed.). Geneva, Switzerland: Author.

World Health Organization. (1996). *Multiaxial classification of child and adolescent psychiatric disorders.* Cambridge, United Kingdom: Cambridge University Press.

Yang, T., & Dunner, D. (2001). Differential sub-typing of depression. *Depression and Anxiety, 13,* 11–17.

Zeanah, C. H. (2010). *Proposal to include child and adolescent manifestations and age related subtypes for PTSD in DSM-V.* Retrieved from http://www.dsm5.org/Proposed%20Revision%20Attachments/DSM-5%20Child%20PTSD%20Review%2012–22–08.pdf

CHAPTER 3

# Genetic and Environmental Influences on Behavior

THEODORE P. BEAUCHAINE AND LISA M. GATZKE-KOPP

## HISTORICAL CONTEXT

THEORIES REGARDING THE CAUSES of psychopathology span much of written history. In the 2nd century A.D., for example, Galen—extending the writings of Hippocrates—attributed temperamental characteristics to individual differences in four bodily humors. According to his account of human behavior, melancholia—or depression—resulted from excess black bile, whereas emotional volatility resulted from excess yellow bile. Although Galen's theory placed the locus of mental illness within the individual, other historically influential accounts of psychopathology emphasized the role of environment in shaping behavior. Perhaps the most famous of these is Freud's psychoanalytic theory, which attributed the causes of mental illness to intrapsychic conflicts among the id, ego, and superego. According to Freud, both the ego and superego derived their relative strength or weakness almost exclusively from early experience.

Although extracted from very different historical epochs, these examples reflect a clear difference in beliefs about the importance of nature vs. nurture in the development of mental illness. Until the 20th century, such differences in opinion were irresolvable because formal scientific methods had not been applied to the study of psychopathology, and because appropriate technological and methodological tools had not been developed to effectively parse the relative contributions of heritable and environmental influences on behavior. Toward the end of the century, however, advances in molecular genetics, along with refinements in both behavioral genetics and statistical modeling, provided the means for resolving longstanding questions about the etiology of psychopathology (see, e.g., Rende & Waldman, 2006). Yet despite these breakthroughs, disagreements over the relative contributions of genes and environment in explaining psychopathology lingered (see, e.g., Albee & Joffe, 2004; Beauchaine, Neuhaus, Brenner, & Gatzke-Kopp, 2008). Indeed, preferred explanations for individual differences in behavior have waxed and waned between

111

genes and environment several times during the past 50 years, often influenced as much by political considerations as by scientific discovery and innovation (see Rutter, Moffitt, & Caspi, 2006b).

In the past 10 to 15 years, a much more balanced perspective has emerged. Theoretical advances, the capacity to conduct genome-wide scans, and more widespread use of the advanced methods noted earlier have revealed that both genetic and environmental influences play significant roles in the expression of almost all behavioral traits—including those linked to psychopathology—and that the nature versus nurture question is misleading because it forces us to choose between influences that are interdependent. Indeed, environment can affect development by altering gene expression—blurring formerly drawn boundaries between the effects of genes and environments in shaping behavior. In fact, although genetic and environmental influences have often been treated as separate, a growing body of research indicates that Gene × Environment interactions may be more important in determining behavior than either factor alone (see Moffitt, Caspi, & Rutter, 2006; Rutter, 2007). It has long been known, for example, that impulsivity is a highly heritable trait (e.g., Hinshaw, 2002, 2003; see also Beauchaine & Gatzke-Kopp, in press; Beauchaine, Hinshaw, & Pang, 2010; Chapter 6), conferring risk for a host of behavioral disorders including delinquency, antisocial behavior, and both alcohol and substance dependencies (e.g., Krueger et al., 2002). However, recent research demonstrates that impulsive boys and girls are more likely to develop these conditions in neighborhoods with high rates of drug use, violence, and criminality (Lynam et al., 2000; Meier, Slutske, Arndt, & Cadoret, 2008), or when maltreated by caretakers (Jaffee et al., 2005; Chapter 5). Furthermore, genetically vulnerable individuals may evoke reactions from others that exacerbate their inherited susceptibilities to psychopathology (e.g., O'Connor, Deater-Deckard, Fulker, Rutter, & Plomin, 1998a). Thus, combinations of genetically conferred vulnerabilities and environmentally mediated risk factors result in worse outcomes than either influence alone. When vulnerability and risk interact in such a way, studying either in isolation causes us to underestimate their combined importance (Beauchaine et al., 2008). Our primary objective in writing this chapter is to provide an integrated account of the interplay of heritable and environmental influences on psychopathology across the lifespan. We focus primarily on broad conceptual issues given that findings specific to particular forms of psychopathology are presented in later chapters. Our approach is informed considerably by the work of Rutter and others, who have written extensively about the mutual interplay of genes and environment in shaping human development and behavior (see, e.g., Moffitt, 2005; Rutter, 2007, 2010; Rutter et al., 2006).

## THE DEVELOPMENTAL PSYCHOPATHOLOGY PERSPECTIVE

As outlined in Chapter 1, the contents of this book are organized primarily around the *developmental psychopathology* perspective, an approach to the study of mental illness that emerged in the past 30 years. The developmental psychopathology framework is advantageous for studying the emergence of behavior disorders because it integrates the strengths of numerous other disciplines, including psychiatric genetics, child clinical psychology, child psychiatry, developmental psychology, epidemiology, and clinical neuroscience, among others. Developmental psychopathologists seek to characterize the course of mental illness as precisely as possible, at as many levels of analysis as possible. Levels of analysis refer to different systems through which a psychopathological trait is expressed, spanning genes to behavior to broad cultural factors (see Beauchaine & Gatzke-Kopp, 2012; Cicchetti, 2008).

The advantage of a multiple-levels-of-analysis approach to understanding psychopathology is exemplified in research on schizophrenia, an oftentimes progressively degenerative disorder in which afflicted individuals experience delusions, exhibit odd behaviors, and become isolated and avolitional (see Chapter 21). Although vulnerability to schizophrenia is heritable, most likely through combinations of vulnerable genes (see Gottesman & Gould, 2003), and/or rare structural genetic variants (Walsh et al., 2008), the exact genetic mechanisms remain uncertain. However, it is important to note that identifying all such genes will not result in a full understanding of the disorder, because genes do not affect behavior directly (see Rutter et al., 2006). Rather, they code for variations in protein expression that lead to structural and functional variations in the central nervous system and other organ systems. Furthermore, traits associated with genetic risk for schizophrenia, including neuromotor abnormalities, eye-tracking dysfunction, and abnormal activity in the prefrontal cortex during working memory tasks, can be present in vulnerable individuals whether they manifest the disorder (Callicott et al., 2003; Erlenmeyer-Kimling, Golden, & Cornblatt, 1989; Glahn et al., 2003; Lenzenweger, McLachlan, & Rubin, 2007; Ross, 2003).

As is the case with many psychiatric conditions, progression from genetic predisposition to manifestation of schizophrenia is affected profoundly by environmental influences (Cannon et al., 2002). Conversely, protective familial environments can improve the course of the disorder and in some cases prevent onset of illness (e.g., Cornblatt, 2001; see also Chapter 21). This example illustrates the importance of incorporating information from genetic, neurological, behavioral, and environmental levels of analysis toward understanding the complexity of debilitating conditions such as schizophrenia. Specifying the determinants of psychopathology across all relevant levels of analysis and understanding interactions and transactions across such levels are therefore primary objectives of developmental psychopathology research (Beauchaine & Gatzke-Kopp, 2012; Cicchetti, 2008).

## TERMINOLOGICAL AND CONCEPTUAL ISSUES

Our main goals in writing this chapter are to (1) describe the interactive roles of heritability and environment in shaping behavior, particularly psychopathology and (2) present important principles for interpreting more specific findings presented in later chapters. Toward addressing these objectives, we first consider important distinctions between *genotypes*, *phenotypes*, and *endophenotypes*, important constructs in genetics research. Although our descriptions are brief, they provide a foundation for understanding contents presented later in this volume.

## GENOTYPES, PHENOTYPES, AND ENDOPHENOTYPES

*Genotype.* The word *genotype* refers to the structural composition of the specific genes within an individual. Genes are comprised of DNA, which guides synthesis of messenger RNA through a process called *transcription*. In turn, messenger RNA guides production of polypeptides through a process called *translation*. These polypeptides are the building blocks of proteins, or *gene products*. Specific genes can be comprised of different *sequences*, or *allelic variants*, which sometimes give rise to individual differences in the volume or functionality of gene products. Some genetic variants give rise to individual differences in the synthesis, reuptake, and catalysis of neurotransmitters subserving mood, self-regulation, and motivation. When functionally compromised, these neurotransmitter systems, including serotonin, dopamine, and norepinephrine (among others), may confer vulnerability to mood disorders, impulse control problems, and asociality, respectively (see Beauchaine, Neuhaus, Zalewski, Crowell, & Potapova, 2011).

In the traditional view, all genetic variation was assumed to be fully inherited and fixed across the life span. It was also believed that heritable genetic variation encoded psychiatric disorders directly, through either single or multiple loci—assumptions referred to as *monogenic* and *polygenic determinism*, respectively. These assumptions imply (at least for serious mental disorders) that particular genes or patterns of genes always result in psychopathology, regardless of environmental input (see Rutter et al., 2006). However, it is now recognized that a number of intervening influences—many of which fall under environmental control—affect gene transcription, translation, and promotion, thereby altering gene expression. Although we discuss some of these intervening influences in later sections, for now it is sufficient to state that (1) both genes and environment are implicated in the expression of almost all forms of psychopathology, (2) there are no genes "for" particular behaviors or disorders, (3) environments can alter gene expression, and (4) many people who are genetically vulnerable never develop mental illness (see Kendler, 2005; Plomin, 1989).

*Phenotype.* The term phenotype refers to observable characteristics—both physical and behavioral—that result from the interplay between an organism's genes and the environment. The phenotype concept stems from early work in Mendelian genetics, where physical characteristics of an organism are reliable, outwardly measurable indicators of underlying genotypes. In Mendel's experiments on flower color and pea pod shape, phenotypes were dictated almost exclusively by inherited pairs of dominant and recessive genes, with limited environmental influence except in cases of severe deprivation (Hartl & Jones, 2002). Such is the case when a phenotype is determined monogenically. In contrast, assumedly polygenic traits such as most forms of psychopathology are influenced by many genes, so the correspondence between genotype and phenotype is far from 1:1. Furthermore, with multiple genetic influences, there are many opportunities for both gene-gene interactions and environmental regulation of gene expression (see below). This limited correspondence between genotypes and behavioral phenotypes presents formidable obstacles for psychiatric genetics (see Gatzke-Kopp, 2011), a topic we return to later.

*Endophenotype.* As defined by Gottesman and Gould (2003), endophenotypes are "measurable components unseen by the unaided eye along the pathway between disease and distal genotype" (Gottesman & Gould, 2003, p. 636). In this sense, endophenotypes are a special case of phenotype, as they too are measurable physical, physiological, or behavioral traits. However, they are closer to the functional output of the gene(s) in question (see Beauchaine, 2009; Gould & Gottesman, 2006; Lenzenweger, 2004). This closer proximity to genes makes carefully chosen endophenotypes quite valuable to psychiatric geneticists in their attempts to identify (1) specific alleles associated with psychopathology, and (2) genetically vulnerable individuals who have not yet developed psychopathology (see Beauchaine & Marsh, 2006; Castellanos & Tannock, 2002; Skuse, 2001).

In psychiatric genetics, it is important to distinguish between endophenotypes and other types of biomarkers. At the broadest level, biomarkers are measureable characteristics that indicate either risk for, or manifestation of, illness. For example, choline concentrations in the anterior cingulate cortex (ACC) correlate with depression severity among patients with bipolar disorder (Moore et al., 2000). Choline concentrations therefore serve as an objective biomarker of both clinical state and treatment response. Although such information may be quite useful in understanding the neural bases of mood and mood state, to qualify as an endophenotype a biomarker must be *state independent*. In other words, an endophenotype must mark genetic risk independent of clinical state to be maximally useful to psychiatric geneticists as they search for genes that contribute vulnerability to mental disorders. To qualify as an endophenotype, a biomarker must (1) segregate with illness in the general population, (2) be heritable, (3) be state independent, (4) co-segregate with disorder within families, (5) be present at higher rates in affected families than in the general population, and (6) be measured reliably and specifically (Gould & Gottesman, 2006). Thus, although the terms biomarker and endophenotype are often used interchangeably, the latter are a subset of the former, with much greater specificity and usefulness in genetics research (Beauchaine, 2009).

To date, a limited number of reliable endophenotypes have been identified in the psychopathology literature. A good example comes from research on schizophrenia. As noted earlier, patients with schizophrenia experience irregularities in smooth-pursuit eye tracking of moving stimuli, as measured by sophisticated eye-tracking devices. Although the pathophysiology of such deficiencies is poorly understood, about 80% of patients with schizophrenia exhibit the trait, as do about 45% of their first-degree relatives, compared with only 10% of those in the general population (see Gottesman & Gould, 2003). Importantly, this 10% figure matches the population prevalence rate of schizophrenia liability (note that only some with genetic liability develop the disorder, a phenomenon known as *incomplete penetrance*). Thus, eye-tracking dysfunction segregates within families, is heritable, is state-independent, cosegregates within families, is observed at higher rates in affected families than in the population, and is specific to schizophrenia liability. It is therefore quite useful in identifying those with a genetic predisposition to the disorder—even if they have not developed outwardly expressed symptoms. Detecting premorbid vulnerability among such individuals may have important implications for prevention, where early identification can improve long-term prognosis considerably (see Beauchaine et al., 2008; Beauchaine & Marsh, 2006).

# PSYCHIATRIC GENETICS

Broadly speaking, there are two overarching objectives of psychiatric genetics. The first is to parse variability in behavioral traits within populations (e.g., impulsivity, aggression, anxiety) into portions accounted for by (a) heritable mechanisms, (b) environmental mechanisms, and sometimes (c) Gene × Environment (G × E) interactions. This is accomplished through *behavioral genetics* research. The second is to identify specific alleles that confer vulnerability to psychopathology. This is accomplished though *molecular genetics* research. Each of these approaches provides unique information to the study of the development of psychopathology.

## BEHAVIORAL GENETICS

Traditionally, behavioral genetics studies have been used to parse sources of variance in behavior into three broad classes, including *additive genetic effects*, *shared environmental effects*, and *nonshared environmental effects*. Additive genetic effects encompass all sources of variance in a behavioral trait that are accounted for by heritable mechanisms within a population. Although potentially confusing, these "genetic effects" can arise from both genetic and nongenetic (although heritable) sources. For example, some genes are activated (turned on) among offspring only when their mothers are exposed to particular environments, oftentimes prenatally (see Rutter et al., 2006). Such *maternal programming* effects may increase risk for or protect against the emergence of psychopathology through *epigenetic* mechanisms described later. These effects are not purely genetic, yet they are often subsumed within the additive genetic component in behavioral genetics studies. Accordingly, to avoid confusion in this chapter we refer to *heritable effects* on behavior when the source of heritability cannot be attributed unambiguously to main effects of genes.

In the shorthand of behavioral genetics, heritable effects are denoted *A*, shared environmental effects are denoted *C*, and nonshared environmental effects are denoted *E* (hence the term ACE model). When squared, each term signifies a proportion of variance in behavior accounted for. In theory, these sources sum to 1.0, accounting for all variance in a particular trait ($A^2 + C^2 + E^2 = 1.0$). For example, averaged across many behavioral genetics studies with participants ranging in age from early childhood through adulthood (Cadoret, Leve, & Devor, 1997), heritable effects account for 44% of the variance in aggression ($A^2$; also denoted $h^2$), shared environmental effects account for 17% of the variance ($C^2$), and nonshared environmental effects account for 38% of the variance ($E^2$). Within rounding error, these sources add to 1.0, indicating that both heredity and environment make important contributions to the expression of violence.

Parsing a behavioral trait into heritable, shared environmental, and nonshared environmental components is accomplished through twin, family, and adoption studies. In the most basic twin design, the following three assumptions are made in estimating A, C, and E:

1. Monozygotic (mz) twins who are raised in the same family share 100% of their genes (A), and 100% common environment (C). Thus, the squared correlation ($r^2$) between phenotypes of mz twins provides an estimate of $A^2 + C^2$ ($r^2_{mz} = A^2 + C^2$).
2. Dizygotic (dz) twins raised in a family share about 50% of their genes (A), and 100% common environment (C). Thus, the squared correlation between phenotypes of dz twins provides an estimate of $\frac{1}{2} A^2 + C^2$. Rearranging algebraically, $A^2 = 2(r^2_{mz} - r^2_{dz})$, and $C^2 = r^2_{mz} - A^2$.
3. $E^2$ is the residual (error) variance not accounted for by $A^2$ and $C^2$. Thus, $E^2 = 1 - (A^2 + C^2)$.

Although variations in behavioral genetics designs are sometimes employed, most are built around these assumptions (interested readers are referred to Rende and Waldman [2006] for a comprehensive account of behavioral genetics in developmental psychopathology research).

*Complexities and limitations of behavioral genetics.* Several complexities and caveats should be considered in any discussion of the behavioral genetics of psychopathology. Perhaps most importantly, heritable vulnerabilities and environmental risk factors often interact to affect both age of onset and severity of psychopathology. For example, in many cases genetic liability is insufficient to result in schizophrenia (see earlier). Rather, vulnerability is translated into illness only when coupled with significant environmental risk (see, e.g., Gottesman & Gould, 2003). When heritable vulnerabilities (G) and environmental risk factors (E) mutually influence the course of psychopathology, a Heritability × Environment (G × E) interaction is observed (see later). Importantly, G × E interactions cannot be disentangled from pure heritability effects in behavioral genetics studies *unless* the specific environmental variable that interacts with genetic vulnerability is quantified precisely. In most behavioral genetics studies, effects of environment are inferred from residual variance, not measured variance (see earlier). Under such conditions, unmeasured G × E interactions are subsumed within the heritability (G) coefficient (see Rutter, 2007). Thus, developmental increases in the heritability of almost all forms of psychopathology (Bergen, Gardner, & Kendler, 2007; see later) in part reflect accumulating effects of environmental risk exposure interacting with genetic vulnerability across the life span. Behavioral genetics studies in which specific environmental influences are not measured therefore overestimate main effects of heritability on emerging mental illness. The likely end result may be a literature-wide overestimation of the main effects of genes in the pathogenesis of psychopathology. This is by no means a trivial point because near uniformly high heritability coefficients of adult psychiatric disorders (e.g., Shih, Belmonte, & Zandi, 2004) are sometimes interpreted as evidence that environment contributes little to the expression of psychopathology. In recognition of this limitation, increasingly sophisticated efforts to quantify G × E interactions have appeared in recent years. These studies, some of which are described later, suggest that G × E interactions may be more common than thought previously (e.g., Caspi et al., 2002, 2003, 2010; Moffitt, 2005). However, most of these G × E interactions have been tested in molecular genetics research (see later), not behavioral genetics research. Moreover, many such findings need to be replicated to confirm their validity (see Duncan & Keller, 2011).

As just noted, it has become apparent in recent years that heritability coefficients of almost all behavioral traits—including those associated with psychopathology—increase substantially from childhood to adulthood (see Beauchaine et al., 2008; Bergen et al., 2007). This general pattern applies to almost all forms of psychopathology that have been assessed at different points in development, including antisocial behavior, anxiety, depression, eating disorders, and substance dependences (Bergen et al., 2007; Hicks et al., 2007; Klump, McGue, & Iacono, 2000; Lyons et al., 1995). Moreover, although environmental effects such as peer influences affect age of onset for smoking and drinking behaviors, both smoking maintenance and heavy drinking are accounted for almost exclusively by heritable effects (e.g., Boomsma, Koopsman, Van Doornen, & Orlebeke, 1994; Koopsman, Slutzke, Heath, Neale, & Boomsma, 1999; Koopsman, Van Doornen, & Boomsma, 1997; McGue, Iacono, Legrand, & Elkins, 2001; Viken, Kaprio, Koskenvuo, & Rose, 1999).

Psychopathology researchers have offered a number of potential explanations for these increasing heritability coefficients. These include suggestions that the nature of psychopathology may be different among children than among adults (e.g., Klein, Torpey, Bufferd, & Dyson, 2008), that different genetic factors operate in childhood versus adolescence (e.g., Kendler, Gardner, & Lichtenstein, 2008), and that differences in heritability may indicate diverse equifinal pathways to psychopathology (e.g., Silberg, Rutter, & Eaves, 2001). Although some or all of these mechanisms are likely at play, important artifactual influences should also be considered. For example, developmental increases in heritability are a mathematical necessity in twin and adoption studies whenever there are individual differences in age of onset, even when underlying causal processes of psychiatric disturbance are similar across members of a population (see Beauchaine et al., 2008). Heritability is estimated from concordance of psychopathology among twin pairs. Differences in age of onset—which could be caused by environmental insults or stochastic (chance, random) effects—necessarily produce increasing concordance and therefore increasing heritability over time. Importantly, even when they are reared in very similar environments, phenotypic variation among twins is observed (Wong, Gottesman, & Petronis, 2005).

It is also important to note that behavioral genetics studies are usually conducted with large samples recruited through twin registries. Ideally, these samples are representative of the population from which they are drawn. As a result, behavioral genetics analyses parse mostly *normal variation* in individual differences. This variation is analyzed by constructing structural models to evaluate linear associations between heritable influences and behavior, and between environmental influences and behavior. However, linear associations do not always represent processes that operate at the extremes of a distribution—the very region where psychopathology is represented (see, e.g., Beauchaine, 2003). According to most definitions, psychopathology is limited to the upper (or lower) extremes of a normal distribution, usually defined as the 95th or 98th percentile (or the 2nd or 5th percentile). Mechanisms of behavior can be quite different at the extremes of a distribution than near the mean of a distribution (see Beauchaine, Lenzeweger, & Waller, 2009). Thus, gene-behavior and environment-behavior relations among those with psychopathology can be swamped in behavioral genetics analyses by mostly normative variation in individual differences, thereby going undetected. Indeed, nearly 90% of a population scores no further than 1.5 *SD* units from the population mean of any normally distributed individual difference. Although this limitation is not specific to behavioral genetics, it has received little attention in the literature.

Finally, behavioral genetics studies are nonspecific, providing broad information about heritable versus environmental risk but yielding no information about particular genes that contribute to phenotypes. As a result, these studies cannot be used to identify disease processes or mechanisms of psychiatric disturbance. Behavioral genetics models contribute most effectively to informing theoretical frameworks from which hypotheses can be derived for testing, a topic discussed in more detail later.

## MOLECULAR GENETICS

*Linkage studies.* In contrast to behavioral genetics, molecular genetics studies identify specific genetic polymorphisms (i.e., allelic variants) that confer vulnerability to psychopathology. There are two types of molecular genetics approaches: *linkage* and *association* studies. Linkage studies scan broad sections of the genome, and require large samples of families with two or more children affected by psychopathology. Genetic data are collected from family members, and searches are conducted for genetic *markers* with known chromosomal locations. For example, the gene responsible for cystic fibrosis was found by "linking" the disease to a genetic variant on the long arm of Chromosome 7 within affected families. This discovery was followed by several subsequent linkage analyses that identified the specific chromosomal location (see Bolsover, Hyams, Jones, Shepard, & White, 1997).

In child psychopathology research, linkage analyses have been applied to families of sibling pairs with autism to identify susceptibility loci for the disorder (see Chapter 20). These studies specify Chromosomes 7 and 9 as likely locations of autism susceptibility genes, with additional markers on Chromosomes 4 and 11 for females and males, respectively (Schellenberg et al., 2006). Specification of multiple susceptibility loci indicates that autism is a polygenic disorder. Although these studies may provide insights into the pathogenesis of autism, specific genes or combinations of genes that are necessary for developing the disorder have yet to be identified conclusively. Nevertheless, information obtained from linkage studies can narrow the list of candidate genes considerably. Linkage studies have also been used to identify several susceptibility loci for externalizing behavior disorders (see, e.g., Jain et al., 2007). To date, however, linkage studies of psychiatric disorders have produced as many or more failures to replicate as replications, with surprisingly few exceptions (see, e.g., Craddock & Forty, 2006; Stein & Gelernter, 2010; Zhou et al., 2008). Thus, much linkage work remains toward identifying genes that confer susceptibility to psychopathology. One potentially promising approach lies in aggregating samples to increase statistical power (e.g., Ng et al., 2009).

*Association studies.* In contrast to linkage studies, genetic association studies begin with a specific candidate gene that is suspected of conferring risk for a psychiatric disorder. Allelic frequencies of this gene are then compared among those with and without the disorder. Results are expressed as *odds ratios*, which compare the likelihood that a person with a candidate polymorphism has a target disorder with the likelihood that a person without a candidate polymorphism has a target disorder. Odds ratios > 1 indicate higher likelihood of illness among those with versus without the candidate allele.

Although there are several types of association studies (see Cordell & Clayton, 2005), two are most common. In *case–control designs*, allelic frequencies of candidate genes are compared among those with and without psychopathology in a population. Although case control studies can provide large numbers of participants and are therefore powerful statistically, they are sensitive to *population stratification*. This refers to differences in allelic frequencies across ethnicities and geographical locales, which can introduce confounds into case–control designs, producing false positive results. Population stratification can be avoided with *family-based designs* in which parents serve as controls. These designs use *transmission disequilibrium tests* and *haploid relative risk analyses* to quantify transmission of genetic alleles from parents to offspring. If a candidate polymorphism confers risk for psychopathology, it should be transmitted from parent to offspring more often in populations with the disorder.

As alluded to earlier, association studies, particularly case–control designs, can detect genetic effects that account for far less variance in behavior than linkage studies can detect. However, well-articulated theories are required to identify candidate genes for analysis. As described in Chapter 6, for example, specific neural theories of impulsivity implicate the mesolimbic and mesocortical dopamine (DA) systems (see Beauchaine & Gatzke-Kopp, 2012; Gatzke-Kopp, 2011; Gatzke-Kopp et al., 2009). Given that impulsivity is a highly heritable trait that confers risk for almost all externalizing disorders (Krueger et al., 2002), genes involved in the synthesis, reuptake, and metabolism of DA should be associated with at least some of these conditions. Consistent with this supposition, association studies have identified several candidate alleles involved in DA neurotransmission, including variations in the DRD4 gene (chromosome 11p15.5) and the DAT1 gene (chromosome 5p15.3), among others (see Castellanos & Tannock, 2002; Gizer, Ficks, & Waldman, 2009).

*Rare structural variants.* A recent development in psychiatric genetics is the use of genome-wide scans to identify *rare structure variants*, or *copy-number variants* (CNVs), including both *microduplications* and *microdeletions*. As these terms imply, such variants result from either more than or less than the normal number of genes being inserted on certain chromosomes. In addition, CNVs can be caused by *inversion* and *translocation* of genes. Rare structural variants can be either inherited or arise *de novo* via mutation, and have been implicated in the pathogenesis of both autism

(Sebat et al., 2007; Chapter 20) and schizophrenia (e.g., Walsh et al., 2008; Chapter 21). In fact, Walsh et al. (2008) demonstrated duplications and deletions of genes among 20% of individuals with early-onset schizophrenia versus 5% of controls. Moreover, the implicated genes disproportionately affected neurodevelopment. In addition to their direct effects, structural variants may interact with other susceptibility genes to "push" certain individuals over the threshold for developing psychopathology.

*Complexities and limitations of molecular genetics.* Even though molecular genetics studies are far more specific than behavioral genetics studies, they are not without limitations. Perhaps the biggest of these is the small amount of variance in behavior that most candidate genes account for. For example, although behavioral genetics studies routinely yield heritability coefficients that explain 80% or more of the variance in impulsivity (see Willcutt, in press), specific genes identified in molecular genetics studies account for a small fraction of this effect. Furthermore, nonreplications across studies are common (Gizer et al., 2009). In part, this is due to the assumedly polygenic nature of most psychiatric disorders, including ADHD (see, e.g., Swanson & Castellanos, 2002). Nevertheless, considerable work remains toward mapping the genetic substrates of almost all behavioral traits that confer vulnerability to psychopathology.

## HETEROGENEITY OF PHENOTYPES

The search for candidate genotypes through selection of homogenous phenotypes presents significant challenges to psychiatric genetics research. Success of this approach is maximized when the association between genotype and phenotype is 1:1, which is infrequently the case (see above). Indeed, most diagnostic criteria are specified solely at the behavioral level of analysis, and are therefore affected by non-genetic influences.

Thus, phenotypic heterogeneity presents a significant obstacle to identifying genetic substrates of psychopathology (see Rende & Waldman, 2006; Skuse, 2001). Such heterogeneity can arise from three sources. First, criteria used for symptom assessment and participant selection often differ across studies. For example, different research laboratories studying the genetics of antisocial behavior sometimes define the construct differently. Some prefer broader definitions that include both aggressive and non-aggressive antisocial activities, whereas others confine their definitions to overtly aggressive and violent offenses. In general, more narrow definitions yield higher heritability coefficients in behavioral genetics studies and more replicable candidate alleles in molecular genetics studies (e.g., Eley, Lichtenstein, & Moffitt, 2003; Waldman et al., 1998). Presumably, this is because narrow phenotypes identify individuals with more similar genetic vulnerabilities.

Second, the same or similar symptoms can develop through different etiological pathways, a phenomenon known as equifinality (Beauchaine & Gatzke-Kopp, 2012; Beauchaine & Marsh, 2006; see Chapter 1). For example, some cases of depression are influenced more by biological vulnerability and less by environmental risk, whereas others are influenced less by biological vulnerability and more by environmental risk (Beauchaine, 2003; Cicchetti, & Rogosch, 2002; Harrington, Rutter, & Fombonne, 1996). Thus, different combinations of liability and risk can give rise to similar behavioral syndromes.

Third, diagnostic syndromes are highly complex and are often defined by a compilation of symptoms. Most diagnostic criteria require only a subset of these symptoms to meet threshold, allowing for a single diagnostic label to apply to a multitude of symptom profiles. Within a given syndrome, a certain set of symptoms may derive from greater genetic influence than another set. For example, evidence suggests that melancholia—a more severe form of depression with a particularly insidious course—is more heritable and results from different genetic vulnerabilities than other forms of mood disorder (Eaves et al., 2005; Willeit et al., 2003). Melancholia also emerges as a discrete subtype of depression in taxometric analyses (Ambrosini, Bennett, Cleland, & Haslam, 2002; Beach & Amir, 2003), is associated with especially high risk of suicide (e.g., Carroll, Greden, & Feinberg, 1980), and confers greater risk for intergenerational transmission of both internalizing and externalizing disorders than other subtypes of depression (Shannon, Beauchaine, Brenner, Neuhaus, & Gatzke-Kopp, 2007).

Despite such indications that melancholia is distinct from other forms of depression, until quite recently most genetic studies of depression—both behavioral and molecular—lumped all participants who met *DSM* criteria into a single group for analysis, with no effort to stratify by subtype. One consequence of commingling participants with different etiologies is to water down and obscure genetic linkages to and associations with specific depression subtypes—resulting in small effect sizes and failures to replicate (see Castellanos & Tannock, 2002; Skuse, 2001). This pattern has led several psychiatric geneticists to advocate for the use of carefully chosen endophenotypes to differentiate between subgroups with distinct heritable vulnerabilities. In the case of melancholia, abnormal hypothalamic-pituitary-adrenal axis reactivity has emerged as a promising endophenotype (see, e.g., Coryell & Schlesser, 2001). This example illustrates why tightened definitions of psychopathology may be required to specify genetic vulnerabilities more precisely.

## GENE-ENVIRONMENT INTERDEPENDENCE

Gene-environment interdependence occurs when heritable and environmental influences either correlate or interact with one another to explain more variance in behavior than their combined main effects (Rutter, 2007). There are several forms of gene-environment interdependence, each of which is outlined later. More comprehensive accounts can be found in Moffitt et al. (2006), Rutter (2006, 2007, 2010), and Rutter et al. (2006).

### GENE-ENVIRONMENT INTERACTION

As mentioned earlier, gene-environment interaction (G × E) refers to situations in which environments moderate the effects of genes on behavior, or in which genes moderate the effects of environments on behavior.[1] Among the most renowned examples of a G × E interaction, demonstrated by Caspi et al. (2003), is the finding that polymorphisms in the promoter region of the serotonin transporter gene (5-HTTLPR) moderate the effects of stressful life events—including maltreatment between ages 3 and 11—on adult depression. Individuals with two copies of the short allele (s/s homozygous) are more likely to experience adult depression following child adversity than individuals with two copies of the long allele (l/l homozygous). Those who are heterozygous (s/l) are at intermediate risk. Similar findings for the 5-HTTLPR gene have since been reported by others (Eley et al., 2004; Kaufman et al., 2004; see also Chapter 17). Polymorphisms in the 5-HTTLPR gene (s/s) also moderate the effects of stressful life events on the development of drinking and drug use (Covault et al., 2007). Although findings of 5-HTTLPR × Stress interactions have been disputed by some (e.g., Risch et al., 2009), consistent findings from well-controlled studies suggest that the s allele indeed confers susceptibility to depression following adversity (Caspi et al., 2010).

Importantly, although the main effect of maltreatment in predicting depression in the Caspi et al. (2003) study was significant, the main effect of 5-HTTLPR variation was not. Thus, had the Gene × Environment interaction not been assessed, variation in the 5-HTTLPR allele would have appeared to be unrelated to adult depression. This example argues strongly for careful consideration of environment in psychiatric genetics research and illustrates how failure to assess interaction effects can lead to incorrect inferences about the importance of heritability in the expression of psychopathology (see Beauchaine et al., 2008; Crowell et al., 2008).

## GENE-ENVIRONMENT CORRELATION

Gene-environment correlation (*r*GE) refers to situations in which (a) heritable traits of parents affect their child's exposure to adverse environments, or (b) heritable traits of children affect their own exposure to adverse environments. Such correlations come in three forms, including *active*, *evocative*, and *passive* effects (Plomin, DeFries, & Loehlin, 1977).

*Active rGE.* Active *r*GE occurs when a child's heritable vulnerabilities influence his or her selection of environments. For example, a primary neural substrate of impulsivity is deficient mesolimbic DA activity (see Beauchaine & Gatzke-Kopp, 2012; Gatzke-Kopp, 2011; Gatzke-Kopp et al., 2009). This DA dysregulation predisposes to sensation-seeking behaviors, including early initiation and sustained use of substances, association with delinquent peers, and other high risk activities

---

1. Deciding whether genes moderate effects of environment on behavior or whether environments moderate effects of genes on behavior is dictated by theoretical considerations. For example, Caspi et al. (2002) demonstrated that maltreated children become violent later in life only if they carry a specific variable number tandem repeat (VNTR) in the promoter region of the monoamine oxidase A (MAOA) gene. This could be viewed as a case of genetic variation moderating effects of maltreatment, or as a case of maltreatment moderating effects of genetic variation. Analytically, the decision is arbitrary since the mathematics are identical. In both cases, the effect of one variable differs as a function of the other—the statistical definition of interaction. Our preference is to consider genetic variation the predictor and environment the moderator because genetic variation precedes maltreatment.

(see Chapter 6). Thus, genetically vulnerable children and adolescents may be predisposed to seek risky environments and experiences, some of which may compound vulnerability. For instance, vulnerable individuals are more likely to engage in high risk behaviors such as substance use. This experience can exacerbate trajectories toward pathology directly through pharmacological effects of drugs on developing mesocortical and mesolimbic systems (Beauchaine et al., 2011; Catlow & Kirstein, 2007), and/or indirectly through exposure to antisocial peer influences and subsequent restriction of access to prosocial peer groups. In this manner, active *r*GE associated with externalizing behavior can feed back to exacerbate pre-existing heritable compromises in motivation and self-control. Similar active *r*GE has been described for other traits including anxiety (Fox, Hane, & Pine, 2007).

*Evocative rGE.* Evocative *r*GE occurs when genetically influenced behaviors elicit reactions from others that interact with and exacerbate existing vulnerabilities. As outlined immediately above, one behavioral trait that can evoke environmental risk is impulsivity. Impulsive children present with challenging behaviors that elicit and reinforce ineffective parenting, which in turn amplifies risk for progression of ADHD to more serious externalizing behaviors (e.g., Patterson, DeGarmo, & Knutson, 2000). O'Connor, Deater-Deckard et al. (1998) reported an evocative *r*GE in a sample of children at high genetic risk for externalizing behaviors who were adopted at birth. Despite being raised by adoptive parents, these children received more negative parenting than those in a matched control group. Because the adoptive parent's behaviors could not be explained by shared genetic risk with the child, these data provide strong evidence for an evocative *r*GE. In a study of parenting behaviors of twin mothers, Neiderhiser et al. (2004) reported a similar evocative effect.

Evoked negative responses from others can then feed back to amplify a child's ineffective self-control, thereby increasing his or her externalizing behaviors and eliciting further negative parental responses. Over time, evoked cycles of negativity may affect developing neural systems through mechanisms of neural plasticity, with potential long-term consequences for adjustment (see Beauchaine et al., 2008; Beauchaine et al., 2011; Pollack, 2005). In this manner, evocative *r*GE may amplify and solidify behavior patterns that were once malleable (see Fishbein, 2000).

*Passive rGE.* Passive *r*GE occurs when genetic factors that are common to both a parent and child influence parenting behaviors or home environments more generally. This process can be associated with either positive or negative outcomes. For example, an intelligent parent may purchase more books for her child and read to him more often than most mothers read to their children. In this case, a genetic advantage is correlated with environmental opportunity. Parents can also confer both genetic vulnerability to their offspring and provide risky rearing environments. For instance, twin studies indicate that genes play a significant role in the intergenerational transmission of depression from mothers to children (e.g., Rice, Harold, & Thapar, 2005), yet overwhelming evidence also demonstrates that maternal depression adversely affects parenting (Lovejoy, Graczyk, O'Hare, & Neuman, 2000; Rutter, 1990).

Given such findings, it may be tempting to infer passive *r*GE as a mechanism of intergenerational transmission of depression. However, passive *r*GE cannot be disentangled from shared environmental effects in ordinary behavioral genetics designs (for a discussion of the difference between *r*GE and shared environmental effects, see Rutter et al., 2006). Rather, sophisticated analyses of data collected from pairs of twin *parents* are required. No such studies have been conducted to demonstrate passive *r*GE for maternal depression. However, Neiderhiser et al. (2004) used a twin parent design to identify passive *r*GE for positive but not negative aspects of maternal parenting behavior in a normative sample. Because these are the only conclusive data demonstrating passive *r*GE for parenting behavior, further research is needed. Notably, however, newly developed statistical models may provide for parsing of passive *r*GE and G × E without twin parent designs (Price & Jaffee, 2008). However, passive *r*GEs have yet to be identified using these techniques.

## Epigenetics

As alluded to earlier, accumulating evidence suggests that a range of both endogenous and exogenous influences—including trauma, adverse rearing conditions, prenatal exposure to stress hormones, and perhaps even cultural factors experienced early in life—can alter gene expression, with later consequences for neural development, neurotransmitter function, and behavior (see, e.g., Beauchaine et al., 2011; Masterpasqua, 2009; Tremblay & Côté, 2009). The term *epigenesis* refers to changes in gene expression that result from alterations in DNA structure (as opposed to sequence, which is heritable) (Hartl & Jones, 2002). These genetic changes are mediated primarily by environmentally triggered methylation processes (i.e., conversion of a cytosine to 5-methylcytosine). Epigenetic effects on behavior have been demonstrated repeatedly in the animal literature. For example, Weaver et al. (2004) reported epigenetically induced genetic variation in hippocampal glucocorticoid receptors among rat pups that experienced high levels of maternal caretaking, including licking, grooming, and arched-back nursing compared with pups that experienced low levels of such behaviors. This epigenetic effect transmits adaptive variations in stress responding to offspring (see Meany, 2007). Rat pups reared in high-risk environments where such maternal caretaking behaviors are altered have more reactive hypothalamic-pituitary-adrenocortical responses and are consequently more fearful, leaving them better prepared for the high-risk environment they are likely to face as they mature. Because low licking/grooming mothers spend just as much time in proximity to and nursing their pups and pups do not differ from peers in any domain of physical development, variations in maternal behavior do not model adversity or neglect. Instead, this form of rat maternal behavior reflects a mechanism through which mothers influence offspring neurodevelopment via epigenesis.

Although epigenetic changes in gene expression clearly occur in humans, unambiguously demonstrating their effects on behavior is difficult because it requires random assignment of groups to different rearing environments (e.g., impoverished versus enriched; see Rutter, 2007), an ethically indefensible practice. However, indirect evidence of epigenetic processes can be gleaned by measuring methylation of target genes. Such studies have become common in recent years following artic-ulation of rich theoretical models invoking epigenetic processes in the expression of several forms of psychopathology, including antisocial behavior (e.g., Tremblay, 2005), schizophrenia (Roth, Lubin, Sodhi, & Kleinman, 2009), autism (e.g., Shulha et al., 2011) and depression (e.g., Schroeder, Krebs, Bleich, & Frieling, 2010). In fact, administration of antidepressants to rodents induces epigenetic changes in the P11 promoter, which regulates a number of cellular processes and has been implicated in the pathophysiology of depression among humans (Melas et al., 2012).

Importantly, mammals are particularly susceptible to environmentally triggered alterations in gene expression (Hartl & Jones, 2002), and increasingly divergent patterns of DNA methylation emerge over the life spans of monozygotic twins (Fraga et al., 2005). Thus, activation and deactivation of genes via epigenetic processes may play important roles in both risk for and resilience to psychopathology (see Kramer, 2005; Rutter, 2005; Rutter et al., 2006).

## GENETICS OF COMORBIDITY

The term comorbidity refers to the co-occurrence of more than one psychiatric disor-der within an individual. Although many subtypes and causes of comorbidity have been described (see Klein & Riso, 1993), two broad forms are important for this dis-cussion. *Homotypic comorbidity* refers to the co-occurrence of multiple externalizing disorders within an individual or the co-occurrence of multiple internalizing disor-ders within an individual. For example, externalizing disorders including ADHD, oppositional defiant disorder (ODD), conduct disorder (CD), antisocial personality disorder (ASPD), and substance use disorders (SUDs) often co-occur, particularly as development proceeds from childhood through adulthood (see Beauchaine et al., 2010; Lewinsohn, Shankman, Gau, & Klein, 2004). Comorbidity of internalizing disorders, including depression, dysthymia, and the anxiety disorders is also high (Angold & Costello, 1993; Brady & Kendall, 1992; Ferdinand, Dieleman, Ormel, & Verhulst, 2007).

In contrast to homotypic comorbidity, *heterotypic comorbidity* refers to the co-occurrence of at least one externalizing disorder and at least one internalizing disorder within an individual (e.g., CD and depression). This form of comorbidity is more perplexing because many (though not all) symptoms appear to overlap minimally (see Sauder, Beauchaine, Gatzke-Kopp, Shannon, & Aylward, 2012; Kopp & Beauchaine, 2007). For example, depression includes symptoms of sadness, anhedonia, and feelings of guilt or worthlessness, whereas CD is characterized by sensation seeking, lying, property destruction, and aggression. Yet despite these apparently distinct presentations, rates of comorbidity of CD and depression are much higher than expected by chance (Angold & Costello, 1993; Essau, 2003).

### BEHAVIORAL GENETICS OF COMORBIDITY

Comorbid disorders have often been treated as distinct yet co-occurring conditions with different etiologies (see Beauchaine, 2003; Kopp & Beauchaine, 2007), yet recent behavioral genetics studies suggest common heritable substrates for both homotypic and heterotypic comorbidity. Biometric modeling of latent associations between assumedly distinct syndromes has advanced our understanding of comorbidity, as described below.

*Homotypic comorbidity*. Behavioral genetics analyses indicated that most disorders within the externalizing spectrum share a common heritable vulnerability, with similar findings reported for disorders within the internalizing spectrum (Baker, Jacobson, Raine, Lozano, & Bezdjian, 2007; Kendler, Prescott, Myers, & Neale, 2003; Krueger et al., 2002; Tambs et al., 2009). For example, about 80% of the variance in disinhibition, conduct problems, antisocial personality, alcohol dependence, and drug dependence is accounted for by a single latent impulsivity trait (Krueger et al., 2002). Yet each specific category of externalizing conduct is influenced strongly by environment. Thus, trait impulsivity arising primarily from heritable predispositions manifests differently depending on environmental opportunities (see Lynam et al., 2000, Chapter 6). Following from these models, molecular genetic and neurobiological research targeting the common heritable vulnerability—as opposed to specific psychiatric syndromes—may provide advances in our understanding of etiology, whereas research on environmental risk mechanisms may be more beneficial if focused on factors that differentially contribute to specific syndromes.

*Heterotypic comorbidity*. Behavioral genetics studies also suggest common heritability across internalizing and externalizing disorders. For example, O'Connor, McGuire, Reiss, Hetherington, and Plomin (1998) reported that 45% of the covariation between depressive and antisocial symptoms was accounted for by a common genetic liability among 10- to 18-year-old twins. Similar findings have since been reported by others in both adolescent and adult samples (Burcusa, Iacono, & McGue, 2003; Kendler et al., 2003). Such findings offer an explanation of comorbidity not as diagnostic co-occurrence, but rather as covariation of related syndromes stemming from common heritable vulnerabilities.

## MOLECULAR GENETICS OF COMORBIDITY

*Homotypic comorbidity*. Recall that molecular genetics studies benefit from, and in some cases require, sound theory to guide the search for candidate genes. As noted earlier, modern accounts of impulsivity implicate mesolimbic DA dysfunction (Beauchaine & Gatzke-Kopp, 2012; Gatzke-Kopp et al., 2009; Chapter 6). In fact, aberrant neural responding in the mesolimbic DA system, including the ventral tegmental area and its projections to the nucleus accumbens, the caudate, and the putamen, is a core neural substrate of risk for all or most externalizing behaviors (Gatzke-Kopp & Beauchaine, 2007; Gatzke-Kopp et al., 2009). Furthermore, studies using both positron emission tomography (PET) and functional magnetic resonance imaging (fMRI) indicate that low levels of neural activity in the DA-mediated primary reward centers of the brain predispose to sensation-seeking, irritability, negative affectivity, and low motivation—core symptoms of externalizing psychopathology (Durston, 2003; Laakso et al., 2003; Leyton et al., 2002; Scheres, Milham, Knutson, & Castellanos, 2007).

As described earlier, these findings suggest that genes involved in the synthesis, catalysis, and reuptake of DA should be candidates in molecular genetics studies of externalizing behavior patterns. In Chapter 6 we summarize studies implicating numerous genes involved in DA neurotransmission (e.g., DAT1, DrD4, dopamine-$\beta$-hydroxylase, monamine oxydase, catechol-o-methyl transferase) in the expression of impulsivity and related externalizing psychopathology. Thus, central DA dysfunction may account for much of the shared vulnerability for externalizing disorders. In contrast, vulnerability for internalizing disorders is conferred largely through trait anxiety, which has been linked closely with serotonin neurotransmission (Gray & McNaughton, 2000; see Chapter 7).

*Heterotypic comorbidity.* Studies of overlapping vulnerabilities for conduct problems and depression provide potential insights into why heterotypic comorbidity is so common. It is important to note that at the symptom level, both disorders are characterized by negative affectivity, irritability, and anhedonia. Neurally, these symptoms are subserved by the same DA deficiencies described earlier (and detailed in Chapter 6) for externalizing disorders (Forbes et al., 2006; Nestler & Carlezon, 2006; Shankman, Klein, Tenke, & Bruder, 2007). In fact, neuroimaging studies reveal blunted activation within DA-mediated brain regions during reward tasks among externalizing children/adolescents and among those with depression (see Durston, 2003; Epstein et al., 2006; Forbes et al., 2006; Scheres et al., 2007). Furthermore, externalizing and internalizing symptoms interact in their association with structural compromises in DA-rich mesolimbic and mesocortical brain regions (Beauchaine et al., 2011). Thus, externalizing and internalizing disorders appear to share a common neural deficiency that accounts at least in part for overlap in symptoms. This conclusion is consistent with results outlined above from behavioral genetics studies indicating a common heritable vulnerability for depression and antisocial behavior (Burcusa et al., 2003; Kendler et al., 2003; O'Connor, Neiderhiser et al., 1998).

Importantly, deficiencies in DA-mediated reward circuitry are moderated by other biologically influenced traits to affect behavior. One such trait is behavioral inhibition (see Figure 3.1), which differentiates between those who present principally with CD

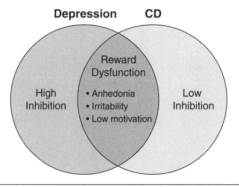

**Figure 3.1** Symptom overlap for depression and conduct disorder.
Both disorders are characterized by heritable deficiencies in dopaminergically mediated reward dysfunction, leading to common symptoms. However, the disorders are differentiated by heritable individual differences in behavioral inhibition. Adapted from Beauchaine et al., 2008.

and those who present principally with depression (Beauchaine, 2001; Chapter 7). In this model, high trait anxiety potentiates depression among those with blunted reward systems, whereas low trait anxiety potentiates delinquency. Trait anxiety is modulated by an entirely different (primarily serotonergic) neural network, often referred to as the *septo-hippocampal system* (Gray & McNaughton, 2000). This provides an example of two heritable traits interacting to affect behavior (i.e., a Trait × Trait interaction; see Derryberry, Reed, & Pilkenton-Taylor, 2003).

## GENETICS OF CONTINUITY

Whereas *homotypic continuity* describes the unfolding of a single class of behavioral/emotional disturbance over time (e.g., aggression), *heterotypic continuity* refers to the sequential development of different internalizing or different externalizing behaviors or disorders across the life span (see Beauchaine et al., 2010; Ferdinand et al., 2007; Rutter, Kim-Cohen, & Maughan, 2006). For example, delinquent adult males are likely to have traversed a developmental pathway that began with hyperactive/impulsive behaviors in toddlerhood, followed by ODD in preschool, early-onset CD in elementary school, SUDs in adolescence, and ASPD in adulthood (see Beauchaine et al., 2010; Loeber & Hay, 1997; Lynam, 1996).[2] Developmental trajectories of internalizing disorders in which infant reactivity and early shyness mark liability for later anxiety and depression have also been described (Kagan, Snidman, Kahn, & Towsley, 2007; see also Rutter et al. 2006; Chapter 7).

Few studies have addressed either the behavioral genetics or the molecular genetics of heterotypic continuity. Although some inferences can be offered from the cross-sectional studies outlined earlier addressing homotypic comorbidity, longitudinal studies are required to make strong statements about the stability of behavior disorders over time or about the heritable versus environmental bases of behavioral stability (see Rutter et al., 2006). In one such behavioral genetics analysis, heritable factors accounted for much of the stability in antisocial behavior, depressive symptoms, and their co-occurrence over a 3-year interval among 10- to 18-year-olds (O'Connor, Neiderhiser et al., 1998). Although molecular genetics studies addressing heterotypic continuity have not appeared in the literature to date, it is quite likely that many of the genes that predispose an individual to early ADHD also predispose the same individual to conduct problems and SUDs in later life, consistent with findings from behavioral genetics research implicating common genes for different externalizing disorders (see earlier). At least one genetic association study demonstrated no additional genetic burden for children with ADHD + conduct disorder compared with those with ADHD alone (e.g., Anney et al., 2008). However, conflicting findings have also been reported (Caspi et al., 2008). Thus, further research into genetic mechanisms of heterotypic continuity is needed.

---

2. This does not mean that all or even most children with ADHD eventually develop antisocial behavior. Although children with ADHD are at risk for more serious externalizing conduct across development, many desist. Nevertheless, most antisocial adult males began as hyperactive-impulsive preschoolers.

As indicated in the latter sections of this chapter, even though much progress has been made toward specifying the behavioral and molecular genetic bases of psychopathology, considerable work remains on questions of comorbidity and continuity (for an extended discussion, see Rutter et al., 2006). Nevertheless, investigations conducted to date suggest that mechanisms of both comorbidity and continuity are likely to result from broad vulnerability *traits* such as impulsivity and anxiety. This supposition is consistent with recent behavioral genetics approaches that have identified general internalizing and externalizing heritable vulnerabilities that account for more variance in psychopathology than do clusters of symptoms specific to any single disorder (e.g., Kendler et al., 2003; Krueger et al., 2002; Skuse, 2001).

## SUMMARY AND CONCLUSIONS

Despite expanded acknowledgment of the importance of both genes and environments in the development of psychopathology, much work remains toward uncovering specific mechanisms through which "nature" and "nurture" interact to affect behavior. Although behavioral genetics studies parse phenotypic variance into that attributed to genes and environment, one must keep in mind that genes are not measured in such studies. Rather, phenotypic similarities between related individuals are used to model heritable effects, which have both genetic and nongenetic origins. The considerable distance between genotypes and phenotypes, along with various interdependencies among genotypes, phenotypes, and environments, can lead to inflated and misleading estimates of heritability. Furthermore, molecular genetics studies aimed at identifying specific allelic variations associated with psychological dysfunction often fail to account for environmental moderators of genetic vulnerability. More mechanistic studies, including experiments with animals, can uncover complex patterns of environmentally mediated gene expression and function. Such epigenetic processes, which have drawn considerable attention in recent years, are likely implicated in the expression of several psychiatric disorders, and may explain some of the "missing" variance unaccounted for by molecular genetics studies compared with behavioral genetics studies. Although epigenetic processes are difficult to study in humans, they should nevertheless be included in emerging models of developmental psychopathology.

Most researchers now reject dichotomizing genetic and environmental influences on behavior (nature versus nurture). Indeed, boundaries between nature and nurture continue to dissolve as we increase our understanding of the interplay between heritable and experiential factors affecting psychopathology. Given the mutual interdependence of genes and environments in affecting behavior, it is no longer tenable to study psychopathology from strictly biological or environmental perspectives (see Beauchaine & Gatzke-Kopp, 2012; Rutter et al., 2006). The next generation of mental health professionals must be facile in their thinking about psychopathology across all relevant levels of analysis including genes, neural systems, environments, and social systems, among others (see Cicchetti, 2008). Breakthroughs in the understanding of and treatment of psychopathology are unlikely to occur by considering these systems in isolation.

# REFERENCES

Albee, G. W., & Joffe, J. M. (2004). Mental illness is NOT "an illness like any other." *Journal of Primary Prevention, 24*, 419–436.

Ambrosini, P. J., Bennett, D. S., Cleland, C. M., & Haslam, N. (2002). Taxonicity of adolescent melancholia: A categorical or dimensional construct? *Journal of Psychiatric Research, 36*, 247–256.

Angold, A., & Costello, E. J. (1993). Depressive comorbidity in children and adolescents: Empirical, theoretical, and methodological issues. *American Journal of Psychiatry, 150*, 1779–1791.

Anney, R. J., Lasky-Su, J., O'Du' shla'ine, C., Kenny, E., Neale, B. M., Mulligan, A., . . . Gill, M. (2008). Conduct disorder and ADHD: Evaluation of conduct problems as a categorical and quantitative trait in the international multicentre ADHD genetics study. *American Journal of Medical Genetics, Neuropsychiatric Genetics, 147B*, 1369–1378.

Baker, L. A., Jacobson, K. C., Raine, A., Lozano, D. I., & Bezdjian, S. (2007). Genetic and environmental bases of child antisocial behavior: A multi-informant twin study. *Journal of Abnormal Psychology, 116*, 219–235.

Beach, S. R. H., & Amir, N. (2003). Is depression taxonic, dimensional, or both? *Journal of Abnormal Psychology, 112*, 228–236.

Beauchaine, T. P. (2003). Taxometrics and developmental psychopathology. *Development and Psychopathology, 15*, 501–527.

Beauchaine, T. P. (2009). The role of biomarkers and endophenotypes in prevention and treatment of psychopathological disorders. *Biomarkers in Medicine, 3*, 1–3.

Beauchaine, T. P. (2012). Physiological markers of emotion and behaviour dysregulation in externalizing psychopathology. *Monographs of the Society for Research in Child Development, 77*, 79–86.

Beauchaine, T. P., & Gatzke-Kopp, L. M. (2012). Instantiating the multiple levels of analysis perspective into a program of study on the development of antisocial behavior. *Development and Psychopathology, 24*, 1003–1018.

Beauchaine, T. P., Hinshaw, S. P., & Pang, K. L. (2010). Comorbidity of attention-deficit/hyperactivity disorder and early-onset conduct disorder: Biological, environmental, and developmental mechanisms. *Clinical Psychology Science and Practice, 17*, 327–336.

Beauchaine, T. P., Lenzenweger, M. F., & Waller, N. (2008). Schizotypy, taxometrics, and disconfirming theories in soft science. *Personality and Individual Differences, 44*, 1652–1662.

Beauchaine, T. P., & Marsh, P. (2006). Taxometric methods: Enhancing early detection and prevention of psychopathology by identifying latent vulnerability traits. In D. Cicchetti & D. Cohen (Eds.), *Developmental psychopathology, Vol. 1. Theory and method* (2nd ed., pp. 931–967). Hoboken, NJ: Wiley.

Beauchaine, T. P., Neuhaus, E., Brenner, S. L., & Gatzke-Kopp, L. (2008). Ten good reasons to consider biological processes in prevention and intervention research. *Development and Psychopathology, 20*, 745–774.

Beauchaine, T. P., Neuhaus, E., Zalewski, M., Crowell, S. E., & Potapova, N. (2011). The effects of allostatic load on neural systems subserving motivation, mood regulation, and social affiliation. *Development and Psychopathology, 23,* 975–999.

Bergen, S. E., Gardner, C. O., & Kendler, K. S. (2007). Age-related changes in heritability of behavioral phenotypes over adolescence and young adulthood: A meta-analysis. *Twin Research and Human Genetics, 10,* 423–433.

Bolsover, S. R., Hyams, J. S., Jones, S., Shepard, E. A., & White, H. A. (1997). *From genes to cells.* New York, NY: Wiley-Liss.

Boomsma, D. I., Koopsman, J. R., Van Doornen, L. J., & Orlebeke, J. F. (1994). Genetic and social influences on starting to smoke: A study of Dutch adolescent twins and their parents. *Addiction, 89,* 219–226.

Brady, E. U., & Kendall, P. C. (1992). Comorbidity of anxiety and depression in children and adolescents. *Psychological Bulletin, 111,* 244–255.

Burcusa, S. L., Iacono, W. G., & McGue, M. (2003). Adolescent twins discordant for major depressive disorder: Shared familial liability to externalizing and other internalizing disorders. *Journal of Child Psychology and Psychiatry, 44,* 997–1005.

Cadoret, R. J., Leve, L. D., & Devor, E. (1997). Genetics of aggressive and violent behavior. *Psychiatric Clinics of North America, 20,* 301–322.

Callicott, J. H., Egan, M. F., Mattay, V. S., Bertolino, A., Bone, A. D., Verchinksi, B., . . . Weinberger, D. R. (2003). Abnormal fMRI response of the dorsolateral prefrontal cortex in cognitively intact siblings of patients with schizophrenia. *American Journal of Psychiatry, 160,* 709–719.

Cannon, T. D., van Erp, T. G. M., Rosso, I. M., Huttunen, M., Lonnqvist, J., Pirkola, T., . . . Standertskjöld-Nordenstam, C. G. (2002). Fetal hypoxia and structural brain abnormalities in schizophrenic patients, their siblings, and controls. *Archives of General Psychiatry, 59,* 35–41.

Carroll, B. J., Greden, J. R., & Feinberg, M. (1980). Suicide, neuroendocrine dysfunction and CSF 5-HIAA concentrations in depression. In B. Angrist (Ed.), *Proceedings of the 12th CINP Congress* (pp. 307–313). Oxford: Pergamon Press.

Caspi, A., Langley, K., Milne, B., Moffitt, T., O'Donovan, M., Owen, M., . . . Thapar, A. (2008). A replicated molecular genetic basis for subtyping antisocial behavior in children with attention-deficit/hyperactivity disorder. *Archives of General Psychiatry, 65,* 203–210.

Caspi, A., McClay, J., Moffitt, T., Mill, J., Martin, J., Craig, I. W., . . . Poulton, R. (2002). Role of genotype in the cycle of violence in maltreated children. *Science, 297,* 851–854.

Caspi, A., Sugden, K., Moffitt, T. E., Taylor, A., Craig, I. W., Harrington, H., . . . Poulton, R. (2003). Influence of life stress on depression: Moderation by a polymorphism in the 5-HTT gene. *Science, 301,* 386–389.

Castellanos, F. X., & Tannock, R. (2002). Neuroscience of attention-deficit/hyperactivity disorder: The search for endophenotypes. *Nature Reviews Neuroscience, 3,* 617–628.

Catlow, B. J., & Kirstein, C. L. (2007). Cocaine during adolescence enhances dopamine in response to a natural reinforcer. *Neurotoxicology and Teratology, 29,* 57–65.

Cicchetti, D. (2008). A multiple-levels-of-analysis perspective on research in developmental psychopathology. In T. P. Beauchaine & S. P. Hinshaw (Eds.), *Child and adolescent psychopathology* (pp. 27–57). Hoboken, NJ: Wiley.

Cicchetti, D., & Rogosch, F. A. (2002). A developmental psychopathology perspective on adolescence. *Journal of Consulting and Clinical Psychology, 70*, 6–20.

Cordell H. J., & Clayton, D. G. (2005). Genetic epidemiology 3: Genetic association studies. *Lancet, 366*, 1121–1131.

Cornblatt, B. A. (2001). Predictors of schizophrenia and preventive intervention. In A. Breier & P. Tran (Eds.), *Current issues in the psychopharmacology of schizophrenia* (pp. 389–406). Philadelphia, PA: Lippincott Williams & Wilkins.

Coryell, W., & Schlesser, M. (2001). The dexamethasone suppression test and suicide prediction. *American Journal of Psychiatry, 158*, 748–753.

Covault, J., Tennen, H., Armeli, S., Conner, T. S., Herman, A. I., Cillessen, A., . . . Hallmayer, M. D. (2007). Interactive effects of the serotonin transporter 5-HTTLPR polymorphism and stressful life events on college student drinking and drug use. *Biological Psychiatry, 61*, 609–616.

Craddock, N., & Forty, L. (2006). Genetics of affective (mood) disorders. *European Journal of Human Genetics, 14*, 660–668.

Crowell, S. E., Beauchaine, T. P., McCauley, E., Smith, C. J., Vasilev, C. A., & Stevens, A. L. (2008). Parent–child interactions, peripheral serotonin, and intentional self-injury in adolescents. *Journal of Consulting and Clinical Psychology, 76*, 15–21.

Derryberry, D., Reed, M. A., & Pilkenton-Taylor, C. (2003). Temperament and coping: Advantages of an individual differences perspective. *Development and Psychopathology, 15*, 1049–1066.

Duncan, L. E., & Keller, M. C. (2011). A critical review of the first 10 years of candidate gene-by-environment interaction research in psychiatry. *American Journal of Psychiatry, 168*, 1041–1049.

Durston, S. (2003). A review of the biological bases of ADHD: What have we learned from imaging studies? *Mental Retardation & Developmental Disabilities Reviews, 9*, 184–195.

Eaves, L., Erkanli, A., Silberg, J., Angold, A., Maes, H. H., & Foley, D. (2005). Application of Bayesian inference using Gibbs sampling to item-response theory modeling of multi-symptom genetic data. *Behavior Genetics, 35*, 765–80.

Eley, T., Lichtenstein, P., & Moffitt, T. E. (2003). A longitudinal behavioral genetic analysis of the etiology of aggressive and nonaggressive antisocial behavior. *Development & Psychopathology, 15*, 383–402.

Eley, T. C., Sugden, K., Corsico, A., Gregory, A. M., Sham, P., McGuffin, P., . . . Craig, I. W. (2004). Gene-environment interaction analysis of serotonin system markers with adolescent depression. *Molecular Psychiatry, 9*, 908–915.

Epstein, J., Hong, P., Kocsis, J. H., Yang, Y., Butler, T., & Chusid, J. (2006). Lack of ventral striatal response to positive stimuli in depressed versus normal subjects. *American Journal of Psychiatry, 163*, 1784–1790.

Erlenmeyer-Kimling, L., Golden, R. R., & Cornblatt, B. A. (1989). A taxometric analysis of cognitive and neuromotor variables in children at risk for schizophrenia. *Journal of Abnormal Psychology, 98*, 203–208.

Essau, C. A. (2003). Epidemiology and comorbidity. In C. A. Essau (Ed.), *Conduct and oppositional defiant disorders: Epidemiology, risk factors, and treatment* (pp. 33–59). Mahwah, NJ: Erlbaum.

Ferdinand, R. F., Dieleman, G., Ormel, J., & Verhulst, F. C. (2007). Homotypic versus heterotypic continuity of anxiety symptoms in adolescents: Evidence for distinction between DSM-IV subtypes. *Journal of Abnormal Child Psychology, 35,* 325–333.

Fishbein, D. (2000). The importance of neurobiological research to the prevention of psychopathology. *Prevention Science, 1,* 89–106.

Forbes, E. E., May, J. C., Siegle, G. J., Ladouceur, C. D., Ryan, N. D., Carter, C. S.,...Dahl, R. E. (2006). Reward-related decision-making in pediatric major depressive disorder: An fMRI study. *Journal of Child Psychology and Psychiatry, 47,* 1031–1040.

Fox, N. A., Hane, A. A., & Pine, D. S. (2007). Plasticity for affective neurocircuitry: How the environment shapes gene expression. *Current Directions in Psychological Science, 16,* 1–5.

Fraga, M. F., Ballestar, E., Paz, M. F., Ropero, S., Setien, F., Ballestar, M. L.,... Esteller, M. (2005). Epigenetic differences arise during the lifetime of monozygotic twins. *Proceedings of the National Academy of Sciences, 102,* 10604–10609.

Gatzke-Kopp, L. M. (2011). The canary in the coalmine: Sensitivity of mesolimbic dopamine to environmental adversity during development. *Neuroscience and Biobehavioral Reviews, 35,* 794–803.

Gatzke-Kopp, L. M., & Beauchaine, T. P. (2007). Central nervous system substrates of impulsivity: Implications for the development of attention-deficit/hyperactivity disorder and conduct disorder. In D. Coch, G. Dawson, & K. Fischer (Eds.), *Human behavior and the developing brain: Atypical development* (pp. 239–263). New York, NY: Guilford Press.

Gatzke-Kopp, L. M., Beauchaine, T. P., Shannon, K. E., Chipman-Chacon, J., Fleming, A. P., Crowell, S. E.,...Aylward, E. (2009). Neurological correlates of reward responding in adolescents with conduct disorder and/or attention-deficit/hyperactivity disorder. *Journal of Abnormal Psychology, 118,* 203–213.

Gizer, I. R., Ficks, C., & Waldman, I. D. (2009). Candidate gene studies of ADHD: A meta-analytic review. *Human Genetics, 126,* 51–90.

Glahn, D. C., Therman, S., Manninen, M., Huttunen, M., Kapiro, J., Lönnqvist, J., & Cannon, T. D. (2003). Spatial working memory as an endophenotype for schizophrenia. *Biological Psychiatry, 53,* 624–626.

Gottesman, I. I., & Gould, T. D. (2003). The endophenotype concept in psychiatry: Etymology and strategic intentions. *American Journal of Psychiatry, 160,* 636–645.

Gould, T. D., & Gottesman, I. I. (2006). Psychiatric endophenotypes and the development of valid animal models. *Genes Brain and Behavior, 5,* 113–119.

Gray, J. A., & McNaughton, N. (2000). *The neuropsychology of anxiety* (2nd ed.). New York, NY: Oxford University Press.

Harrington, R., Rutter, M., & Fombonne, E. (1996). Developmental pathways in depression: Multiple meanings, antecedents, and endpoints. *Development and Psychopathology, 8,* 601–616.

Hartl, D. L., & Jones, E. W. (2002). *Essential genetics: A genomics perspective.* Boston, MA: Jones & Bartlett.

Hicks, B. M., Blonigen, D. M., Kramer, M. D., Krueger, R. F., Patrick, C. J., Iacono, W. G., & McGue, M. (2007). Gender differences and developmental change in externalizing disorders from late adolescence to early adulthood: A longitudinal twin study. *Journal of Abnormal Psychology, 116,* 433–447.

Hinshaw, S. P. (2002). Is ADHD an impairing condition in childhood and adolescence? In P. S. Jensen & J. R. Cooper (Eds.), *Attention deficit hyperactivity disorder* (pp. 5-1-5–21). Kingston, NJ: Civic Research Institute.

Hinshaw, S. P. (2003). Impulsivity, emotion regulation, and developmental psychopathology: Specificity vs. generality of linkages. *Annals of the New York Academy of Sciences, 1008,* 149–159.

Jain, M., Palacio, L. G., Castellanos, F. X., Palacio, J. D., Pineda, D., Restrepo, M. I., . . . Muenke, M. (2007). Attention-deficit/hyperactivity disorder and comorbid disruptive behavior disorders: Evidence of pleiotropy and new susceptibility loci. *Biological Psychiatry, 61,* 1329–1339.

Kagan, J., Snidman, N., Kahn, V., & Towsley, S. (2007). The preservation of two infant temperaments into adolescence. *Monographs of the Society for Research in Child Development, 72,* 1–75.

Kaufman, J., Yang, B., Douglas-Palumberi, H., Houshyar, S., Lipschitz, D., Krystal, & Gelernter, J. (2004). Social supports and serotonin transporter gene moderate depression in maltreated children. *Proceedings of the National Academy of Sciences, 101,* 17316–17421.

Kendler, K. S. (2005). "A gene for . . ." The nature of gene action in psychiatric disorders. *American Journal of Psychiatry, 162,* 1243–1252.

Kendler, K. S., Gardner, C. O., & Lichtenstein, P. (2008). A developmental twin study of symptoms of anxiety and depression: Evidence for genetic innovation and attenuation. *Psychological Medicine, 38,* 1567–1575.

Kendler, K. S., Prescott, C. A., Myers, J., & Neale, M. C. (2003). The structure of genetic and environmental risk factors for common psychiatric and substance use disorders in men and women. *Archives of General Psychiatry, 60,* 929–937.

Klein, D. N., & Riso, L. P. (1993). Psychiatric disorders: Problems of boundaries and comorbidity. In C. G. Costello (Ed.), *Basic issues in psychopathology* (pp. 19–66). New York, NY: Guilford Press.

Klein, D. N., Torpey, D. C., Bufferd, S. J., & Dyson, M. W. (2008). Depressive disorders. In T. P. Beauchaine & S. P. Hinshaw (Eds.), *Child and adolescent psychopathology* (pp. 477–509). Hoboken, NJ: Wiley.

Klump, K. L., McGue, M., & Iacono, W. G. (2000). Differential heritability of eating attitudes and behaviors in prepubertal versus pubertal twins. *International Journal of Eating Disorders, 33,* 287–292.

Koopsman, J. R., Slutzke, W. S., Heath, A. C., Neale, M. C., & Boomsma, D. I. (1999). The genetics of smoking initiation and quantity smoked in Dutch adolescent and young adult twins. *Behavior Genetics, 29,* 383–393.

Koopsman, J. R., van Doornen, L. J., & Boomsma, D. I. (1997). Association between alcohol use and smoking in adolescent and young adult twins: A bivariate genetic analysis. *Alcoholism: Clinical and Experimental Research, 21,* 537–546.

Kopp, L. M., & Beauchaine, T. P. (2007). Patterns of psychopathology in the families of children with conduct problems, depression, and both psychiatric conditions. *Journal of Abnormal Child Psychology, 35*, 301–312.

Kramer, D. A. (2005). Commentary: Gene-environment interplay in the context of genetics, epigenetics, and gene expression. *Journal of the American Academy of Child and Adolescent Psychiatry, 44*, 19–27.

Krueger, R. F., Hicks, B. M., Patrick, C. J., Carlson, S. R., Iacono, W. G., & McGue, M. (2002). Etiologic connections among substance dependence, antisocial behavior, and personality: Modeling the externalizing spectrum. *Journal of Abnormal Psychology, 111*, 411–424.

Laakso, A., Wallius, E., Kajander, J., Bergman, J., Eskola, O., Solin, O., . . . Hietala, J. (2003). Personality traits and striatal dopamine synthesis capacity in healthy subjects. *American Journal of Psychiatry, 160*, 904–910.

Lenzenweger, M. (2004). Consideration of the challenges, complications, and pitfalls of taxometric analysis. *Journal of Abnormal Psychology, 113*, 10–23.

Lenzenweger, M. F., McLachlan, G., & Rubin, D. B. (2007). Resolving the latent structure of schizophrenia endophenotypes using expectation-maximization-based finite mixture modeling. *Journal of Abnormal Psychology, 116*, 16–29.

Lewinsohn, P. M., Shankman, S. A., Gau, J. M., & Klein, D. N. (2004). The prevalence and co-morbidity of subthreshold psychiatric conditions. *Psychological Medicine, 34*, 613–622.

Leyton, M., Boileau, I., Benkelfat, C., Diksic, M., Baker, G., & Dagher, A. (2002). Amphetamine-induced increases in extracellular dopamine, drug wanting and novelty seeking: A PET/[$^{11}$C]Raclopride study in healthy men. *Neuropsychopharmacology, 27*, 1027–1035.

Loeber, R., & Hay, D. (1997). Key issues in the development of aggression and violence from childhood to early adulthood. *Annual Review of Psychology, 48*, 371–410.

Lovejoy, M. C., Graczyk, P. A., O'Hare, E., & Neuman, G. (2000). Maternal depression and parenting behavior: A meta-analytic review. *Clinical Psychology Review, 20*, 561–592.

Lynam, D. R. (1996). The early identification of chronic offenders: Who is the fledgling psychopath? *Psychological Bulletin, 120*, 209–234.

Lynam, D. R., Caspi, A., Moffitt, T. E., Wikström, P. H., Loeber, R., & Novak, S. (2000). The interaction between impulsivity and neighborhood context on offending: The effects of impulsivity are stronger in poorer neighborhoods. *Journal of Abnormal Psychology, 109*, 563–574.

Lyons, M. J., True, W. R., Eisen, S. A., Goldberg, J., Meyer, J. M., Faraone, S. V., . . . Tsuang, M. T. (1995). Effects of genes and environment on antisocial traits. *Archives of General Psychiatry, 52*, 906–915.

Masterpasqua, F. (2009). Psychology and epigenetics. *Review of General Psychology, 13*, 194–201.

McGue, M., Iacono, W. G., Legrand, L. N., & Elkins, I. (2001). Origins and consequences of age at first drink. II. Familial risk and heritability. *Alcoholism: Clinical and Experimental Research, 25*, 1166–1173.

Meany, M. J. (2007). Maternal programming of defensive responses through sustained effects on gene expression. In D. Romer & E. F. Walker (Eds.), *Adolescent psychopathology and the developing brain* (pp. 148–172). Oxford, United Kingdom: Oxford University Press.

Meier, M. H., Slutske, W. S., Arndt, S., & Cadoret, R. J. (2008). Impulsive and callous traits are more strongly associated with delinquent behavior in higher risk neighborhoods among boys and girls. *Journal of Consulting and Clinical Psychology, 117*, 377–385.

Melas, P. A., Rogdaki, M., Lennartsson, A., Björk, K., Qi, H., Witasp, A., . . . Lavebratt, C. (2012). Antidepressant treatment is associated with epigenetic alterations in the promoter of P11 in a genetic model of depression. *International Journal of Neuropsychopharmacology, 15*, 669–679.

Moffitt, T. E. (2005). The new look of behavioral genetics in developmental psychopathology: Gene-environment interplay in antisocial behaviors. *Psychological Bulletin, 131*, 533–554.

Moffitt, T. E., Caspi, A., & Rutter, M. (2006). Measured gene-environment interactions in psychopathology: Concepts, research strategies, and implications for research, intervention, and public understanding of genetics. *Perspectives on Psychological Science, 1*, 5–27.

Moore, C. M., Breeze, J. L., Gruber, S. A., Babb, S. M., Frederick, B. B., Villafuerte, R. A., . . . Renshaw, P. F. (2000). Choline, myo-inositol and mood in bipolar disorder: A proton magnetic resonance spectroscopic imaging study of the anterior cingulate cortex. *Bipolar Disorders, 2*, 207–216.

Neiderhiser, J. M., Reiss, D., Pedersen, N. L., Lichtenstein, P., Spotts, E. L., Hansson, K., . . . Ellhammer, O. (2004). Genetic and environmental influences on mothering of adolescents: A comparison of two samples. *Developmental Psychology, 40*, 335–351.

Nestler, E. J., & Carlezon, W. A. (2006). The mesolimbic dopamine reward circuit in depression. *Biological Psychiatry, 59*, 1151–1159.

Ng, M. Y. M., Levinson, D. F., Faraone, S. V., Suarez, B. K., DeLisi, L. E., Arinami, T., . . . Lewis, C. M. (2009). Meta-analysis of 32 genome-wide linkage studies of schizophrenia. *Molecular Psychiatry, 14*, 774–785.

O'Connor, T. G., Deater-Deckard, K., Fulker, D., Rutter, M., & Plomin, R. (1998a). Genotype-environment correlations in late childhood and adolescence: Antisocial behavior problems and coercive parenting. *Developmental Psychology, 34*, 970–981.

O'Connor, T. G., McGuire, S., Reiss, D., Hetherington, E., & Plomin, R. (1998b). Co-occurrence of depressive symptoms and antisocial behavior in adolescence: A common genetic liability. *Journal of Abnormal Psychology, 107*, 27–37.

O'Connor, T. G., Neiderhiser, J. M., Reiss, D., Hetherington, E. M., & Plomin, R. (1998c). Genetic contributions to continuity, change, and co-occurrence of antisocial and depressive symptoms in adolescence. *Journal of Child Psychology and Psychiatry, 39*, 323–336.

Patterson, G. R., DeGarmo, D. S., & Knutson, N. M. (2000). Hyperactive and antisocial behaviors: Comorbid or two points in the same process? *Development and Psychopathology, 12*, 91–107.

Plomin, R. (1989). Environment and genes. *American Psychologist, 44*, 105–111.

Plomin, R., DeFries, J. C., & Loehlin, J. C. (1977). Genotype-environment interaction and correlation in the analysis of human behavior. *Psychological Bulletin, 84*, 309–322.

Pollack, S. D. (2005). Early adversity and mechanisms of plasticity: Integrating effective neuroscience with developmental approaches to psychopathology. *Development and Psychopathology, 17*, 735–752.

Price, T. S., & Jaffee, S. R. (2008). Effects of the family environment: Gene–environment interaction and passive gene–environment correlation. *Developmental Psychology, 44*, 305–315.

Rende, R., & Waldman, I. (2006). Behavioral and molecular genetics and developmental psychopathology. In D. Cicchetti & D. Cohen (Eds.), *Developmental psychopathology, Vol. 2. Developmental neuroscience* (2nd ed., pp. 427–464). Hoboken, NJ: Wiley.

Rice, F., Harold, G. T., & Thapar, A. (2005). The link between depression in mothers and offspring: An extended twin analysis. *Behavior Genetics, 35*, 565–577.

Risch, N., Herrell, R., Lehner, T., Liang, K-Y., Eaves, L., & Hoh, J, . . . Merikangas, K. R. (2009). Interaction between the serotonin transporter gene (*5-HTTLPR*), stressful life events, and risk of depression. *Journal of the American Medical Association, 301*, 2462–2471.

Ross, R. G. (2003). Early expression of a pathophysiological feature of schizophrenia: Saccadic intrusions into smooth-pursuit eye movements in school-age children vulnerable to schizophrenia. *Journal of the American Academy of Child and Adolescent Psychiatry, 42*, 468–476.

Roth, T. L., Lubin, F. D., Sodhi, M., & Kleinman, J. E. (2009). Epigenetic mechanisms in schizophrenia. *Biochimica et Biophysica Acta General Subjects, 1790*, 869–877.

Rutter, M. (1990). Commentary: Some focus and process considerations regarding effects of parental depression on children. *Developmental Psychology, 26*, 60–67.

Rutter, M. (2005). Environmentally mediated risk for psychopathology: Research strategies and findings. *Journal of the American Academy of Child and Adolescent Psychiatry, 44*, 3–18.

Rutter, M. (2006). *Genes and behavior: Nature-nurture interplay explained*. Oxford, United Kingdom: Blackwell.

Rutter, M. (2007). Gene-environment interdependence. *Developmental Science, 10*, 12–18.

Rutter, M. (2010) Gene-environment interplay. *Depression and Anxiety, 27*, 1–4.

Rutter, M., Kim-Cohen, J., & Maughan, B. (2006). Continuities and discontinuities in psychopathology between childhood and adult life. *Journal of Child Psychology and Psychiatry, 47*, 276–295.

Rutter, M., Moffitt, T. E., & Caspi, A. (2006). Gene-environment interplay and psychopathology: Multiple varieties but real effects. *Journal of Child Psychology and Psychiatry, 47*, 226–261.

Sauder, C., Beauchaine, T. P., Gatzke-Kopp, L. M., Shannon, K. E., & Aylward, E. (2012). Neuroanatomical correlates of heterotypic comorbidity in externalizing youth. *Journal of Clinical Child and Adolescent Psychology, 41*, 346–352.

Schellenberg, G. D., Dawson, G., Sung, Y. J., Estes, A., Munson, J., Rosenthal, E.,...Wijsman E. M. (2006). Evidence for multiple loci from a genome scan of autism kindreds. *Molecular Psychiatry, 11*, 1049–1060.

Scheres, A., Milham, M. P., Knutson, B., & Castellanos, F. X. (2007). Ventral striatal hyporesponsiveness during reward anticipation in attention-deficit/hyperactivity disorder. *Biological Psychiatry, 61*, 720–724.

Schroeder, M., Krebs, M. O., Bleich, S., & Frieling, H. (2010). Epigenetics and depression: Current challenges and new therapeutic options. *Current Opinion in Psychiatry, 23*, 588–592.

Sebat, J., Lakshmi, B., Malhotra, D., Troge, J., Lese-Martin, C., Walsh, T.,...Wigler, M. (2007). Strong association of de novo copy number mutations with autism. *Science, 316*, 445–449.

Shankman, S. A., Klein, D. N., Tenke, C. E., & Bruder, G. E. (2007). Reward sensitivity in depression: A biobehavioral study. *Journal of Abnormal Psychology, 116*, 95–104.

Shannon, K. E., Beauchaine, T. P., Brenner, S. L., Neuhaus, E., & Gatzke-Kopp, L. (2007). Familial and temperamental predictors of resilience in children at risk for conduct disorder and depression. *Development & Psychopathology, 19*, 701–727.

Shih, R. A., Belmonte, P. L., & Zandi, P. P. (2004). A review of the evidence from family, twin, and adoption studies for a genetic contribution to adult psychiatric disorders. *International Review of Psychiatry, 16*, 260–283.

Shulha, H. P., Cheung, I., Whittle, C., Wang, J., Virgil, D., Lin, C. L.,...Weng, Z. (2011). Epigenetic signatures of autism: Trimethylated H3K4 landscapes in prefrontal neurons. *Archives of General Psychiatry, 69*, 314–324.

Silberg, J. L., Rutter, M., & Eaves, L. (2001). Genetic and environmental influences on the temporal association between earlier anxiety and later depression in girls. *Biological Psychiatry, 49*, 1040–1049.

Skuse, D. H. (2001). Endophenotypes in child psychiatry. *British Journal of Psychiatry, 178*, 395–396.

Stein, M. B., & Gelernter, J. (2010). Genetic basis of social anxiety disorder. In S. G. Hofmann & P. M. DiBartololo (Eds.), *Social anxiety* (2nd. ed., pp. 313–322). Oxford, United Kingdom: Elsevier.

Swanson, J. M., & Castellanos, F. X. (2002). Biological bases of ADHD— Neuroanatomy, genetics, and pathophysiology. In P. S. Jensen & J. R. Cooper (Eds.), *Attention deficit hyperactivity disorder* (pp. 7-1–7-20). Kingston, NJ: Civic Research Institute.

Tambs, K., Czajkowsky, N., Røysamb, E., Neale, M. C., Reichborn-Kjennerud, T., Aggen, S. H.,...Kendler, K. S. (2009). Structure of genetic and environmental risk factors for dimensional representations of DSM–IV anxiety disorders. *British Journal of Psychiatry, 195*, 301–307.

Tremblay, R. E. (2005). Towards an epigenetic approach to experimental criminology: The 2004 Joan McCord Prize Lecture. *Journal of Experimental Criminology, 1*, 397–415.

Tremblay, R. E., & Côté, S. (2009). Development of sex differences in physical aggression: The maternal link to epigenetic mechanisms. *Behavioral and Brain Sciences, 32*, 290–291.

Viken, R. J., Kaprio, J., Koskenvuo, M., & Rose, R. J. (1999). Longitudinal analyses of the determinants of drinking and of drinking to intoxication in adolescent twins. *Behavior Genetics, 29*, 455–461.

Waldman, I. D., Rowe, D. C., Abramowitz, A., Kozel, S. T., Mohr, J. H., Sherman, S. L., . . . Stever, C. (1998). Association and linkage of dopamine transporter gene and attention-deficit/ hyperactivity disorder in children: Heterogeneity owing to diagnostic subtype and severity. *American Journal of Human Genetics, 63*, 1767–1776.

Walsh, T., McClellan, J. M., McCarthy, S. E., Addington, A. M., Pierce, S. B., Cooper, G. M., . . . Sebat, J. (2008). Rare structural variants disrupt multiple genes in neurodevelopmental pathways in schizophrenia. *Science, 320*, 539–543.

Weaver, I. C. G., Cervoni, N., Champagne, F. A., D'Alessio, A. C., Sharma, S., Seckl, J. R., . . . Meaney, M. J. (2004). Epigenetic programming by maternal behavior. *Nature Neuroscience, 7*, 847–854.

Willcutt, E. G. (in press). Genetics of ADHD. In D. Barch (Ed.), *Cognitive and affective neuroscience of psychopathology.* New York, NY: Oxford University Press.

Willeit, M., Praschak-Rieder, N., Neumeister, A., Zill, P., Leisch, F., Stastny, J., . . . Kasper, S. (2003). A polymorphism (5-HTTLPR) in the serotonin transporter promoter is associated with DSM-IV depression subtypes in seasonal affective disorder. *Molecular Psychiatry, 8*, 942–946.

Wong, A. H. C., Gottesman, I. I., & Petronis, A. (2005). Phenotypic differences in genetically identical organisms: The epigenetic perspective. *Human Molecular Genetics, 14*, 11–18.

Zhou, K., Dempfle, A., Arcos-Burgos, M., Bakker, S. C., Banaschewski, T., Biederman, J., . . . Asherson, P. (2008). Meta-analysis of genome-wide linkage scans of attention deficit hyperactivity disorder. *American Journal of Medical Genetics, 147B*, 1392–1398.

# PART II

# VULNERABILITIES AND RISK FACTORS FOR PSYCHOPATHOLOGY

# CHAPTER 4

# Risk and Resilience in Child and Adolescent Psychopathology

## Processes of Stress, Coping, and Emotion Regulation

BRUCE E. COMPAS AND CHARISSA ANDREOTTI

## HISTORICAL CONTEXT

PROCESSES OF RISK AND resilience are central to understanding the nature and etiology of psychopathology during childhood and adolescence. Understanding risk factors and processes of risk is important in the identification of those children/adolescents most in need of early intervention, whereas clarification of protective factors and processes of resilience can inform characteristics of interventions to strengthen those at greatest risk (e.g., Cicchetti & Blender, 2006; Compas & Reeslund, 2009; Luthar & Cicchetti, 2000). Two constructs, exposure to *stress* and the ways that individuals *cope* with stress, have a long history in risk and resilience research and theory in developmental psychopathology (e.g., Garmezy & Rutter, 1983) and remain central constructs after more than four decades of research. However, recent work has led to more refined and nuanced views on stress and coping that have made these long-standing constructs even more relevant to understanding the development of psychopathology. In this chapter we first consider the concepts of risk and resilience in developmental psychopathology more broadly. We then briefly review processes related to stress and coping—central constructs for understanding risk and resilience. Next, we examine recent work that can enhance our understanding of stress and coping processes, including research on allostatic load, exposure to adversity early in development, and emotion regulation as a process closely related to coping. Finally, we examine research on depression during adolescence as an exemplar of progress and continued challenges to research on risk and resilience during adolescence.

## TERMINOLOGICAL AND CONCEPTUAL ISSUES

Research and theory on processes of risk and resilience as they relate to psychopathology in childhood and adolescence have a long and rich history. However, there has been considerable confusion and debate about the definitions of these constructs. We begin by briefly summarizing several recent attempts to bring clarity to risk and resilience for child and adolescent psychopathology.

### RISK AND RESILIENCE

*Risk.* The term *risk* refers to increased probability of a negative developmental outcome in a specified population (Kraemer et al., 1997; Kraemer, Stice, Kazdin, Offord, & Kupfer, 2001). Thus, risk (or *degree of risk*) is a quantitative concept that is reflected as either an odds ratio (see Chapter 3) when outcomes are measured categorically, or as some variant of a regression weight when outcomes are continuous or quantitative. For example, the odds of developing a mood disorder (major depressive disorder or dysthymic disorder) or a disruptive behavior disorder (oppositional defiant disorder or conduct disorder) can be calculated as a function of characteristics of the individual (e.g., age, sex), family factors (e.g., harsh parenting, parental psychopathology), and neighborhood characteristics (e.g., violence, inadequate housing). A *risk factor* is an agent or characteristic of the individual or the environment that is related to the increased probability of a negative outcome. The degree of risk associated with a given risk factor can be calculated at various levels, including the degree of risk for an individual person, a family, or a community. A landmark report by the National Research Council and the Institute of Medicine (NRC/IOM, 2009) further distinguished between risk factors that are specific to a particular outcome (e.g., depression) as opposed to nonspecific risk factors that are related to a number of outcomes (e.g., depression, anxiety, eating disorders).

   In addition to distinguishing levels of risk, temporal precedence must be established between risks and outcomes; that is, the presence of or exposure to the risk factor must precede evidence of the development of the outcome. Kraemer et al. (2001) address the issue of temporal precedence within a typology of risk factors. If a factor is simply associated with an outcome at a single point in time, it is identified as a *correlate*. A correlate that precedes an outcome is a *risk factor*, and a risk factor that can be changed or changes with development is a *variable risk factor*. Finally, if manipulation of the risk factor changes an outcome, it is a *causal risk factor*. In human research the final step in risk research is likely to involve preventive interventions designed to change established risk factors to determine their possible causal role. *Cumulative risk* refers to the co-occurrence of more than one risk factor for a given individual or within a population (Sameroff, 2006). For example, poverty and economic hardship are associated with multiple additional risks factors, including neighborhood crime and violence, lack of access to quality schools, single parenthood, and family conflict (e.g., Chen, 2007; Evans & Kim, 2007; Evans & Wachs, 2010; Miller, Chen, & Parker, 2011). Similarly, parental psychopathology, another important risk factor throughout childhood and adolescence, is linked with family conflict and discord and possible genetic risk for psychopathology (e.g., Goodman et al., 2011; see Chapter 3). The probability of negative outcomes may increase additively or exponentially as the number of risk factors increases.

The effects of risk factors can also be nonlinear. Kraemer et al. (2001) spell out conditions in which one risk factor (A) moderates the effects of a second risk factor (B) on an outcome (O). For A to function as a moderator of B, A must precede B, A and B must not be correlated, and A cannot influence B directly. However, the strength of the effect of B on O must be affected by the level of A. For example, there is an interaction between sex and pubertal timing in predicting depression in adolescence, such that girls with early onset puberty have an increased likelihood of a major depressive episode (Negriff & Susman, 2011). Following the principles outlined by Kraemer et al. (2001), in this case sex (A) precedes pubertal timing (B), sex is uncorrelated with pubertal timing, and both are related to depression (O). However, the strength of the association between early onset puberty and depression is greater for girls than for boys; that is, pubertal timing moderates the relation between sex and depression. Thus, pubertal timing is a source of increased vulnerability to depression among girls but not among boys. Greater precision of the relations among risk factors and their moderating effects will contribute to greater clarity in distinguishing between risk factors and sources of vulnerability.

*Resilience.* The concept of resilience is closely linked to risk. Luthar and Cicchetti (2000) define resilience as a "dynamic process wherein individuals display positive adaptation despite experiences of significant adversity or trauma" (p. 858). Similarly, Masten (2001) defines resilience as "a class of phenomena characterized by good outcomes in spite of threats to adaptation or development" (p. 228). Resilience does not merely imply a personality trait or an attribute of the individual; rather, it is intended to reflect a process of positive adaptation in the presence of risk that may be the result of individual factors, environmental factors, or the interplay of the two (Luthar, 2006; Luthar & Cicchetti, 2000). Resilience research is concerned with identifying mechanisms or processes that might underlie evidence of positive adaptation in the presence of risk. Masten (2001) distinguished among several models of resilience. Variable-focused models of resilience test relations among quantitative measures of risk, outcomes, and potential characteristics of the individual or the environment that may serve a protective function against the adverse effects of risk. Within this approach, researchers can test for mediators and moderators of risk that can provide evidence of protection or resilience. Person-focused models of resilience examine individuals in an attempt to identify and compare those who display patterns of resilience (as evidenced by positive outcomes) and those who succumb to risk (as reflected in negative outcomes).

*Risk and resilience.* Although there is merit to distinguishing between risk and resilience, there are challenges in the conceptualization of these factors and processes (Compas & Reeslund, 2009). Foremost is the difficulty of determining whether risk and resilience are distinct constructs, or whether they exist along a continuum. In some instances, high levels of a factor protect individuals from risk whereas low levels of the same factor amplify risk (Luthar, Sawyer, & Brown, 2006). For example, high IQ may serve as a protective factor in the face of socioeconomic adversity, whereas low IQ may increase the potency of the effects of poverty. Thus, IQ may both increase and decrease risk associated with socioeconomic hardship. In other instances, high levels of a factor are protective, but low levels may be neutral or benign in relation to the source of risk. For example, temperamental characteristics of negative affectivity and positive affectivity, respectively, are risk and resilience factors for emotional problems (Compas, Connor-Smith, & Jaser, 2004). However, these two traits are independent, as low negative affectivity does not denote positive affectivity. Thus, low negative affectivity indicates the absence of this vulnerability factor, but it does not necessarily serve as a protective factor.

The situation is further complicated because some risk and protective factors are stable, whereas others change with development. For example, some temperamental characteristics emerge in infancy and remain stable throughout childhood and adolescence. Stable individual differences in temperament may function as either risk or protective factors in adolescence, depending on the characteristic in question. Similarly, some features of the environment may be stable sources of risk or protection throughout childhood and adolescence (e.g., chronic poverty, a supportive and structured family environment). Other factors may emerge during adolescence as sources of risk and protection and can be defined as developmental risk and protective factors. For example, some aspects of cognitive and brain development change dramatically during early adolescence and mark this as a period of heightened risk for many adolescents (Casey, Getz, & Galvan, 2008; Spear, 2011; Steinberg, 2005, 2008). Similarly, it appears that the effects of certain types of stressful events are relatively benign during childhood but are much more likely to be associated with negative outcomes during adolescence (Hankin & Abramson, 2001).

## STRESS AND COPING: UNIFYING CONCEPTS FOR UNDERSTANDING RISK AND RESILIENCE

Research on exposure to stressful events and circumstances and the ways in which children and adolescents respond to and cope with stress are central to understanding processes of risk and resilience for psychopathology in young people. Specifically, exposure to stressful events and circumstances, including the generation of stressors in neighborhood, school, peer, and family environments, are primary risk factors that exert effects on child and adolescent mental (and physical) health. Furthermore, individual differences in coping and related processes of stress reactivity and emotion regulation are crucial sources of resilience in the face of both distal and proximal sources of stress.

### STRESS

In spite of strong criticisms of the construct (e.g., Lazarus, 1993), stress remains a centrally important factor in understanding risk for psychopathology. Prevailing definitions of stress all include environmental circumstances or conditions that threaten, challenge, exceed, or harm the psychological or biological capacities of the individual (see Chapter 8). Definitions of stress differ, however, in the degree to which processes of cognitive appraisal are implicated in determining what is and is not stressful to a given individual. Transactional approaches suggest that the occurrence of stress is dependent on the degree to which individuals *perceive* environmental demands as threatening, challenging, or harmful (Lazarus & Folkman, 1984). Alternatively, environmental perspectives have emphasized the importance of *objectively* documenting the occurrence of environmental events and conditions independent of the potential confounds of cognitive appraisals (Cohen, Kessler, & Gordon, 1995).

Although the transactional definition of stress continues to be widely embraced, it poses problems for stress research with children and adolescents. For example, research on stress during infancy and early childhood indicates clear negative effects of maternal separation, abuse, and neglect on infants (e.g., Miskovic, Schmidt, Goergiades, & Boyle, 2010; Pollak et al., 2010). Whether these events are subjectively experienced as stressful, it is clear that adverse effects can occur in young children without the complex cognitive appraisals that are central to the transactional approach. In addition, research indicates that cognitive appraisal processes do not interact with stressful events in the prediction of symptoms until late childhood or early adolescence and that appraisals increase in significance during this period (e.g., Cole et al., 2008).

Given limitations of transactional definitions of stress for research with children and adolescents, other developmental perspectives on stress focus on objective external, environmental events or circumstances. Grant, Compas, Stuhlmacher, Thurm, and McMahon (2003) proposed a definition of stressors that emphasizes objective environmental events or chronic conditions that threaten adolescents' physical and/or psychological health or well being of youth. This definition is consistent with traditional stimulus-based definitions of stress and more recent definitions of stressors and objective measures of stress (e.g., Rudolph & Hammen, 2000). Events or chronic circumstances can threaten the well-being of an individual without leading to a negative outcome. Thus, stressful events and conditions are defined independent of their effects or outcomes. This definition allows for positive outcomes in the face of objectively threatening circumstances; that is, it allows for resilience.

The study of stressful events and circumstances remains central to current etiological theories of child and adolescent psychopathology. This is evident in the more than 1,500 empirical investigations of the relation between stressors and psychological symptoms among youth identified by Grant, Compas, Thurm, McMahon, and Gipson (2004). However, the level of interest in the relation between stressors and psychological problems in adolescence has not been matched by progress in the field. Variability in the conceptualization and operationalization of stress and stressors has created significant problems (Grant et al., 2003). Underlying these specific measurement concerns is the broader issue that most studies of relations between stressors and psychological problems in children and adolescents have not been theory-driven beyond the general notion that stressors pose risk for psychopathology (Grant et al., 2003; Steinberg & Avenevoli, 2000).

In a series of reviews, Grant and colleagues (Grant et al., 2003, 2004, 2006; McMahon, Grant, Compas, Thurm, & Ey, 2003) identified several overarching findings from research on stress and psychopathology in children and adolescents. First, as noted above, Grant et al. (2003) suggest that stress is best conceptualized in terms of the occurrence of acute events or chronic conditions or circumstances (referred to as *stressors*) that threaten the physical or mental health of the child or adolescent. The nature of events (e.g., parental divorce, family move) and chronic conditions (e.g., poverty, chronic parental conflict and discord) that constitute sources of stress vary as a function of children's development and social context. Second, more than 50 prospective longitudinal studies have provided evidence that exposure to stressful events and chronic adversity predict *increases* in both internalizing and externalizing symptoms over time (Grant et al., 2004). Most importantly, there is substantial evidence that stressful events and adversities at one point in time predict increases in both internalizing and externalizing symptoms of psychopathology at a later time point, suggesting that stressors may play a causal role in the development of both types of symptoms (although see Chapter 3 for alternative Gene x Environment interaction and gene-environment correlation models). Thus, stressful events in the lives of children and adolescents meet criteria for risk factors as outlined by Kraemer et al. (2001). Third, consistent with a heuristic model proposed by Nolen-Hoeksema and Watkins (2011), exposure to stressful life events functions as a distal risk factor whose association with internalizing and externalizing symptoms is mediated by more proximal family characteristics, including disrupted parenting and parent–child relationships (Grant et al., 2003, 2006; Chapter 14). Evidence is particularly strong for poverty and economic disadvantage as distal risk factors that affect child/adolescent internalizing and externalizing symptoms through their effects on positive and negative parenting (Grant et al., 2003).

Finally, McMahon et al. (2003) concluded exposure to stressful events and chronic sources of adversity appears to operate as a nonspecific risk factor that places children and adolescents at risk for the full range of internalizing and externalizing forms of psychopathology. These authors reviewed studies of the effects of a wide range of stressors in childhood and adolescence including exposure to violence, physical and sexual abuse, divorce/marital conflict, poverty, physical illness, and cumulative life events across multiple domains. Exposure to stressful events and adversity plays a role in virtually all types of psychopathology including total internalizing and externalizing problems, as well as symptoms of depression, anxiety, eating disorders, aggressive behavior problems, conduct problems, substance use and abuse, and somatization. McMahon et al. (2003) note that across the various stressors examined, the most consistent evidence for specificity was found in the association of sexual abuse with internalizing symptoms, PTSD, and sexual acting out symptoms across several studies. Subsequent research indicates specificity among a wider set of psychosocial risk factors that include but are not limited to stressful events (Shanahan, Copeland, Costello, & Angold, 2008). On the other hand, recent evidence from the National Comorbidity Survey Replication (Green et al., 2010) suggests that childhood adversities, including interpersonal loss (parental death, parental divorce, and other separation from parents or caregivers), parental maladjustment (mental illness, substance abuse, criminality, and violence), maltreatment (physical abuse, sexual abuse, and neglect), life-threatening childhood physical illness, and extreme childhood family economic adversity are associated with all types of psychopathology in adulthood. Thus, current evidence suggests that exposure to stressful life events and circumstances of adversity are broad, non-specific risk factors for a wide range of co-occurring patterns of symptoms and disorders in childhood and adolescence.

## NEW DIRECTIONS IN RESEARCH ON STRESS

The large body of evidence on the role of stressors in child and adolescent psychopathology could suggest that research in this area has reached its zenith and that there is little new to be learned. However, several new perspectives have emerged that have the potential to expand on the decades of research on stressful life events, including the construct of allostatic load and the importance of exposure to early adversity. Allostatic load refers to the cost or wear and tear on biological and psychological systems as a result of chronic or repeated exposure to significant stress (McEwen, 2003; Chapter 8). Underlying biological systems can become dysregulated as a result of prolonged exposure to stressful events or conditions leading to behavioral, emotional, and biological dysfunction (Juster, McEwen, Bruce, & Lupien, 2010). The concept of allostatic load has added value for understanding the role of stress in developmental psychopathology in part because unlike traditional research on stressful life events it emphasizes the integration of multiple levels of analyses, including genetic and neurobiological processes, developmental history, and current context and experience (Cicchetti, 2011). Drawing on both human and animal research, these multiple levels of analyses hold promise for delineating some of the processes through which exposure to stressful events and circumstances contribute the development of psychopathology.

Research guided by an allostatic load model has generated a number of findings that are potentially important to child and adolescent psychopathology. For example, initial conceptualizations of allostatic load emphasized the effects of chronic stress on activation and dysregulation of the hypothalamic-pituitary-adrenal axis and the production of cortisol. However, Beauchaine, Neuhaus, Zalewski, Crowell, and Potapova (2011) have noted the importance of dysregulation in monoamine neural systems including dopamine, norepinephrine, and serotonin. For example, repeated and prolonged exposure to stress often alters central serotonin expression through epigenetic mechanisms, conferring lifelong risk for anxiety, depression, and other adverse outcomes. Research on allostatic load highlights the important role of chronic exposure to stress as a major source of risk for other biological systems and behaviors as well. For example, repeated exposure to violence alters neurodevelopment in the hippocampus and prefrontal cortex, conferring risk for learning and memory difficulties, disrupted social affiliation, and substance use and abuse (Mead, Beauchaine, & Shannon, 2010).

Research on the effects of stressful life events has typically focused on the occurrence of events within a specified and relatively recent period of time (e.g., the prior 6 months). In contrast, recent research on stress has placed greater emphasis on the developmental timing of exposure to stress, with increasing evidence accumulating for the long-term significance of early exposure to stress and adversity. For example, work by Evans and colleagues has documented long-term effects of growing up with the chronic stress engendered by poverty on later psychological and physical health (e.g., Evans et al., 2010; Evans & Schamberg, 2009). Extensive research also indicates that exposure to abuse and neglect early in development is related to increased risk for subsequent psycholopathology in childhood and adolescence (e.g., Mead et al., 2010).

## COPING

Given the significant role of stress in psychopathology during childhood and adolescence, it is somewhat axiomatic that the ways that individuals attempt to cope with stress in their lives is a potential source of resilience. The most widely cited definition of coping is that of Lazarus and Folkman (1984), which is derived from their appraisal-based model of stress and coping. Lazarus and Folkman define coping as "constantly changing cognitive and behavioral efforts to manage specific external and/or internal demands that are appraised as taxing or exceeding the resources of the person" (p. 141). Coping is viewed as an ongoing dynamic process that changes in response to the changing demands of a stressful encounter or event. Furthermore, coping is conceptualized as purposeful responses that are directed toward resolving the stressful relationship between the self and the environment (problem-focused coping) or toward palliating negative emotions that arise as a result of stress (emotion-focused coping).

Perspectives on coping that are more explicitly concerned with childhood and adolescence include those outlined by Weisz and colleagues (Rudolph, Dennig, & Weisz, 1995; Weisz, McCabe, & Dennig, 1994), Skinner and colleagues (e.g., Skinner & Zimmer-Gembeck, 2007), and Eisenberg and colleagues (e.g., Eisenberg, Fabes, & Guthrie, 1997; see Compas, Connor-Smith, Saltzman, Thomsen, & Wadsworth, 2001, for a review of these perspectives). A central issue in defining coping during adolescence (and childhood) is whether coping includes all responses to stress, particularly both controlled and automatic responses. Skinner's (1995) original definition of coping included both volitional and involuntary or automatic responses to manage threats to competence, autonomy, and relatedness, and although Eisenberg et al. (1997) acknowledge that coping and emotional regulation are processes that typically involve effort, coping is not always conscious and intentional.

Consensus has slowly emerged regarding the nature and dimensions or types of coping in childhood and adolescence. Skinner, Edge, Altman, and Sherwood (2003) identified more than 400 categories or types of coping that have been represented in research on this construct. Previous categories include problem- versus emotion-focused coping as described earlier, approach versus avoidance, and active versus passive coping. Although the problem- and emotion-focused distinction may be important historically, an alternative three-factor control-based model of coping (Compas et al., 2001, in press; Connor-Smith, Compas, Thomsen,

Wadsworth, & Saltzman, 2000; Rudolph et al., 1995) has been validated successfully in several samples. Within this model, responses to stress are first distinguished along the dimension of automatic versus controlled processes. Coping responses are considered controlled, volitional efforts to regulate cognition, behavior, emotion, and physiological processes, as well as aspects of the environment in response to stress. Coping responses are further distinguished as primary control engagement (problem solving, emotional modulation, emotional expression), secondary control engagement (acceptance, cognitive reappraisal, positive thinking, distraction), or disengagement (cognitive and behavioral avoidance, denial, wishful thinking). This model has been supported in at least seven confirmatory factor analytic studies with children, adolescents, and adults coping with a wide range of stressors (e.g., peer stressors, war-related stressors, family stressors, economic stressors, chronic pain, cancer), from diverse socioeconomic and cultural backgrounds and international samples (e.g., Euro-American, Native American Indian, Spanish, Bosnian, Chinese), using multiple informants (Benson et al., 2011; Compas et al., 2006a; Compas et al., 2006b; Connor-Smith et al., 2000; Connor-Smith & Calvete, 2004; Wadsworth, Reickmann, Benson, & Compas, 2004; Yao et al., 2010).

## NEW DIRECTIONS IN RESEARCH ON COPING

In addition to recent progress in research on coping in childhood and adolescence, processes of adaptation to stress are also reflected in recent research on the closely related construct of emotion regulation (Chapter 11). In spite of considerable overlap in the conceptualization and measurement of coping and emotion regulation, the literatures on these two constructs have developed quite independently, with the former largely preceding the latter (Compas, 2009). We see this as problematic, as a richer understanding of adaptation to stress will result from an integration of these lines of work. To that end, we now consider recent work on emotion regulation and coping. To examine processes involved in the regulation of emotion, it is first necessary to define what is meant by the terms *emotion* and *emotion regulation*. Emotion is broadly defined as a person-environment interaction requiring attention that involves considerable personal significance and evokes a complex, continuously evolving response (Gross & Thompson, 2007). The environment may include external stimuli or internal representations involving thoughts and memories. Emotions have historically been divided into primary emotions (including anger, sadness, fear, happiness, disgust, surprise) and secondary emotions (e.g., shame, pride). Whereas primary emotions are direct responses to environmental stimuli and constitute a biological preparation for appraisal and response (Izard, 2002), secondary emotions occur as a result of primary emotions. Seminal work by Zajonc (1980, p. 151) posited the primacy of emotions in human thought and behavior patterns, stating that, "preferences need no inferences." That is, personal beliefs about one's likes and dislikes are based in automatic affective responses and do not require higher-order cognitive processes.

A widely accepted definition of emotion-regulation has been offered by Thompson (1994): "The extrinsic and intrinsic processes responsible for monitoring, evaluating, and modifying emotional reactions, especially their intensive and temporal feature, to accomplish one's goals" (pp. 27–28). This definition includes the set of processes that allow for the increase, decrease, or maintenance of an affective state (Davidson, Putnam, & Larson, 2000). Although some behaviors may be performed to alter the emotions of others, emotion regulation generally refers to processes focused on the self and one's own emotions. This definition includes the child and her or his social context as part of the regulatory process, both of which are of central importance in the development of emotion-regulation. Young children rely on parents and other adult caregivers to soothe and manage negative emotions, but during adolescence emotion-regulation may become more internal and autonomous. Thompson also points to the multiple facets of emotion-regulation that range from recognizing and understanding one's emotions to taking steps to try to alter or modify their intensity and duration. Cole, Martin, and Dennis (2004; Chapter 11) further distinguish between two types of regulation—emotion as *regulating* and emotion as *regulated*. In the former, changes are observed in other domains (e.g., behavior or cognition) as a result of an emotion, whereas the latter refers to changes in the valence, intensity, or time course of an emotion that may occur within an individual or between individuals.

A multistage process model of the generation and modulation of emotions maintains that regulation can occur during several sequential steps in the generation of an emotion (Gross, 1998). At any of these stages, emotion regulation can be an automatic or controlled process (Gross & Thompson, 2007). Conscious, controlled strategies of emotion regulation have received the greatest attention in research. These strategies require effort, and studies have shown that individuals are able to accurately report their own use of such effortful strategies in daily functioning (Connor-Smith et al., 2000; Connor-Smith & Compas, 2004). However, emotion regulation can also be automatic, and an individual may be unaware when such a strategy is employed (Masters, 1991; Mauss, Bunge, & Gross, 2007). An example of an automatic emotion-regulation strategy is the unconscious diversion of attention away from a negative stimulus. Further, emotion regulation includes both the up-regulation of positive emotions and the down-regulation of negative emotions (Gross, 1998). However, research by Gross and colleagues indicates that adolescents and young adults down-regulate negative emotions more often than they up-regulate positive ones (Gross & Thompson, 2007).

Although coping and emotion regulation overlap significantly in that both involve volitional efforts to reduce negative emotions associated with stressful experiences and circumstances, there have traditionally been some differences between these two constructs. Whereas coping typically refers to the down-regulation of a negative emotion, emotion regulation also includes the maintenance or augmentation of a positive emotion (Eisenberg et al., 1997). However, recent conceptualizations of coping have included the regulation of both negative and positive emotions in response to stress (Folkman & Moskowitz, 2000). For example, Austenfeld and Stanton (2004) have used the term *emotional approach coping*, to describe coping that involves acknowledging, expressing, and understanding emotions in response to stressors. Their conceptualization of emotional approach coping provides an alternative to emotion-focused coping, which has been previously associated with poorer psychological and health-related outcomes. In addition, Jaser et al. (2011) found that secondary control coping is related to both the down-regulation of negative affect (sadness) and up-regulation of positive affect.

Several strategies have been discussed widely across the literatures as means of both affect regulation and coping with stress. For example, cognitive restructuring, as viewed in the context of coping as efforts to actively reinterpret stressful or negative events in more neutral or positive terms, overlaps heavily with the cognitive reappraisal form of emotion regulation. Implementation of this strategy is linked to reduced physiological and emotional arousal when an individual is presented with an emotional stimulus (e.g., Oschner, Bunge, Gross, & Gabrieli, 2002), and it is used clinically as part of evidence-based cognitive behavioral therapy treatments for several disorders (e.g., Stark, Krumholz, Ridley, & Hamilton, 2009).

Although taking actions to act directly on a source of stress in the environment, including addressing or solving the problem eliciting negative affect, has historically been unique to the construct of coping (Compas et al., 2009; Compas, Connor, Thomsen, Saltzman, & Wadsworth, 1999), some recent work has posited problem solving as a means of emotion regulation as well (Nolen-Hoeksema, in press). The inclusion of problem solving as a form of emotion regulation begs the question of whether the act of problem solving is actually undertaken to specifically regulate negative emotions. The need to regulate negative emotion before attempting to address a problem in order to more adeptly engage with the stressor and the use of problem solving strategies to achieve goals other than the regulation of one's emotions are important processes to consider.

In contrast to strategies such as cognitive reappraisal and problem solving, often considered adaptive means of coping with stress, other less adaptive strategies and responses to stress such as rumination and the suppression of both negative cognitions and emotions have been linked to emotion dysregulation. Rumination, the repetitive deliberation of the cause, experience, and consequence of negative emotions, increases negative affect and may actually hinder problem solving abilities (Aldo, Nolen-Hoeksema, & Schweizer, 2010). Furthermore, according to Roemer and Borkovec (1994), active attempts to suppress a negative thought may result in the formation of an association between the thought and a negative emotion. The intrusive qualities of the thought may be increased due to the relationship with negative emotionality, and increased thought intrusion may lead to heightened attempts to suppress the thought. As effective suppression requires additional distraction through neutral or positive stimuli (e.g., Wegner & Erber, 1992), suppression of negative thoughts may be significantly less effective as a coping mechanism, especially in depressed or chronically stressed populations. In several studies (Aldo et al., 2010), the use of such maladaptive strategies was significantly more strongly related to development of symptoms of psychopathology, including depression, anxiety, and eating disorders, than the use of adaptive strategies was related to more positive outcomes.

Deficits in the use of adaptive strategies in response to stress have been tied to significant emotional and behavioral problems including mood and anxiety disorders in adults (e.g., Campbell-Sills & Barlow, 2007), as well as depressive symptoms and disorders in children and adolescents (Compas et al., 2010). Deficits in emotion regulation specifically in the presence of stress have been tied to many *DSM* Axis I diagnoses in adults, including mood, anxiety, eating, and substance use disorders, as well as Axis II personality disorders (e.g., Campbell-Sills & Barlow, 2007; Gross & Levenson, 1997; Miller, Rathus, & Linehan, 2007). In addition, a deficiency in regulating negative emotions has been linked to depressive symptoms and disorders in children and adolescents (Compas, Jaser, & Benson, 2009). The biological and psychological mechanisms underlying these relationships continue to remain unclear, however. For example, several possibilities have emerged to explain the role of emotion regulation deficits in major depressive disorder (Rottenberg, Gross, & Gotlib, 2005). One hypothesis links depression to a decreased ability to experience positive emotions. This notion stems from a series of past findings describing decreased positive affect in individuals suffering from major depressive disorder (Watson & Tellegen, 1985). Research has expanded on this view by examining the underlying neurobiology of this phenomenon. For example, Davidson and Tomarken (1989) found evidence for frontal laterality in the experience of positive and negative affect. Specifically, left anterior frontal regions have been associated with approach behaviors, and Henriques and Davidson (1991) found that hypoactivation in left anterior frontal regions in depressed individuals.

## RISK AND RESILIENCE: EXAMPLES FROM RESEARCH ON STRESS, COPING, AND DEPRESSION

To further exemplify stress and coping processes in child and adolescent risk and resilience for psychopathology, we focus here on examples from research on the development of depression during childhood and adolescence. Depression provides a useful example of risk and resilience because it increases dramatically in prevalence over the course of childhood and adolescence and there is now a substantial body of work identifying stress as a significant source of risk, stress reactivity as a potential vulnerability factor, and coping as a source of resilience. Specifically, children and adolescents whose parents experience one or more episodes of depression are exposed to a significant source of risk for depression and other mental health problems.

The high prevalence of depression in the general population represents a significant mental health problem in the United States (see Chapter 17). As reported in the National Comorbidity Survey Replication, Kessler et al. (2003) found the lifetime prevalence of major depressive disorder to be 16.9%. It is expected that 32 to 35 million adults in the United States will experience an episode of depression over the course of their lifetime. Depression increases significantly from childhood to adolescence. Longitudinal studies suggest that middle adolescence (age 15 to 16 years old) is the peak time for the onset of major depression (e.g., Hankin et al., 1998). Depression is also a highly recurrent disorder, as more than 80% of depressed individuals experience more than one episode and about 50% of those who undergo an episode experience a recurrence within 2 years of recovery (Belsher & Costello,

1988). An initial onset of depression during adolescence predicts a more severe and recurrent course of the disorder and higher levels of impairment (e.g., Hammen, Brennan, Kennan-Miller, & Herr, 2008).

Rates of depression in women are highest in young adulthood, during childbearing years, and among women with children (Kessler et al., 1994, 2003). In a similar pattern, rates of depression are higher in males younger than age 45 than men age 45 and older (Blazer, Kessler, McGonagle, & Swartz, 1994). As Kane and Garber (2004) noted, this age group of men is also likely to have children. Thus, it is quite apparent that a significant number of children and adolescents are repeatedly exposed to symptoms of depression—both when their parents are in and out of episode. The significant number of mothers who experience clinical depression during their children's lifetimes is particularly problematic, as maternal depression is linked to significant negative developmental outcomes in children (Goodman, 2007).

Children of depressed parents are at high risk for *both* internalizing and externalizing psychopathology, including a two- to threefold increased risk of developing depressive disorders (England & Sim, 2009). As many as 50% to 80% of offspring of depressed parents (i.e., 7.5 to 12 million children) will likely meet criteria for a psychiatric disorder by young adulthood (England & Sim, 2009). Adolescence marks a particularly important developmental period for increased depression risk, as rates are relatively low during childhood and increase significantly by mid-adolescence (e.g., Hankin et al., 1998). Thus, early to middle adolescent offspring (10 to 15 years old) of depressed parents are an ideal target for prevention, given their high risk for the development of depression, anxiety, and externalizing behavior problems (England & Sim, 2009). Risk and protective factors for children of depressed parents include biological, psychological, and interpersonal processes (Goodman & Gotlib, 1999).

Having established that parental depression is a significant risk factor for depression in children and adolescents, it is important to understand the mechanisms and processes by which this risk affects offspring. In addition, as not all offspring of depressed parents develop psychopathology, understanding the protective processes that lead to resilience are also important to consider.

*Risk processes.* The effects of parental depression on offspring are likely transmitted through multiple mechanisms, including the heritability of depression; innate dysfunctional neuroregulatory mechanisms; exposure to negative maternal cognitions, behaviors, and affect; and the stressful context of the adolescent's life (Goodman & Gotlib, 1999; Chapter 17). Of particular relevance to this chapter are the disrupted interpersonal interactions that depressed individuals experience, as they may contribute to high levels of stress for children and adolescents in families of depressed parents. Parenting is a complex form of social interaction that is significantly impaired by depression. Parent–child interactions serve as critical mechanisms through which children are exposed to risk factors associated with parental depression—particularly negative parental affect and cognitions, as well as stressful family exchanges (Lovejoy, Graczyk, O'Hare, & Neuman, 2000). In addition, coping may be a particularly important protective factor in shielding against the effects of psychosocial risk processes associated with parental depression.

Exposure to stressful parent–child interactions is one of the primary psychosocial mechanisms through which parental depression exerts its effects on children (e.g., Jaser et al., 2005, 2007, 2008; Langrock, Compas, Keller, Merchant, & Copeland, 2002). For example, Hammen, Brennan, and Shih (2004) found that, in a community sample, adolescents with mothers meeting criteria for current depression, past depression, or dysthymia all experienced increased levels of conflict and stress when compared to children of women without psychopathology. Furthermore, when examining adolescents exposed to similar levels of parent–child conflict, rates of depression were higher in offspring of depressed mothers than nondepressed mothers. Therefore, not only do offspring of depressed parents experience more stressful parent–child relationships, these children also may be more reactive to or affected by stressful circumstances (Hammen et al., 2004). Children of depressed parents tend to experience more negative exchanges with their parents, either through verbal communication (e.g., criticism or blaming) or actions (e.g., ignoring or punishing), contributing to a chronically stressful environment. For example, Cummings and Davies (1994) found that dysfunctional parenting skills, particularly inconsistent discipline, displayed by depressed parents may be perceived as stressful and are likely to result in a negative cycle of child behavior problems.

Depression significantly impairs parents' ability to effectively provide support, nurturance, and structure for their children, leading to disruptions in parenting. Most of the research on parenting in depressed parents has concentrated on parenting difficulties associated with the physical, cognitive, and emotional symptoms of depression (e.g., sad mood, irritability, lack of interest, fatigue, or difficulty concentrating; Lovejoy et al., 2000). Studies have documented parental withdrawal (e.g., avoidance or unresponsiveness to their children's needs) and parental intrusiveness (e.g., irritability toward their children or excessive involvement in their children's lives) as characteristic of depressed parents in their interactions with their children (e.g., Cummings, DeArth-Pendley, DuRocher-Schudlich, & Smith, 2001).

Exposure to hostile, disengaged, and inconsistent parenting, as opposed to nurturing parenting, contributes to a chronically stressful and unpredictable environment for children and tends to result in increased symptoms in offspring of depressed parents. Recent studies have shown that children exposed to higher levels of parental intrusiveness/irritability and withdrawal have higher internalizing and externalizing symptoms. For example, Langrock et al. (2002) found that both parental intrusiveness and withdrawal were significantly correlated with higher levels of offspring anxiety/depression and aggression, according to parent reports. Jaser et al. (2005) extended those findings by using adolescent reports of family stress and adolescent psychological symptoms in combination with parent reports. Cross-informant correlations showed that adolescent reports of parental intrusive behaviors were significantly correlated with parent reports of adolescent internalizing and externalizing symptoms. Specifically, parental intrusiveness was correlated positively with anxiety/depression and aggression. Thus, when using cross-informant analyses of parent and adolescent reports to control for shared method variance in the measurement of parenting and adolescent adjustment, parental intrusiveness is associated with increased levels of psychological symptoms in offspring of depressed parents.

Through several risk processes, offspring of depressed parents are at increased risk for depression and other forms of psychopathology. However, research suggests that even under the stressful circumstances of having a parent with depression, some or even most children are resilient and adapt successfully. Attempts to explain resilience have focused on potential moderators. For some children and adolescents, the effect of parental depression may be significant, while for others the effect may be negligible. The ways that adolescents react to and cope with the stress of living with a depressed parent may serve as both mediators and moderators of the effects of this stress.

*Coping and emotion regulation as sources of resilience in children of depressed parents.* The way in which individuals respond to and deal with stress plays a critical role in the impact that stress has on their emotional and psychological well-being (Compas et al., 2001). The proposition that coping functions as a mediator or moderator between parental depression and child psychopathology leads to a series of questions regarding the ways in which children in these families of depressed parents may respond to and cope with stress, and how coping helps to buffer the stress of parental depression. First, how do children cope with the stress associated with parental depression? Second, how does depression in a parent constrain or alter the ways that children cope with stress related to parents' depression? Third, how do children's coping responses moderate the relationship between stress and children's adjustment in families of depressed parents?

Our research group has studied coping and stress responses in three samples of adolescent offspring of depressed parents (Fear et al., 2009; Jaser et al., 2005, 2007, 2008, 2011; Langrock et al., 2002). First, we examined these processes in a sample of adolescents whose mother or father had a history of depression, and who had experienced at least one episode of depression in the adolescent's lifetime (Jaser et al., 2005, 2007; Langrock et al., 2002). We found that adolescents' use of secondary control coping (i.e., positive thinking, distraction, acceptance, and cognitive restructuring) was related to lower symptoms of anxiety and depression, both within and across adolescents' and parents' reports of adolescents' coping and symptoms. Furthermore, higher levels of stress reactivity (emotional and physiological arousal, intrusive thoughts) were related to higher symptoms of anxiety/depression. A troubling pattern was identified in these adolescents. As levels of stress (parental withdrawal and parental intrusiveness) increased, adolescents used less secondary control coping and reported higher levels of stress reactivity (Jaser et al., 2005; Langrock et al., 2002). That is, as stress increases and adaptive coping becomes more important, adolescents use less secondary control coping and experience higher levels of reactivity. This is consistent with the notion that stress contributes to dysregulation (heightened stress reactivity) and interferes with controlled self-regulation and coping, both of which lead to increased risk for depressive symptoms (Compas, 2006).

Second, we have examined coping and stress responses in adolescents whose mothers had a history of depression and compared them with a demographically matched sample of adolescents whose mothers did not have a history of depression (Jaser et al., 2008). As expected, adolescents of mothers with a history of depression were higher in depressive symptoms and externalizing problems than adolescents whose mothers did not have a history of depression. Further, adolescent children of mothers with a history of depression reported higher levels of stress reactivity (e.g., emotional and physiological arousal, intrusive thoughts) than children of mothers with no history of depression. Mothers' reports of their current depressive symptoms and observations of maternal sadness during parent–child interactions in the laboratory were both related to higher levels of adolescents' depressive symptoms and externalizing problems, higher stress reactivity, and lower levels of secondary control coping. Finally, adolescents' use of secondary control coping and stress reactivity accounted for the relation between maternal history of depression and adolescents' depressive symptoms. These findings replicate those found by Jaser et al. (2005) and Langrock et al. (2002) but extend the previous studies by using direct observations to assess parental depressive symptoms and parent–adolescent interactions.

Third, we have examined stress and coping in adolescent offspring of mothers and fathers with a history of depression (Fear et al., 2009). In this sample our focus was on adolescents' coping with interparental conflict, and a similar pattern of findings emerged. Once again, we found support for secondary control coping as a predictor of lower internalizing and externalizing symptoms, after accounting for method variance in adolescent and parent reports of coping and symptoms. Further, secondary control coping partially or fully accounted for the association between interparental conflict and adolescent symptoms (Fear et al., 2009).

Researchers have also begun to examine emotion regulation, a concept closely related to coping (Compas et al., 2009; see earlier) in children of depressed parents; however, studies with this population have not yet examined emotion-regulation in adolescents. The most extensive work has been conducted by Kovacs, Forbes, Silk and colleagues and has used direct observation methods to assess young children's (age 3 to 7 years old) emotion regulation in response to laboratory stress tasks and examined the relation between children's emotion regulation and their depressive symptoms (Forbes, Fox, Cohn, Galles, & Kovacs, 2006a; Forbes et al., 2006b; Silk, Shaw, Forbes, Lane, & Kovacs, 2006a; Silk, Shaw, Skuban, Oland, & Kovacs, 2006b). Because of the relevance of understanding emotion regulation and depression in young people, these studies will be reviewed here. These studies are noteworthy for several reasons, including inclusion of a particularly high-risk sample, children whose mothers had themselves first experienced depression during childhood, and the use of direct observations and physiological measures of emotion regulation.

Silk et al. (2006a) observed children's responses to a delay of gratification task as an example of an emotionally arousing (frustration) context for children and their mothers. Silk et al. found that children of mothers with childhood-onset depression were more likely to focus on a delay object (a response that is similar to rumination in that it is a form of passive engagement with the source of stress or source of emotional arousal) than children of mothers without a history of depression. Furthermore, the use of positive reward anticipation (displays of joy and information gathering, a component of problem solving, a form of primary control engagement coping) was related to fewer internalizing symptoms in children of mothers with childhood-onset depression and current depressive symptoms, but not for children of mothers without a history of depression (Silk et al., 2006b). These studies suggest that processes of coping and emotion regulation may develop during childhood and carry over into adolescence.

*Prevention of psychopathology in children of depressed parents.* Drawing on evidence for the importance of stress and coping in families of depressed parents, Compas, Forehand, Keller and colleagues developed and tested the initial efficacy of a family group cognitive-behavioral (FGCB) preventive intervention for parents with a history of depression and their children (Compas, Forehand, & Keller, 2011; Compas, Keller, & Forehand, 2011; Compas, Langrock, Keller, Merchant, & Copeland, 2001). The preventive intervention is designed to reduce stressful parent–child interactions that are associated with parental withdrawal and irritability/intrusiveness and enhance children's and parents' use of secondary control engagement coping strategies to reduce the risk for symptoms and disorder in these children.

The FGCB intervention is a manualized 12-session program (8 weekly and 4 monthly follow-up sessions) that is designed to teach coping skills to families with a parent who has a history of a depressive disorder in a small family group format. Each family group includes four families and is co-led by a mental health professional with extensive training in group facilitation and a doctoral student in clinical psychology. The program is designed for participation by both parents and children. Goals are to educate families about depressive disorders, increase family awareness of the impact of stress and depression on functioning, help families recognize and monitor stress, facilitate the development of children's adaptive coping responses to stress, and improve parenting skills. Information is presented to group members during eight weekly sessions, practice and discussion of skills are facilitated during the sessions, and all members are given weekly at-home practice exercises. Four monthly follow-up booster sessions are included to provide additional practice and support in continued development and refinement of the skills learned in the initial weekly sessions.

The intervention is designed to address the hypothesized mediators of the effects of parental depression on children: parental depressive symptoms and negative affect, stressful parent–child interactions, and children's coping with these stressors. The intervention sessions include separate modules targeting parenting skills and children's coping skills. The parenting component of the intervention includes building skills to increase parental warmth and involvement with their children, as well as increasing structure and consequences for children's problem behavior. Children are taught skills to cope with their parents' depression, including the use of acceptance, distraction, and cognitive reappraisal.

The coping skills that are taught and practiced as part of the program are designed to enhance the development of secondary control coping strategies (cognitive restructuring, acceptance, distraction) in participants. The research summarized above shows that these strategies are effective in coping with stressful parent–child interactions associated with parental depression. One goal of the FGCB intervention is to increase these skills in the children and adolescents coping with depression in their family. Parents are taught to support their children's use of these skills, and they also are encouraged to practice these skills themselves.

The parenting modules of this intervention are drawn from well-established, empirically supported programs for parenting training designed to address issues of oppositional behavior in children and adolescents (e.g., Forehand & McMahon, 1981; McMahon & Forehand, 2003), and are similar to modules used in parenting interventions for the treatment of childhood anxiety (e.g., Barrett, Dadds, & Rapee, 1996; Dadds et al., 1999; Dadds, Spence, Holland, Barrett, & Laurens, 1997). The parenting sessions focus on the teaching of basic parenting skills, with an emphasis on areas that are likely to be impacted by depression such as consistency, structure, parental responsiveness, parent–child communication, and involvement in family activities.

The initial efficacy of the intervention has been tested in a clinical trial in which families were randomized to the FGCB intervention or to a written information (WI) comparison condition in which parents and children received information about the nature of depression and its effects on families but did not participate in the group intervention and were not taught coping or parenting skills. Significant effects on children's (ages 9 to 15 years) mental health favoring the FGCB intervention were found at 2-, 6-, and 12-month follow-ups (Compas et al., 2009), effects that were generally maintained at 18 months, although some effects dissipated at 24 months (Compas, Forehand, Thigpen et al., 2011). The FGCB intervention led to significantly lower levels of Youth Self-Report (YSR) internalizing symptoms at 2, 6, 12, and 18 months and significantly lower externalizing symptoms at 12, 18, and 24 months. There was also an effect for the intervention on a specific youth self-report measure of depressive symptoms at 12 months and mixed anxiety-depression symptoms at 2, 6, 12, and 18 months. Effects on parents' reports of their children's symptoms were quite limited, with the only significant effect occurring for externalizing symptoms on the CBCL at 12 months. Finally, the FGCB intervention had a significant effect on children's episodes of major depression as measured with diagnostic interviews with the parents and children. Over the 24 months from baseline, fewer children in the FGCB intervention experienced a major depressive episode (14.3%) than children in the WI comparison condition (32.7%).

Mediational analyses examined whether changes in children's coping and changes in parenting behaviors accounted for the effects of the FGCB on children's mental health outcomes. Specifically, changes in coping from baseline to the 6-month follow-up were examined as mediators of the effects of the intervention on children's internalizing and externalizing symptoms at 12 months (Compas et al., 2010). This design allowed for a test of the temporal precedence of changes in coping and parenting in relation to children's mental health. Significant effects were found for changes in children's coping as a mediator of the intervention, as changes in secondary control coping from baseline to 6-months mediated intervention effects on changes in children's depression, mixed anxiety-depression, internalizing, and externalizing symptoms from baseline to 12-month follow-up. We also tested for possible effects of the intervention on children's primary control coping and there were no significant findings. The intervention was specific in its effects on secondary control coping, and strong evidence was found for secondary control coping as a protective factor for both internalizing and externalizing symptoms. These findings support the role of children's coping and impaired parenting skills in parents suffering from depression as possible causal factors as outlined by Kraemer et al. (2001).

## CONCLUSIONS

Exposure to stress and adversity and the ways that individuals cope with stress are venerable and well-tested constructs that are central to understanding sources of risk and resilience to psychopathology in children and adolescents. Stressful life events and chronic adversity, most notably poverty and chronic abuse during development, are powerful, nonspecific predictors of internalizing and externalizing symptoms and disorders. These risk factors are balanced by the resilient qualities of the use of ways of coping with stress. Recent research supports a control-based model of coping in children and adolescents, with protective effects associated with the use of primary and secondary control coping methods. The foundation of research on stress and coping is now being built on by research on new iterations on these themes, including the importance of processes of allostatic load, the long-term effects of exposure to adversity early in development, and the elucidation of specific emotion regulation processes as part of overall efforts to cope with stress. Advances in research on children and adolescents at high risk for depression provides salient examples of risk and resilience processes in this population. And perhaps most importantly, recent evidence suggests that these processes can inform the development of promising interventions to prevent depression in children at high risk. The field is now poised to extend research on stress, allostatic load, coping, and emotion regulation to other types of symptoms and disorders to inform the development of preventive interventions and treatments.

## REFERENCES

Aldo, A., Nolen-Hoeksema, S., & Schweizer, S. (2010). Emotion regulation strategies across psychopathology: A meta-analytic review. *Clinical Psychology Review, 30,* 217–237.

Austenfeld, J. L., & Stanton, A. L. (2004). Coping through emotional approach: A new look at emotion, coping, and health-related outcomes. *Journal of Personality,* 72(6), 1335–1363.

Beauchaine, T. P., Neuhaus, E., Zalewski, M., Crowell, S. E., & Potapova, N. (2011). The effects of allostatic load on neural systems subserving motivation, mood regulation, and social affiliation. *Development and Psychopathology, 23,* 975–999.

Belsher, G., & Costello, C. G. (1988). Relapse after recovery from unipolar depression: A critical review. *Psychological Bulletin, 104,* 84–96.

Benson, M. A., Compas, B. E., Layne, C. M., Vandergrift, N., Pasalic, H., Katalinski, R., & Pynoos, R. S. (2011). Measurement of post-war coping and stress responses:

A study of Bosnian adolescents. *Journal of Applied Developmental Psychology, 32,* 323–335.

Blazer, D. G., Kessler, R. C., McGonagle, K. A., & Swartz, M. S. (1994). The prevalence and distribution of depression of major depression in a national community sample. *American Journal of Psychiatry, 151,* 979–986.

Campbell-Sills, K., & Barlow, D. H. (2007). Incorporating emotion regulation into conceptualization and treatment of anxiety and mood disorders. In J. J. Gross (Ed.), *Handbook of emotion regulation* (pp. 542–560). New York, NY: Guilford Press.

Casey, B. J., Getz, S., & Galvan, A. (2008). The adolescent brain. *Developmental Review, 28,* 62–77.

Chen, E. (2007). Impact of socioeconomic status on physiological health in adolescents: An experimental manipulation of psychosocial factors. *Psychosomatic Medicine, 69,* 348–355.

Cicchetti, D. (2011). Allostatic load. *Development and Psychopathology, 23,* 723–724.

Cicchetti, D., & Blender, J. A. (2006). A multiple-levels-of analysis perspective on resilience: Implications for the developing brain, neural plasticity, and preventive interventions. *Annals of the New York Academy of Sciences, 1094,* 248–258.

Cohen, S., Kessler, R. C., & Gordon, L. U. (1995). *Measuring stress.* New York, NY: Oxford University Press.

Cole, D. A., Ciesla, J. A., Dallaire, D. H., Jacquez, F. M., Pineda, A. Q., LaGrange, B., et al. (2008). Emergence of attributional style and its relation to depressive symptoms. *Journal of Abnormal Psychology, 117,* 16.

Cole, D. A., Nolen-Hoeksema, S., Girgus, J., & Paul, G. (2006). Stress exposure and stress generation in child and adolescent depression: A latent trait–state–error approach to longitudinal analyses. *Journal of Abnormal Psychology, 115,* 40–51.

Cole, P. M., Martin, S. E., & Dennis, T. A. (2004). Emotion regulation as a specific construct: Methodological challenges and directions for child development research. *Child Development, 75,* 317–333.

Cole, P. M., & Deater-Deckard, K. (2009). Emotion regulation, risk and psychopathology. *Journal of Child Psychology and Psychiatry, 50,* 1327–1330.

Compas, B. E. (2006). Psychobiological processes of stress and coping: Implications for resilience in childhood and adolescence. *Annals of the New York Academy of Sciences, 1094,* 226–234.

Compas, B. E. (2009). Coping, regulation and development during childhood and adolescence. In E. Skinner & M. J. Zimmer-Gembeck (Eds.), *Coping and the development of regulation* (a volume for the series). (R. W. Larson & L. A. Jensen, Eds.-in-Chief.) *New directions in child and adolescent development,* San Francisco, CA: Jossey-Bass.

Compas, B. E., Beckjord, E., Agocha, B., Sherman, M. L., Langrock, A., Grossman, C., . . . Luecken, L. (2006a). Measurement of coping and stress responses in women with breast cancer. *Psycho-Oncology, 15,* 1038–1054.

Compas, B. E., Boyer, M. C., Stanger, C., Colletti, R. B., Thomsen, A. H., Dufton, L. M., & Cole, D. A. (2006b). Latent variable analysis of coping, anxiety/depression, and somatic symptoms in adolescents with chronic pain. *Journal of Consulting and Clinical Psychology, 74,* 1132–1142.

Compas, B. E., Champion, J. E., Forehand, R., Cole, D. A., Reeslund, K. L., Fear, J., . . . Roberts, L. (2010). Coping and parenting: Mediators of 12-month outcomes of a family group cognitive-behavioral preventive intervention with families of depressed parents. *Journal of Consulting and Clinical Psychology, 78,* 623–634.

Compas, B. E., Connor-Smith, J. K., & Jaser, S. S. (2004). Temperament, stress reactivity, and coping: Implications for depression in childhood and adolescence. *Journal of Clinical Child and Adolescent Psychology, 33,* 21–31.

Compas, B. E., Connor-Smith, J. K., Saltzman, H., Thomsen, A. H., & Wadsworth, M. E. (2001). Coping with stress during childhood and adolescence: Progress, problems, and potential in theory and research. *Psychological Bulletin, 127,* 87–127.

Compas, B. E., Connor, J. K., Thomsen, A., Saltzman, H., & Wadsworth, M. E. (1999). Getting specific about coping: Effortful and involuntary responses to stress in development. In M. Lewis & D. Ramsey (Eds.), *Stress and soothing* (pp. 229–256). Mahwah, NJ: Erlbaum.

Compas, B. E., Forehand, R., & Keller, G. (2011). Preventive intervention in families of depressed parents: A family cognitive-behavioral intervention. In T. J. Strauman, P. R. Costanzo, J. Garber, & L. Y. Abramson (Eds.), *Preventing depression in adolescent girls: A multidisciplinary approach.* New York, NY: Guilford Press.

Compas, B. E., Forehand, R., Keller, G., Champion, A., Reeslund, K. L., McKee, L., . . . Cole, D. A. (2009). Randomized clinical trial of a family cognitive-behavioral preventive intervention for children of depressed parents. *Journal of Consulting and Clinical Psychology, 77,* 1009–1020.

Compas, B. E., Forehand, R., Thigpen, J. C., Keller, G., Hardcastle, E. J., Cole, D. A., . . . Roberts, L. (2011). Family group cognitive-behavioral preventive intervention for families of depressed parents: 18- and 24-month outcomes. *Journal of Consulting and Clinical Psychology, 79,* 488–499.

Compas, B. E., Jaser, S. S., & Benson, M. (2009). Coping and emotion regulation: Implications for understanding depression during adolescence. In S. Nolen-Hoeksema & L. Hilt (Eds.), *Handbook of adolescent depression.* New York, NY: Wiley.

Compas, B. E., Langrock, A. M., Keller, G., Merchant, M. J., & Copeland, M. E. (2001). Children coping with parental depression: Processes of adaptation to family stress. In S. Goodman & I. Gotlib (Eds.), *Children of depressed parents: Alternative pathways to risk for psychopathology.* Washington, DC: American Psychological Association.

Compas, B. E., & Reeslund, K. L. (2009). Processes of risk and resilience: Linking contexts and individuals. In R. M. Lerner & L. Steinberg (Eds.), *Handbook of adolescence* (3rd ed.). New York, NY: Wiley.

Connor-Smith, J. K., & Calvete, E. (2004). Cross-cultural equivalence of coping and involuntary responses to stress in Spain and the United States. *Anxiety, Stress and Coping: An International Journal, 17,* 163–185.

Connor-Smith, J. K., & Compas, B. E. (2004). Coping as a moderator of relations between reactivity to interpersonal stress, health status, and internalizing problems. *Cognitive Therapy and Research, 38,* 347–368.

Connor-Smith, J. K., Compas, B. E., Thomsen, A. H., Wadsworth, M. E., & Saltzman, H. (2000). Responses to stress: Measurement of coping and reactivity in children and adolescents. *Journal of Consulting and Clinical Psychology, 68,* 976–992.

Cummings, M. E., & Davies, P. T. (1994). Maternal depression and child development. *Journal of Child Psychology and Psychatry and Allied Disciplines, 35,* 73–112.

Cummings, M. E., DeArth-Pendley, G., DuRocher-Schudlich, T., & Smith, D. A. (2001). Parental depression and family functioning: Toward a process-oriented model of children's adjustment. In S. R. Beach (Ed.), *Marital and family processes in depression: A scientific foundation for clinical practice* (pp. 89–110). Washington, DC: American Psychological Association.

Dadds, M. R., Holland, D. E., Laurens, K. R., Mullins, M., Barrett, P. M., & Spence, S. (1999). Early intervention and prevention of anxiety disorders in children: Results at 2-year follow-up. *Journal of Consulting and Clinical Psychology, 67,* 145–150.

Dadds, M. R., Spence, S. H., Holland, D., Barrett, P. H., & Laurens, K. (1997). Early intervention and prevention of anxiety disorders: A controlled trial. *Journal of Consulting and Clinical Psychology, 65,* 627–635.

Davidson, R. J., Putnam, K. M., & Larson, C. L. (2000). Dysfunction in the neural circuitry of emotion regulation—A possible prelude to violence. *Science, 289,* 591–594.

Davidson, R. J., & Tomarken, A. J. (1989). Laterality and emotion: An electrophysiological approach. In F. Boller & J. Grafman (Eds.), *Handbook of neuropsychology* (pp. 419–441). Amsterdam, Netherlands: Elsevier.

Eisenberg, N., Fabes, R. A., & Guthrie, I. (1997). Coping with stress: The roles of regulation and development. In J. N. Sandler & S. A. Wolchik (Eds.), *Handbook of children's coping with common stressors: Linking theory, research, and intervention.* New York, NY: Plenum Press.

England, M. J., & Sim, L. J. (Eds.). (2009). *Depression in parents, parenting, and children: Opportunities to improve identification, treatment, and prevention.* Washington, DC: National Academies Press.

Evans, G. W., & Kim, P. (2007). Childhood poverty and health: Cumulative risk exposure and stress dysregulation. *Psychological Science, 18,* 953–957.

Evans, G. W., Ricciuti, H. N., Hope, S., Schoon, I., Bradley, R. H., Corwyn, R. F., & Hazan, C. (2010). Crowding and cognitive development: The mediating role of maternal responsiveness among 36-month old children. *Environment and Behavior, 42,* 135–148.

Evans, G. W., & Schamberg, M. A. (2009). Childhood poverty, chronic stress, and adult working memory. *Proceedings of the National Academy of Sciences, 106,* 6545–6549.

Evans, G. W., & Wachs, T. D. (2010). *Chaos and its influence on children's development: An ecological perspective.* Washington, DC: American Psychological Association.

Fear, J. M., Champion, J. E., Reeslund, K. L., Forehand, R., Colletti, C., Roberts, L., & Compas, B. E. (2009). Parental depression and interparental conflict: Adolescents' self-blame and coping responses. *Journal of Family Psychology, 23,* 762–766.

Folkman, S., & Moskowitz, J. T. (2000). Positive affect and the other side of coping. *American Psychologist*, 55, 647–654.

Forbes, E. E., Fox, N. A., Cohn, J. F., Galles, S. F., & Kovacs, M. (2006a). Children's affect regulation during disappointment: Psychophysiological responses and relation to parent history of depression. *Biological Psychology*, 71, 264–277.

Forbes, E. E., Shaw, D. S., Fox, N. A., Cohn, J. F., Silk, J. S., & Kovacs, M. (2006b). Maternal depression, child frontal asymmetry, and child affective behavior as factors in child behavior problems. *Journal of Child Psychology and Psychiatry*, 47, 79–87.

Forehand, R., & McMahon, R. J. (1981). *Helping the noncompliant child*. New York: Guilford Press.

Garmezy, N., & Rutter, M. (Eds.) (1983). *Stress, coping, and development in children* (pp. 43–84). Baltimore, MD: Johns Hopkins University Press.

Goodman, S. H. (2007). Depression in mothers. *Annual Review of Clinical Psychology*, 3, 107–135.

Goodman, S. H., & Gotlib, I. H. (1999). Risk for psychopathology in the children of depressed mothers: A developmental model for understanding mechanisms of transmission. *Psychological Review*, 106(3), 458–490.

Goodman, S. H., Rouse, M. H., Connell, A. M., Broth, M. R., Hall, C. M., & Heyward, D. (2011). *Clinical Child and Family Psychology Review*, 14, 1–27.

Grant, K. E., Compas, B. E., Stuhlmacher, A., Thurm, A. E., & McMahon, S. D. (2003). Stressors and child/adolescent psychopathology: Moving from markers to mechanisms of risk. *Psychological Bulletin*, 129, 447–476.

Grant, K. E., Compas, B. E., Thurm, A. E., McMahon, S. D., & Gipson, P. Y. (2004). Stressors and child/adolescent psychopathology: Measurement issues and prospective effects. *Journal of Clinical Child and Adolescent Psychology*, 33, 412–425.

Grant, K. E., Compas, B. E., Thurm, A. E., McMahon, S. D., Gipson, P. Y., Campbell, A. J., . . . Westerholm, R.I. (2006). Stressors and child and adolescent psychopathology: Evidence of moderating and mediating effects. *Clinical Psychology Review*, 26, 257–283.

Green, J. G., McLaughlin, K. A., Berglund, P. A., Gruber, M. J., Sampson, N. A., Zaslavsky, A. M., & Kessler, R. C. (2010). Childhood adversities and adult psychiatric disorders in the national comorbidity survey replication I: Associations with first onset of DSM-IV disorders. *Archives of General Psychiatry*, 67, 113–123.

Gross, J. J. (1998). The emerging field of emotion regulation: An integrative review. *Review of General Psychology*, 2, 271–299.

Gross, J. J., & Levenson, R. W. (1997). Hiding feelings: The acute effects of inhibiting negative and positive emotion. *Journal of Abnormal Psychology*, 106, 95–103.

Gross, J. J., & Thompson, R. A. (2007). Emotion regulation: Conceptual foundations. In J. J. Gross (Ed.), *Handbook of emotion regulation* (pp. 3–24). New York, NY: Guilford Press.

Hammen, C., Brennan, P. A., Kennan-Miller, D., & Herr, N. R. (2008). Early onset recurrent subtype of adolescent depression: Clinical and psychosocial correlates. *Journal of Child Psychology and Psychiatry*, 49, 433–440.

Hammen, C., Brennan, P. A., & Shih, J. H. (2004). Family discord and stress predictors of depression and other disorders in adolescent children of depressed and nondepressed women. *Journal of the American Academy of Child and Adolescent Psychiatry, 43,* 994–1002.

Hankin, B. L., & Abramson, L. Y. (2001). Development of gender differences in depression: An elaborated cognitive vulnerability-transactional stress theory. *Psychological Bulletin, 127,* 773–796.

Hankin, B. L., Abramson, L. Y., Moffitt, T. E., McGee, R., Silva, P. A., & Angell, K. E. (1998). Development of depression from preadolescence to young adulthood: Emerging gender differences in a 10-year longitudinal study. *Journal of Abnormal Psychology, 107,* 128–140.

Hasking, P. A., Coric, S. J., Swannell, S., Martin, G., Thompson, H. K., & Frost, A. D. J. (2010). Brief report: Emotion regulation and coping as moderators in the relationship between personality and self-injury. *Journal of Adolescence, 33*(5), 767–773.

Henriques, J. B., & Davidson, R. J. (1991). Left frontal hypoactivation in depression. *Journal of Abnormal Psychology, 100,* 535–545.

Izard, C. E. (2002). Translating emotion theory and research into preventive interventions. *Psychological Bulletin, 128,* 796–824.

Jaser, S. S., Champion, J. E., Dharamsi, K. R., Reising, M. M., & Compas, B. E. (2011). Coping and positive affect in adolescents of mothers with and without a history of depression. *Journal of Child and Family Studies, 20,* 353–360.

Jaser, S. S., Champion, J. E., Reeslund, K., Keller, G., Merchant, M. J., . . . Compas, B.E. (2007). Cross-situational coping with peer and family stressors in adolescent offspring of depressed parents. *Journal of Adolescence, 30,* 917–932.

Jaser, S. S., Fear, J. M., Reeslund, K. L., Champion, J. E. Reising, M. M., & Compas, B. E. (2008). Maternal sadness and adolescents' responses to stress in offspring of mothers with and without a history of depression. *Journal of Clinical Child and Adolescent Psychology, 37,* 736–746.

Jaser, S. S., Langrock, A. M., Keller, G., Merchant, M. J., Benson, M., Reeslund, K., . . . Compas, B.E. (2005). Coping with the stress of parental depression II: Adolescent and parent reports of coping and adjustment. *Journal of Clinical Child and Adolescent Psychology, 34,* 193–205.

Juster, R. P., McEwen, Bruce S., & Lupien, S. J. (2010). Allostatic load biomarkers of chronic stress and impact on health and cognition. *Neuroscience & Biobehavioral Reviews, 35*(1), 2–16.

Kane, P., & Garber, J. (2004). The relations among depression in fathers, children's psychopathology, and father–child conflict: A meta-analysis. *Clinical Psychology Review, 24,* 339–360.

Kessler, R. C., Berglund, P., Demler, O., Jin, R., Koretz, D., Merikangas, K. R., . . . Wang, P. S. (2003). The epidemiology of major depressive disorder: Results from the national comorbidity survey replication (NCS-R). *Journal of the American Medical Association, 289,* 3095–3105.

Kessler, R. C., McGonagle, K. A., Zhao, S., & Nelson, C. B. (1994). Lifetime and 12-month prevalence of DSM-III-R psychiatric disorders in the United States: Results from the national comorbidity study. *Archives of General Psychiatry, 51,* 8–19.

Kraemer, H. C., Kazdin, A. E., Offord, D. R., Kessler, R. C., Jensen, P. S., & Kupfer, D. J. (1997). Coming to terms with the terms of risk. *Archives of General Psychiatry, 54,* 337–343.

Kraemer, H. C., Stice, E., Kazdin, A., Offord, D., & Kupfer, D. (2001). How do risk factors work together? Mediators, moderators, and independent, overlapping, and proxy risk factors. *American Journal of Psychiatry, 158,* 848–856.

Langrock, A. M., Compas, B. E., Keller, G., Merchant, M. J., & Copeland, M. E. (2002). Coping with the stress of parental depression: Parents' reports of children's coping, emotional, and behavioral problems. *Journal of Clinical Child and Adolescent Psychology, 31,* 312–324.

Lazarus, R. S. (1993). From psychological stress to the emotions: A history of changing outlooks. *Annual Review of Psychology, 44,* 1–21.

Lazarus, R. S., & Folkman, S. (1984). *Stress, appraisal and coping.* New York, NY: Springer.

Lovejoy, M. C., Graczyk, P. A., O'Hare, E., & Neuman, G. (2000). Maternal depression and parenting: A meta-analytic review. *Clinical Psychology Review, 20,* 561–592.

Luthar, S. S. (2006). Resilience in development: A synthesis of research across five decades. In D. J. Cohen & D. Cicchetti (eds.), *Developmental psychopathology, vol. 3: Risk, disorder and adaptation,* 2nd ed. (pp/ 739–795). Hoboken, NJ: Wiley.

Luthar, S. S., & Cicchetti, D. (2000). The construct of resilience: Implications for interventions and social policy. *Development and Psychopathology, 12,* 857–885.

Luthar, S. S., Sawyer, J. A., & Brown, P J. (2006). Conceptual issues in studies of resilience: Past, present and future research. *Annals of the New York Academy of Sciences, 1094,* 105–115.

Masten, A. S. (2001). Ordinary magic: Resilience processes in development. *American Psychologist, 56,* 227–238.

Masters, J. C. (1991). The development of emotional regulation and dysregulation. In J. Garber & K. A. Dodge (Eds.), *Strategies and mechanisms for the personal and social control of emotion.* Cambridge, United Kingdom: Cambridge University Press.

Mauss, I. B., Bunge, S. A., & Gross, J. J. (2007). Automatic emotion regulation. *Social and Personality Psychology Compass, 1,* 1–22.

McEwen, B. S. (2003). Mood disorders and medical illness: Mood disorders and allostatic load. *Biological Psychiatry, 54,* 200–207.

McMahon, R. J., & Forehand, R. (2003). *Helping the noncompliant child: Family based treatment for oppositional behavior* (2nd ed.). New York: Guilford Press.

McMahon, S. D., Grant, K. E., Compas, B. E., Thurm, A. E., & Ey, S. (2003). Stress and psychopathology in children and adolescents: Is there evidence for specificity? *Journal of Child Psychology and Psychiatry, 44,* 1–27.

Mead, H. K., Beauchaine, T. P., & Shannon, K. E. (2010). Neurobiological adaptations to violence across development. *Development and Psychopathology, 22,* 1–22.

Miller, A. L., Rathus, J. H., & Linehan, M. (2007). *Dialectical behavior therapy for suicidal adolescents.* New York, NY: Guilford Press.

Miller, G. E., Chen, E., & Parker, K. J. (2011). Psychological stress in childhood and susceptibility to the chronic diseases of aging: Moving toward a model of behavioral and biological mechanisms. *Psychological Bulletin, 137,* 959–997.

Miskovic, V., Schmidt, L. A., Goergiades, K., & Boyle, M. (2010). Adolescent females exposed to child maltreatment exhibit atypical EEG coherence and psychiatric impairment: Linking early adversity, the brain, and psychopathology. *Development and Psychopathology, 22,* 419–432.

National Research Council and Institute of Medicine (2009). *Preventing mental, emotional and behavioral disorders among young people: Progress and possibilities.* Washington, DC: National Academies Press.

Negriff, S., & Susman, E. J. (2011). Pubertal timing, depression, and externalizing problems: A framework, review, and examination of gender differences. *Journal of Research on Adolescence, 21,* 717–746.

Nolen-Hoeksema, S. (in press). Emotion regulation and psychopathology: The role of gender. *Annual Review of Clinical Psychology.*

Nolen-Hoeksema, S., & Watkins, E. R. (2011). A heuristic for developing trans-diagnostic models of psychopathology: Explaining multifinality and divergent trajectories. *Perspectives on Psychological Science, 6*(6), 589–609.

Oschner, K. N., Bunge, S. A., Gross, J. J., & Gabrieli, J. D. E. (2002). Rethinking feelings: An fMRI study of the cognitive regulation of emotion. *Journal of Cognitive Neuroscience, 14,* 1215–1229.

Pollak, S. D., Nelson, C. A., Schlaak, M. F., Roeber, B. J., Wewerka, S. S., Wiik, K. L.,...Gunnar, M. R. (2010). Neurodevelopmental effects of early deprivation in post-institutionalized children. *Child Development, 81*(1), 224–236.

Roemer, L., & Borkovec, T. D. (1994). Effects of suppressing thoughts about emotional material. *Journal of Abnormal Psychology, 103,* 467–474.

Rottenberg, J., Gross, J. J., & Gotlib, I. H. (2005). Emotion context insensitivity in major depressive disorder. *Journal of Abnormal Psychology, 114,* 627–639.

Rudolph, K. D., Dennig, M. D., & Weisz, J. R. (1995). Determinants and consequences of children's coping in the medical setting: Conceptualization, review, and critique. *Psychological Bulletin, 118,* 328–357.

Rudolph, K. D., & Hammen, C. (2000). Age and gender determinants of stress exposure, generation, and reactions in youngsters: A transactional perspective. *Child Development, 70,* 660–677.

Sameroff, A. (2006). Identifying risk and protective factors for healthy child development. In A. Sameroff (ed.), *Families count: Effects on child and adolescent development,* 53–76. New York, NY, US: Cambridge University Press.

Shanahan, L., Copeland, W., Costello, E. J., & Angold, A. (2008). Specificity of putative psychosocial risk factors for psychiatric disorders in children and adolescents. *Journal of Child Psychiatry and Psychology, 49,* 34–42.

Silk, J. S., Shaw, D. S., Forbes, E. E., Lane, T. L., & Kovacs, M. (2006a). Maternal depression and child internalizing: The moderating role of child emotion regulation. *Journal of Clinical Child and Adolescent Psychology, 35,* 116–126.

Silk, J. S., Shaw, D. S., Skuban, E. M., Oland, A. A., & Kovacs, M. (2006b). Emotion regulation strategies of childhood-onset depressed mothers. *Journal of Child Psychology and Psychiatry, 47,* 69–78.

Skinner, E. A. (1995). *Perceived control, motivation, & coping.* Thousand Oaks, CA, US: Sage Publications, Inc., 1995.

Skinner, E. A., Edge, K., Altman, J., & Sherwood, H. (2003). Searching for the structure of coping: A review and critique of category systems for classifying words of coping. *Psychological Bulletin, 129,* 216–269.

Skinner, E. A., & Zimmer-Gembeck, M. J. (2007). The development of coping. *Annual Review of Psychology, 58,* 119–144.

Spear, L. P. (2000). Neurobehavioral changes in adolescence. *Current Directions in Psychological Science, 9,* 111–114.

Spear, L. P. (2011). Adolescent neurobehavioral characteristics, alcohol sensitivities, and intake: Setting the stage for alcohol use disorders? *Child Development Perspectives, 5,* 231–238.

Stark, K. D., Krumholz, L. S., Ridley, K. P., & Hamilton, A. (2009). Cognitive behavioral therapy for youth depression: The ACTION treatment program. In S. Nolen-Hoeksema & L. M. Hilt (Eds.), *Handbook of depression in adolescence* (pp. 475–510). New York, NY: Routledge.

Steinberg, L. (2005). Cognitive and affective development in adolescence. *Trends in Cognitive Sciences, 9,* 69–74.

Steinberg, L. (2008). A social neuroscience perspective on adolescent risk-taking. *Developmental Review, 28,* 78–106.

Steinberg, L., & Avenevoli, S. (2000). The role of context in the development of psychopathology: A conceptual framework and some speculative propositions. *Child Development, 71,* 66–74.

Thompson, R. A. (1994). Emotion regulation: A theme in search of a definition. The development of emotion regulation: Biological and behavioral considerations. *Monographs of the Society for Research in Child Development, 59,* 25–52.

Wadsworth, M. E., Reickmann, T., Benson, M., & Compas, B. E. (2004). Coping and responses to stress in Navajo adolescents: Psychometric properties of the responses to stress questionnaire. *Journal of Community Psychology, 32,* 391–411.

Watson, D., & Tellegen, A. (1985). Toward a consensual structure of mood. *Psychological Bulletin, 98,* 219–235.

Wegner, D. M., & Erber, R. (1992). The hyperaccessibility of suppressed thoughts. *Journal of Personality and Social Psychology, 63,* 903–912.

Weisz, J. R., McCabe, M. A., & Dennig, M. D. (1994). Primary and secondary control among children undergoing medical procedures: Adjustment as a function of coping style. *Journal of Consulting and Clinical Psychology, 62,* 324–332.

Yao, S., Xiao, J., Zhu, X., Zhang, C., Auerbach, R. P., Mcwhinnie, C. M., . . . Wang, C. (2010). Coping and involuntary responses to stress in Chinese university students: Psychometric properties of the responses to stress questionnaire. *Journal of Personality Assessment, 92*(4), 356.

Zajonc, R. B. (1980). Feeling and thinking: Preferences need no inferences. *American Psychologist, 35,* 151–175.

# CHAPTER 5

# Child Maltreatment and Risk for Psychopathology

SARA R. JAFFEE AND ANDREA KOHN MAIKOVICH-FONG

E ACH YEAR WITHIN THE United States alone more than 770,000 children are victimized by abuse and neglect (U.S. Department of Health and Human Services, 2011). Our aims in writing this chapter are to review the literature on the relationship between child maltreatment and children's mental health; to describe possible mechanisms through which child maltreatment contributes to compromised mental health; to describe factors at the levels of child, family, and community that moderate risk for psychopathology; and to describe treatment approaches to helping maltreated children.

## TERMINOLOGICAL AND CONCEPTUAL ISSUES

Child Protective Services (CPS) agencies in the United States typically receive more than 3 million reports of abuse and neglect annually, of which 60% to 65% are investigated. Approximately 20% of investigations result in the substantiation of at least one child as an abuse or neglect victim (U.S. Department of Health and Human Services, 2011). More than 1,500 annual child deaths are attributed to child abuse or neglect (U.S. Department of Health and Human Services, 2011).

The most common reason for substantiation in 2010—and the reason in approximately 78% of cases—was physical neglect. Neglect comprises failures to meet children's basic physical needs with respect to clothing, hygiene, food, and safety (U.S. Department of Health and Human Services, 2011). Approximately 18% of victims in 2010 were substantiated due to physical abuse, defined as harm by a caregiver or someone who has responsibility for the child resulting in nonaccidental physical injury (from minor bruises to severe fractures or death) (Leeb, Paulozzi, Melanson, Simon, & Arias, 2008). Sexual abuse was the documented cause for substantiation in 9% of cases, and approximately 8% of maltreatment victims were substantiated for emotional abuse, sometimes referred to as *psychological abuse*. The core feature of this form of maltreatment is a pattern of behavior that impairs a child's emotional development or sense of self-worth (Leeb et al., 2008). Finally, approximately 10% of substantiated maltreatment victims were classified in an "other" category (e.g., congenital drug addiction and medical neglect). Note that these totals add up to more than 100%, which reflects the fact that some youth are substantiated for more than one category of maltreatment.

According to official estimates, approximately 2.4% of children in the United States were investigated for allegations of abuse or neglect in 2010, although only about 20% of these allegations were substantiated (U.S. Department of Health and Human Services, 2011). This is likely to be a gross underestimate of the actual prevalence of maltreatment in the population. For example, the National Survey of Children's Exposure to Violence was conducted to estimate the past-year incidence and prevalence of children's exposure to various forms of violence in a nationally representative U.S. sample (Finkelhor, Turner, Ormrod, Hamby, & Cracke, 2009). Of youth surveyed, 10.2% reported having experienced maltreatment in the past 12 months, more than 4 times the rate of investigated cases and approximately 17 times the rate of substantiated cases. The lifetime prevalence of maltreatment among youth under 18 years of age was 18.6%.

## Prevalence Rates of Maltreatment Among Subgroups

Maltreatment rates are approximately equal for boys and girls, although some types of maltreatment are more common in one sex than the other. Maltreatment is most prevalent among children under the age of 4 years, who represent approximately one third of victims (U.S. Department of Health and Human Services, 2011). Maltreatment rates are highest among African American, Native American/Alaska Native, and multiethnic youth, and lowest among Asian youth. Rates for Hispanic and white youth fall in between (U.S. Department of Health and Human Services, 2011). Recent analyses of national data support the hypothesis that minority children are disproportionately represented in the child welfare system because minority families experience high rates of poverty and other social stressors rather than pervasive bias in the child welfare system (Drake et al., 2011).

# MALTREATMENT AND CHILDREN'S RISK
# FOR PSYCHOPATHOLOGY

In this section we describe studies that have tested whether maltreated children are at elevated risk for psychopathology. We focus our review on the most method-ologically rigorous studies that include the following features: (1) a prospective research design wherein maltreatment predated the onset of psychopathology, (2) a demographically matched control sample or statistical adjustments for variables that could confound the association between maltreatment and risk for psychopathol-ogy, and (3) psychometrically valid measures of psychopathology, including (but not limited to) diagnostic measures. In the majority of these studies, information about maltreatment came from child protective services records, although in some studies maltreatment was reported by caregivers.

## Maltreatment and Risk for Externalizing Psychopathology

Victims of maltreatment are at elevated risk for a range of externalizing problems in childhood and adolescence, including attention deficit/hyperactivity disorder, conduct disorder, oppositional defiant disorder (Cohen, Brown, & Smailes, 2001; Famularo, Kinscherff, & Fenton, 1992), delinquency (Lansford et al., 2007; Stouthamer-Loeber, Loeber, Homish, & Wei, 2001; Widom, 1989; Williams, Van Dorn, Bright, Jonson-Reid, & Nebbitt, 2010), and antisocial behavior (Jaffee, Caspi, Moffitt, & Taylor, 2004; Jonson-Reid et al., 2010; Lansford et al., 2002; Manly, Kim, Rogosch, & Cicchetti, 2001; Moylan et al., 2010). Some studies have identified elevated symptoms of substance use in maltreated versus nonmaltreated youth (Lansford, Dodge, Pettit, & Bates, 2010), but others have not observed this pattern (Cohen et al., 2001).

Risk for externalizing problems extends into adulthood, where victims have significantly elevated rates of antisocial personality disorder (Johnson, Cohen, Brown, Smailes, & Bernstein, 1999; Luntz & Widom, 1994), self-reported crime (Thornberry, Henry, Ireland, & Smith, 2010), and criminal arrests (Maxfield & Widom, 1996). Findings with respect to drug and alcohol use have been mixed, with some studies identifying elevated rates of drug and alcohol use among young adults with a history of maltreatment versus those without such a history (Cohen et al., 2001; Noll, Trickett, Harris, & Putnam, 2009; Scott, Smith, & Ellis, 2010; Thornberry et al., 2010), and others finding that the relationship between these problems and child maltreatment varies as a function of age and sex (Widom, Ireland, & Glynn, 1995; Widom, Marmorstein, & White, 2006).

## Maltreatment and Risk for Internalizing Psychopathology

Victims of maltreatment are at risk for a range of internalizing problems in childhood as well, including major depressive disorder (Brown, Cohen, Johnson, & Smailes, 1999), anxiety disorders (Cohen et al., 2001), posttraumatic stress disorder (PTSD) and trauma symptoms (Crusto et al., 2010; Famularo et al., 1992; Milot, Ethier, St-Laurent, & Provost, 2010; Putnam, Helmers, & Horowitz, 1995), and internalizing symptoms (Bolger & Patterson, 2001; Lansford et al., 2002; Manly et al., 2001; Moylan et al., 2010). Risk for internalizing disorders associated with child maltreatment extends into adulthood. Victims have significantly elevated rates of major depressive disorder (Brown et al., 1999; Noll et al., 2009; Scott et al., 2010; Widom, DuMont, & Czaja, 2007), depressive symptoms (Thornberry et al., 2010), anxiety disorders (Cohen et al., 2001; Scott et al., 2010), and PTSD (Scott et al., 2010; Widom, 1999) compared to adults without a history of child maltreatment.

## Maltreatment and Risk for Personality Disorders, Psychotic Symptoms, and Suicide

As adults, victims of child maltreatment are at risk for borderline personality disorder (Johnson et al., 1999; Widom, Czaja, & Paris, 2009), with one study also showing risk for Cluster B (dramatic, emotional, erratic) and C (anxious, fearful) personality disorders more broadly (Johnson et al., 1999). At least one study demonstrated that child victims of maltreatment have elevated rates of psychotic symptoms in early adolescence compared with non-maltreated youth (Arseneault et al., 2011). In addition, victims of child maltreatment are at elevated risk for suicide in adolescence and adulthood (Brown et al., 1999; Thornberry et al., 2010) and engage in elevated rates of self-injury (Yates, Carlson, & Egeland, 2008).

## Does the Association Between Maltreatment and Psychopathology Reflect Reverse Causation?

Although the literature showing that maltreatment is a risk factor for various forms of psychopathology is largely based on epidemiological data, the findings are typically interpreted to mean that maltreatment causes children to become aggressive, hyperactive, depressed, or anxious. For example, researchers have hypothesized that physically abused children engage in antisocial behavior because they learn that aggression is an acceptable form of expressing anger or frustration (e.g., Straus, Gelles, & Steinmetz, 1980). An alternative explanation is that parents become abusive in response to a child's perceived difficult behavior or other characteristics that are difficult to manage (Belsky, 1993). For example, children with physical disabilities are at elevated risk for physical abuse (Sullivan & Knutson, 2000) as are children with behavior problems (Helton & Cross, 2011). Using data from a prospective study of twins, Jaffee et al. (2004) provided four pieces of evidence consistent with the hypothesis that maltreatment was a cause of children's antisocial behavior rather than the reverse: (1) abuse was associated with changes over time in children's antisocial behavior, (2) there was a dose–response relationship between the severity of the abuse and the severity of children's antisocial behavior, (3) genetic factors accounted for a small and statistically nonsignificant portion of the variation (7%) in children's experience of abuse, suggesting that genetic factors related to children's behavior did not provoke abusive discipline, and (4) abuse remained a significant predictor of children's antisocial behavior controlling for parental antisocial behavior. Thus, these data were consistent with the hypothesis that characteristics of the parents and the family, but not the child, explained why some children were more likely than others to be abused. In all likelihood, the relationship between child, maternal, and family predictors of abuse is likely to be complex and "main effects" models will not capture the possibility that children's difficult behavior is likely to provoke abusive discipline when, for example, caregivers experience many other sources of stress and lack the internal or external resources to cope adequately with a stressful environment (Belsky, 1993). Prospective, longitudinal data are needed to capture developmental pathways whereby temperamental precursors of psychiatric disorder increase the risk—under certain conditions—that children will experience maltreatment and whereby maltreatment increases the risk that these temperamental precursors will develop into full-blown disorder.

## ETIOLOGICAL FORMULATIONS

Potential mechanisms explaining the link between maltreatment and psychopathology range from the biological to the cognitive to the behavioral. These different levels of analysis fit within an overarching theoretical framework, wherein early adversities trigger a chain of biobehavioral events starting at the cellular level which, over time, result in dysregulation of multiple, interacting biological and behavioral systems. A number of integrative reviews of early adversity and physical and mental health over the life course are available (e.g., Miller, Chen, & Parker, 2011; Shonkoff, Boyce, & Mcewen, 2009). We review these different levels of investigation in the following sections. We note that a review of the extensive animal literature on the biological sequelae of early adversity is beyond the scope of this chapter. Interested readers are referred elsewhere for such accounts (e.g., Beauchaine, Neuhaus, Zalewski, Crowell, & Potapova, 2011; Mead, Beauchaine, & Shannon, 2010).

### Biological Mechanisms

*Epigenetic effects of maltreatment.* Abusive experiences may lead to psychopathology by triggering epigenetic mechanisms that regulate gene expression in the central nervous system. Epigenetic mechanisms involve processes such as DNA methylation and histone deacetylation, both of which alter the physical structure of DNA (see Chapter 3), making it more or less receptive to extracellular events triggering gene expression, such as changes in diet, hormonal exposures, or experiences such as abuse (Zhang & Meaney, 2010). At least two studies have compared adults with and without a history of maltreatment and shown methylation differences in glucocorticoid genes (McGowan et al., 2009) and in the serotonin transporter gene (SLC6A4) (Beach, Brody, Todorov, Gunter, & Philibert, 2010). In the latter sample, SLC6A4 methylation levels accounted for the association between a childhood history of sexual abuse and adult antisocial personality disorder in women (Beach, Brody, Todorov, Gunter, & Philibert, 2011). Findings must be interpreted with caution, however, because epigenetic profiles are highly tissue-specific, and it is not clear whether methylation profiles identified in peripheral tissues (which are commonly sampled in studies of humans) will be identified in brain tissue where genes involved in mental illness are more likey to be expressed.

*Maltreatment and limbic-hypothalamic pituitary adrenal (LHPA) axis function.* The LHPA axis is activated in response to physical and psychosocial stressors such as maltreatment, resulting in release of corticotropin releasing factor (CRF), adrenocorticotropic hormone (ACTH), and glucocorticoids (cortisol in humans and primates), which terminate the stress response through feedback at the level of the hypothalamus and the pituitary (Gunnar & Vazquez, 2006). Chronic activation of the system in response to an ongoing stressor such as maltreatment contributes to decreased energy, decreased ability to concentrate, and depressed mood (Gunnar & Vazquez, 2006). LHPA axis dysregulation has been implicated in a range of mental disorders including depression, anxiety disorders (Arborelius, Owens, Plotsky, & Nemeroff, 1999) and conduct disorder (van Goozen, Fairchild, Snoek, & Harold, 2007).

The literature on LHPA axis function and maltreatment is complex, and we refer interested readers to Tarullo and Gunnar (2006) for a more extensive review. Broadly speaking, however, there is evidence that among women who have a history of maltreatment, the LHPA axis becomes hypersensitized as evidenced by pituitary overreactivity to pharmacological and psychosocial challenge, which releases ACTH (Heim et al., 2000; Heim, Newport, Bonsall, Miller, & Nemeroff, 2001). Counterregulatory mechanisms in the periphery may result in hyporeactivity of the adrenal gland, which releases cortisol (Carpenter, Shattuck, Tyrka, Geracioti, & Price, 2011; Heim et al., 2001). Similar to cortisol findings from adults, maltreated youth often exhibit a blunted cortisol response to psychosocial challenge compared with nonmaltreated youth (Gunnar, Frenn, Wewerka, & Van Ryzin, 2009; MacMillan et al., 2009; Ouellet-Morin et al., 2008). One study has shown that cortisol hyporeactivity accounts for the association between childhood victimization and subsequent emotional and behavioral problems (Ouellet-Morin et al., 2008). Under conditions of ongoing stress—as might be observed among women who have a history of maltreatment and who are currently depressed—pharmacological challenge produces a blunted ACTH response (De Bellis et al., 1994; Heim et al., 2001; but see Kaufman et al., 1997 for an exception), suggesting that ongoing stress may result in down-regulation of CRF receptors in the anterior pituitary (Heim et al., 2001).

Tarullo and Gunnar (2006) hypothesize that the prepubertal period constitutes a stress hyporesponsive phase wherein the LHPA axis is relatively unresponsive to stressful events—a process that is mediated by adequate caregiving. In animals (and potentially in humans) puberty represents the start of a stress responsive phase wherein the LHPA axis is responsive to events that did not previously elicit a response. Thus, maltreated children are hypothesized to have high levels of basal cortisol because they tend to lack the social supports that would buffer the stress response. In contrast, adults with a history of maltreatment in childhood are expected to have low levels of basal cortisol, perhaps reflecting habituation of the LHPA axis to chronic activation throughout childhood. Although longitudinal data are scarce, support for this developmental hypothesis has been reported (see Tarullo & Gunnar, 2006). Cross-sectional data are typically consistent with the hypothesis that basal cortisol levels are elevated in maltreated versus nonmaltreated children (e.g., Carrion et al., 2002; Cicchetti & Rogosch, 2001; De Bellis et al., 1999a; Fries, Shirtcliff, & Pollak, 2008), but blunted in maltreated versus nonmaltreated adults (Heim et al., 2001; Yehuda, Halligan, & Grossman, 2001; van der Vegt, van der Ende, Kirschbaum, Verhulst, & Tiemeier, 2009).

LHPA axis dysregulation may result in chronic inflammation because glucocorticoids control the immune system through a negative feedback loop (Chrousos, 1995). Chronic inflammation—as evidenced by elevated levels of C-reactive protein—has been linked with physical and mental health problems, notably depression (Evans et al., 2005). C-reactive protein levels are elevated in adults with a history of maltreatment (Danese, Pariante, Caspi, Taylor, & Poulton, 2007) and are most pronounced among children (Danese et al., 2011) and adults (Danese et al., 2008) who are currently depressed and who have a history of maltreatment. Early adverse experiences are also associated with an increasingly pronounced cytokine response to *in vitro* bacterial challenge (Miller & Chen, 2010), resistance to the anti-inflammatory properties of cortisol (Miller & Chen, 2010), failure of the immune system to limit viral reactivation (Shirtcliff, Coe, & Pollak, 2009), and elevated secretion of pro-inflammatory cytokines in response to psychosocial stressors (Carpenter et al., 2011). Preliminary evidence suggests that early adversities such as abuse may exacerbate effects of current stress on inflammatory processes (Kiecolt-Glaser et al., 2011).

*Structural and functional changes in the brain.* A number of structural differences have been detected between the brains of individuals who were maltreated as children and the brains of individuals who were not maltreated. For details, we direct interested readers to reviews by McCrory, De Brito, and Viding (2010) and Woon and Hedges (2008). Here we note that differences have been detected in brain regions implicated in the development of psychopathology, including the hippocampus (Bremner et al., 1997; Bremner et al., 2003; Stein, Koverola, Hanna, Torchia, & McClarty, 1997; Thomaes et al., 2010), the corpus callosum (e.g., De Bellis et al., 1999b; De Bellis et al., 2002; Kitayama et al., 2007; Teicher et al., 2004), the prefrontal cortex (Carrion et al., 2009; Hanson et al., 2010; Richert, Carrion, Karchemskiy, & Reiss, 2006), and the cerebellum (Bauer, Hanson, Pierson, Davidson, & Pollak, 2009; Carrion et al., 2009), but not the amygdala (Woon & Hedges, 2008).

Differences between maltreated and nonmaltreated children have also been identified in functional imaging studies. In general, these studies support the hypothesis that maltreatment increases risk for depression by altering dopaminergic circuitry projecting to the basal ganglia, thus producing a relatively weak response to cues for reward and subsequently increasing risk for anhedonia and depression (Dillon et al., 2009). A large body of evidence also suggests that maltreated versus non-maltreated children are selectively attentive to cues for anger, as evidenced, for example, by greater activation of the right amygdala and anterior insula bilaterally to angry faces (but not sad faces) versus neutral faces (McCrory et al., 2011). Event related potential methodologies indicate that children with a history of physical abuse are more attentive to angry cues (versus other negatively valenced cues) and have more difficulty disengaging from angry versus happy cues (Cicchetti & Curtis, 2005; Curtis & Cicchetti, 2011; Pollak, Klorman, Thatcher, & Cicchetti, 2001; Pollak & Tolley-Schell, 2003; Shackman, Shackman, & Pollak, 2007). Such hyperattention to threat mediates the association between a history of maltreatment and current symptoms of anxiety (Shackman et al., 2007).

Together, these studies suggest that children who are victims of maltreatment may be hypervigilant to perceived threat in the form of angry stimuli, and although this response may be adaptive in the context of an abusive environment (Mead et al., 2010), it may predispose children to anxiety and reactive aggression if the response is generalized. Moreover, changes in dopaminergic circuitry may result in a relatively weak response to positive stimuli, thus increasing risk for depression.

## Cognitive, Behavioral, and Socioemotional Processes

*Externalizing problems.* As just described, physically abused youth selectively attend to angry stimuli compared with nonabused youth. Consistent with these findings, physically abused youth have a tendency to attribute hostile intent to others' behavior and to respond accordingly (Dodge, Bates, & Pettit, 1990), which can make youth susceptible to chronic aggression. In addition, maltreated youth have difficulty regulating their own emotions (as captured by appropriate displays of emotion, emotional awareness, and empathy). Such emotion dysregulation, in turn, is associated with peer rejection and, consequently, increased externalizing problems over time (Kim & Cicchetti, 2006). Maltreated preschoolers also have difficulty with emotion understanding, as evidenced by inability to match positive, negative, and neutral events with positive and negative emotions (Perlman, Kalish, & Pollak, 2008). This deficit may affect their ability to predict the reactions that their own negative behaviors elicit from others. Maltreated youth also have more positive beliefs about violence, which leads them to antisocial peer groups and increases their risk for violent behavior in adolescence (Herrenkohl, Huang, Tajima, & Whitney, 2003).

Maltreatment may also lead to a high-risk behavioral trajectory. For example, youth who run away from home to escape abuse are likely to drop out of school and may become homeless (Paradise & Cauce, 2002; Stein, Leslie, & Nyamathi, 2002). With nowhere to live and no formal education, some of these youth may resort to prostitution (Wilson & Widom, 2008) and other criminal behaviors as a means of supporting themselves (Kim, Tajima, Herrenkohl, & Huang, 2009). This constellation of problem behaviors emerging in adolescence and young adulthood accounts for the association between child maltreatment and women's illicit drug use in middle age (Wilson & Widom, 2009).

*Internalizing problems.* Childhood sexual abuse in particular has been linked with a range of problems in self-functioning, defined in terms of self-coherence, self-continuity, self-affectivity, and self-agency (Stern, 1985). Some studies show that abused and neglected youth report elevated symptoms of dissociation compared with nonmaltreated youth (Macfie, Cicchetti, & Toth, 2001), particularly among those who feel shame and blame themselves for the abuse (Feiring, Taska, & Lewis, 1996; Feiring, Cleland, & Simon, 2010). Moreover, when combined with high levels of arousal and avoidant coping, symptoms of dissociation account for substantial variation in symptoms of PTSD among sexually abused youth (Kaplow, Dodge, Amaya-Jackson, & Saxe, 2005). The tendency to feel shame and to self-blame is also associated with internalizing and externalizing problems (Feiring & Cleland, 2007; McGee, Wolfe, & Olson, 2001) and, in the short term, low self-esteem (Feiring, Taska, & Lewis, 2002). Others have found that sexually abused and neglected children are more likely than nonabused children to develop an external locus of control, with perceived external control accounting substantially for their elevated symptoms of internalizing problems (Bolger & Patterson, 2001).

## MODERATORS OF MALTREATMENT ON RISK FOR PSYCHOPATHOLOGY

Although maltreated children are, on average, at elevated risk for psychopathology, some are affected more severely than others. In studies where resilience to maltreatment is stringently defined as competence that is sustained over time across more than one domain, between 12% and 22% of individuals who were maltreated as children are defined as resilient (Cicchetti, Rogosch, Lynch, & Holt, 1993; Jaffee & Gallop, 2007; Kaufman, Cook, Arny, Jones, & Pittinsky, 1994; McGloin & Widom, 2001). Researchers have examined characteristics of the maltreatment, characteristics of the individual, and characteristics of the child's environment in an effort to explain this heterogeneity.

## CHARACTERISTICS OF THE MALTREATMENT

*Maltreatment subtype.* There is some evidence that children who experience certain types of maltreatment are affected differently or more adversely than children who experience other types of maltreatment. In one study, even though all maltreated children were at elevated risk for externalizing problems compared with non-maltreated children, only physically neglected children were at elevated risk for internalizing problems (Manly et al., 2001). In another investigation, children who experienced multiple forms of abuse and neglect had more externalizing problems than children who experienced fewer forms of maltreatment, whereas children who experienced only supervisory neglect and emotional maltreatment had lower levels of internalizing problems compared with children who experienced more types of maltreatment (Pears et al., 2008). Finally, sexual abuse (controlling for neglect and harsh parenting) was found to be uniquely predictive of children's internalizing problems (Bolger & Patterson, 2001).

Interpretation of these findings is hampered by the fact that even when the overall sample is relatively large, many subgroups are small. Thus, low statistical power could generate a pattern of findings wherein children who experience one type of maltreatment have elevated levels of problem behaviors compared with nonmaltreated children, but children who experience other types of maltreatment do not. Moreover, cross-study comparisons are complicated by the fact that researchers use different methods to group maltreated children. In summary, although child victims of maltreatment vary in terms of what forms of maltreatment they experience, no clear picture has emerged as to whether this heterogeneity is meaningfully and consistently associated with children's mental health over time.

*Maltreatment chronicity.* In contrast to the literature on maltreatment subtypes, maltreatment chronicity has consistently been related to child psychopathology. There is ample evidence that children who are chronically maltreated—that is, children who are subject to ongoing maltreatment over time—have higher levels of psychopathology than children who are not maltreated or who experience more transitory maltreatment (e.g., English, Graham, Litrownik, Everson, & Bangdiwala, 2005; Jaffee & Maikovich-Fong, 2011; Manly et al., 2001; Thornberry, Ireland, & Smith, 2001). At least one study has shown, however, that differences between children who experience chronic versus transitory maltreatment can be partly accounted for by elevated levels of other risk factors to which chronically maltreated children are exposed, including caregiver depression and antisocial behavior, as well as residence in dangerous neighborhoods (Jaffee & Maikovich-Fong, 2011).

*Developmental timing.* Organizational theories of development propose that the effects of maltreatment on children's health and behavior are more detrimental the earlier in development maltreatment begins, because the experience undermines the mastery of early developmental tasks, thus depriving children of the skills required to master subsequent developmental challenges (Sroufe & Rutter, 1984). Studies of children and adolescents are generally consistent with this hypothesis. These studies have found that early experiences of maltreatment (e.g., prior to school age) are more strongly associated with risk for internalizing and externalizing problems than are later experiences of maltreatment (Keiley, Howe, Dodge, Bates, & Pettit, 2001; Manly et al., 2001). Studies of adults maltreated as children have also found that the earlier in childhood maltreatment started, the more internalizing problems adults report (Kaplow & Widom, 2007; Thornberry et al., 2010). In contrast, studies of adults who were maltreated as children report the opposite pattern of findings with respect to externalizing problems measured in adulthood: the later the maltreatment started—particularly if it started in adolescence—the more externalizing problems adults report (Kaplow & Widom, 2007; Thornberry et al., 2010). It is possible that a later onset of maltreatment may be associated specifically with more severe forms of externalizing psychopathology measured in adulthood (e.g., antisocial personality disorder, violent crime, and arrest or incarceration) as opposed to the more general forms of externalizing psychopathology measured by the Child Behavior Checklist (Achenbach & Rescorla, 2001) or similar measures of child problem behaviors.

## Characteristics of the Individual

*Sex.* Firm conclusions about sex differences are difficult to make because of differences across studies in the type of maltreatment studied, outcomes, and populations (e.g., nationally representative samples versus selected samples). We restrict our review to studies that involved large, representative samples (many of which assessed maltreatment retrospectively) or studies in which maltreatment and subsequent psychopathology were assessed prospectively.

One nationally representative survey of adults who retrospectively reported physical abuse in childhood found that a history of abuse increased risk for adult mental health problems for women, but not men (Thompson, Kingree, & Desai, 2004). Two prospective, longitudinal studies have found that females, but not males with a history of childhood abuse or neglect are at risk for alcohol use problems in adolescence (Lansford et al., 2010) and adulthood (Widom et al., 1995), although sex differences in the effects of childhood maltreatment on other forms of psychopathology were not evident in either study. Other large, representative samples have failed to identify sex differences in the effects of childhood maltreatment on adult mental health (Arnow, Blasey, Hunkeler, Lee, & Hayward, 2011; Kessler, Davis, & Kendler, 1997; Molnar, Buka, & Kessler, 2001). Prospective, longitudinal studies of maltreated children have generally not identified strong sex differences in the effects of maltreatment on risk for psychopathology (Maikovich, Koenen, & Jaffee, 2009), although there is evidence from some studies (Maxfield & Widom, 1996), but not others (Lansford et al., 2007), that a history of maltreatment increases the risk of arrest for violent offenses more dramatically in women than in men. In summary, there is not strong evidence that women are more severely affected by maltreatment than men or the reverse, although there is evidence that maltreated girls may be more at risk for alcohol use problems than maltreated boys.

*Race.* Data from the National Epidemiologic Survey of Alcohol and Related Conditions found that African American adults who experience child maltreatment are more likely than whites to develop PTSD, although this race effect is not large (Roberts, Gilman, Breslau, Breslau, & Koenen, 2011). In addition, two studies indicate that differences between maltreated and nonmaltreated youth in risk for violent offending (particularly as measured by official records) are more pronounced among African Americans versus whites (Lansford et al., 2007; Maxfield et al., 1996), but this finding may reflect racial differences in arrest and conviction rates in general (Rivera & Widom, 1990).

*Personality characteristics.* Children who are resilient to maltreatment (in the sense that they are doing better than expected considering their histories of abuse or neglect) tend to be characterized by high ego control and ego resiliency, high self-esteem, high self-reliance, and the tendency to attribute successes to their own efforts (Cicchetti et al., 1993; Feiring et al., 2002; Moran & Eckenrode, 1992). Above-average intelligence has been identified as a protective factor in some studies (Herrenkohl, Herrenkohl, & Egolf, 1994; Jaffee, Caspi, Moffitt, Polo-Tomas, & Taylor, 2007), but not others (Cicchetti & Rogosch, 1997; Widom et al., 2007). These individual characteristics may only be protective as long as children are not exposed to a multitude of stressors in addition to maltreatment (Widom et al., 2007; Jaffee et al., 2007).

*Genotype.* Recently, evidence has accumulated that genotype moderates the effect of maltreatment (Genotype × Environment interaction, or G × E), although there is considerable controversy surrounding the replicability of G × E (e.g., Caspi, Hariri, Holmes, Uher, & Moffitt, 2010; Duncan & Keller, 2011; Risch et al., 2009; see Chapter 3). An extensive review of this literature is beyond the scope of the chapter, but we note briefly that several genes may be implicated in Genotype × Maltreatment interactions. These include monoamine oxidase A, the low-activity variant of which has been found to increase risk for antisocial behavior in the context of maltreatment (Caspi et al., 2002; Edwards et al., 2010; Kim-Cohen et al., 2006; Widom & Brzustowicz, 2006) and the serotonin transporter linked promoter region gene variant (5HTTLPR; SLC6A4), the short form of which has been shown to increase risk for depression in the context of maltreatment (e.g., Caspi et al., 2003; Kaufman et al., 2004; Kumsta et al., 2010; Taylor et al., 2006).

Although there is not consistent replication of the findings on Genotype × Maltreatment interactions involving MAOA and 5HTTLPR (Jaffee, 2012), there is plausible biological evidence from animals and humans that these Genotype × Environment interactions capture real biological processes (for a review, see Caspi et al., 2010). MAOA is involved in the metabolism of monoamines in the brain and other organs (Shih & Thompson, 1999) and 5HTTLPR is involved in the reuptake of serotonin at brain synapses (Heils et al., 1995). Results of studies that either knock out or functionally excise these genes support the involvement of MAOA in aggressive traits (Cases et al., 1995; Shih, 2004) and 5HTTLPR in anxious traits (Murphy & Lesch, 2008). Experimental studies of nonhuman primates provide evidence of G × E that is consistent with the human findings (Caspi et al., 2010), and 5HTTLPR and MAOA have been associated with brain activity in regions implicated in depression and aggression in response to negative stimuli (Buckholtz & Meyer-Lindenberg, 2008; Munafo, Brown, & Hariri, 2008).

There is also evidence of Genotype × Maltreatment interactions involving genes that affect LHPA axis function, including glucocorticoid receptor variants (Bet et al., 2009), variants of the corticotropin-releasing hormone receptor 1 (CRHR1) gene (e.g., Bradley et al., 2008; Polanczyk et al., 2009), and FK506 binding protein 5 (e.g., Appel et al., 2011; Bevilacqua et al., 2012; Binder et al., 2008; Bradley et al., 2008; Xie et al., 2010; Zimmermann et al., 2011). These Genotype × Maltreatment interactions have been shown to increase risk for aggression (Bevilacqua et al., 2012), depression (Appel et al., 2011; Bradley et al., 2008, Polanczyk et al., 2009; Zimmermann et al., 2011), and PTSD (Binder et al., 2008; Xie et al., 2010).

A major challenge for the field is to identify mechanisms that explain why maltreatment increases risk for psychopathology only in specific genetic subgroups. Hypothesized mechanisms include epigenetic processes (Mill, 2011), endocrine dysregulation (Tyrka et al., 2009), and alterations in brain structure, function, and functional connectivity that underlie social evaluations and the processing of emotions (e.g., Buckholtz & Meyer-Lindenberg, 2008). For example, one study of adults found that a history of maltreatment was associated with increased cortisol levels in response to the dexamethasone/CRH test, but only for individuals who were homozygous for the G allele in two different single nucleotide polymorphisms in the CRHR1 gene (Tyrka et al., 2009). A second study of children (Cicchetti, Rogosch, & Oshri, 2011) genotyped a haplotype in the CRHR1 gene that had been found to buffer individuals with a history of maltreatment against depression (Bradley et al., 2008; Polanczyk et al., 2009). Cicchetti et al. (2011) found that among individuals who carried two copies of the haplotype, childhood maltreatment was associated with an attenuated diurnal slope in cortisol, whereas individuals who carried 0 or 1 copy of the haplotype showed the typical decrease in cortisol across the day regardless of maltreatment status.

## CHARACTERISTICS OF THE ENVIRONMENT

A child's environment can both diminish and enhance the likelihood of resilience to maltreatment. For example, children whose parents have substance use problems and who live in neighborhoods characterized by low levels of social efficacy (i.e., neighbors do not share values, trust one another, or act to ensure each other's welfare) are less likely to be resilient to maltreatment than they are to be non-resilient (Jaffee et al., 2007). In contrast, stable family environments are associated with resilience (Widom et al., 2007; Herrenkohl et al., 1994), although this effect may not extend to resilience in young adulthood (Widom et al., 2007). Socially supportive relationships promote resilience (Widom et al., 2007; Ezzell, Swenson, & Brondino, 2000), even among children who are otherwise genetically vulnerable (Kaufman et al., 2004).

Again, the degree to which characteristics of the environment can buffer children from the adverse effects of maltreatment may depend on the overall level of risk to which the child is exposed. For example, a recent study of maltreated children found that those who reported more (vs. less) socially supportive relationships had lower levels of depression, but this protective effect was most pronounced for children with less complex maltreatment histories (Salazar, Keller, & Courtney, 2011).

A major challenge for researchers is to determine whether these features of the child's environment play a *causal* role in exacerbating or buffering risk associated with maltreatment. For example, some children are more likely than others to receive social support because they are more socially skilled, do better in school, and tend to experience lower levels of depression in the first place (Dingfelder, Jaffee, & Mandell, 2010). These qualities—rather than social support per se—may explain why children with high levels of social support subsequently experience lower levels of depression than children with low levels of social support. An experimental design could easily rule out such a challenge to causal inference by randomly assigning maltreated children to relationships characterized by high versus low social support. In practice, such an approach would be unethical (although randomized control trials in which the intervention group received high social support and the control group experienced treatment as usual might effectively accomplish the same thing). Therefore, to make stronger causal inferences about risk and protective factors in the development of psychopathology, researchers must adopt quasi-experimental and other statistically innovative approaches that accomplish by design or by statistical matching methods what experimental designs accomplish by random assignment to treatment and control conditions (Jaffee, Strait, & Odgers, 2012).

## CLINICAL TREATMENT OF MALTREATED CHILDREN

Although child maltreatment is often associated with a range of negative developmental sequelae, there has been a significant amount of research to evaluate interventions and treatments designed to help mitigate these outcomes. This growing body of research has provided consistent empirical support for some treatments, while suggesting that other treatments may actually be harmful (i.e., iatrogenic) to already-vulnerable children.

Common components of trauma-focused interventions include psycho-education, trauma narration, enhancing emotion regulation skills, developing parenting skills, addressing grief and loss, promoting safety skills, and maximizing patient and family engagement while addressing barriers to service-seeking. As reviewed by Saunders, Berliner, and Hanson (2004), many trauma-focused interventions are deemed empirically supported and acceptable. These include, for example, cognitive-behavioral and dynamic play therapy for children with sexual behavior problems and their caregivers (group therapies); cognitive processing therapy; eye-movement desensitization and reprocessing therapy; multisystemic therapy; and parent–child interaction therapy. The strongest empirical support is for trauma-focused cognitive behavioral therapy, which is grounded in behavioral principles that assume learned behavioral responses and maladaptive cognitions facilitate symptom development and maintenance (Brewin, 1989; Deblinger, Mannarino, Cohen, & Steer, 2006). In contrast, attachment therapy (the Evergreen Model) was deemed concerning and potentially harmful.

## CONCLUSIONS

Maltreatment is a significant public health problem. From a basic research perspective, there is a need for more prospective, longitudinal data on maltreatment to better understand the course of resilience and dysfunction over time and the long-term effects of maltreatment on mental and physical health. A mix of research strategies and research models are needed to understand the mechanisms by which neglect and abuse influence basic biological and psychological processes. Research on the biology of maltreatment would benefit from larger and more representative samples, whereas research on the psychological sequelae of maltreatment would benefit from research designs that allow for stronger causal inferences about potential mediators of maltreatment. An integrative, multi-level perspective is needed to trace the effects of maltreatment on pathways from genes to brain to behavior. From a clinical perspective, more research is needed to better evaluate treatment efficacy for maltreated children, to improve access to services and the quality of services for maltreated children, and to understand why some maltreated children respond better to treatment than others.

## REFERENCES

Achenbach, T. M., & Rescorla, L. A. (2001). *Manual for the ASEBA school-age forms & profiles*. Burlington, VT: University of Vermont, Research Center for Children, Youth, and Families.

Appel, K., Schwahn, C., Mahler, J., Schulz, A., Spitzer, C., Fenske, K, . . . Grabe, H. J. (2011). Moderation of adult depression by a polymorphism in the *FKBP5* gene and childhood physical abuse in the general population. *Neuropsychopharmacology, 36*, 1982–1991.

Arborelius, L., Owens, M. J., Plotsky, P. M., & Nemeroff, C. B. (1999). The role of corticotropin-releasing factor in depression and anxiety disorders. *Journal of Endocrinology, 160*, 1–12.

Arnow, B. A., Blasey, C. M., Hunkeler, E. M., Lee, J., & Hayward, C. (2011). Does gender moderate the relationship between childhood maltreatment and adult depression? *Child Maltreatment, 16*, 175–183.

Arseneault, L., Cannon, M., Fisher, H. L., Polanczyk, G., Moffitt, T. E., & Caspi, A. (2011). Childhood trauma and children's emerging psychotic symptoms: A genetically sensitive longitudinal cohort study. *American Journal of Psychiatry, 168*, 65–72.

Bauer, P. M., Hanson, J. L., Pierson, R. K., Davidson, R. J., & Pollak, S. D. (2009). Cerebellar volume and cognitive functioning in children who experienced early deprivation. *Biological Psychiatry, 66*, 1100–1106.

Beach, S. R. H., Brody, G. H., Todorov, A. A., Gunter, T. D., & Philibert, R. A. (2010). Methylation at *SLC6A4* is linked to family history of child abuse: An examination of the Iowa Adoptee Sample. *American Journal of Medical Genetics Part B-Neuropsychiatric Genetics, 153B,* 710–713.

Beach, S. R. H., Brody, G. H., Todorov, A. A., Gunter, T. D., & Philibert, R. A. (2011). Methylation at 5HTT mediates the impact of child sex abuse on women's antisocial behavior: An examination of the Iowa adoptee sample. *Psychosomatic Medicine, 73,* 83–87.

Beauchaine, T. P., Neuhaus, E., Zalewski, M., Crowell, S. E., & Potapova, N. (2011). The effects of allostatic load on neural systems subserving motivation, mood regulation, and social affiliation. *Development and Psychopathology, 23,* 975–999.

Belsky, J. (1993). Etiology of child maltreatment: A developmental-ecological analysis. *Psychological Bulletin, 114,* 413–434.

Bet, P. M., Penninx, B. W. J. H., Bochdanovits, Z., Uitterlinden, A. G., Beekman, A. T. F., van Schoor, N. M., . . . Hoogendijk, W. J. G. (2009). Glucocorticoid receptor gene polymorphisms and childhood adversity are associated with depression: New evidence for a gene-environment interaction. *American Journal of Medical Genetics Part B-Neuropsychiatric Genetics, 150B,* 660–669.

Bevilacqua, L., Carli, V., Sarchiapone, M., George, D. K., Goldman, D., Roy, A., . . . Enoch, M. A. (2012). Interaction between *FKBP5* and childhood trauma and risk of aggressive behavior. *Archives of General Psychiatry, 69,* 62–70.

Binder, E., B., Bradley, R. G., Liu, W., Epstein, M. P., Deveaux, T. C., Mercer, K. B., . . . Ressler, K. J. (2008). Association of FKBP5 polymorphisms and childhood abuse with posttraumatic stress disorder symptoms in adults. *JAMA, 299,* 1291–1305.

Bolger, K. E., & Patterson, C. J. (2001). Pathways from child maltreatment to internalizing problems: Perceptions of control as mediators and moderators. *Development and Psychopathology, 13,* 913–940.

Bradley, R. G., Binder, E. B., Epstein, M. P., Tang, Y., Nair, H. P., Liu, W., . . . Ressler, K. J. (2008). Influence of child abuse on adult depression—Moderation by the corticotropin-releasing hormone receptor gene. *Archives of General Psychiatry, 65,* 190–200.

Bremner, J. D., Randall, P., Vermetten, E., Staib, L., Bronen, R. A., Mazure, C., . . . Charney, D. S. (1997). Magnetic resonance imaging-based measurement of hippocampal volume in posttraumatic stress disorder related to childhood physical and sexual abuse - A preliminary report. *Biological Psychiatry, 41,* 23–32.

Bremner, J. D., Vythilingam, M., Vermetten, E., Southwick, S. M., McGlashan, T., Nazeer, A., . . . Charney, D. S. (2003). MRI and PET study of deficits in hippocampal structure and function in women with childhood sexual abuse and posttraumatic stress disorder. *American Journal of Psychiatry, 160,* 924–932.

Brewin, C. R. (1989). Cognitive change processes in psychotherapy. *Psychological Review, 96,* 379–394.

Brown, J., Cohen, P., Johnson, J. G., & Smailes, E. M. (1999). Childhood abuse and neglect: Specificity of effects on adolescent and young adult depression and suicidality. *Journal of the American Academy of Child and Adolescent Psychiatry, 38,* 1490–1496.

Buckholtz, J. W., & Meyer-Lindenberg, A. (2008). MAOA and the neurogenetic architecture of human aggression. *Trends in Neurosciences, 31,* 120–129.

Carpenter, L. L., Shattuck, T. T., Tyrka, A. R., Geracioti, T. D., & Price, L. H. (2011). Effect of childhood physical abuse on cortisol stress response. *Psychopharmacology, 214,* 367–375.

Carrion, V. G., Weems, C. F., Ray, R. D., Glaser, B., Hessl, D., & Reiss, A. L. (2002). Diurnal salivary cortisol in pediatric posttraumatic stress disorder. *Biological Psychiatry, 51,* 575–582.

Carrion, V. G., Weems, C. F., Watson, C., Eliez, S., Menon, V., & Reiss, A. L. (2009). Converging evidence for abnormalities of the prefrontal cortex and evaluation of midsagittal structures in pediatric posttraumatic stress disorder: An MRI study. *Psychiatry Research-Neuroimaging, 172,* 226–234.

Cases, O., Seif, I., Grimsby, J., Gaspar, P., Chen, K., Pournin, S., . . . De Maeyer, E. (1995). Aggressive behavior and altered amounts of brain serotonin and nore-pinephrine in mice lacking MAOA. *Science, 268,* 1763–1766.

Caspi, A., Hariri, A. R., Holmes, A., Uher, R., & Moffitt, T. E. (2010). Genetic sensitivity to the environment: The case of the serotonin transporter gene and its implications for studying complex diseases and traits. *American Journal of Psychiatry, 167,* 509–527.

Caspi, A., McClay, J., Moffitt, T. E., Mill, J., Martin, J., Craig, I. W., . . . Poulton, R. (2002). Role of genotype in the cycle of violence in maltreated children. *Science, 297,* 851–854.

Caspi, A., Sugden, K., Moffitt, T. E., Taylor, A., Craig, I. W., Harrington, H., . . . Poulton, R. (2003). Influence of life stress on depression: Moderation by a poly-morphism in the 5-HTT gene. *Science, 31,* 386–389.

Chrousos, G. P. (1995). Seminars in medicine of the Beth Israel Hospital, Boston—The hypothalamic-pituitary-adrenal axis and immune-mediated inflammation. *New England Journal of Medicine, 332,* 1351–1362.

Cicchetti, D., & Curtis, W. J. (2005). An event-related potential study of the processing of affective facial expressions in young children who experienced maltreatment during the first year of life. *Development and Psychopathology, 17,* 641–677.

Cicchetti, D., & Rogosch, F. A. (1997). The role of self-organization in the promotion of resilience in maltreated children. *Development and Psychopathology, 9,* 797–815.

Cicchetti, D., & Rogosch, F. A. (2001). The impact of maltreatment and psy-chopathology on neuroendocrine functioning. *Development and Psychopathology, 13,* 783–804.

Cicchetti, D., Rogosch, F. A., Lynch, M., & Holt, K. D. (1993). Resilience in maltreated children: Processes leading to adaptive outcome. *Development and Psychopathology, 5,* 629–647.

Cicchetti, D., Rogosch, F. A., & Oshri, A. (2011). Interactive effects of corticotropin releasing hormone receptor 1, serotonin transporter linked polymorphic region, and child maltreatment on diurnal cortisol regulation and internalizing symp-tomatology. *Development and Psychopathology, 23,* 1125–1138.

Cohen, P., Brown, J., & Smailes, E. (2001). Child abuse and neglect and the development of mental disorders in the general population. *Development and Psychopathology, 13,* 981–999.

Crusto, C. A., Whitson, M. L., Walling, S. M., Feinn, R., Friedman, S. R., Reynolds, J., . . . Kaufman, J. S (2010). Posttraumatic stress among young urban children exposed to family violence and other potentially traumatic events. *Journal of Traumatic Stress, 23,* 716–724.

Curtis, W., & Cicchetti, D. (2011). Affective facial expression processing in young children who have experienced maltreatment during the first year of life: An event-related potential study. *Development and Psychopathology, 23,* 373–395.

Danese, A., Caspi, A., Williams, B., Ambler, A., Sugden, K., Mika, J., . . . Arseneault, L. (2011). Biological embedding of stress through inflammation processes in childhood. *Molecular Psychiatry, 16,* 244–246.

Danese, A., Moffitt, T. E., Pariante, C. M., Ambler, A., Poulton, R., & Caspi, A. (2008). Elevated inflammation levels in depressed adults with a history of childhood maltreatment. *Archives of General Psychiatry, 65,* 409–416.

Danese, A., Pariante, C. M., Caspi, A., Taylor, A., & Poulton, R. (2007). Childhood maltreatment predicts adult inflammation in a life-course study. *PNAS, 104,* 1319–1324.

De Bellis, M. D., Baum, A. S., Birmaher, B., Keshavan, M. S., Eccard, C. H., Boring, A. M., . . . Ryan, N. D. (1999a). Developmental traumatology Part I: Biological stress systems. *Biological Psychiatry, 45,* 1259–1270.

De Bellis, M. D., Chrousos, G. P., Dorn, L. D., Burke, L., Helmers, K., Kling, M. A., . . . Putnam, F. W. (1994). Hypothalamic-pituitary-adrenal axis dysregulation in sexually abused girls. *Journal of Clinical Endocrinology & Metabolism, 78,* 249–255.

De Bellis, M. D., Keshavan, M. S., Clark, D. B., Casey, B. J., Giedd, J. N., Boring, A. M., . . . Ryan, N. D. (1999b). Developmental traumatology Part II: Brain development. *Biological Psychiatry, 45,* 1271–1284.

De Bellis, M. D., Keshavan, M. S., Shifflett, H., Iyengar, S., Beers, S. R., Hall, J., . . . Moritz, G. (2002). Brain structures in pediatric maltreatment-related posttraumatic stress disorder: A sociodemographically matched study. *Biological Psychiatry, 52,* 1066–1078.

Deblinger, E., Mannarino, A. P., Cohen, J. A., & Steer, R. A. (2006). A follow-up study of a multisite, randomized, controlled trial for children with sexual abuse-related PTSD symptoms. *Journal of the American Academy of Child and Adolescent Psychiatry, 45,* 1474–1484.

Dillon, D. G., Holmes, A. J., Birk, J. L., Brooks, N., Lyons-Ruth, K., & Pizzagalli, D. A. (2009). Childhood adversity is associated with left basal ganglia dysfunction during reward anticipation in adulthood. *Biological Psychiatry, 66,* 206–213.

Dingfelder, H. E., Jaffee, S. R., & Mandell, D. S. (2010). The impact of social support on depressive symptoms among adolescents in the child welfare system: A propensity score analysis. *Children and Youth Services Review, 32,* 1255–1261.

Dodge, K. A., Bates, J. E., & Pettit, G. S. (1990). Mechanisms in the cycle of violence. *Science, 250,* 1678–1683.

Drake, B., Jolley, J. M., Lanier, P., Fluke, J., Barth, R. P., & Jonson-Reid, M. (2011). Racial bias in child protection? A comparison of competing explanations using national data. *Pediatrics, 127,* 471–478.

Duncan, L. E., & Keller, M. C. (2011). A critical review of the first 10 years of candidate gene-by-environment interaction research in psychiatry. *American Journal of Psychiatry, 168,* 1041–1049.

Edwards, A. C., Dodge, K. A., Latendresse, S. J., Lansford, J. E., Bates, J. E., Pettit, G. S., . . . Dick, D. M. (2010). MAOA-uVNTR and early physical discipline interact to influence delinquent behavior. *Journal of Child Psychology and Psychiatry, 51,* 679–687.

English, D. J., Graham, J. C., Litrownik, A. J., Everson, M., & Bangdiwala, S. I. (2005). Defining maltreatment chronicity: Are there differences in child outcomes? *Child Abuse & Neglect, 29,* 575–595.

Evans, D. L., Charney, D. S., Lewis, L., Golden, R. N., Gorman, J. M., Krishnan, K. R. R., . . . Valvo, W. J. (2005). Mood disorders in the medically ill: Scientific review and recommendations. *Biological Psychiatry, 58,* 175–189.

Ezzell, C. E., Swenson, C. C., & Brondino, M. J. (2000). The relationship of social support to physically abused children's adjustment. *Child Abuse & Neglect, 24,* 641–651.

Famularo, R., Kinscherff, R., & Fenton, T. (1992). Psychiatric diagnoses of maltreated children: Preliminary findings. *Journal of the American Academy of Child and Adolescent Psychiatry, 31,* 863–867.

Feiring, C., & Cleland, C. (2007). Childhood sexual abuse and abuse-specific attributions of blame over 6 years following discovery. *Child Abuse & Neglect, 31,* 1169–1186.

Feiring, C., Cleland, C. M., & Simon, V. A. (2010). Abuse-specific self-schemas and self-functioning: A prospective study of sexually abused youth. *Journal of Clinical Child and Adolescent Psychology, 39,* 35–50.

Feiring, C., Taska, L., & Lewis, M. (1996). A process model for understanding adaptation to sexual abuse: The role of shame in defining stigmatization. *Child Abuse & Neglect, 20,* 767–782.

Feiring, C., Taska, L., & Lewis, M. (2002). Adjustment following sexual abuse discovery: The role of shame and attributional style. *Developmental Psychology, 38,* 79–92.

Finkelhor, D., Turner, H., Ormrod, R., Hamby, S., & Kracke, K. (2009). Children's exposure to violence: A comprehensive national survey. Retrieved from https://www.ncjrs.gov/pdffiles1/ojjdp/227744.pdf

Fries, A. B., Shirtcliff, E. A., & Pollak, S. D. (2008). Neuroendocrine dysregulation following early social deprivation in children. *Developmental Psychobiology, 50,* 588–599.

Gunnar, M. R., & Vazquez, D. (2006). Stress neurobiology and developmental psychopathology. In D. Cicchetti & D. J. Cohen (Eds.), *Developmental psychopathology. Volume 2. Developmental Neuroscience* (2nd ed., pp. 533–577). Hoboken, NJ: Wiley.

Gunnar, M. R., Frenn, K., Wewerka, S. S., & Van Ryzin, M. J. (2009). Moderate versus severe early life stress: Associations with stress reactivity and regulation in 10–12-year-old children. *Psychoneuroendocrinology, 34*, 62–75.

Hanson, J. L., Chung, M. K., Avants, B. B., Shirtcliff, E. A., Gee, J. C., Davidson, R. J., . . . Pollak. S. D. (2010). Early stress is associated with alterations in the orbitofrontal cortex: A tensor-based morphometry investigation of brain structure and behavioral risk. *Journal of Neuroscience, 30*, 7466–7472.

Heils, A., Teufel, A., Petri, S., Seemann, M., Bengel, D., Balling, U., . . . Lesch, K. P. (1995). Functional promoter and polyadenylation site mapping of the human serotonin (5-HT) transporter gene. *Journal of Neural Transmission, 102*, 247–254.

Heim, C., Newport, D. J., Bonsall, R., Miller, A. H., & Nemeroff, C. B. (2001). Altered pituitary-adrenal axis responses to provocative challenge tests in adult survivors of childhood abuse. *American Journal of Psychiatry, 158*, 575–581.

Heim, C., Newport, D. J., Heit, S., Graham, Y. P., Wilcox, M., Bonsall, R., . . . Nemeroff, C. B. (2000). Pituitary-adrenal and autonomic responses to stress in women after sexual and physical abuse in childhood. *JAMA–Journal of the American Medical Association, 284*, 592–597.

Helton, J. J., & Cross, T. P. (2011). The relationship of child functioning to parental physical assault: Linear and curvilinear models. *Child Maltreatment, 16*, 126–136.

Herrenkohl, E. C., Herrenkohl, R., & Egolf, M. (1994). Resilient early school-age children from maltreating homes: Outcomes in late adolescence. *American Journal of Orthopsychiatry, 64*, 301–309.

Herrenkohl, T. I., Huang, B., Tajima, E. A., & Whitney, S. D. (2003). Examining the link between child abuse and youth violence—An analysis of mediating mechanisms. *Journal of Interpersonal Violence, 18*, 1189–1208.

Jaffee, S. R. (2012). Teasing out the role of genotype in the development of psychopathology in maltreated children. In C. S. Widom (Ed.), *Trauma, psychopathology, and violence: Causes, consequences, or correlates?* (pp. 49–75). New York, NY: Oxford University Press.

Jaffee, S. R., Caspi, A., Moffitt, T. E., Polo-Tomas, M., & Taylor, A. (2007). Individual, family, and neighborhood characteristics promote resilience to physical maltreatment. *Child Abuse & Neglect, 31*, 231–253.

Jaffee, S. R., Caspi, A., Moffitt, T. E., & Taylor, A. (2004). Physical maltreatment victim to antisocial child: Evidence of an environmentally mediated process. *Journal of Abnormal Psychology, 113*, 44–55.

Jaffee, S. R., & Gallop, R. (2007). Social, emotional, and academic competence among children who have had contact with child protective services: Prevalence and stability estimates. *Journal of the American Academy of Child & Adolescent Psychiatry, 46*, 757–765.

Jaffee, S. R., & Maikovich-Fong, A. K. (2011). Effects of chronic maltreatment and maltreatment timing on children's behavior and cognitive abilities. *Journal of Child Psychology and Psychiatry, 52*, 184–194.

Jaffee, S. R., Strait, L. B., & Odgers, C. L. (2012). From correlates to causes: Can quasi-experimental studies and statistical innovations bring us closer to identifying the causes of antisocial behavior? *Psychological Bulletin, 138,* 272–295.

Johnson, J. G., Cohen, P., Brown, J., Smailes, E. M., & Bernstein, D. P. (1999). Childhood maltreatment increases risk for personality disorders during early adulthood. *Archives of General Psychiatry, 56,* 600–606.

Jonson-Reid, M., Presnall, N., Drake, B., Fox, L., Bierut, L., Reich, W., . . . Constantino, J. N. (2010). Effects of child maltreatment and inherited liability on antisocial development: An official records study. *Journal of the American Academy of Child and Adolescent Psychiatry, 49,* 321–332.

Kaplow, J. B., Dodge, K. A., Amaya-Jackson, L., & Saxe, G. N. (2005). Pathways to PTSD, Part II: Sexually abused children. *American Journal of Psychiatry, 162,* 1305–1310.

Kaplow, J. B., & Widom, C. S. (2007). Age of onset of child maltreatment predicts long-term mental health outcomes. *Journal of Abnormal Child Psychology, 116,* 176–187.

Kaufman, J., Yang, B. Z., Douglas-Palumberi, H., Houshyar, S., Lipschitz, D., Krystal, J. H., . . . Gelernter, J. (2004). Social supports and serotonin transporter gene moderate depression in maltreated children. *PNAS, 101,* 17316–17321.

Kaufman, J., Birmaher, B., Perel, J., Dahl, R. E., Moreci, P., Nelson, B., . . . Ryan, N. D (1997). The corticotropin-releasing hormone challenge in depressed abused, depressed nonabused, and normal control children. *Biological Psychiatry, 42,* 669–679.

Kaufman, J., Cook, A., Arny, L., Jones, B., & Pittinsky, T. (1994). Problems defining resiliency: Illustrations from the study of maltreated children. *Development and Psychopathology, 6,* 215–229.

Keiley, M. K., Howe, T. R., Dodge, K. A., Bates, J. E., & Pettit, G. S. (2001). The timing of child physical maltreatment: A cross-domain growth analysis of impact on adolescent externalizing and internalizing problems. *Development and Psychopathology, 13,* 891–912.

Kessler, R. C., Davis, C. G., & Kendler, K. S. (1997). Childhood adversity and adult psychiatric disorder in the US national comorbidity survey. *Psychological Medicine, 27,* 1101–1119.

Kiecolt-Glaser, J. K., Gouin, J. P., Weng, N. P., Malarkey, W. B., Beversdorf, D. Q., & Glaser, R. (2011). Childhood adversity heightens the impact of later-life caregiving stress on telomere length and inflammation. *Psychosomatic Medicine, 73,* 16–22.

Kim, J. & Cicchetti, D. (2006). Longitudinal trajectories of self-system processes and depressive symptoms among maltreated and nonmaltreated children. *Child Development, 77,* 624–639.

Kim, M. J., Tajima, E. A., Herrenkohl, T. I., & Huang, B. (2009). Early child maltreatment, runaway youths, and risk of delinquency and victimization in adolescence: A mediational model. *Social Work Research, 33,* 19–28.

Kim-Cohen, J., Caspi, A., Taylor, A., Williams, B., Newcombe, R., Craig, I. W., . . . Moffitt, T. E. (2006). MAOA, maltreatment, and gene-environment interaction predicting children's mental health: New evidence and a meta-analysis. *Molecular Psychiatry, 11,* 903–913.

Kitayama, N., Brummer, M., Hertz, L., Quinn, S., Kim, Y., & Bremner, J. (2007). Morphologic alterations in the corpus callosum in abuse-related posttraumatic stress disorder. *Journal of Nervous and Mental Disease, 195,* 1027–1029.

Kumsta, R., Stevens, S., Brookes, K., Schlotz, W., Castle, J., Beckett, C., . . . Sonuga-Barke, E. (2010). 5HTT genotype moderates the influence of early institutional deprivation on emotional problems in adolescence: Evidence from the English and Romanian Adoptee (ERA) study. *Journal of Child Psychology and Psychiatry, 51,* 755–762.

Lansford, J. E., Dodge, K. A., Pettit, G. S., Bates, J. E., Crozier, J., & Kaplow, J. (2002). Long-term effects of early child physical maltreatment on psychological, behavioral, and academic problems in adolescence: A 12-year prospective study. *Archives of Pediatrics and Adolescent Medicine, 156,* 824–830.

Lansford, J. E., Dodge, K. A., Pettit, G. S., & Bates, J. E. (2010). Does physical abuse in early childhood predict substance use in adolescence and early adulthood? *Child Maltreatment, 15,* 190–194.

Lansford, J. E., Miller-Johnson, S., Berlin, L. J., Dodge, K. A., Bates, J. E., & Pettit, G. S. (2007). Early physical abuse and later violent delinquency: A prospective longitudinal study. *Child Maltreatment, 12,* 233–245.

Leeb, R. T., Paulozzi, L., Melanson, C., Simon, T., & Arias, I. (2008). *Child maltreatment surveillance: Uniform definitions for public health and recommended data elements, version 1.0.* Atlanta, GA: Centers for Disease Control and Prevention, National Center for Injury Prevention and Control.

Luntz, B. K., & Widom, C. S. (1994). Antisocial personality disorder in abused and neglected children grown up. *American Journal of Psychiatry, 151,* 670–674.

Macfie, J., Cicchetti, D., & Toth, S. L. (2001). The development of dissociation in maltreated preschool-aged children. *Development and Psychopathology, 13,* 233–254.

MacMillan, H. L., Georgiades, K., Duku, E. K., Shea, A., Steiner, M., Niec, A., . . . Schmidt, L. A. (2009). Cortisol response to stress in female youths exposed to childhood maltreatment: Results of the Youth Mood Project. *Biological Psychiatry, 66,* 62–68.

Maikovich, A. K., Koenen, K. C., & Jaffee, S. R. (2009). Posttraumatic stress symptoms and trajectories in child sexual abuse victims: An analysis of sex differences using the National Survey of Child and Adolescent Well-Being. *Journal of Abnormal Child Psychology, 37,* 727–737.

Manly, J. T., Kim, J. E., Rogosch, F. A., & Cicchetti, D. (2001). Dimensions of child maltreatment and children's adjustment: Contributions of developmental timing and subtype. *Development and Psychopathology, 13,* 759–782.

Maxfield, M. G., & Widom, C. S. (1996). The cycle of violence—Revisited 6 years later. *Archives of Pediatrics & Adolescent Medicine, 150,* 390–395.

McCrory, E., De Brito, S. A., Sebastian, C. L., Mechelli, A., Bird, G., Kelly, P. A., . . . Viding, E. (2011). Heightened neural reactivity to threat in child victims of family violence. *Current Biology, 21,* R947–R948.

McCrory, E., De Brito, S. A., & Viding, E. (2010). Research review: The neurobiology and genetics of maltreatment and adversity. *Journal of Child Psychology and Psychiatry, 51,* 1079–1095.

McGee, R., Wolfe, D., & Olson, J. (2001). Multiple maltreatment, attribution of blame, and adjustment among adolescents. *Development and Psychopathology, 13,* 827–846.

McGloin, J. M., & Widom, C. S. (2001). Resilience among abused and neglected children grown up. *Development and Psychopathology, 13,* 1021–1038.

McGowan, P. O., Sasaki, A., D'Alessio, A. C., Dymov, S., Labonte, B., Szyf, M., . . . Meaney, M. J. (2009). Epigenetic regulation of the glucocorticoid receptor in human brain associates with childhood abuse. *Nature Neuroscience, 12,* 342–348.

Mead, H. K., Beauchaine, T. P., & Shannon, K. E. (2010). Neurobiological adaptations to violence across development. *Development and Psychopathology, 22,* 1–22.

Mill, J. (2011). Epigenetic effects on gene function and their role in mediating gene-environment interactions. In K. S. Kendler, S. R. Jaffee, & D. Romer (Eds.), *The dynamic genome and mental health: The role of genes and environments in youth development* (pp. 145–171). New York, NY: Oxford University Press.

Miller, G. E., & Chen, E. (2010). Harsh family climate in early life presages the emergence of a proinflammatory phenotype in adolescence. *Psychological Science, 21,* 848–856.

Miller, G. E., Chen, E., & Parker, K. J. (2011). Psychological stress in childhood and susceptibility to the chronic diseases of aging: Moving toward a model of behavioral and biological mechanisms. *Psychological Bulletin, 137,* 959–997.

Milot, T., Ethier, L. S., St-Laurent, D., & Provost, M. A. (2010). The role of trauma symptoms in the development of behavioral problems in maltreated preschoolers. *Child Abuse & Neglect, 34,* 225–234.

Molnar, B. E., Buka, S. L., & Kessler, R. C. (2001). Child sexual abuse and subsequent psychopathology: Results from the national comorbidity survey. *American Journal of Public Health, 91,* 753–760.

Moran, P. B., & Eckenrode, J. (1992). Protective personality characteristics among adolescent victims of maltreatment. *Child Abuse & Neglect, 16,* 743–754.

Moylan, C. A., Herrenkohl, T. I., Sousa, C., Tajima, E. A., Herrenkohl, R. C., & Russo, M. J. (2010). The effects of child abuse and exposure to domestic violence on adolescent internalizing and externalizing behavior problems. *Journal of Family Violence, 25,* 53–63.

Munafo, M. R., Brown, S. M., & Hariri, A. R. (2008). Serotonin transporter (5-HTTLPR) genotype and amygdala activation: A meta-analysis. *Biological Psychiatry, 63,* 852–857.

Murphy, D. L., & Lesch, K. P. (2008). Targeting the murine serotonin transporter: Insights into human neurobiology. *Nature Reviews Neuroscience, 9,* 85–96.

Noll, J. G., Trickett, P. K., Harris, W. W., & Putnam, F. W. (2009). The cumulative burden borne by offspring whose mothers were sexually abused as children: Descriptive results from a multigenerational study. *Journal of Interpersonal Violence, 24,* 424–449.

Ouellet-Morin, I., Boivin, M., Dionne, G., Lupien, S. J., Arsenault, L., Barr, R. G., . . . Tremblay, R. E. (2008). Variations in heritability of cortisol reactivity to stress as a function of early familial adversity among 19-month-old twins. *Archives of General Psychiatry, 65,* 211–218.

Paradise, M., & Cauce, A. M. (2002). Home street home: The interpersonal dimensions of adolescent homelessness. *Analyses of Social Issues and Public Policy, 2*, 238.

Pears, K. C., Kim, H. K., & Fisher, P. A. (2008). Psychosocial and cognitive functioning of children with specific profiles of maltreatment. *Child Abuse & Neglect, 32*, 958–971.

Perlman, S. B., Kalish, C. W., & Pollak, S. D. (2008). The role of maltreatment experience in children's understanding of the antecedents of emotion. *Cognition & Emotion, 22*, 651–670.

Polanczyk, G., Caspi, A., Williams, B., Price, T. S., Danese, A., Sugden, K., . . . Moffitt, T. E (2009). Protective effect of CRHR1 gene variants on the development of adult depression following childhood maltreatment: Replication and extension. *Archives of General Psychiatry, 66*, 978–985.

Pollak, S. D., Klorman, R., Thatcher, J. E., & Cicchetti, D. (2001). P3b reflects maltreated children's reactions to facial displays of emotion. *Psychophysiology, 38*, 267–274.

Pollak, S. D., & Tolley-Schell, S. A. (2003). Selective attention to facial emotion in physically abused children. *Journal of Abnormal Psychology, 112*, 323–338.

Putnam, F. W., Helmers, K., & Horowitz, L. A. (1995). Hypnotizability and dissociativity in sexually abused girls. *Child Abuse & Neglect, 19*, 645–655.

Richert, K. A., Carrion, V. G., Karchemskiy, A., & Reiss, A. L. (2006). Regional differences of the prefrontal cortex in pediatric PTSD: An MRI study. *Depression and Anxiety, 23*, 17–25.

Risch, N., Herrell, R., Lehner, T., Liang, K. Y., Eaves, L., Hoh, J. et al. (2009). Interaction between the serotonin transporter gene (5-HTTLPR), stressful life events, and risk of depression: A meta-analysis. *JAMA–Journal of the American Medical Association, 301*, 2462–2471.

Rivera, B., & Widom, C. S. (1990). Childhood victimization and violent offending. *Violence and Victims, 5*, 19–35.

Roberts, A. L., Gilman, S. E., Breslau, J., Breslau, N., & Koenen, K. C. (2011). Race/ethnic differences in exposure to traumatic events, development of post-traumatic stress disorder, and treatment-seeking for post-traumatic stress disorder in the United States. *Psychological Medicine, 41*, 71–83.

Salazar, A. M., Keller, T. E., & Courtney, M. E. (2011). Understanding social support's role in the relationship between maltreatment and depression in youth with foster care experience. *Child Maltreatment, 16*, 102–113.

Saunders, B. E., Berliner, L., & Hanson, R. F. (Eds.) (2004). *Child physical and sexual abuse: Guidelines for treatment* (revised report: April 26, 2004). Charleston, SC: National Crime Victims Research and Treatment Center.

Scott, K. M., Smith, D. R., & Ellis, P. M. (2010). Prospectively ascertained child maltreatment and its association with DSM-IV mental disorders in young adults. *Archives of General Psychiatry, 67*, 712–719.

Shackman, J. E., Shackman, A. J., & Pollak, S. D. (2007). Physical abuse amplifies attention to threat and increases anxiety in children. *Emotion, 7*, 838–852.

Shih, J. C. (2004). Cloning, after cloning, knock-out mice, and physiological functions of MAO A and B. *Neurotoxicology, 25*, 21–30.

Shih, J., & Thompson, R. (1999). Monoamine oxidase in neuropsychiatry and behavior. *American Journal of Human Genetics, 65*, 593–598.

Shirtcliff, E. A., Coe, C. L., & Pollak, S. D. (2009). Early childhood stress is associated with elevated antibody levels to herpes simplex virus type 1. *Proceedings of the National Academy of Sciences of the United States of America, 106*, 2963–2967.

Shonkoff, J. P., Boyce, W. T., & Mcewen, B. S. (2009). Neuroscience, molecular biology, and the childhood roots of health disparities: Building a new framework for health promotion and disease prevention. *JAMA–Journal of the American Medical Association, 301*, 2252–2259.

Sroufe, L. A., & Rutter, M. (1984). The domain of developmental psychopathology. *Child Development, 55*, 17–29.

Stein, J. A., Leslie, M. B., & Nyamathi, A. (2002). Relative contributions of parent substance use and childhood maltreatment to chronic homelessness, depression, and substance abuse problems among homeless women: Mediating roles of self-esteem and abuse in adulthood. *Child Abuse & Neglect, 26*, 1011–1027.

Stein, M. B., Koverola, C., Hanna, C., Torchia, M. G., & McClarty, B. (1997). Hippocampal volume in women victimized by childhood sexual abuse. *Psychological Medicine, 27*, 951–959.

Stern, D. (1985). *The interpersonal world of the infant: A view from psychoanalysis and developmental psychology.* New York, NY: Basic Books.

Stouthamer-Loeber, M., Loeber, R., Homish, D. L., & Wei, E. (2001). Maltreatment of boys and the development of disruptive and delinquent behavior. *Development and Psychopathology, 13*, 941–955.

Straus, M. A., Gelles, R. J., & Steinmetz, S. K. (1980). *Behind closed doors: Violence in the American family.* New York, NY: Anchor Press/Doubleday.

Sullivan, P. M., & Knutson, J. F. (2000). Maltreatment and disabilities: A population-based epidemiological study. *Child Abuse & Neglect, 24*, 1257–1273.

Tarullo, A. R., & Gunnar, M. R. (2006). Child maltreatment and the developing HPA axis. *Hormones and Behavior, 50*, 632–639.

Taylor, S. E., Way, B. M., Welch, W. T., Hilmert, C. J., Lehman, B. J., & Eisenberger, N. I. (2006). Early family environment, current adversity, the serotonin transporter promoter polymorphism, and depressive symptomatology. *Biological Psychiatry, 60*, 671–676.

Teicher, M. H., Dumont, N. L., Ito, Y., Vaituzis, C., Giedd, J. N., & Andersen, S. L. (2004). Childhood neglect is associated with reduced corpus callosum area. *Biological Psychiatry, 56*, 80–85.

Thomaes, K., Dorrepaal, E., Draijer, N., de Ruiter, M. B., van Balkom, A. J., Smit, J. H., . . . Veltman, D. J. (2010). Reduced anterior cingulate and orbitofrontal volumes in child abuse-related complex PTSD. *Journal of Clinical Psychiatry, 71*, 1636–1644.

Thompson, M. P., Kingree, J. B., & Desai, S. (2004). Gender differences in long-term health consequences of physical abuse of children: Data from a nationally representative survey. *American Journal of Public Health, 94*, 599–604.

Thornberry, T. P., Henry, K. L., Ireland, T. O., & Smith, C. A. (2010). The causal impact of childhood-limited maltreatment and adolescent maltreatment on early adult adjustment. *Journal of Adolescent Health, 46*, 359–365.

Thornberry, T. P., Ireland, T. O., & Smith, C. A. (2001). The importance of timing: The varying impact of childhood and adolescent maltreatment on multiple problem outcomes. *Development and Psychopathology*, *13*, 957–979.

Tyrka, A. R., Price, L. H., Gelernter, J., Schepker, C., Anderson, G. M., & Carpenter, L. L. (2009). Interaction of childhood maltreatment with the corticotropin-releasing hormone receptor gene: Effects on hypothalamic-pituitary-adrenal axis reactivity. *Biological Psychiatry*, *66*, 681–685.

U.S. Department of Health and Human Services (2011). *Child Maltreatment 2010*. Retrieved from http://www.acf.hhs.gov/programs/cb/stats_research/index .htm#can

van der Vegt, E. J. M., van der Ende, J., Kirschbaum, C., Verhulst, F. C., & Tiemeier, H. (2009). Early neglect and abuse predict diurnal cortisol patterns in adults: A study of international adoptees. *Psychoneuroendocrinology*, *34*, 660–669.

van Goozen, S. H. M., Fairchild, G., Snoek, H., & Harold, G. T. (2007). The evidence for a neurobiological model of childhood antisocial behavior. *Psychological Bulletin*, *133*, 149–182.

Widom, C. S. (1989). The cycle of violence. *Science*, *244*, 160–166.

Widom, C. S. (1999). Posttraumatic stress disorder in abused and neglected children grown up. *American Journal of Psychiatry*, *156*, 1223–1229.

Widom, C. S., & Brzustowicz, L. M. (2006). MAOA and the "cycle of violence": Childhood abuse and neglect, MAOA genotype, and risk for violent and antisocial behavior. *Biological Psychiatry*, *60*, 684–689.

Widom, C. S., Czaja, S. J., & Paris, J. (2009). A prospective investigation of borderline personality disorder in abused and neglected children followed up into adulthood. *Journal of Personality Disorders*, *23*, 433–446.

Widom, C. S., DuMont, K., & Czaja, S. J. (2007). A prospective investigation of major depressive disorder and comorbidity in abused and neglected children grown up. *Archives of General Psychiatry*, *64*, 49–56.

Widom, C. S., Ireland, T., & Glynn, P. J. (1995). Alcohol abuse in abused and neglected children followed-up: Are they at increased risk? *Journal of Studies on Alcohol*, *56*, 207–217.

Widom, C. S., Marmorstein, N. R., & White, H. R. (2006). Childhood victimization and illicit drug use in middle adulthood. *Psychology of Addictive Behaviors*, *20*, 394–403.

Williams, J. H., Van Dorn, R. A., Bright, C. L., Jonson-Reid, M., & Nebbitt, V. E. (2010). Child maltreatment and delinquency onset among African American adolescent males. *Research on Social Work Practice*, *20*, 253–259.

Wilson, H., & Widom, C. S. (2008). An examination of risky sexual behavior and HIV among victims of child abuse and neglect: A thirty-year follow-up. *Health Psychology*, *27*, 149–158.

Wilson, H. W., & Widom, C. S. (2009). A prospective examination of the path from child abuse and neglect to illicit drug use in middle adulthood: The potential mediating role of four risk factors. *Journal of Youth and Adolescence*, *38*, 340–354.

Woon, F. L., & Hedges, D. W. (2008). Hippocampal and amygdala volumes in children and adults with childhood maltreatment-related posttraumatic stress disorder: A meta-analysis. *Hippocampus*, *18*, 729–736.

Xie, P., Kranzler, H. R., Poling, J., Stein, M. B., Anton, R. F., Farrer, L. A., . . . Gelernter, J. (2010). Interaction of FKBP5 with childhood adversity on risk for post-traumatic stress disorder. *Neuropsychopharmacology, 35*, 1684–1692.

Yates, T. M., Carlson, E. A., & Egeland, B. (2008). A prospective study of child maltreatment and self-injurious behavior in a community sample. *Development and Psychopathology, 20*, 651–671.

Yehuda, R., Halligan, S. L., & Grossman, R. (2001). Childhood trauma and risk for PTSD: Relationship to intergenerational effects of trauma, parental PTSD, and cortisol excretion. *Development and Psychopathology, 13*, 733–753.

Zhang, T. Y., & Meaney, M. J. (2010). Epigenetics and the environmental regulation of the genome and its function. *Annual Review of Psychology, 61*, 439–466.

Zimmermann, P., Brueckl, T., Nocon, A., Pfister, H., Binder, E. B., Uhr, M., . . . Ising, M. (2011). Interaction of FKBP5 gene variants and adverse life events in predicting depression onset: Results from a 10-year prospective community study. *American Journal of Psychiatry, 168*, 1107–1116.

# CHAPTER 6

# Impulsivity and Vulnerability to Psychopathology

EMILY NEUHAUS AND THEODORE P. BEAUCHAINE

TERMS SUCH AS IMPULSIVE, disinhibited, and hyperactive have long been used to describe individuals with deficient control over their behaviors. Although some degree of such traits is developmentally appropriate for young children, those who display extreme impulsivity or fail to acquire age-appropriate self-regulation as they mature are vulnerable to a host of maladaptive outcomes. According to developmental psychopathology models of externalizing behavior, extreme impulsivity expressed in the preschool years may represent the first stage in a trajectory that can progress via potentiating and mediating variables to early onset delinquency and other antisocial behaviors (Beauchaine, Hinshaw, & Pang, 2010; Beauchaine, Gatzke-Kopp, & Mead, 2007; Campbell, Shaw, & Gilliom, 2000; Hinshaw, Lahey, & Hart, 1993; Patterson, DeGarmo, & Knutson, 2000). Indeed, trait impulsivity likely underlies a range of disorders falling along the externalizing spectrum, including attention-deficit/hyperactivity disorder (ADHD), conduct disorder (CD), antisocial personality disorder (ASPD), and substance use disorders (see Barkley, 1997; Beauchaine, Klein, Crowell, Derbidge, & Gatzke-Kopp, 2009; Krueger et al., 2002). In other cases, temperamental disinhibition marks the beginning stages of a developmental trajectory that culminates in self-harm, depression, and other forms of internalizing psychopathology (Beauchaine et al., 2009; Hirshfeld-Becker et al., 2002). Thus, impulsivity observed very early in life may indicate considerable risk for a wide range of adverse, multifinal outcomes.

## HISTORICAL CONTEXT

As with nearly all psychological phenomena, ideas about the nature and etiology of disinhibition have evolved considerably over the 19th and 20th centuries. Early neurobiological theories of behavioral control focused on frontal regions of the brain. These theories derived largely from observations of altered behavior among those who suffered from traumatic brain injuries, such as Phineas Gage. In 1848, Gage, a railroad foreman, suffered a severe brain injury when a blasting charge propelled an iron rod through his eye socket and out the frontal part of his skull. Despite full recovery of motor and sensory functions, Gage's personality transformed radically as a result of his injury (Macmillan, 1992). Whereas Gage had been "quiet and respectful" prior to the accident, he became "gross, profane, coarse, and vulgar to such a degree that his society was intolerable to decent people" (Bigelow, 1850, cited in Macmillan, 1992, p. 86). He was further described as "impatient of restraint or advice when it conflicts with his desires, at times pertinaciously obstinate, yet capricious and vacillating, devising many plans of future operation, which are no sooner arranged than they are abandoned in turn for others appearing more feasible" (Harlow, 1868, cited in Macmillan, 2004). Thus, the most striking result of Gage's injuries was marked behavioral disinhibition that contrasted starkly with his socially appropriate demeanor prior to the injury.

Consistent with theories of the time, explanations of Gage's behavior relied on two assumptions. First, particular brain regions located in the frontal lobe were assumed to support specific behavioral traits. When these regions were damaged, those traits were no longer supported. In Gage's case, the shift in behavior was attributed to the rod having injured the "regions of the organs of BENEVOLENCE and VENERATION" (Harlow, 1868, cited in Macmillan, 1992). Second, it was assumed that competing factors were at work within the mind, with behavior resulting from the equilibrium established between them. When this equilibrium was disrupted by damage to parts of the brain, the changing balance affected behavior. In the absence of the inhibiting influence of the damaged areas, the balance between Gage's "intellectual faculties and his animal propensities" was destroyed (Harlow, 1868, cited in Macmillan, 2004), resulting in disinhibited behavior. As later sections of this chapter reveal, this theme—that behavior derives from a relative equilibrium between self-gratifying and cautious motivations—has influenced most major theories of impulsivity and continues to do so today.

Twentieth-century conceptualizations of impulsivity and disinhibition continued to look toward imbalances in competing neurobiological systems. Eppinger and Hess (1915) argued that vagotonia, an imbalance within the autonomic nervous system favoring the parasympathetic over the sympathetic division, accounted for a number of medical and psychological phenomena. They described vagotonia as an "abnormal irritability of all or only a few autonomic nerves" (p. 39), including the 10th cranial (vagus) nerve, and portrayed it as a chronic disposition as opposed to an acute disorder. Occurring more frequently in young individuals, vagotonia was hypothesized to cause neurasthenia, hysteria, and nervousness. Eppinger and Hess described patients with vagotonia as "hasty and precipitous" (p. 40), foreshadowing the links that would later be made between the condition and hyperactivity. Although the vagotonia hypothesis has since been refuted (see Beauchaine, 2001), by the mid-20th century, it was a candidate cause of restlessness and hyperactivity in children, and was considered a possible predictor of later antisocial behavior (e.g., Venables, 1988). More recent sources indicate compromised sympathetic *and* parasympathetic functioning in impulsive children and adolescents (Beauchaine &

Gatzke-Kopp, 2012; Beauchaine, Katkin, Strassberg, & Snarr, 2001; Beauchaine et al., 2007; Crowell et al., 2006).

At about the same time the vagotonia hypothesis emerged, the encephalitis epidemics of 1918 yielded a group of children who displayed marked impulsivity, hyperactivity, inattention, aggression, and impairments in judgment (Carlson & Rapport, 1989; Schachar, 1986). Neurologists of the time attributed these behaviors (even in the absence of encephalitic infection) to some kind of underlying neurological disturbance, and the term minimal brain dysfunction (MBD) came to describe such children, as well as those with learning disabilities and other problems (Hässler, 1992). Theories varied with respect to which region(s) of the brain were injured, but it was assumed that impulsivity and hyperactivity resulted from brain damage of some sort, even among children with no documented history of head trauma or illness (Lyon, Fletcher, & Barnes, 2003). Although the problem behaviors included under MBD shifted over the next few decades, variations of the term and concept remained popular until recently (Hässler, 1992). It was not until the *DSM-III* emerged in 1980 that the category of MBD was dropped, and children with learning difficulties were distinguished officially from those with behavioral difficulties (Lyon et al., 2003).

## TERMINOLOGICAL AND CONCEPTUAL ISSUES

Despite the centrality of trait impulsivity to current theories of ADHD, conduct disorder (CD), antisocial behavior, and substance use disorders, the construct lacks both a consistent operational definition and a standard method of measurement. Although impulsivity has been defined traditionally by behavioral symptoms, some researchers have attempted to refine these definitions based on results from neuropsychological tests. For example, reaction time during verbal tasks has been used to assess the degree of "short-circuiting of analytic or reflective thought processes" (Oas, 1985, p. 141). Alternatively, errors in maze solving have been suggested to reflect impulsivity, as they may represent poor attention to detail as well as carelessness and lack of planning (Porteus, 1965). Perseverative errors during set-shifting tasks such as the Wisconsin Card Sorting Test have also been attributed to impulsivity (e.g., Avila, Cuenca, Félix, Parcet, & Miranda, 2004), as have errors due to overly quick responding and lack of reflection during match-to-sample tasks such as the Matching Familiar Figures Test (Oas, 1984). Among the most popular measures of impulsivity in neuropsychology are drawing tasks such as the Bender Gestalt (Bender, 1938) and the Draw-A-Person test (Koppitz, 1968). In such tests, impulsivity is assessed by scoring drawings on the basis of variables such as completion time, overall quality, omissions, asymmetry, detailing, and shading (Oas, 1984). Continuous performance tests (e.g., Conners & MHS Staff, 2000; Gordon, 1988) are also purported to assess impulsivity by indexing errors of commission—when participants fail to inhibit inappropriate responses.

Although measures such as these provide various means of operationalizing impulsivity, they do not speak to the neural mechanisms underlying the construct, nor do they fully explain relations between impulsivity and psychopathology (see

Gatzke-Kopp, 2011). Many of these formulations describe impulsivity in highly cognitive terms, likening it to executive functions such as inhibitory control (the ability to interrupt an ongoing action or prevent a prepotent reaction; Kenemans et al., 2005) or effortful control (the ability to control attentional processes and behavior to inhibit a dominant response in favor of a nondominant response; Rothbart & Bates, 1998), two closely related constructs. Although it remains to be determined how cognitive constructs such as these relate to behavioral or trait disinhibition, they are likely to show some overlap, as different measures of inhibitory and effortful control correlate with various facets of impulsivity and problem behavior (e.g., Enticott, Ogloff, & Bradshaw, 2006; Murray & Kochanska, 2002).

More recent cognitive models of disinhibition integrate multiple components of the trait, suggesting several alternative brain mechanisms that may be responsible for impulsive behavior, exemplifying equifinality (see Chapter 1). Nigg (2000, 2005; Chapter 12), for example, has suggested that disinhibition results from dysfunction in at least one of two inhibitory systems. He distinguishes between motivational inhibition, which results from behavioral suppression in the context of anxiety-provoking cues, and executive inhibition, or the deliberate process of stopping or suppressing a response that is prepotent but task-inappropriate. Barkley (1997) has also characterized disinhibition as faulty inhibition, positing a hierarchical inhibitory structure in which behavioral inhibition consists of three subprocesses (inhibition of prepotent responses, halting of ongoing responses, and control of interfering stimuli), each supporting a number of executive functions that allow for effective goal-directed behavior.

Behaviorally, impulsivity has been described as actions that are "socially inappropriate or maladaptive and quickly emitted without forethought" (Oas, 1984, 1985). This behavioral rather than neuropsychological definition has a number of strengths. Although it is distinct from the more heavily cognitive formulations of disinhibition, it does not rule out cognitively mediated mechanisms. Furthermore, it emphasizes disinhibition as a maladaptive trait, distinguishing it from other qualities such as spontaneity that are frequently viewed more positively. Finally, it does not include causal assumptions regarding the etiology of disinhibition, allowing for both psychological and biological contributions.

At present, the most widely used definition of impulsivity/disinhibition is likely that described in the *DSM-IV* (2000). As a component of attention-deficit/hyperactivity disorder (ADHD), impulsivity is demonstrated by "impatience, difficulty in delaying responses, blurting out answers before questions have been completed, difficulty awaiting one's turn, and frequently interrupting or intruding on others" (p. 86). Similarly, Sagvolden, Johansen, Aase, and Russell (2005) describe impulsivity as taking action without forethought and failing to plan ahead, linking it to such related concepts as risk taking, novelty-seeking, sensation-seeking, over-rapid responding, and susceptibility to the pull of immediate rewards (see also Hirshfeld-Becker et al., 2002). These behaviors are considered pathological when they are performed to the point that they interfere with social, academic, and/or occupational functioning, consistent with Oas's (1985) theme of disinhibition as maladaptive and socially inappropriate.

## ETIOLOGICAL FORMULATIONS

As should be apparent from this discussion, behavioral (phenotypic) expression of impulsivity may derive from one or more of several sources (see also Sonuga-Barke, 2005). Well-characterized influences on impulsive behavior include brain injuries, which may result from head trauma, hypoxia, or other central nervous system insults (Chapter 10); exposure to teratogens such as alcohol, stimulant drugs of abuse, and/or lead (Chapter 9); early traumatic experiences including social deprivation, child abuse, and neglect (Lucas et al., 2004; Poeggel et al., 1999; Chapter 5); or genetic vulnerabilities that give rise to deficient executive control over behavior (Chapter 12). Although this list is certainly not exhaustive, it illustrates the heterogeneous nature of broad behavioral traits such as impulsivity (see Beauchaine et al., 2010; Beauchaine & Marsh, 2006).

### HETEROGENEITY IN THE IMPULSIVITY PHENOTYPE

Rather than describing each of these mechanisms in detail, we begin by focusing on particular neurobiological substrates of disinhibition that (a) give rise to individual differences in impulsivity that are temperamental, present very early in life, and emerge before ADHD can be diagnosed; (b) are supported by voluminous literatures derived from both animal models and humans; and (c) confer vulnerability to externalizing disorders across the lifespan, particularly in the context of high risk environments characterized by violence, trauma, and emotional lability. This focus on temperamental impulsivity is consistent with our main objective in writing this chapter: to describe early-onset impulsivity as a *vulnerability* for later psychopathology. Readers should note, however, that it may be difficult in clinical practice to distinguish between children who are impulsive due to an inherited temperamental trait versus children who are impulsive due to other etiological influences such as prenatal stimulant exposure (see, e.g., Beauchaine, Neuhaus, Zalewski, Crowell, & Potapova, 2011).

Most modern accounts of temperamental disinhibition emphasize structural and functional abnormalities in phylogenetically old brain regions including the mesolimbic dopamine system and the basal ganglia, overlapping neural networks that mature very early in life and are likely to subserve individual differences in impulsivity among young children (see Beauchaine et al., 2001, 2010, 2012; Gatzke-Kopp, 2011; Gatzke-Kopp & Beauchaine, 2007; Sagvolden et al., 2005). Accordingly, heritable compromises in the functioning of these brain regions and associated risk for psychopathology provide the foundations of this chapter. In contrast, frontal theories of disinhibition are not considered "foundational," because these brain regions mature late in adolescence (or beyond) and are therefore less likely to underlie the early expression of trait impulsivity (Halperin & Schulz, 2006). Nevertheless, the neurodevelopment of frontal regions may be affected—through mechanisms of neural plasticity, programming, and pruning—by early experiences that are themselves a product of impulsivity (Beauchaine, Neuhaus, Brenner, & Gatze-Kopp, 2008; Sagvolden et al., 2005; see also Shannon, Sauder, Beauchaine,

& Gatzke-Kopp, 2009). In other words, heritable compromises in the functioning of early maturing brain regions that give rise to impulsivity are likely to alter the neurodevelopment of later maturing brain regions that are responsible for executive functioning and planning—especially in high-risk environments. This model highlights the transactional nature of the brain in affecting behavior, and of behavior in affecting subsequent brain development. Recognition and description of such transactions between the individual and the environment are tenets of the developmental psychopathology perspective (see Beauchaine & Gatzke-Kopp, 2012; Cicchetti, 2006; Rutter & Sroufe, 2000; Sroufe & Rutter, 1984; Chapter 1). In later sections, we therefore describe neurodevelopmental mechanisms through which early impulsivity may potentiate vulnerability for deficient executive functioning later in life.

## Temperamental Impulsivity and Central Dopamine Functioning

Theories advanced to explain individual differences in impulsivity have long focused on the mesolimbic dopamine (DA) system, including the ventral tegmental area and its projections to the nucleus accumbens (Swartz, 1999), and on other dopaminergic networks within the central nervous system (Beauchaine & Gatzke-Kopp, 2012; Castellanos, 1999; Gatzke-Kopp, 2011; Gatzke-Kopp & Beauchaine, 2007, Kalivas & Nakamura, 1999; Sagvolden et al., 2005). Many of these theories follow from seminal research on reinforcement motivation and substance dependence conducted with rodents and nonhuman primates. This research demonstrates that (a) electrical and pharmacological stimulation of dopaminergically mediated mesolimbic structures is reinforcing, such that trained animals will engage in prolonged periods of operant behaviors (e.g., lever pressing) to obtain these incentives (see Milner, 1991); (b) neural activity increases within mesolimbic structures during both reward anticipation and reward-seeking behaviors, and following administration of DA agonists (see Knutson, Fong, Adams, Varner, & Hommer, 2001; Phillips, Blaha, & Fibiger, 1989; Schott et al., 2008); and (c) DA antagonists attenuate—and in extreme cases block—the rewarding properties of food, water, and stimulant drugs of abuse (e.g., Rolls et al., 1974).

Based on this set of observations, several authors have offered theories of impulsivity and personality that explain individual differences in approach behavior as variations in activity of mesolimbic structures. The most prominent of these theories is that offered by Gray (1987a, 1987b), in which he proposed a mesolimbic behavioral approach system (BAS) as the neural substrate of appetitive motivation. Soon afterward, clinical scientists interested in impulsivity co-opted dopaminergic theories of approach motivation to explain the unbridled reward-seeking behaviors observed in ADHD, CD, and related externalizing disorders (e.g., Fowles, 1988; Quay, 1993; Rogeness, Javors, & Pliszka, 1992).

Although these early theories correctly identified mesolimbic neural structures implicated in the expression of impulsivity, most researchers at the time subscribed to the face-valid assumption that excessive dopaminergic activity led to impulsive behavior. In other words, they assumed a positive correspondence between neural responding and behavior. This assumption is evident in the formulation of measures such as the BIS/BAS scales (Carver & White, 1994), which presuppose a direct relation between impulsive behaviors and BAS activity (see Brenner, Beauchaine, & Sylvers, 2005). However, several clear and consistent findings present intractable problems for theories linking excessive mesolimbic DA activity to impulsivity.

First, several studies indicate reduced sympathetic nervous system (SNS)-linked cardiac reactivity to reward among impulsive preschoolers, middle-schoolers, and adolescents (Beauchaine et al., 2001, 2007; Crowell et al., 2006). These findings are significant because (a) SNS-linked cardiac reactivity to incentives serves as a peripheral index of central DA responding (Brenner et al., 2005; Brenner & Beauchaine, 2011) and (b) infusions of DA into mesolimbic structures produce SNS-mediated increases in cardiac output (van den Buuse, 1998). Thus, reduced cardiac reactivity to reward among impulsive children is likely to mark attenuated DA responding—directly opposite to expectations based on the excessive DA theory.

Second, studies using both single photon emission computed tomography (SPECT) and positron emission tomography (PET) demonstrate that the primary mechanism of action of methylphenidate and related DA agonists is increased neural activity in the striatum, a structure located within the mesolimbic reward pathway (e.g., Vles et al., 2003; Volkow, Fowler, Wang, Ding, & Gatley, 2002). Thus, pharmacological interventions that *increase* mesolimbic DA activity by inhibiting reuptake *decrease* hyperactivity, impulsivity, and related aggressive behaviors (e.g., Hinshaw, Henker, Whalen, Erhardt, & Dunnington, 1989; MTA Cooperative Group, 1999). Theories of excessive DA as a mechanism of impulsivity predict the opposite effect (i.e., increasing striatal DA activity should exacerbate impulsivity).

Finally, infusions of DA into mesolimbic structures are experienced as pleasurable, and individual differences in central DA expression predict trait positive affectivity (see Ashby, Isen, & Turken, 1999; Berridge, 2003; Forbes & Dahl, 2005). In contrast, PET studies indicate that low levels of striatal DA activity are associated with trait irritability (Laakso et al., 2003). When interpreted in the context of positive relations between externalizing behaviors and both negative affectivity and irritability (e.g., Martel & Nigg, 2006; Mick, Spencer, Wozniak, & Biederman, 2005), these findings suggest diminished rather than excessive DA functioning among at least some impulsive individuals.

These converging sources of evidence for reduced DA functioning as a neural substrate of impulsivity have led to a reformulation of first-generation models. We and others have suggested that underactivation of striatal DA leads to increased behavioral responding, which functions to raise activation levels within the mesolimbic system (Beauchaine et al., 2007; Beauchaine et al., 2012; Gatzke-Kopp, 2011; Gatzke-Kopp & Beauchaine, 2007; Sagvolden et al., 2005; Volkow et al., 2009). Thus, what has been assumed to be reward hypersensitivity is more likely to be reward *insensitivity*, which results in increased impulsive and perseverative responding to up-regulate a chronically aversive mood state—the affective consequence of an underactive mesolimbic DA system (Ashby et al., 1999; Forbes & Dahl, 2005; Laakso et al., 2003). In addition to the literature cited above, this interpretation is supported by research indicating (a) associations between low basal DA activity/blunted DA reactivity and a propensity to use DA agonist drugs of abuse (De Witte, Pinto, Ansseau, & Verbanck, 2003; Laine, Ahonen, Räsänen, & Tiihonen, 2001; Martin-Soelch et al., 2001; Martinez et al., 2007); (b) significant correlations between blunted DA responses to amphetamine administration and the personality trait of novelty seeking (Leyton et al., 2002); and (c) recent neuroimaging studies indicating reduced striatal activity during reward tasks among children and adolescents with ADHD and CD (Carmona et al., 2011; Durston et al., 2003; Vaidya et al., 1998). Thus, accumulating evidence now supports the hypothesis that trait impulsivity results at least in part from abnormally low central DA activity.

## GENETICS AND HERITABILITY

There are two general approaches to studying the genetic bases and heritability of any behavioral trait—behavioral genetics and molecular genetics (see Chapter 3)—each of which contributes differently but significantly to our understanding of impulsivity.

### BEHAVIORAL GENETICS OF IMPULSIVITY

Behavioral genetics studies are used to parse variability in a behavioral trait into heritable (both genetic and nongenetic) and nonheritable (environmental) components. Overwhelming evidence indicates that impulsivity is among the most highly heritable of all behavioral traits. Behavior genetics studies comparing concordance rates of impulsivity and ADHD for monozygotic and dizygotic twins produce heritability estimates ($h^2$) approaching and exceeding .8, indicating that as much as 80% of the variance in impulsive behavior is accounted for by heritable factors (e.g., Levy, Hay, McStephen, Wood, & Waldman, 1997; Price, Simonoff, Waldman, Asherson, & Plomin, 2001; Sherman, Iacono, & McGue, 1997; Willcutt, in press; Wood, Rijsdijk, Saudino, Asherson, & Kuntsi, 2008). Furthermore, Krueger et al. (2002) identified a common vulnerability for a wide range of externalizing symptoms including disinhibition, conduct problems, antisocial personality, alcohol dependence, and drug dependence among a sample of 1,048 participants in the Minnesota Twin Family Study. This latent vulnerability for externalizing disorders, which likely reflects trait impulsivity (Beauchaine & Marsh, 2006), was 81% heritable. Similar findings have since been reported in child samples (Tuvblad, Zheng, Raine, & Baker, 2009). However, each specific category of externalizing behavior was influenced strongly by environmental effects. This finding is important because it demonstrates that a common genetic vulnerability can result in divergent multifinal outcomes depending on environmental experience (Beauchaine et al., 2010; 2012), a point to which we return later.

### MOLECULAR GENETICS OF IMPULSIVITY

Molecular genetics approaches, including both linkage and association studies, are designed to identify specific genes that contribute to the expression of a trait or disorder (see Chapter 3). Linkage studies search for chromosomal regions that are shared more often than expected among large numbers of families with two or more affected children (Faraone & Mick, 2010). Using this approach, the gene responsible for cystic fibrosis was found by 'linking' the disease to a DNA variant on the long arm of Chromosome 7 within affected families. This discovery was followed by a number of additional linkage studies that specified the location on Chromosome 7 in greater detail (see Bolsover, Hyams, Jones, Shepard, & White, 1997). Because linkage analyses scan broad sections of the genome, the approach works best when very few genes with large effects contribute to a behavioral trait or disease—a rare precondition for psychiatric disorders, which are usually determined polygenically. Nonetheless, a recent genome scan meta-analysis combining 7 datasets supported a significant linkage for ADHD on Chromosome 16, with possible linkages within a number of other regions (Zhou et al., 2008). However, no specific gene has yet been identified through linkage analysis, and failures to replicate plague psychiatric genetics research (see Chapter 3).

In contrast to linkage studies, genetic association studies begin with a candidate gene that is thought to play an etiological role in the expression of a disorder (see Chapter 3). Using this approach, allelic frequencies of specific genetic polymorphisms are compared among those with and without the condition under study. Association studies can be used to detect genes that account for much smaller amounts of variance in behavior. Given well-articulated theories specifying altered DA functioning as a pathophysiological determinant of impulsivity (see above), association studies are well suited for use with this behavioral trait (Galili-Weisstub & Segman, 2003).

Not surprisingly, association studies far outnumber linkage studies of impulsivity and ADHD. Although the consistency of results and effect sizes from these studies have been mixed, meta-analyses suggest a small but significant role for the DRD4 gene (Chromosome 11p15.5), which codes for DA receptors located throughout the central and peripheral nervous systems (Benjamin et al., 1996; Faraone & Mick, 2010; Li, Sham, Owen, & He, 2006). The DAT1, or dopamine transporter gene (Chromosome 5p15.3), regulates synaptic levels of DA, the principal target of psychostimulants used to treat ADHD (Grace, 2002). Although allelic status appears to correlate with volume and activation within mesolimbic structures (Durston, 2010), the precise role of DAT1 in the pathophysiology of ADHD is unclear. Early findings varied considerably across studies and samples (Castellanos & Tannock, 2002; Yang, Chan, Jing, Li, Sham, & Chen, 2007). However, recent data suggest that DAT1 may be more influential in combination with specific environment risk factors such as prenatal substance exposure (Faraone & Mick, 2010; Laucht et al., 2007; Neuman et al., 2007). Other DA genes have been studied as well, but evidence for their roles in the pathophysiology of impulsivity is less consistent (see also Chapter 12).

In addition to genes that are involved directly in DA expression, association studies have also been conducted to evaluate the effects of genes that are involved in the synthesis and metabolism of DA, as these processes also influence synaptic activity and reuptake. Candidate genes include those that encode for dopamine-$\beta$-hydroxylase (DBH), which converts DA to norepinephrine; and both monoamine oxydase (MAO) and catechol-o-methyl transferase (COMT), enzymes involved in DA (and other monoamine neurotransmitter) degradation. Association studies involving these genes have been few and conflicting. With regard to DBH, allelic status has been linked with ADHD within some child and adult samples (Hess et al., 2009), but meta-analyses cast doubt on the reliability and strength of these links (Gizer, Ficks, & Waldman, 2009). Current evidence suggests that polymorphisms in both the MAOA gene (Xp11.23–11.4) and the COMT gene are associated with antisocial behavior among impulsive individuals, particularly in the context of environmental adversity (Caspi et al., 2002; Qian et al., 2009; Thapar et al., 2005). However, direct associations between these genes and ADHD are less consistent in direction and effect size (see Faraone & Mick, 2010), and MAO may have differential effects on impulsivity according to sex (indeed, it is X-linked; see Biederman et al., 2008). Taken together, this set of genes (DBH, MAO, and COMT) may have little effect on the core trait of impulsivity but larger effects on externalizing sequelae, reflecting the effects of Gene × Environment interactions on the development of externalizing behavior (see Beauchaine et al., 2009).

To summarize, behavioral genetics studies of trait impulsivity indicate impressively high heritability estimates and suggest that disinhibition contributes to a number of externalizing behavior patterns. Yet despite this high heritability, candidate genes identified to date account for little variance in impulsive behavior. This state of affairs suggests that considerable work remains in the attempt to understand the genetic bases of impulsivity, which extends to research on most behavioral traits (see Chapter 3).

## IMPULSIVITY AND VULNERABILITY TO PSYCHOPATHOLOGY

In developmental psychopathology, a distinction is often made between vulnerabilities and risk factors for psychiatric disorders (e.g., Luthar, 2006; Shannon, Beauchaine, Brenner, Neuhaus, & Gatzke-Kopp, 2007). Vulnerabilities are usually assumed to be biologically based traits that render individuals susceptible to psychopathology, whereas risk factors are environmental influences that interact with vulnerabilities to potentiate psychopathology. For example, it is now known that distressing experiences (risk factors) elicit post-traumatic stress disorder mainly in genetically predisposed (vulnerable) individuals (e.g., Orr et al. 2003; Stein, Jang, Taylor, Vernon, & Livesley, 2002). Although the distinction between vulnerabilities and risk factors breaks down when we consider the interactive roles that genetically determined traits play in eliciting specific environments (evocative effects) and that environments play in the expression of genes (see Moffitt, 2005; Shannon et al., 2007), we maintain traditional use of the terms in upcoming sections, where we outline factors that amplify the likelihood of psychopathology among impulsive and therefore vulnerable individuals.

Before proceeding, however, it should be noted that temperamental impulsivity is usually not enough (except in perhaps the most extreme cases) to result in psychopathology in the absence of additional vulnerabilities and/or risk factors. Research with impulsive preschoolers indicates that at least half progress into later childhood without developing significant behavior problems (see Beauchaine et al., 2010; Campbell et al., 2000). In the sections to follow we summarize several additional vulnerabilities and risk factors that interact with temperamental disinhibition to increase the probability of later psychopathology.

## BEHAVIORAL INHIBITION

In addition to impulsivity, a second well characterized temperamental trait is behavioral *inhibition*. This term refers to a general tendency to be wary in novel situations, to be "slow to warm up," and to avoid overly stimulating environments. Kagan, Reznick, and Snidman (1988) identified a group of 3-year-olds who displayed high degrees of behavioral inhibition in unfamiliar laboratory settings. These children avoided approaching and interacting with unfamiliar children and adults, remained in close proximity to their mothers, and ceased vocalizing in the presence of strangers. When they were reassessed at age 7, they remained quiet, cautious, and socially avoidant. Thus, like trait impulsivity, behavioral inhibition can be detected very early in life and is stable (although not invariant) across development. It is also mediated largely by genetic factors (see Chapter 7).

It has often been assumed that trait inhibition and impulsivity mark extremes along a continuum of behavioral control, yet the neural substrates of the two traits are almost completely non-overlapping. In contrast to impulsivity, behavioral inhibition, which renders individuals vulnerable to anxiety disorders, is mediated by the septo-hippocampal system, a primarily serotonergic network (see Gray & McNaughton, 2000). Moreover, the two systems evolved to subserve distinct functions: approach behaviors promote survival by ensuring engagement in activities such as eating, drinking, and copulating; whereas avoidance behaviors promote survival by reducing exposure to danger. In fact, Gray and others (Gray & McNaughton, 2000; McNaughton & Corr, 2004) have argued convincingly that the functional role of the septo-hippocampal system is to *suppress* approach behaviors under conditions of threat.

This conceptualization, in which approach tendencies are actively suppressed by avoidance tendencies, is supported by a large literature on experiments with animals and has direct implications for psychopathology (see Beauchaine, 2001; Beauchaine et al., 2011). Given that the approach and avoidance systems operate with substantial independence, one can be high or low on either or both dimensions. A person who is temperamentally impulsive due to a heritable DA deficiency may be protected from severe psychopathology *if* he or she is also high on behavioral inhibition. Although this might seem implausible at first glance, symptoms of anxiety are surprisingly common among impulsive children with ADHD (Angold, Costello, & Erkanli, 1999; MTA Cooperative Group, 1999), and in the absence of additional comorbidities, such children are more responsive to behavioral interventions than their non-anxious counterparts (Jensen et al., 2001). Furthermore, older externalizing youth with comorbid anxiety are less physically aggressive, regarded less negatively by peers, and experience fewer police contacts than those without anxiety symptoms (Walker et al., 1991). Such findings are precisely what would be expected from a more responsive septo-hippocampal system. Consistent with this interpretation, in a recent structural neuroimaging study, interactions between trait anxiety and trait impulsivity predicted individual differences in gray matter volumes in both septo-hippocampal and mesolimbic brain regions among children with ADHD (Sauder, Beauchaine, Gatzke-Kopp, Shannon, & Aylward, 2012). Those with ADHD who experienced comorbid anxiety showed normal gray matter volumes in these brain regions compared with controls, whereas those who experienced low levels of anxiety exhibited reduced gray matter volumes.

As this discussion implies, an impulsive person who is low on trait anxiety may be especially vulnerable to developing more serious externalizing disorders. Psychopathy, a behavior pattern characterized by manipulation of others, superficial charm, callousness, and lack of remorse, is probably the most intractable form of externalizing conduct (see Lykken, 2006). As several authors have noted, individuals high in psychopathy exhibit excessive approach behaviors that are *coupled with* a disturbing lack of anxiety and fear (see Fowles & Dindo, 2006). Thus, their impulsive tendencies are not inhibited by impending consequences, presumably because they are very low on behavioral inhibition. As a result, the condition is largely unresponsive to treatment.

Given that temperamental impulsivity and inhibition are both largely heritable, individuals with psychopathy appear to be "doubly vulnerable" to psychopathology. This situation might best be considered a Trait × Trait interaction, with two largely independent heritable attributes contributing to behavioral functioning (see also Derryberry, Reed, & Pilkenton-Taylor, 2003). Although such models are rare in psychopathology research, recent advances in molecular genetics make it much easier to study interactions among underlying genes that potentiate psychiatric morbidity (see, e.g., Beauchaine et al., 2009).

## ENVIRONMENTAL RISK

There is also considerable evidence that environmental risk can lead to more severe psychopathology among impulsive children, including those with ADHD. These youth are more likely than their non-ADHD peers to develop oppositional defiant disorder (ODD), conduct disorder (CD), and antisocial personality disorder (Barkley, 2003). Longitudinal studies suggest that for many children, hyperactivity/impulsivity constitutes the first stage in a trajectory that progresses via mediating risk factors to antisocial behaviors, eventually culminating in early-onset delinquency (see Beauchaine et al., 2010). We outline some of these risk factors below.

*Parenting.* One of the most thoroughly studied environmental correlates of externalizing behavior is parenting. Numerous studies have demonstrated that the parents of impulsive and aggressive children are more negative, lax, verbose, and over-reactive in their discipline practices than the parents of control children (Arnold, O'Leary, Wolff, & Acker, 1993; Barkley, Karlsson, & Pollard, 1985). In a longitudinal study of impulsive boys, Patterson et al. (2000) demonstrated that the relation between hyperactivity and antisocial behavior was mediated fully by coercive parental discipline. Thus, hyperactivity led to more serious externalizing behaviors only when parents consistently nagged their children and were explosive in their discipline practices. Similarly, Biederman et al. (1996) demonstrated that hyperactive children who developed conduct disorder were more likely to be reared by antisocial parents than hyperactive children who did not develop conduct disorder. Exposure to parental psychopathology more broadly has a similar effect on emerging externalizing symptoms among children with ADHD (Biederman et al., 1995).

Consistent with these findings, coercive family interaction patterns in which both children and their parents escalate aversive behaviors and negative affect in order to assert their respective wills promote physical aggression, conduct problems, and delinquency (Snyder, Edwards, McGraw, Kilgore, & Holton, 1994; Snyder, Schrepferman, & St. Peter, 1997). Developmental models suggest that these repeated episodes of affective and behavioral escalation, which are enacted thousands of times in the families of at risk children, promote emotion dysregulation and emotional lability, which in turn increase risk for more severe conduct problems (Beauchaine et al., 2007; Crowell, Beauchaine, & Linehan, 2009; Chapter 18). Moreover, interventions that successfully reduce such parenting behaviors also reduce delinquency (e.g., Hartman, Stage, & Webster-Stratton, 2003; Martinez & Forgatch, 2001; Piquero, Farrington, Welsh, Tremblay, & Jennings, 2009). This coercive model has recently been extended to the development of self-inflicted injury, particularly among female adolescents (Beauchaine et al., 2009), which highlights the potential moderating role of sex in the developmental trajectory of impulsivity. Although this body of findings has been interpreted by some as evidence of direct environmental effects, it is possible that heritable genetic vulnerabilities are driving the coercive behaviors observed by both parties (an example of a gene-environment correlation; see Chapter 3). Such genetic versus environmental hypotheses cannot be disambiguated without true experiments in which impulsive children are assigned randomly to coercive and noncoercive caretakers—an ethically indefensible practice. Nevertheless, in a randomized clinical trial, Hinshaw et al. (2000) found that reductions in negative/ineffective discipline in parents of youth with ADHD mediated school-based reductions in disruptive behavior and improvements in social skills, with effects most pronounced for families receiving the multimodal combination of medication and intensive behavior therapy. Similarly, a recent randomized clinical trial demonstrated improved parenting and reduced externalizing behavior among preschool children with ADHD following an empirically supported parent intervention (Webster-Stratton, Reid, & Beauchaine, 2011, 2012).

*Child abuse and neglect.* Although associated with parenting practices (Azar, 2002), a second risk factor that we consider separately is child abuse and neglect. Those who study child maltreatment have traditionally considered social mechanisms of risk and intergenerational transmission (see Cicchetti & Valentino, 2006). We have therefore included child abuse and neglect under environmental risk factors. However, evidence also suggests that genetic and temperamental factors play roles in determining who engages in child abuse and neglect, and in influencing the likelihood that a person who experiences abuse will become a future offender (Farrington, Jolliffe, Loeber, Stouthamer-Loeber, & Kalb, 2001; Chapter 5). Although the direction of effects is unclear, maltreated children are more impulsive than nonmaltreated children (Famularo, Kinscherff, & Fenton, 1992), and histories of abuse are associated with higher levels of externalizing symptoms among children with ADHD (Briscoe-Smith & Hinshaw, 2006). Furthermore, behavior genetics studies indicate that physical abuse often plays a direct role in the development of antisocial behavior among children at risk (Trouton, Spinath, & Plomin, 2002). Abuse is also more likely to lead to conduct disorder among children who are genetically vulnerable—as determined in part by impulsive characteristics of family members (Jaffee et al., 2004). Thus, impulsive children may be at higher risk for child abuse and neglect, which then amplifies risk for conduct problems and delinquency. As noted above, one possible mechanism for this effect is a Gene × Environment interaction involving a polymorphism of the MAOA gene, which is associated with high risk for antisocial behavior among males who were maltreated as children (Caspi et al., 2002). This variant in MAOA is likely to affect behavior in part through altered DA turnover.

*Neighborhood effects.* A third environmental risk factor that interacts with trait impulsivity is neighborhood context. Several studies indicate that impulsive children who are reared in high-risk neighborhoods (typically defined by such factors as low socioeconomic status, high rates of violence and criminality, and low community involvement) are more prone to engage in antisocial behavior than impulsive children reared in low-risk neighborhoods (Meier, Slutske, Arndt, & Cadoret, 2008; Trentacosta, Hyde, Shaw, & Cheong, 2009; Zalot, Jones, Kincaid, & Smith, 2009). For example, Lynam et al. (2000) found that impulsive boys, as assessed by a number of neuropsychological tests and self-report measures, were at higher risk than nonimpulsive boys for engaging in both status offenses and violent crimes, yet only when they lived in neighborhoods of low socioeconomic status and high delinquency. No such effects were observed in high SES neighborhoods (see Zimmerman, 2010, for a different pattern of findings). Taken together, these findings exemplify a Trait × Environment interaction, and illustrate the importance of environmental opportunities in the expression of temperamental risk.

## Epigenetic and Other Experience-Dependent Effects

*Epigenetic effects.* Epigenetic effects refer to alterations in gene expression that result from changes in DNA structure rather than changes in DNA sequence (Hartl & Jones, 2002; see Chapter 3). Such alterations are mediated by methylation processes that are triggered by environmental events. For example, Weaver et al. (2004) demonstrated epigenetically transmitted differences in the glucocorticoid receptor gene promoter in the hippocampi of rat pups that received high levels of maternal licking, grooming, and arched-back nursing compared with pups that experienced low levels of these maternal behaviors. This epigenetic effect transmits adaptive variations in stress responding to offspring. Rat pups reared in hazardous environments where maternal behaviors are compromised have more reactive hypothalamic-pituitary-adrenocortical (HPA) responses, and are consequently more fearful and wary. Thus, they are better prepared for the hazardous environment that they are likely to face.

Although evidence of epigenetic effects on psychopathology has only begun to emerge, mammals are particularly susceptible to such alterations in gene expression (Hartl & Jones, 2002), and increasingly divergent patterns of DNA methylation emerge over the lifetimes of monozygotic twin pairs (Fraga et al., 2005). Accordingly, several authors have emphasized the importance of epigenetic effects for child psychopathology research (e.g., Beauchaine et al., 2011; Kramer, 2005; Rutter, 2005), and theoretical models of antisocial behavior that include epigenetic effects have begun to appear (Tremblay, 2005).

Several recent empirical findings are relevant to our understanding of these effects with regard to impulsivity. The expression of brain-derived neurotrophic factor (BDNF), which is involved in the differentiation of DA neurons in developing mesolimbic structures and has been implicated in the pathogenesis of impulsivity, may be susceptible to paternally-mediated epigenetic effects (Kent et al., 2005). Similarly, animal studies suggest that prenatal exposure to synthetic glucocorticoids leads to overactivity and ADHD-like behaviors, suggesting such exposure may influence the "programming" of nascent DA systems (Kapoor, Petropoulos, & Matthews, 2008). Moreover, brain tissue from spontaneously hypertensive rats (a well-characterized animal model of ADHD) exposed to polychlorinated biphenyls (PCBs) evidenced differences in mRNA, suggesting an epigenetic effect of PCB on gene expression (DasBanerjee et al., 2008). In addition, although the precise mechanism remains to be described, the DRD4*7 allele, which has been linked with ADHD (see earlier), is less likely to be transmitted to offspring born in the autumn and winter months than to offspring born in the spring or summer (Seeger, Schloss, Schmidt, Rüter-Jungfleisch, & Henn, 2004). In the future, greater understanding of the processes and timing of epigenetic effects may help in formulating targeted interventions for vulnerable children.

*Neural plasticity.* In addition to epigenetic effects, several other mechanisms of neural programming are relevant for models linking early impulsivity to later psychopathology. Neural plasticity refers to experience-dependent functional changes in neural networks, including their efficiency, sensitivity, and time course of responding (Pollak, 2005). Such experience-dependent changes occur in several neural systems including mesolimbic DA structures (see Beauchaine et al., 2011). For example, Lucas et al. (2004) reported decreased DA transporter densities in mesolimbic brain regions of male rats that were exposed repeatedly to more dominant males in a stress-inducing paradigm. Similarly, repeated episodes of maternal separation early in the lives of rat pups produce long-term decreases in DA transporter expression (Meaney, Brake, & Gratton, 2002). Of particular significance, these effects result in greater sensitivity to the behavioral effects of cocaine and amphetamines later in life. Although similar experiments clearly cannot be conducted with humans, these findings illustrate the exquisite sensitivity of the mesolimbic DA system to early experience and suggest the possibility that experience-dependent changes in DA functioning may predispose affected individuals to stimulant use and/or abuse.

Perhaps more troubling, strong stimulants themselves induce experience-dependent changes in neural function that are similar to those observed following stress exposure. Through this mechanism, alterations in DA expression lead to sensitization and addiction to stimulants including nicotine, amphetamines, and cocaine (e.g., Saal, Dong, Bonci, & Malenka, 2003; Taylor & Jentsch, 2001; Thomas, Beurrier, Bonci, & Malenka, 2001). Chronic elevation of DA neural firing in the nucleus accumbens by strong stimulants has two other problematic effects. First, it down-regulates basal DA activity (Scafidi et al., 1996), which may exacerbate impulsive tendencies that emerge from mesolimbic hypo-responding (see above). Second, it suppresses the strength of connections from the mesolimbic system to the prefrontal cortex (Thomas et al., 2001), which may alter development of executive functioning and long-term planning. In normally developing adolescents, mesolimbic structures are recruited during reward-seeking behaviors in much the same way as observed in children. In contrast, adults depend more on frontal regions in responding to reward (Galvin et al., 2006). This shift reflects a developmental migration from dependence on "bottom-up" neural processing in phylogenetically old limbic structures to "top-down" neural processing in phylogenetically newer cortical structures. Once developed, these frontal (mesocortical) structures inhibit reward-related behaviors when it is advantageous to do so (Taylor & Jentsch, 2001). Environmental risks including stress and drug exposure may prevent this maturational process from unfolding, resulting in an underdeveloped mesocortical DA system that predisposes the individual to further stimulant use and abuse (Prasad, Hochstatter, & Sorg, 1999), and to the potential long-term sequelae of early impulsivity, including conduct problems, delinquency, and antisocial personality development.

It is important to note, however, that sensitization appears to be limited to early exposure to drugs of abuse, and does not extend to the therapeutic use of stimulant medications among children with ADHD. Although animal models prompted suggestions that the use of stimulants such as methylphenidate during childhood might increase the likelihood of substance abuse later in life (Schenk & Davidson, 1997), this has not been supported by analogous research, which has uncovered little evidence of increased risk of substance abuse following stimulant treatment of ADHD (e.g., Barkley, Fischer, Smallish, & Fletcher, 2003; Biederman, Wilens, Mick, Spencer, & Faraone, 1999; Volkow & Swanson, 2008). Instead, increased substance abuse among individuals with ADHD is accounted for by the presence of comorbid antisocial behaviors (Mannuzza et al., 2008), rather than a history of receiving stimulant medications.

## Implications for Learning

As many readers are probably aware, the same mesolimbic and mesocortical structures that have been discussed in this chapter are also recruited for associative learning processes (see Berridge & Robinson, 2003; Sagvolden et al., 2005). Thus, alterations in DA responding that arise from genetic, epigenetic, and experience-dependent effects are likely to influence the efficiency of knowledge acquisition. This might occur through at least three mechanisms: (1) sensation-seeking tendencies that reduce motivation for learning "mundane" information; (2) reduced efficacy of associative learning due to dampened activation of mesolimbic structures; and (3) compromised executive functioning. Although we do not have space to review the learning literature in further detail, these findings underscore the importance of early intervention for impulsive children who may be on an externalizing trajectory.

## SYNTHESIS AND FUTURE DIRECTIONS

In this chapter, we have described (a) heritable biological mechanisms of vulnerability that lead to impulsivity among affected children, (b) environmental risk factors that can potentiate vulnerability, leading to more serious externalizing behaviors that are especially difficult to treat, and (c) the potential importance of gene-environment correlations and Gene × Environment interactions in the expression and development of externalizing behaviors among impulsive and therefore vulnerable children. Although discussion of environmental, epigenetic, and experience-dependent risk factors for delinquency is sobering, it is worth repeating that only about half of impulsive preschool children develop more serious externalizing behaviors (Campbell et al., 2000). Furthermore, progress over the past decade in the specification of mechanisms through which impulsive behaviors escalate has been truly astounding.

Modern neuroscientific methods have provided insights into the development of externalizing behaviors that were unimaginable just a few years ago. When considered in conjunction with findings from more traditional approaches, it becomes apparent that some children face a cascade of cumulative vulnerability and risk that is increasingly difficult to reverse across development. In the worst cases, impulsive children are reared by impulsive parents who, in addition to conferring genetic liability, transmit risk through inconsistent and stressful caretaking during infancy, child maltreatment, and coercive, labile parenting (see Beauchaine et al., 2011). Further accumulation of risk may occur via exposure to violence in high-risk neighborhoods, early escalation of substance use, low motivation, and learning difficulties. By middle childhood and adolescence, exposure to stimulant drugs of abuse compromises the development of executive functions and self-regulation, compounding problem behaviors.

In contrast, an impulsive child who is reared in a maximally protective environment faces few or none of these additional risk factors, and may develop both psychological and biological resilience given enriched educational experiences and competent parenting that teaches strong emotion regulation skills (Beauchaine et al., 2007; Raine et al., 2001; see also Chapter 11). Parenting interventions have proven quite effective in reversing risk for conduct problems, especially when delivered early in childhood (Beauchaine, Webster-Stratton, & Reid, 2005; Nock, 2003; Piquero et al., 2009). Thus, there is reason to be optimistic. It is our hope that our knowledge of risk and resilience will continue to grow, and that science will influence public policy such that more children on externalizing trajectories receive preventive services.

# REFERENCES

American Psychiatric Association. (1980). *Diagnostic and statistical manual of mental disorders* (3rd ed.). Washington, DC: Author.

American Psychiatric Association. (2000). *Diagnostic and statistical manual of mental disorders* (4th ed., text revision). Washington, DC: Author.

Angold, A., Costello, E. J., & Erkanli, A. (1999). Comorbidity. *Journal of Child Psychology and Psychiatry, 40*, 57–87.

Arnold, D. S., O'Leary, S. G., Wolff, L. S., & Acker, M. M. (1993). The parenting scale: A measure of dysfunctional discipline practices. *Psychological Assessment, 5*, 137–144.

Ashby, F. G., Isen, A. M., & Turken, A. U. (1999). A neuropsychological theory of positive affect and its influence on cognition. *Psychological Review, 106*, 529–550.

Avila, C., Cuenca, I., Félix, V., Parcet, M. A., & Miranda, A. (2004). Measuring impulsivity in school-aged boys and examining its relationship with ADHD and ODD ratings. *Journal of Abnormal Child Psychology, 32*, 295–304.

Azar, S. (2002). Parenting and child maltreatment. In M. H. Bornstein (Ed.), *Handbook of parenting: Vol. 4. Social conditions and applied parenting* (2nd ed., pp. 361–388). Mahwah, NJ: Erlbaum.

Barkley, R. A. (1997). Behavioral inhibition, sustained attention, and executive functions: Constructing a unifying theory of ADHD. *Psychological Bulletin, 121*, 65–94.

Barkley, R. A. (2003). Attention-deficit/hyperactivity disorder. In E. J. Mash & R. A. Barkley (Eds.), *Child psychopathology* (2nd ed., pp. 75–143). New York, NY: Guilford Press.

Barkley, R. A., Fischer, M., Smallish, L., & Fletcher, K. (2003). Does the treatment of attention-deficit/hyperactivity disorder with stimulants contribute to drug use/abuse? A 13-year prospective study. *Pediatrics, 111*, 97–109.

Barkley, R. A., Karlsson, J., & Pollard, S. (1985). Effects of age on the mother-child interactions of ADD-H and normal boys. *Journal of Abnormal Child Psychology, 13*, 631–637.

Beauchaine, T. P. (2001). Vagal tone, development, and Gray's motivational theory: Toward an integrated model of autonomic nervous system functioning in psychopathology. *Development and Psychopathology, 13*, 183–214.

Beauchaine, T. P., & Gatzke-Kopp, L. M. (2012). Instantiating the multiple levels of analysis perspective into a program of study on the development of antisocial behavior. *Development and Psychopathology, 24*, 1003–1018.

Beauchaine, T. P., Gatzke-Kopp, L., & Mead, H. K. (2007). Polyvagal theory and developmental psychopathology: Emotion dysregulation and conduct problems from preschool to adolescence. *Biological Psychology, 74*, 174–184.

Beauchaine, T. P., Hinshaw, S. P., & Pang, K. L. (2010). Comorbidity of attention-deficit/hyperactivity disorder and early-onset conduct disorder: Biological, environmental, and developmental mechanisms. *Clinical Psychology: Science and Practice, 17*, 327–336.

Beauchaine, T. P., Katkin, E. S., Strassberg, Z., & Snarr, J. (2001). Disinhibitory psychopathology in male adolescents: Discriminating conduct disorder from attention-deficit/hyperactivity disorder through concurrent assessment of multiple autonomic states. *Journal of Abnormal Psychology, 110,* 610–624.

Beauchaine, T. P., Klein, D. N., Crowell, S. E., Derbidge, C., & Gatzke-Kopp, L. M. (2009). Multifinality in the development of personality disorders: A biology x sex x environment interaction model of antisocial and borderline traits. *Development and Psychopathology, 21,* 735–770.

Beauchaine, T. P., & Marsh, P. (2006). Taxometric methods: Enhancing early detection and prevention of psychopathology by identifying latent vulnerability traits. In D. Cicchetti & D. Cohen (Eds.), *Developmental psychopathology, Vol. 1. Theory and method* (2nd ed., pp. 931–967). Hoboken, NJ: Wiley.

Beauchaine, T. P., Neuhaus, E., Brenner, S. L., & Gatzke-Kopp, L. (2008). Ten good reasons to consider biological processes in prevention and intervention research. *Development and Psychopathology, 20,* 745–774.

Beauchaine, T. P., Neuhaus, E., Zalewski, M., Crowell, S. E., & Potapova, N. (2011). The effects of allostatic load on neural systems subserving motivation, mood regulation, and social affiliation. *Development and Psychopathology, 23,* 975–999.

Beauchaine, T. P., Webster-Stratton, C., & Reid, M. J. (2005). Mediators, moderators, and predictors of one-year outcomes among children treated for early-onset conduct problems: A latent growth curve analysis. *Journal of Consulting and Clinical Psychology, 73,* 371–388.

Benjamin, J., Lin, L., Patterson, C., Greenberg, B. D., Murphy, D. L., & Hamer, D. H. (1996). Population and familial association between the D4 dopamine receptor gene and measures of novelty seeking. *Nature Genetics, 12,* 81–84.

Bender, L. (1938). *A visual-motor Gestalt test and its clinical use.* New York, NY: American Orthopsychiatric Association.

Berridge, K. C. (2003). Pleasures of the brain. *Brain and Cognition, 52,* 106–128.

Berridge, K. C., & Robinson, T. E. (2003). Parsing reward. *Trends in Neuroscience, 26,* 507–513.

Biederman, J., Faraone, S. V., Milberger, S., Jetton, J. G., Chen, L., Mick, F., . . . Russell, R. L. (1996). Is childhood oppositional defiant disorder a precursor to adolescent conduct disorder? Findings from a four-year follow-up of children with ADHD. *Journal of the American Academy of Child and Adolescent Psychiatry, 35,* 1193–1204.

Biederman, J., Kim, J. W., Doyle, A. E., Mick, E., Fagerness, J. Smoller, J. W., & Faraone, S. V. (2008). Sexually dimorphic effects of four genes (COMT, SLC6A2, MAOA, SLC6A4) in genetic associations of ADHD. *American Journal of Medical Genetics Part B (Neuropsychiatric Genetics), 147B,* 1511–1518.

Biederman, J., Milberger, S., Faraone, S. V., Kiely, K., Guite, J, Mick, E., . . . Davis, S. G. (1995). Impact of adversity on functioning and comorbidity in children with attention-deficit hyperactivity disorder. *Journal of the American Academy of Child and Adolescent Psychiatry, 34,* 1495–1503.

Biederman, J., Wilens, T., Mick, E., Spencer, T., & Faraone, S. V. (1999). Pharmacotherapy of attention-deficit/hyperactivity disorder reduces risk for substance use disorder. *Pediatrics, 104,* e20.

Bigelow, J. J. (1850). Dr. Harlow's case of recovery from the passage of an iron bar through the head. *American Journal of the Medical Sciences, 19,* 13–22.

Bolsover, S. R., Hyams, J. S., Jones, S., Shepard, E. A., & White, H. A. (1997). *From genes to cells.* New York, NY: Wiley-Liss.

Brenner, S. L., & Beauchaine, T. P. (2011). Cardiac pre-ejection period reactivity and psychiatric comorbidity prospectively predict substance use initiation among middle-schoolers: A pilot study. *Psychophysiology, 48,* 1587–1595.

Brenner, S. L., Beauchaine, T. P., & Sylvers, P. D. (2005). A comparison of psychophysiological and self-report measures of BAS and BIS activation. *Psychophysiology, 42,* 108–115.

Briscoe-Smith, A. M., & Hinshaw, S. P. (2006). Linkages between child abuse and attention-deficit/hyperactivity disorder in girls: Behavioral and social correlates. *Child Abuse and Neglect, 30,* 1239–1255.

Campbell, S. B., Shaw, D. S., & Gilliom, M. (2000). Early externalizing behavior problems: Toddlers and preschoolers at risk for later maladjustment. *Development and Psychopathology, 12,* 467–488.

Carlson, G. A., & Rapport, M. D. (1989). Diagnostic classification issues in attention-deficit hyperactivity disorder. *Psychiatric Annals, 19,* 576–583.

Carmona, S., Hoekzema, E., Ramos-Quiroga, J. A., Richarte, V., Canals, C., Bosch, R., . . . Vilarroya, O. (2011). Response inhibition and reward anticipation in medication-naïve adults with attention-deficit/hyperactivity disorder: A within-subject case–control neuroimaging study. *Human Brain Mapping.* doi: 10.1002/hbm.21368 (ePub ahead of print)

Carver, C. S., & White, T. L. (1994). Behavioral inhibition, behavioral activation, and affective responses to impending reward and punishment: The BIS/BAS scales. *Journal of Personality and Social Psychology, 67,* 319–333.

Caspi, A., McClay, J., Moffitt, T. E., Mill, J., Martin J., Craig, I. W., . . . Poulton, R. (2002). Role of genotype in the cycle of violence in maltreated children. *Science, 297,* 851–854.

Castellanos, F. X. (1999). The psychobiology of attention-deficit/hyperactivity disorder. In H. C. Quay & A. E. Hogan (Eds.), *Handbook of disruptive behavior disorders* (pp. 179–198). New York, NY: Kluwer/Plenum.

Castellanos, F. X., & Tannock, R. (2002). Neuroscience of attention-deficit/hyperactivity disorder: The search for endophenotypes. *Nature Reviews Neuroscience, 3,* 617–628.

Cicchetti, D. (2006). Development and psychopathology. In D. Cicchetti & D. J. Cohen (Eds.), *Developmental psychopathology, Vol. 1. Theory and method* (2nd ed., pp. 1–24). New York, NY: Wiley.

Cicchetti, D., & Valentino, K. (2006). An ecological-transactional perspective on child maltreatment: Failure of the average expected environment and its influence on child development. In D. Cicchetti & D. J. Cohen (Eds.), *Developmental psychopathology, Vol. 3. Risk, disorder, and adaptation* (2nd ed., pp. 129–201). New York, NY: Wiley.

Conners, C. K., & MHS Staff. (2000). *Conners' continuous performance test II (CPT II).* North Tonawanda, NY: Multi-Health Systems.

Crowell, S., Beauchaine, T. P., Gatzke-Kopp, L., Sylvers, P., Mead, H., & Chipman-Chacon, J. (2006). Autonomic correlates of attention-deficit/hyperactivity disorder and oppositional defiant disorder in preschool children. *Journal of Abnormal Psychology, 115,* 174–178.

Crowell, S. E., Beauchaine, T. P., & Linehan, M. (2009). A biosocial developmental model of borderline personality: Elaborating and extending Linehan's theory. *Psychological Bulletin, 135*, 495–510.

DasBanerjee, T., Middleton, F. A., Berger, D. F., Lombardo, J. P., Sagvolden, T., & Faraone, S. V. (2008). A comparison of molecular alterations in environmental and genetic rat models of ADHD: A pilot study. *American Journal of Medical Genetics Part B (Neuropsychiatric Genetics), 147B*, 1554–1563.

De Witte, Ph., Pinto, E., Ansseau, M., & Verbanck, P. (2003). Alcohol and withdrawal: From animal research to clinical issues. *Neuroscience and Biobehavioral Reviews, 27*, 189–197.

Derryberry, D., Reed, M. A., & Pilkenton-Taylor, C. (2003). Temperament and coping: Advantages of an individual differences perspective. *Development and Psychopathology, 15*, 1049–1066.

Durston, S. (2010). Imaging genetics in ADHD. *NeuroImage, 53*, 832–838.

Durston, S., Tottenham, N. T., Thomas, K. M., Davidson, M. C., Eigsti, I-M., Yang, Y.,...Casey, B. J. (2003). Differential patterns of striatal activation in young children with and without ADHD. *Biological Psychiatry, 53*, 871–878.

Enticott, P. G., Ogloff, J. R. P., & Bradshaw, J. L. (2006). Associations between laboratory measures of executive inhibitory control and self-reported impulsivity. *Personality and Individual Differences, 41*, 285–294.

Eppinger, H., & Hess, L. (1915). *Vagotonia; A clinical study in negative neurology* (W. M. Kraus & S. E. Jelliffe, Trans.). New York, NY: Nervous and Mental Disease. (Original work published 1910)

Famularo, R., Kinscherff, R., & Fenton, T. (1992). Psychiatric diagnoses of mal-treated children: Preliminary findings. *Journal of the American Academy of Child and Adolescent Psychiatry, 31*, 863–867.

Faraone, S. V., & Mick, E. (2010). Molecular genetics of attention deficit hyperactivity disorder. *Psychiatric Clinics of North America, 33*, 159–180.

Farrington, D. P., Jolliffe, D., Loeber, R., Stouthamer-Loeber, M., & Kalb, L. M. (2001). The concentration of offenders in families, and family criminality in predicting boys' delinquency. *Journal of Adolescence, 24*, 579–596.

Forbes, E. E., & Dahl, R. E. (2005). Neural systems of positive affect: Relevance to understanding child and adolescent depression? *Development and Psychopathology, 17*, 827–850.

Fowles, D. C. (1988). Psychophysiology and psychopathology: A motivational approach. *Psychophysiology, 25*, 373–391.

Fowles, D. C., & Dindo, L. (2006). A dual-deficit model of psychopathy. In C. J. Patrick (Ed.), *Handbook of psychopathy* (pp. 14–34). New York, NY: Guilford Press.

Fraga, M. F., Ballestar, E., Paz, M. F., Ropero, S., Setien, F., Ballestar, M. L.,...Esteller, M. (2005). Epigenetic differences arise during the lifetime of monozygotic twins. *Proceedings of the National Academy of Sciences, 102*, 10604–10609.

Galili-Weisstub, E. & Segman, R. H. (2003). Attention deficit and hyperactivity disorder: Review of genetic association studies. *Israel Journal of Psychiatry and Related Sciences, 40*, 57–66.

Galvin, A., Hare, T. A., Parra, C. E., Penn, J., Voss, H., Glover, G., & Casey, B. J. (2006). Earlier development of the accumbens relative to orbitofrontal cortex might underlie risk-taking behavior in adolescents. *Journal of Neuroscience, 26,* 6885–6892.

Gatzke-Kopp, L. M. (2011). The canary in the coalmine: Sensitivity of mesolimbic dopamine to environmental adversity during development. *Neuroscience and Biobehavioral Reviews, 35,* 794–803.

Gatzke-Kopp, L., & Beauchaine, T. P. (2007). Central nervous system substrates of impulsivity: Implications for the development of attention-deficit/hyperactivity disorder and conduct disorder. In D. Coch, G. Dawson, & K. Fischer (Eds.), *Human behavior and the developing brain: Atypical development* (pp. 239–263). New York, NY: Guilford Press.

Gizer, I. R., Ficks, C., & Waldman, I. D. (2009). Candidate gene studies of ADHD: A meta-analytic review. *Human Genetics, 126,* 51–90.

Gordon, M. (1988). *The Gordon diagnostic system.* Dewitt, NY: Gordon Systems.

Grace, A. A. (2002). Dopamine. In K. L. Davis, D. Charney, J. T. Coyle, & C. Nemeroff (Eds.), *Neuropsychopharmacology: The fifth generation of progress* (pp. 119–132). Nashville, TN: American College of Neuropsychopharmacology.

Gray, J. A. (1987a). The neuropsychology of emotion and personality. In S. M. Stahl, S. D. Iversen, & E. C. Goodman (Eds.). *Cognitive neurochemistry.* (pp. 171–190). Oxford, United Kingdom: Oxford University Press.

Gray, J. A. (1987b). Perspectives on anxiety and impulsivity: A commentary. *Journal of Research in Personality, 21,* 493–509.

Gray, J. A., & McNaughton, N. (2000). *The neuropsychology of anxiety* (2nd ed.). New York, NY: Oxford University Press.

Halperin, J. M., & Schulz, K. P. (2006). Revisiting the role of the prefrontal cortex in the patho-physiology of attention-deficit/hyperactivity disorder. *Psychological Bulletin, 132,* 560–581.

Harlow, J. M. (1868). Recovery from the passage of an iron bar through the head. *Publications of the Massachusetts Medical Society, 2,* 327–347.

Hartl, D. L., & Jones, E. W. (2002). *Essential genetics: A genomics perspective* (3rd ed.). Boston, MA: Jones and Bartlett.

Hartman, R. R., Stage, S. A., & Webster-Stratton, C. (2003). A growth curve analysis of parent training outcomes: Examining the influence of child risk factors (inattention, impulsivity, and hyperactivity problems), parental and family risk factors. *Journal of Child Psychology and Psychiatry, 44,* 388–398.

Hässler, F. (1992). The hyperkinetic child: A historical review. *Acta Paedopsychiatrica, 55,* 147–149.

Hess, C., Reif, A., Strobel, A., Boreatti-Hummer, A., Heine, M., Lesch, K.-P., & Jacob, C. P. (2009). A functional dopamine-$\beta$-hydroxylase gene promoter polymorphism is associated with impulsive personality styles but not with affective disorders. *Journal of Neural Transmission, 116,* 121–130.

Hinshaw, S. P., Henker, B., Whalen, C. K., Erhardt, D., & Dunnington, R. E. (1989). Aggressive, prosocial, and nonsocial behavior in hyperactive boys: Dose effects of methylphenidate in naturalistic settings. *Journal of Consulting and Clinical Psychology, 57,* 636–643.

Hinshaw, S. P., Lahey, B. B., & Hart, E. L. (1993). Issues of taxonomy and comorbidity in the development of conduct disorder. *Development and Psychopathology, 5,* 31–49.

Hinshaw, S. P., Owens, E. B., Wells, K. C., Kraemer, H. C., Abikoff, H. B., Arnold, L. E., ... Wigal, T. (2000). Family processes and treatment outcome in the MTA: Negative/ineffective parenting practices in relation to multimodal treatment. *Journal of Abnormal Child Psychology, 28,* 555–568.

Hirshfeld-Becker, D. R., Biederman, J., Faraone, S. V., Violette, H., Wrightsman, J., & Rosenbaum, J. F. (2002). Temperamental correlates of disruptive behavior disorders in young children: Preliminary findings. *Biological Psychiatry, 50,* 563–574.

Jaffee, S. R., Caspi, A., Moffitt, T. E., Polo-Tomas, M., Price, T. S., & Taylor, A. (2004). The limits of child effects: Evidence for genetically mediated child effects on corporal punishment but not on physical maltreatment. *Developmental Psychology, 40,* 1047–1058.

Jensen, P. S., Hinshaw, S. P., Kraemer, H. C., Lenora, N., Newcorn, J. H., Abikoff, H. B., ... Vitiello, B. (2001). ADHD comorbidity findings from the MTA study: Comparing comorbid subgroups. *Journal of the American Academy of Child and Adolescent Psychiatry, 40,* 147–158.

Kagan, J., Reznick, J. S., & Snidman, N. (1988). Biological bases of childhood shyness. *Science, 240,* 167–171.

Kalivas, P. W., & Nakamura, M. (1999). Neural systems for behavioral activation and reward. *Current Opinion in Neurobiology, 9,* 223–227.

Kapoor, A., Petropoulos, S., & Matthews, S. G. (2008). Fetal programming of hypothalamic-pituitary-adrenal (HPA) axis function and behavior by synthetic glucocorticoids. *Brain Research Reviews, 57,* 586–595.

Kenemans, J. L., Bekker, E. M., Lijffijt, M., Overtoom, C. C. E., Jonkman, L. M., & Verbaten, M. N. (2005). Attention deficit and impulsivity: Selecting, shifting, and stopping. *International Journal of Psychophysiology, 58,* 59–70.

Kent L., Green, E., Hawi, Z., Kirley, A., Dudbridge, F., Lowe, N., ... Craddock, N. (2005). Association of the paternally transmitted copy of common valine allele of the Val66Met polymorphism of the brain-derived neurotrophic factor (BDNF) gene with susceptibility to ADHD. *Molecular Psychiatry, 10,* 939–943.

Knutson, B., Fong, G. W., Adams, C. M., Varner, J. L., & Hommer, D. (2001). Dissociation of reward anticipation and outcome with event-related fMRI. *Brain Imaging, 12,* 3683–3687.

Koppitz, E. M. (1968). *Psychological evaluation of children's human figure drawings.* New York, NY: Grune & Stratton.

Kramer, D. A. (2005). Commentary: Gene-environment interplay in the context of genetics, epigenetics, and gene expression. *Journal of the American Academy of Child and Adolescent Psychiatry, 44,* 19–27.

Krueger, R. F., Hicks, B. M., Patrick, C. J., Carlson, S. R., Iacono, W. G., & McGue, M. (2002). Etiologic connections among substance dependence, antisocial behavior, and personality: Modeling the externalizing spectrum. *Journal of Abnormal Psychology, 111,* 411–424.

Laakso, A., Wallius, E., Kajander, J., Bergman, J., Eskola, O. Solin, O., . . . Hietala, J. (2003). Personality traits and striatal dopamine synthesis capacity in healthy subjects. *American Journal of Psychiatry, 160*, 904–910.

Laine, T., Ahonen, A., Räsänen, P., & Tiihonen, J. (2001). Dopamine transporter density and novelty seeking among alcoholics. *Journal of Addictive Diseases, 20*, 95–100.

Laucht, M., Skowronek, M. H., Becker, K., Schmidt, M. H., Esser, G., Schulze, T. G., & Rietschel, M. (2007). Interacting effects of the dopamine transporter gene and psychosocial adversity on attention-deficit/hyperactivity disorder symptoms among 15-year-olds from a high-risk community sample. *Archives of General Psychiatry, 64*, 585–590.

Levy, F., Hay, D. A., McStephen, M., Wood, C., & Waldman, I. (1997). Attention-deficit hyperactivity disorder: A category or a continuum? Genetic analysis of a large-scale twin study. *Journal of the American Academy of Child and Adolescent Psychiatry, 36*, 737–744.

Leyton, M., Boileau, I., Benkelfat, C., Diksic, M., Baker, G., & Dagher, A. (2002). Amphetamine-induced increases in extracellular dopamine, drug wanting and novelty seeking: A PET/[$^{11}$C]Raclopride study in healthy men. *Neuropsychopharmacology, 27*, 1027–1035.

Li, D., Sham, P. C., Owen, M. J., & He, L. (2006). Meta-analysis shows significant association between dopamine system genes and attention deficit hyperactivity disorder (ADHD). *Human Molecular Genetics, 15*, 2276–2284.

Lucas, L., Celen, Z., Tamashiro, K., Blanchard, R., Blanchard, D., Markham, C., Sakai, R., & McEwen, B. (2004). Repeated exposure to social stress has long term effects on indirect markers of dopaminergic activity in brain regions associated with motivated behavior. *Neuroscience, 124*, 449–457.

Luthar, S. S. (2006). Resilience in development: A synthesis of research across five decades. In D. Cicchetti & D. Cohen (Eds.), *Developmental psychopathology, Vol. 3. Risk, disorder, and adaptation* (2nd ed., pp. 739–795). Hoboken, NJ: Wiley.

Lykken, D. T. (2006). Psychopathic personality. In C. J. Patrick (Ed.), *Handbook of psychopathy* (pp. 3–13). New York, NY: Guilford Press.

Lynam, D., Caspi, A., Moffitt, T. E., Wikström, P-O. H., Loeber, R., & Novak, S. (2000). The interaction between impulsivity and neighborhood context on offending: The effects of impulsivity are stronger in poorer neighborhoods. *Journal of Abnormal Psychology, 109*, 563–574.

Lyon, G. R., Fletcher, J. M., & Barnes, M. C. (2003). Learning disabilities. In E. J. Mash & R. A. Barkley (Eds.), *Child psychopathology* (2nd ed., pp. 520–586). New York, NY: Guilford Press.

Macmillan, M. (1992). Inhibition and the control of behavior: From Gall to Freud via Phineas Gage and the frontal lobes. *Brain and Cognition, 19*, 72–104.

Macmillan, M. (2004). Inhibition and Phineas Gage: Repression and Sigmund Freud. *Neuro-Psychoanalysis, 6*, 181–192.

Mannuzza, S., Klein, R. G., Truong, N. L., Moulton, J. L., Roizen, E. R., Howell, K. H., & Castellanos, F. X. (2008). Age of methylphenidate treatment initiation in children with ADHD and later substance abuse: Prospective follow-up into adulthood. *American Journal of Psychiatry, 165,* 604–609.

Martel, M. N., & Nigg, J. T. (2006). Child ADHD and personality/temperament traits of reactive and effortful control, resiliency, and emotionality. *Journal of Child Psychology and Psychiatry, 47,* 1175–1183.

Martin-Soelch, C., Leenders, K. L., Chevalley, A. F., Missimer, J., Künig, G., Magyar, S., . . . Schultz, W. (2001). Reward mechanisms in the brain and their role in dependence: Evidence from neurophysiological and neuroimaging studies. *Brain Research Reviews, 36,* 139–149.

Martinez, C. R., & Forgatch, M. S. (2001). Preventing problems with boys' noncompliance: Effects of a parent training intervention for divorcing mothers. *Journal of Consulting and Clinical Psychology, 69,* 416–428.

Martinez, D., Narendran, R., Foltin, R. W., Slifstein, M., Hwang, D. R., Broft, A., . . . Laruelle, M. (2007). Amphetamine-induced dopamine release: Markedly blunted in cocaine dependence and predictive of the choice to self-administer cocaine. *American Journal of Psychiatry, 164,* 622–627.

McNaughton, N., & Corr, P. J. (2004). A two-dimensional neuropsychology of defense: Fear/anxiety and defensive distance. *Neuroscience and Biobehavioral Reviews, 28,* 285–305.

Meaney, M. J., Brake, W., & Gratton, A. (2002). Environmental regulation of the development of mesolimbic dopamine systems: A neurobiological mechanism for vulnerability to drug abuse? *Psychoneuroendocrinology, 27,* 127–138.

Meier, M. H., Slutske, W. S., Arndt, S., & Cadoret, R. J. (2008). Impulsive and callous traits are most strongly associated with delinquent behavior in higher risk neighborhoods among boys and girls. *Journal of Abnormal Psychology, 117,* 377–385.

Mick, E., Spencer, T., Wozniak, J., & Biederman, J. (2005). Heterogeneity of irritability in attention-deficit/hyperactivity disorder subjects with and without mood disorders. *Biological Psychiatry, 58,* 576–582.

Milner, P. M. (1991). Brain stimulation reward: A review. *Canadian Journal of Psychology, 45,* 1–36.

Moffitt, T. E. (2005). A new look at behavioral genetics in developmental psychopathology: Gene-environment interplay in antisocial behaviors. *Psychological Bulletin, 131,* 533–554.

MTA Cooperative Group (1999). A 14-month randomized clinical trial of treatment strategies for attention-deficit/hyperactivity disorder. *Archives of General Psychiatry, 56,* 1073–1086.

Murray, K. T., & Kochanska, G. (2002). Effortful control: Factor structure and relation to externalizing and internalizing behaviors. *Journal of Abnormal Child Psychology, 30,* 503–514.

Neuman, R. J., Lobos, E., Reich, W., Henderson, C. A., Sun, L.-W., & Todd, R. D. (2007). Prenatal smoking exposure and dopaminergic genotypes interact to cause a severe ADHD subtype. *Biological Psychiatry, 61,* 1320–1328.

Nigg, J. T. (2000). On inhibition/disinhibition in developmental psychopathology: Views from cognitive and personality psychology and a working inhibition taxonomy. *Psychological Bulletin, 126*, 220–246.

Nigg, J. T. (2005). Reinforcement gradient, response inhibition, genetic versus experiential effects, and multiple pathways to ADHD. *Behavioral and Brain Sciences, 28*, 437–438.

Nock, M. K. (2003). Progress review of the psychosocial treatment of child conduct problems. *Clinical Psychology Science and Practice, 10*, 1–28.

Oas, P. (1984). Validity of the draw-a-person and Bender gestalt tests as measures of impulsivity with adolescents. *Journal of Consulting and Clinical Psychology, 52*, 1011–1019.

Oas, P. (1985). The psychological assessment of impulsivity: A review. *Journal of Psychoeducational Assessment, 3*, 141–156.

Orr, S. P., Metzger, L. J., Lasko, N. B., Macklin, M. L., Hu, F. B., Shalev, A. Y., & Pitman, R. K. (2003). Physiologic responses to sudden, loud tones in monozygotic twins discordant for combat exposure: Association with posttraumatic stress disorder. *Archives of General Psychiatry, 60*, 283–288.

Patterson, G. R., DeGarmo, D. S., & Knutson, N. (2000). Hyperactive and antisocial behaviors: Comorbid or two points in the same process? *Development and Psychopathology, 12*, 91–106.

Phillips, A. G., Blaha, C. D., & Fibiger, H. C. (1989). Neurochemical correlates of brain-stimulation reward measured by ex vivo and in vivo analyses. *Neuroscience and Biobehavioral Reviews, 13*, 99–104.

Piquero, A. R., Farrington, D. P., Welsh, B. C., Tremblay, R., & Jennings, W. G. (2009). Effects of early family/parent training programs on antisocial behavior and delinquency. *Journal of Experimental Criminology, 5*, 83–120.

Poeggel, G., Lange, E., Hase, C., Metzger, M., Gulyaeva, N., & Braun, K. (1999). Maternal separation and early social deprivation in Octodon degus: Quantitative changes in nicotinamide adenine dinucleotide phosphate-diaphorase-reactive neurons in the prefrontal cortex and nucleus accumbens. *Neuroscience, 94*, 497–504.

Pollak, S. (2005). Early adversity and mechanisms of plasticity: Integrating affective neuroscience with developmental approaches to psychopathology. *Development and Psychopathology, 17*, 735–752.

Porteus, S. D. (1965). *Porteus maze tests: Fifty years application*. Palo Alto, CA: Pacific Books.

Prasad, B. M., Hochstatter, T., & Sorg, B. A. (1999). Expression of cocaine sensitization: Regulation by the medial prefrontal cortex. *Neuroscience, 88*, 765–774.

Price, T. S., Simonoff, E., Waldman, I., Asherson, P., & Plomin, R. (2001). Hyperactivity in pre-school children is highly heritable. *Journal of the American Academy of Child and Adolescent Psychiatry, 40*, 1342–1364.

Qian, Q.-J., Liu, J., Wang, Y.-F., Yang, L., Guan, L.-L., & Faraone, S. V. (2009). Attention deficit hyperactivity disorder comorbid oppositional defiant disorder and its predominately inattentive type: Evidence for an association with COMT but not MAOA in a Chinese sample. *Behavioral and Brain Functions, 5*: 8.

Quay, H. C. (1993). The psychobiology of undersocialized aggressive conduct disorder: A theoretical perspective. *Development and Psychopathology, 5*, 165–180.

Raine, A., Venables, P. H., Dalais, C., Mellingen, K., Reynolds, C., & Mednick, S. A. (2001). Early educational and health enrichment at age 3–5 years is associated with increased autonomic and central nervous system arousal and orienting at age 11 years: Evidence from the Mauritius Child Health Project. *Psychophysiology, 38*, 254–266.

Rogeness, G., Javors, M., & Pliszka, S. (1992). Neurochemistry and child and adolescent psychiatry. *Journal of the American Academy of Child and Adolescent Psychiatry, 31*, 765–781.

Rolls, E. T., Rolls, B. J., Kelly, P. H., Shaw, S. G., Wood, R. J., & Dale, R. (1974). The relative attenuation of self-stimulation, eating, and drinking produced by dopamine receptor blockade. *Psychopharmacologia, 38*, 219–230.

Rothbart, M. K., & Bates, J. E. (1998). Temperament. In W. Damon (Series Ed.) & N. Eisenberg (Vol. Ed.), *Handbook of child psychology. Vol. 3. Social, emotional, and personality development* (pp. 105–176). New York, NY: Wiley.

Rutter, M. (2005). Environmentally mediated risk for psychopathology: Research strategies and findings. *Journal of the American Academy of Child and Adolescent Psychiatry, 44*, 3–18.

Rutter, M., & Sroufe, L. A. (2000). Developmental psychopathology: Concepts and challenges, *Development and Psychopathology, 12*, 265–296.

Saal, D., Dong, Y., Bonci, A., & Malenka, R. C. (2003). Drugs of abuse and stress trigger a common synaptic adaptation in dopamine neurons. *Neuron, 37*, 577–582.

Sagvolden, T., Johansen, E. B., Aase, H., & Russell, V. A. (2005). A dynamic developmental theory of attention-deficit/hyperactivity disorder (ADHD) predominantly hyperactive/impulsive and combined subtypes. *Behavioral and Brain Sciences, 28*, 397–468.

Sauder, C., Beauchaine, T. P., Gatzke-Kopp, L. M., Shannon, K. E., & Aylward, E. (2012). Neuroanatomical correlates of heterotypic comorbidity in externalizing youth. *Journal of Clinical Child and Adolescent Psychology, 41*, 346–352.

Scafidi, F. A., Field, T. M., Wheeden, A., Schanberg, S., Kuhn, C., Symanski, R., . . . Bandstra, E. S. (1996). Cocaine-exposed preterm neonates show behavioral and hormonal differences. *Pediatrics, 97*, 851–855.

Schachar, R. (1986). Hyperkinetic syndrome: Historical development of the concept. In E. A. Taylor (Ed.), *The overactive child* (pp. 19–40). London, United Kingdom: MacKeith.

Schenk, S., & Davidson, E. S. (1997). Stimulant preexposure sensitizes rats and humans to the rewarding effects of cocaine. *NIDA Research Monograph, 169*, 56–82.

Schott, B. H., Minuzzi, L., Krebs, R. M., Elmenhorst, E., Lang, M., Winz, O. H., . . . Bauer, A. (2008). Mesolimbic functional magnetic resonance imaging activations during reward anticipation correlate with reward-related ventral striatal dopamine release. *Journal of Neuroscience, 28*, 14311–14319.

Seeger, G., Schloss, P., Schmidt, M. H., Rüter-Jungfleisch, A., & Henn, F. A. (2004). Gene-environment interaction in hyperkinetic conduct disorder (HD + CD) as indicated by season of birth variations in dopamine receptor (DRD4) gene poly-morphism. *Neuroscience Letters, 366*, 282–286.

Shannon, K. E., Beauchaine, T. P., Brenner, S. L., Neuhaus, E., & Gatzke-Kopp, L. (2007). Familial and temperamental predictors of resilience in children at risk for conduct disorder and depression. *Development and Psychopathology, 19*, 701–727.

Shannon, K. E., Sauder, C., Beauchaine, T. P., & Gatzke-Kopp, L. (2009). Disrupted effective connectivity between the medial frontal cortex and the caudate in ado-lescent boys with externalizing behavior disorders. *Criminal Justice and Behavior, 36*, 1141–1157.

Sherman, D., Iacono, W., & McGue, M. (1997). Attention deficit hyperactivity disorder dimensions: A twin study of inattention and impulsivity hyperactivity. *Journal of the American Academy of Child and Adolescent Psychiatry, 36*, 745–753.

Snyder, J., Edwards, P., McGraw, K., Kilgore, K., & Holton, A. (1994). Escalation and reinforcement in mother-child conflict: Social processes associated with the development of physical aggression. *Development and Psychopathology, 6*, 305–321.

Snyder, J., Schrepferman, L., & St. Peter, C. (1997). Origins of antisocial behavior: Negative reinforcement and affect dysregulation of behavior as socialization mechanisms in family interaction. *Behavior Modification, 21*, 187–215.

Sonuga-Barke, E. J. S. (2005). Causal models of attention-deficit/hyperactivity disor-der: From common simple deficits to multiple developmental pathways. *Biological Psychiatry, 57*, 1231–1238.

Sroufe, L. A., & Rutter, M. (1984). The domain of developmental psychopathology. *Child Development, 55*, 17–29.

Stein, M. B., Jang, K. L., Taylor, S., Vernon, P. A., & Livesley, W. J. (2002). Genetic and environmental influences on trauma exposure and posttraumatic stress disorder symptoms: A twin study. *American Journal of Psychiatry, 159*, 1675–1681.

Swartz, J. R. (1999). Dopamine projections and frontal systems function. In B. L. Miller & J. L. Cummings (Eds.), *The human frontal lobes: Functions and disorders* (pp. 159–173). New York, NY: Guilford Press.

Taylor, J. R., & Jentsch, J. D. (2001). Stimulant effects on striatal and cortical dopamine systems involved in reward-related behavior and impulsivity. In M. V. Salanto, A. F. T. Arnsten, & F. X. Castellanos (Eds.), *Stimulant drugs and ADHD: Basic and clinical neuroscience* (pp. 104–133). New York, NY: Oxford University Press.

Thapar, A., Langley, K., Fowler, T., Rice, F., Turic, D., Whittinger, N., . . . O'Donovan, M. (2005). Catechol-o-methyltransferase gene variant and birth weight predict early-onset antisocial behavior in children with attention-deficit/hyperactivity disorder. *Archives of General Psychiatry, 62*, 1275–1278.

Thomas, M. J., Beurrier, C., Bonci, A., & Malenka, R. C. (2001). Long-term depression in the nucleus accumbens: A neural correlate of behavioral sensitization to cocaine. *Nature Neuroscience, 4*, 1217–1223.

Tremblay, R. E. (2005). Towards an epigenetic approach to experimental criminol-ogy: The 2004 Joan McCord prize lecture. *Journal of Experimental Criminology, 1*, 397–415.

Trentacosta, C. J., Hyde, L. W., Shaw, D. S., & Cheong, J. (2009). Adolescent disposi-tions for antisocial behavior in context: The roles of neighborhood dangerousness and parental knowledge. *Journal of Abnormal Psychology, 118*, 564–575.

Trouton, A., Spinath, F. M., & Plomin, R. (2002). Twins early development study (TEDS): A multivariate, longitudinal genetic investigation of language, cognition and behavior problems in childhood. *Twin Research, 5*, 444–448.

Tuvblad, C., Zheng, M., Raine, A., & Baker, L. A. (2009). A common genetic factor explains the covariation among ADHD, ODD, and CD symptoms in 9–10-year-old boys and girls. *Journal of Abnormal Child Psychology, 37*, 153–167.

Vaidya, C., Austin, G., Kirkorian, G., Ridlehuber, H. W., Desmond, J. E., Glover, G. H., & Gabrieli, J. D. (1998). Selective effects of methylphenidate in attention deficit hyperactivity disorder: A functional magnetic resonance study. *Proceedings of the National Academy of Sciences, 95*, 14494–14499.

van den Buuse, M. (1998). Role of the mesolimbic dopamine system in cardiovascular homeostasis: Stimulation of the ventral tegmental area modulates the effect of vasopressin in conscious rats. *Clinical Experimental Pharmacology and Physiology, 25*, 661–668.

Vazsonyi, A. T., Cleveland, H. H., & Wiebe, R. P. (2006). Does the effect of impulsivity on delinquency vary by level of neighborhood disadvantage? *Criminal Justice and Behavior, 33*, 511–541.

Venables, P. H. (1988). Psychophysiology and crime. In T. E. Moffit & S. A. Mednick (Eds.), *Biological contributions to crime causation* (pp. 3–13). Boston, MA: Martinus Nijhoff.

Vles, J., Feron, F., Hendriksen, J., Jolles, J., van Kroonenburgh, M., & Weber, W. (2003). Methylphenidate down-regulates the dopamine receptor and transporter system in children with attention deficit hyperkinetic disorder. *Neuropediatrics, 34*, 77–80.

Volkow, N. D., Fowler, J. S., Wang, G., Ding, Y., & Gatley, S. J. (2002). Mechanism of action of methylphenidate: Insights from PET imaging studies. *Journal of Attention Disorders, 6*, S31–S43.

Volkow, N. D., & Swanson, J. M. (2008). Does childhood treatment of ADHD with stimulant medication affect substance abuse in adulthood? *American Journal of Psychiatry, 165*, 553–555.

Volkow, N. D., Wang, G.-J., Kollins, S. H., Wigal, T. L., Newcorn, J. H., Telang, F., ... Swanson, J. (2009). Evaluating dopamine reward pathway in ADHD. *Journal of the American Medical Association, 302*, 1084–1091.

Walker, J. L., Lahey, B. B., Russo, M. F., Frick, P. J., Christ, M. A. G., McBurnett, K., ... Green, S. M. (1991). Anxiety, inhibition, and conduct disorder in children: I. Relations to social impairment. *Journal of the American Academy of Child and Adolescent Psychiatry, 30*, 187–191.

Weaver, I. C. G., Cervoni, N., Champagne, F. A., D'Alessio, A. C., Sharma, S., Seckl, J. R., ... Meaney, M. J. (2004). Epigenetic programming by maternal behavior. *Nature Neuroscience, 7*, 847–854.

Webster-Stratton, C., Reid, M. J., & Beauchaine, T. P. (2011). Combining parent and child training for young children with attention-deficit/hyperactivity disorder. *Journal of Clinical Child and Adolescent Psychology, 40*, 191–203.

Webster-Stratton, C., Reid, M. J., & Beauchaine, T. P. (2012). *One-year follow-up of combined parent and child intervention for young children with ADHD*. Manuscript submitted for publication.

Willcutt, E. G. (in press). Genetics of ADHD. In D. Barch (Ed.), *Cognitive and affective neuroscience of psychopathology*. New York, NY: Oxford University Press.

Wood, A. C., Rijsdijk, F., Saudino, K. J., Asherson, P., & Kuntsi, J. (2008). High heritability for a composite index of children's activity level measures. *Behavior Genetics, 38*, 266–276.

Yang, B., Chan, R. C. K., Jing, J., Li, T., Sham, P., & Chen, R. Y. L. (2007). A meta-analysis of association studies between the 10-repeat allele of a VNTR polymorphism in the 3'-UTR of dopamine transporter gene and attention deficit hyperactivity disorder. *American Journal of Medical Genetics Part B (Neuropsychiatric Genetics), 144B*, 541–550.

Zalot, A., Jones, D. J., Kincaid, C., & Smith, T. (2009). Hyperactivity, impulsivity, inattention (HIA) and conduct problems among African American youth: The roles of neighborhood and gender. *Journal of Abnormal Child Psychology, 37*, 535–549.

Zhou, K., Dempfle, A., Arcos-Burgos, M., Bakker, S. C., Banaschewski, T., Bieder-man, J., . . . Asherson, P. (2008). Meta-analysis of genome-wide linkage scan of attention deficit hyperactivity disorder. *American Journal of Medical Genetics Part B (Neuropsychiatric Genetics), 147B*, 1392–1398.

Zimmerman, G. M. (2010). Impulsivity, offending, and the neighborhood: Investigating the person-context nexus. *Journal of Quantitative Criminology, 26*, 301–332.

# CHAPTER 7

# Behavioral Inhibition as a Temperamental Vulnerability to Psychopathology

JEROME KAGAN

## HISTORICAL CONTEXT

BOTH THE EXPLICIT AND implicit meanings of psychopathology undergo serious changes as a result of historical events. The pace of these changes has accelerated over the past 200 years. Americans and Europeans during the 18th and most of the 19th centuries restricted the referent for psychopathology to a small number of deviant profiles, usually those currently called schizophrenia, bipolar disorder, or autism, that disrupted community harmony and/or prevented individuals from carrying out their expected responsibilities. Most of these troubled individuals were regarded as biologically distinct from the rest of the population. This frame of mind is easy to understand. Most families during these years lived in small communities and implemented relatively similar child-rearing practices. Hence, if a 15-year-old in a village became unusually aggressive, suicidal, or fearful, it was reasonable to assume that the cause had a foundation in an atypical biological constitution.

Freud introduced three seminal changes in this perspective. First, he inserted the vague notion of anxiety between the biology that was presumed to be the primary foundation of symptoms and the individual's thoughts, behaviors, and emotions. Second, he insisted that the child's early experiences, especially those within the family, made an important contribution to psychological symptoms. Finally, Freud argued that any child exposed to experiences that generated anxiety was potentially vulnerable to acquiring a neurosis. Thus, according to Freud, anyone could acquire symptoms of mental illness.

Freud's assumptions were concordant with the strong egalitarian ethic held by many Americans who wanted to believe that the quality of psychological adaptation had experiential origins. This assumption implied that America could assimilate the large number of poor, often illiterate European immigrants who arrived in large numbers between 1880 and 1910. When this ethical ideal was combined with the emphasis on environmental causation promoted by both Freud and behaviorists, psychologists and physicians sought to prove that children's socialization was the major determinant of later problems.

Importantly, at the center of this mission was the belief that a mother's care for and love of her infant and young child were the most important protections against future pathology. This assumption, which had a critical origin in 18th-century Europe, was widely disseminated by John Bowlby, who published a landmark trilogy of books on attachment (Bowlby, 1969, 1973, 1980). The confluence of these events persuaded psychologists and psychiatrists who were active during the half-century between 1910 and 1960 that children and adults who developed a mental illness, including autism, must have suffered, along with other experiences, insufficient maternal affection.

This narrative was interrupted rather abruptly by a confident cohort of behavioral geneticists, followed quickly by neuroscientists and molecular biologists, armed with novel methods to study genes and the molecules that affect a material brain, who asserted that inherited biological conditions were the causes of most forms of psychopathology. This suggestion found a receptive audience because social scientists who had advocated a formative role for early experience, without the help of biology, had failed to prove that experience alone could create a variety of disabling symptoms.

Equally significant, Americans have always been friendly to the premise that material entities are the foundation of all natural phenomena. This view suggests that one day physicians will be able to correct the biological pathologies that create symptoms with medicines, thereby doing away with the need for prolonged psychotherapy or changes in children's social conditions. These factors catapulted biological processes to an alpha position in psychological science, over the complaints of psychoanalysts and developmental psychologists with more psychodynamic orientations. The dominant consensus at present is that the emergence of psychopathology requires a biological vulnerability, usually but not always inherited, combined with an acute trauma, chronic stress, or disadvantaged position in society. In the majority of cases, specific genes or experiences acting alone are unlikely to precipitate anxiety, depression, antisocial acts, restlessness, inattention, or inability to regulate a variety of impulses to act inappropriately.

## CONCEPTUAL ISSUES

At least four conceptual issues penetrate research on the conditions that lead to pathology. They include, in abbreviated form, (1) the number and exact nature of biological vulnerabilities (diatheses), (2) the number and types of experiential risks (stressors) encountered, (3) the most fruitful categories for psychopathology, and (4) the evidence used to infer the constructs for risk and pathology. All four provoke controversy. For example, experts remain uncertain over which genes contribute to a vulnerability to any particular symptom profile. This issue is complicated by the fact that a small number of putatively genetic contributions are actually epigenetic (environmentally induced; Chapter 3) alterations in gene expression that can be reversible and need not be heritable. In addition, genes influence proteins, some of which alter neurotransmitter levels; yet they cannot produce specific behavioral symptoms that define a disorder without being combined with a life history and specific current circumstances.

Experiential risks belong to two different categories. Most investigators emphasize events that a child experiences directly, such as parental abuse, neglect, or lack of affection; peer rejection; and traumata such as rape, serious illness, or various forms of threat or physical attack. This approach ignores events that affect large segments of the population, such as persistent membership in an economically disadvantaged or minority group, a widespread form of child rearing, or historical changes in social conditions that potentiate the level of competition for status or increase the frequency of betrayals. I believe, for example, that a majority of the generation of U.S. middle-class, white children born between 1945 and 1970 experienced a relatively gentle childhood marked by parental indulgence and encouragement in both sexes for perfection of the self. Compared to many in the generation born between 1920 and 1945, who suffered through the Great Depression and World War II, this generation of adolescents and young adults escaped the serious stressors of war, harsh socialization, demeaning acts of prejudice, and economic hardship. As a result, many were not well prepared to cope with the worries created by gaining admission to college, maintaining high grades, peer gossip, and betrayal by close friends or lovers. They were therefore more vulnerable to a bout of anxiety and depression when any of these events occurred.

Most individuals must meet two criteria before being assigned to a category of psychopathology. First, the symptom profile must be deviant statistically. More than 50% of Americans live in dense urban and suburban communities with many strangers. As a result, anger is a frequent experience, either because a stranger violates an ethical norm or frustrates another more directly on highways, in movie queues, on buses, and so on. Because anger is an expected and common emotion in contemporary life, it is not treated as a sign of pathology. The same is true for the varied forms of sexual behavior practiced by many adolescents, and the binge drinking and drug use by some high school students. These behaviors were uncommon among the youth of ancient Athens and colonial New England and these communities would have regarded these acts as signs of mental disturbance.

Second, the symptoms must compromise the individual's capacity for pleasure and/or hinder his or her ability to meet daily responsibilities. A woman who cleaned her home daily, washed her hands hourly, and hoarded string, but reported feeling good as she engaged in these rituals and met all her other responsibilities effectively might not be diagnosed with OCD; whereas, a woman who was unhappy over her inability to control the same compulsive habits would receive this diagnosis.

McHugh (2008) suggested that symptoms of pathology should be assigned to one of four families based on the nature of the symptoms together with their presumed origin. One family is defined by serious compromises in logic and affect, often due to one of many possible anomalies in the genome. This family contains the schizophrenia and bipolar spectra. The second contains the internalizing symptoms of depression and one or more anxiety disorders stemming from specific biological vulnerabilities. The third family comprises the externalizing spectrum, which includes patients with ADHD, conduct disorder, or weak executive control due to a different set of biological vulnerabilities. Finally, the fourth family includes individuals who display the same symptoms of Families 2 or 3, but in the absence of the same biological vulnerabilities present in those families. In these cases, life histories, especially rearing in a disadvantaged social class, are primary origins of the disabling properties. At the moment, rearing by a disadvantaged family remains the best predictor of anxiety and depression (Kagan, 2012). Recall from Chapter 3, however, that genes may be correlated with environments ($r$GE); hence, it is usually difficult to prove that environmental events made the major contribution to the emergence of psychopathology.

Unfortunately, most of the evidence used for inferences about experiential conditions contributing to pathology comes from verbal reports, usually on questionnaires but occasionally from interviews, without direct behavioral or biological measures. This strategy poses a serious problem because every verbal description of a personality trait, mood, or memory of a past experience can originate in different biological states and life histories. One of the most robust facts in psychopathology is that women who grew up in disadvantaged homes are at a high risk for an anxiety disorder (Kagan, 2012). Yet, when one team of investigators asked a large number of New England mothers from varied class and ethnic groups to rate their daughter's anxiety level, the girls growing up in the most economically disadvantaged homes were described as less anxious than the girls from more affluent families (Mian, Wainwright, Briggs-Gowan, & Carter, 2011).

I note later that adolescents with distinct temperaments and life histories can report similar descriptions of depression or social anxiety. In addition, adults vary in the tendency to exaggerate or to minimize a stressful event that occurred in the past (Diekelmann, Wilhelm, Wagner, & Born, 2011; Raczka et al., 2010). Thus the frequency of past stressors, when based only on fallible recall, may not correspond with what a camera would have recorded or the person would have described at the time. A mother's verbal descriptions of the traits of her child, as well as an adult's verbal descriptions of his or her memories of past adversities—without any corroboration—are phenomena to be understood rather than the obvious "cause" of current problems. The popularity of the Rorschach inkblots and the Thematic Apperception Test, from about 1930 to 1960, was attributable to the general recognition that verbal replies to direct questions were not accurate measures of what investigators needed to know. Unfortunately, these techniques also proved wanting. But rather than try to invent more sensitive procedures, many psychologists, unaware of the earlier disappointment with this evidence and eager to begin their inquiries, returned to verbal answers on questionnaires or in interviews.

## THE ETIOLOGICAL ROLE OF TEMPERAMENTS

The theme of the remainder of this chapter is that heritable brain structures and functions render some children susceptible to feelings and actions that, on occasion, become symptoms of psychopathology. These biases favoring certain feeling and action states are called *temperaments*. Temperaments are not brain structures or functions. They are consistent patterns of behavioral/emotional response tendencies, usually appearing early in development, that are sculpted by experience into a large, but nonetheless limited, number of profiles that define a personality trait or type. Consistent display of sociability with strangers, conscientiousness with important tasks, and impulsive decisions, for example, are the joint products of a temperamental bias and a personal history. The temperamental contribution to a trait or a symptom is not easily detected in older children or adults with currently available methods. No questionnaire administered in adulthood can provide an accurate index of a human temperament. Temperamental biases in adolescents can be likened to drops of black ink that become invisible after being stirred in a vessel of clear glycerine.

It is generally assumed, but not yet proven, that heritable patterns of neurochemistry are the biological foundations for many but not all human temperaments. This hypothesis, which was anticipated more than a century ago (McDougall, 1908; Rich, 1928), was present in the writings of the ancients who posited melancholic, sanguine, choleric, and phlegmatic temperamental types derived from the balance of the four body humors within each person.

### GENES, NEUROCHEMISTRY, AND TEMPERAMENTS

There are at least 150 different molecules that, along with the density and locations of their receptors, have the potential to influence the feelings and behaviors that define human temperaments. These include norepinephrine, dopamine, epinephrine, serotonin, corticotropin releasing hormone (CRH), glutamate, gamma aminobutyric acid (GABA), opioids, vasopressin, oxytocin, prolactin, monoamine oxidase (MAO), neuropeptide S, and the sex hormones androgen and estrogen (Hartl & Jones, 2005). The genes that code for concentrations of these molecules and their receptor distributions and densities often have a number of polymorphisms in one or more of the gene's exons, introns, or regulatory sequences, called *promoters* and *enhancers*. Promoters control the level of transcription of the exon into messenger RNA; enhancers determine where and when transcriptions will occur (see also Chapter 3).

If each gene, consisting of exons, introns, enhancers, and promoters, that influenced brain activity had an average of 5 polymorphisms, there can be about $3 \times 10^{750}$ possible neurochemical combinations that potentially could be the foundation of a temperamental bias (Irizarry & Galbraith, 2004). Even if a majority of these neurochemical profiles had no relevance for temperament, which is likely to be the case, the large number of remaining patterns implies that future scientists will discover many hundreds of temperaments that remain undetected. The immaturity in our current understanding of the relations among genes, brain chemistry, experience, and behavior frustrates scientists seeking reliable relations between a gene, or set of genes, and any known temperamental bias. Hence, at present, most definitions of a temperament have to be based primarily on behaviors, preferably observed directly, rather than based on verbal reports by the person or one or more informants.

## Reactions to the Unexpected or Unfamiliar

Two biases that have been studied more extensively than others refer to the contrast between children who show restrained, cautious, avoidant reactions to unfamiliar objects, people, or settings—called *behaviorally inhibited*—and those displaying spontaneous approach to the same events, called *uninhibited* (Asendorpf, 1989, 1991; Bates, 1989; Buss, 2011; Kagan, 1994; Volbrecht & Goldsmith, 2010). Both biases can be observed reliably by the first birthday, are modestly stable over time, relatively easy to measure, have moderate heritabilities, and are present in every mammalian species studied (Bartels et al., 2004; Kagan & Saudino, 2001; Schneirla, 1959; Scott & Fuller, 1965; Sussman & Ha, 2011; Wirtschafter, 2005). The behaviors that define these contrasting biases are correlated, but only moderately, with theoretically expected peripheral physiological measures, including changes in heart rate, blood pressure, and muscle tension to challenge (Kagan & Snidman, 2004).

Particular genetic polymorphisms make small contributions to behavioral inhibition, especially when combined with particular experiences. The short versus long form of the gene for 5-HTTLPR (serotonin transporter) in the promoter region has been a popular target of study (Battaglia et al., 2005; Bethea et al., 2004; Lakatos et al., 2003). For example, Taiwanese adults who reported experiencing many past stressors were more likely to be homozygous for the short allele of the serotonin transporter gene (Yeh et al., 2009). Unfortunately, these relations are not always replicated across laboratories because scientists use different measures of the behavioral construct; the samples are stratified (i.e., vary by gender, ethnicity, social class, and/or age) and/or the investigators quantify only one polymorphism rather than a pattern of several alleles (Arbelle et al., 2003). When several alleles of the same gene or of different genes are examined in the same sample, relations between the short or long forms of 5-HTTLPR and a psychological outcome are often altered (Kaufman et al., 2006). One of the many reasons is that the serotonin transporter clears dopamine as well as serotonin from select synapses (Larsen et al., 2011). Therefore, possession of the short or long alleles of 5-HTTLPR can also influence functions affected by dopamine (see Chapter 6).

Experts agree that both acute experiences and chronic exposure to particular settings select the specific psychological phenotype that will develop from these and other temperamental profiles. Children's social class, a proxy for a host of experiences, represents one of the most important environmental influences. Upper-middle-class adults with 2 or 5 rather than 7 repeats in the DRD4 receptor gene are high in novelty seeking but, surprisingly, individuals from economically disadvantaged backgrounds with the same polymorphisms are not (Caspi et al., 2003; Eley et al., 2004; Lahti et al., 2006; Kaufman et al., 2004). As noted earlier, social class remains the best predictor of developing an anxiety, depressive, conduct, or addictive disorder as defined by *DSM-IV-TR* (2000), far better than any gene or Gene ×

Experience interaction detected to date (Pickett & Wilkinson, 2010; Werner & Smith. 1982; Xin, Zhang, & Liu, 2010). Among children who suffered from maltreatment, those who possess different risk alleles (homozygous for the s allele in the dopamine transporter [DAT] gene and valine rather than methionine in codon 66 in the brain derived neurotrophic factor [BDNF] gene), but also reported many social supports, more characteristic of advantaged environments, were less likely to be diagnosed with a depressive disorder than maltreated children who enjoyed little or no social support (Kaufman et al., 2006).

It is possible that careful attention to the person's social class can help resolve the continuing controversy surrounding the claim by Caspi et al. (2003) that possession of the s allele of the 5-HTTLPR gene, combined with the experience of stress during childhood/adolescence, especially severe maltreatment, increases by a small amount the risk for persistent adult depression (Karg, Burmeister, Shedden & Sen, 2011; Uher et al., 2011). The least controversial fact is that possession of the s allele lowers the threshold for psychological states of uncertainty and vigilance in animals and humans. Therefore, young children with the s allele might be more difficult to rear than those with the l allele. Less well-educated parents with low incomes and unskilled jobs are more likely than educated parents to maltreat irritable children. Third, adults with a low threshold for uncertainty and vigilance who spent their lives in lower class homes and correlated settings are at the highest risk for depression. Thus, it remains a possibility, albeit speculative, that the presumed interaction between the s allele and maltreatment increasing the risk for depression is a gene-environment correlation (rGE). That is, young children who are irritable and anxious because they possess the short allele are more likely to be maltreated by lower class parents, and if they remain in a less advantaged setting as adolescents and young adults they will be at a higher risk for depression.

Perhaps the most accurate way to summarize the evidence is as follows. Possession of the s allele on both chromosomes creates a specific pattern of brain function that, in developed societies, is likely to generate a psychological state that individuals interpret as anxiety or uncertainty. The accompanying personality traits will depend on one's social class and past history. Although most will not acquire symptoms that meet *DSM-IV-TR* (2000) criteria for a disorder, adults reared in economically disadvantaged homes who do develop symptoms are likely to emphasize a chronic mood of depression because of their compromised status, frustrated sense of agency, financial worries, health problems, and fragile social supports. The occurrence of severe maltreatment among a small proportion of these persons is probably less critical than their class position over several decades. This may explain why British adults homozygous for the l allele who report severe maltreatment are also at higher than average risk for depression (Uher et al., 2011). In contrast, s allele homozygotes who enjoy economic and social advantage are probably at a slightly higher risk for general anxiety, social phobia, or perhaps OCD. Some may become workaholics if their vocation allows them to gain status and/or money through overwork. In this explanation the most important phenomenon to explain in those with the s allele is their private interpretations of the feeling state that penetrates consciousness. The s allele does not lead to one dominant emotional state. Rather, because social class affects such interpretations in many contemporary societies, the critical interaction is between possession of the s allele and social class rather than between the allele and maltreatment. If we knew the genomes and primary symptoms of the respected clerics in Catholic French villages or Muslim towns in the Otttoman empire in the 14th century, I suspect, but cannot prove, that depression would not be the major symptom among those with the s allele.

## High- and Low-Reactive Infants

My colleagues and I have been following a large longitudinal cohort of middle-class, healthy, Caucasian children from their first assessment at 16 weeks through 18 years. The initial aim of this research was to discover patterns of infant behaviors that might predict the inhibited and uninhibited profiles that appear after the first birthday (see earlier). The central hypothesis guiding the infant assessments was that inherited variation in the excitability of the amygdala would be accompanied by distinct patterns of motor activity and distress to unexpected familiar or unfamiliar events if the infants were assessed early in life before brain maturation provides them some control over their actions.

The amygdala consists of a number of neuronal clusters, called the lateral, basal, cortical, medial, intercalated, and central regions. Each cluster has a distinctive set of connections, neurochemistries, and functions (Stefanacci & Amaral, 2002). The threshold of excitability in each region of the amygdala can be influenced by any of a large number of molecules, including GABA, glutamate, opioids, CREB, norepinephrine, dopamine, vasopressin, and oxytocin (Kirsch et al., 2005). The balance among these molecules and their appropriate receptors, as well as modulating inputs from other brain sites, determines the neural state in each neuronal cluster.

The primary functions of the amygdala are to respond to all unfamiliar or unexpected events and to generate an initial state of vigilance and preparation for action when the event poses a threat (Fitzgerald et al., 2006). Hence, infants with excitable amygdalae should be more likely than others to become inhibited children. Newborn infants whose rate of sucking increases dramatically following an unexpected change in taste sensation from water to sweet are more inhibited during the second year than infants who show a minimal increase in sucking rate following the same change in taste (LaGasse, Gruber, & Lipsitt, 1989). The unexpected change in taste sensation activated the central nucleus of the amygdala, which was followed by activation of the motor centers that control sucking. Infants with more excitable central nuclei should have larger increase in sucking rates. The more critical fact for our purposes is that activation of the amygdala of many species is accompanied by vigorous limb movements, back arching, and distress cries (Pitkanen, 2000). Human infants display all three behaviors.

The corpus of evidence implies that young infants who inherit a neurochemistry that renders one or more regions of the amygdala excitable display more vigorous motor activity, especially arches of the back, and more frequent crying to unfamiliar events, compared with infants born with a different neurochemistry that renders the amygdala less excitable. This hypothesis is in accord with Rothbart's (1989) emphasis on variation in reactivity as one basis of temperament.

We coded from film records the frequency of vigorous limb movements, back arching, fretting, and crying, along with babbling, smiling, and heart rate, in over 450 healthy, 16-week-old Caucasian, middle-class infants during a battery that included presentation of small, unfamiliar, colorful objects moving back and forth in front of the face, recordings of speech emanating from a schematic face with no human present, and a cotton swab that had been dipped in dilute alcohol applied to the nostrils. Twenty percent of the infants showed a pattern that combined high levels of limb activity, back arching, and crying. These children were called high reactive. Forty percent showed a pattern of minimal motor activity, few arches, and little crying. These infants were called low reactive. I do not believe we would have detected these two groups of infants as accurately if we had interviewed the mothers or given them a questionnaire. Two other groups, defined by low motor activity with frequent crying or high motor activity with minimal crying represent two other distinct temperaments. Indeed, Degnan et al. (2011) report that a small group of 4-month-old infants with combined high levels of limb activity with babbling and smiling, but very little crying, are biased to become exuberant 5-year-olds.

We assessed the high- and low-reactive infants on seven occasions through 18 years of age. Detailed results of these evaluations are summarized elsewhere (Kagan, 1994; Kagan & Snidman, 2004; Kagan, Snidman, Kahn, & Towsley, 2007). A brief summary follows.

*Child and early adolescent evaluations.* High reactives assessed at 14 and 21 months were significantly more avoidant of and fearful to a series of unfamiliar social and nonsocial incentives than low reactives. However, about 20% of the high reactives were not highly fearful at both ages because, we presume, their experiences allowed them to gain some control of the public expression of signs of fear. In addition, high reactives had significantly narrower faces than low reactives at these ages (Arcus & Kagan, 1995). Because variation in the neural crest cells in the young embryo influence facial width, it is possible that genes that affect the neurochemical profiles of neural crest cells, which include the 5-HT and 5-HTTLPR genes, also contribute to the differences between high and low reactive infants.

At age 7 years about half of the high reactives possessed fears of animals, the dark, thunderstorms, and/or unfamiliar people and places, compared with fewer than 10% of low reactives. At 11 and 15 years high reactives were not only quieter and emotionally more subdued, but they also showed few spontaneous smiles during laboratory sessions designed to measure four biological reactions that are indirect signs of a more excitable amygdala. Specifically, more high than low reactives displayed greater activation of the right compared with the left frontal lobe. Right frontal activation, measured by less alpha power in the right compared with the left hemisphere, is modestly correlated with an unpleasant state in infants, a more anxious mood in adults, and with behavioral signs of fear in animals (Adamec, Blundell & Burton, 2005; Blackhart, Minnix, & Kline, 2006; Davidson, 2003; Davidson, Jackson, & Kalin, 2000; Fox et al., 2005; Fox, Calkins, & Bell, 1994; Schmidt, 2008). Among a group of exuberant toddlers, as assessed by behavioral observations, only those who also showed left frontal activation at three years were described by their mothers at age five as being highly energetic, sociable, and joyful, called high in surgency, or simply exuberant. Exuberant toddlers with right frontal activation were not described this way (Degnan et al., 2011).

Because the amygdala projects ipsilaterally to sites in the frontal cortex, greater activity in the right amygdala should be accompanied by greater activation in the right frontal area (Cameron, 2002). Visceral feedback from the body to the central nucleus of the amygdala is greater to the right than to the left amygdala. Therefore, children who experience more frequent visceral activity should have a more active right amygdala and display right, rather than left, frontal activation.

More high than low reactives showed a larger brain stem auditory evoked response from the inferior colliculus at both 11 and 15 years. Because the amygdala primes the inferior colliculus, this result also suggests that high reactives possess a more excitable amygdala (Baas, Milstein, Donlevy & Grillon, 2006; Brandao, Coimbra, & Osaki, 2001). High-reactive adolescents also showed larger N400 waveforms to discrepant visual scenes (for example, a chair with one leg) and greater sympathetic rather than parasympathetic tone in the cardiovascular system (Kagan & Snidman, 2004). These results are in accord with reports of others (Fox et al., 2005; Schmidt, Fox, Schulkin, & Gold, 1999).

High reactives interviewed at home at age 15 smiled and talked less often and showed more restless activity than low reactives. Interviewers asked several questions designed to discover the targets of each adolescent's primary worries. Although almost all adolescents reported concerns with the quality of their performances in school and when engaged in extracurricular activities, more high than low reactives also confessed to worrying over encountering crowds, strangers, unfamiliar situations, and their futures. Two thirds of high reactives, but only 20% of low reactives, nominated one or more of these less realistic worries.

Every one of the 11 high reactive adolescents for whom the 4-month infant assessment was terminated early because they became extremely distressed and could not be soothed nominated at least one unrealistic worry. Verbatim excerpts illustrate their concern with unpredictable situations: "In a crowd I feel isolated and left out, I don't know what to pay attention to because it is also ambiguous"; "I worry about the future, over not knowing what will happen next"; "I wanted to be a doctor but decided against it because I felt it would be too much of a strain"; "I like being alone and, therefore, horses are my hobby, I don't have to worry about fitting in with others when I am with my horses"; "I get nervous before every vacation because I don't know what will happen." Similar statements were rare among the low reactives.

The high reactives were also less likely on a Q-sort procedure to rank "Most of the time I'm happy" as a salient characteristic of their personality, and were more likely to describe themselves as serious and desiring a more relaxed mood. Adolescents who possess this mood are at a higher risk for a later mental illness (Colman et al., 2007).

Youth in the contemporary United States are trying to establish their personal philosophy at a time when there is little if any consensus on the meaning of life or the ethical standards that demand unquestioned loyalty. This state of affairs creates high levels of uncertainty in high-reactive adolescents. These youth might be expected to seek a means of muting their angst. A religious commitment is one effective strategy because it provides a partial answer to these questions and assures each believer of his or her essential virtue when disappointments, failures, or frustrations occur. Forty-five percent of the adolescents who had been high-reactive infants said they were very religious, compared with only 25% of the low reactives, despite no difference in the religious commitment of their parents. High reactives said that their religious commitment diluted their level of tension when unexpected challenges occurred.

*Age 18 assessments.* Carl Schwartz, a psychiatrist at Massachusetts General Hospital, measured the anatomy and functional brain activity in 135 high- and low-reactive 18-year-olds. In addition, a clinician who was blind to each youth's earlier history administered a standard psychiatric interview and assigned *DSM-IV-TR* (2000) categories to those who met relevant criteria. This section presents an integration of the biological and psychiatric measures.

The high and low reactives differed significantly on three biological measures. First, the high reactives had a thicker cortex in a small region in the ventromedial prefrontal cortex (vmPFC) of the right hemisphere (Schwartz et al., 2010). This area is connected reciprocally with the amygdala and projects to sites in the central gray that are responsible for the back arching displayed by high-reactive infants. It is of interest that adults with lesions in this general area are bothered less by moral violations (Moretto, Ladavas, Mattioli, & di Pelligrino, 2010) (see also Hill et al., 2010; Welborn et al., 2009; Young et al., 2010). High reactives are especially vulnerable to anxiety and guilt over moral errors. Furthermore, adolescent males who are high in the trait called surgency (see earlier), which is infrequent among high reactives, show less activity in this area when, in the presence of friends, they make errors in a game (Segalowitz et al., 2011).

The thicker cortex in the small area in the right vmPFC of high reactives seems, on the surface, to be inconsistent with many reports suggesting that this area modulates the amygdala and mutes its excitability. Yet high reactives possess a more excitable amygdala. This paradox might be resolved by noting that the high reactives do not possess a thicker cortex in the left vmPFC and it is possible that the projections from the left hemisphere are more effective in silencing the amygdala. This suggestion is supported by the observation that adults with a thicker left vmPFC show less activation of the amygdala when judging emotional faces (Foland-Ross et al., 2010).

Second, high reactives showed a larger surge of blood flow (the BOLD signal) to the right amygdala the first time they saw a set of angry faces they did not expect (the episode contained four presentations of angry, fear, and neutral faces appearing in random order). Third, high reactives showed a shallower slope of habituation of the BOLD signal to the left amygdala to repeated presentations of ecologically invalid scenes (for example, an infant's head on an animal's body) and to the right amygdala to repeated presentations of unfamiliar faces with neutral expressions (Schwartz et al., in press) (see also Blackford et al., 2010; Eley, 2011).

The clinician's diagnoses revealed a significantly higher prevalence of depression, social phobia, and/or general anxiety disorder among high reactives than low reactives (42% versus 26%). More than half of the high-reactive females and close to one third of high-reactive males received one of these diagnoses. The value for high-reactive females is twice the prevalence of lifetime diagnoses of anxiety and depression among large representative groups of American adolescents (unpublished data). These diagnoses are high in adolescents perhaps because projections from the prefrontal cortex to limbic sites, which modulate the latter, are not yet fully mature (Brendgen et al., 2005; Eley, 2011; Gladstone & Parker; 2006; Mick & Telch, 1998). This result is also in accord with the fact that French adults with social anxiety disorder and comorbid depression had the highest scores on a 30-item questionnaire asking them to recall how shy, timid, and fearful they were as children (odds ratio of 1.9; Rotge et al., 2011).

The low-reactive males who as children were the least fearful on every assessment, had the lowest prevalence of depression or anxiety (13%) and the highest proportion with no *DSM-IV-TR* (2000) symptoms (60% reported no depression, no anxiety, drug or alcohol problems, no conduct disorder, and no ADHD). The combination of a low-reactive temperament and a male sex produces an unusually relaxed and fearless adolescent.

Equally important, the biological measures distinguished clearly between low-reactives who reported a bout of depression or anxiety, mainly girls, and high reactives given the same diagnoses. Specifically, among the adolescents diagnosed with depression, general anxiety, or social anxiety significantly more high than low reactives showed a thick vmPFC, a large surge of blood flow to the initial appearance of the angry faces, and/or a shallow habituation of the BOLD signal to the invalid scenes. For example, 71% of anxious/depressed high reactives, but only 23% of depressed/anxious low reactives, had their maximal BOLD signal to the first set of angry faces.

In addition, more high reactives given one of these diagnoses showed very frequent back arches at 4 months and/or high fear scores in the laboratory at 14 months compared with high reactives who had none of these diagnoses and low reactives with one of the diagnoses. Ninety percent of the high reactives with a diagnosis of social anxiety or depression had either frequent arches or a high fear score or both, whereas not one low reactive with one of these diagnoses met either criterion (these data reveal a sensitivity of 90% and a specificity of 100%). Finally, a pattern that combined the display of many fears to unfamiliar events at 14 months with a thick vmPFC in the right hemisphere at age 18 years also separated the high and low reactives given exactly the same diagnoses. Two-thirds of the high reactives who were fearful at 14 months and had a thick vmPFC received diagnoses of depression, general anxiety, or social anxiety disorder. Not one low reactive diagnosed with depression or anxiety possessed both features. These results imply that these *DSM-IV-TR* (2000) diagnostic categories can be the product of different physiologies and life histories. Hence, clinicians and investigators should gather biological and behavioral evidence on all potential patients in order to parse those with the same symptoms into theoretically more fruitful categories that might profit best from different therapeutic regimens (see e.g., Beauchaine, Neuhaus, Brenner, & Gatzke-Kopp, 2008).

## SYNTHESIS

The evidence reviewed thus far has two important implications for the study of psychopathology. First, investigators should be sensitive to the contexts of observation, a requirement that applies to the source of evidence used for inferences. High-reactive children are cautious and subdued in unfamiliar settings that do not seem to bother most children; they are not cautious or timid in familiar ones (Buss, 2011). Thus, parent or teacher reports of shy or timid behavior are not always accurate proxies for direct observations of inhibited behavior.

Second, investigators should base their inferences on patterns of variables, not single measures (Kagan, 2011). Some high-reactive and many low-reactive 15-year-olds denied being shy on a Q-sort and interview. Yet only the high reactives who denied shyness and described themselves as sociable frequently looked away from the interviewer. Low reactives did not.

The high frequency of unrealistic worries about future encounters with unfamiliar settings reported by high reactives provides a clue to the processes responsible for their profile. These adolescents are chronically uncertain of the qualities by which others will judge them or how they will react; they believe there is not much they can do to reduce the probability of an incorrect or socially inappropriate response. Their state of uncertainty differs from the state of those who are concerned only with the quality of their performances.

A survey of the fears of college students from seven different societies revealed minimal cultural or sex differences in the prevalence of realistic fears (e.g., dangerous animals), but significant cultural and sex differences in the incidence of less realistic fears (e.g., small animals; Davey et al., 1998). The self-reported unrealistic fears of monozygotic twins and their spouses (an accident while boating or walking in a dark place) had higher heritability values than more realistic, and more probable fears of illness, a car accident, or criticism for a mistake (Sundet, Skre, Okkenhaug, & Tambs, 2003). Thus, a high-reactive temperament makes a greater contribution to level of worry over less-realistic, low-probability threats than to anxiety over serious realistic threats.

All adolescents meet new people, visit unfamiliar places, and know they are unable to control future events. Thus, it is appropriate to ask why high reactives are most likely to name these events as a primary source of worry. One possible contribution to this vulnerability is their greater susceptibility to detecting the unexpected visceral feedback from targets in the gut, muscle, and autonomic nervous system. When these sensations pierce consciousness they create uncertainty because they are unexpected and their origin is ambiguous. This psychological state resembles the one evoked when they encountered unfamiliar objects, people, or situations during childhood and can function as a conditioned stimulus to provoke a state of uncertainty to any unexpected incentive.

High-reactive youth in our culture are biased to interpret the feeling evoked by the visceral feedback as implying that they are worried about encounters with strangers, unexpected challenges, and new places because these events are the most frequent novelties in their lives, and because the folk theory they learned implied that their uncertainty was due to a compromise in their psychological characteristics. Members of other cultures might impose different interpretations on the same visceral feedback. Cambodian refugees living in Massachusetts, for example, interpret an unexpected bout of tachycardia as implying a weak heart produced by a loss of energy following lack of sleep or diminished appetite (Hinton, Pich, Safren, Pollack, & McNally, 2005a; Hinton, Pich, Chhean, Pollack, & McNally, 2005b).

If the uncertainty produced by unexpected visceral feedback over unfamiliar events were frequent or intense during childhood, the amygdala-hippocampal pathway could become sensitized—the technical term is kindled—so these children might remain vulnerable to anxiety over the anticipation of unfamiliar contexts for a long time (Pape & Stork, 2003). Rat strains differ in the ease of amygdala kindling due in part to inherited genetic and neurochemical profiles (Kelly, McIntosh, McIntyre, Merali, & Anisman, 2003). Resulting alterations in amygdalar function following adversity may be lifelong (for a review see Beauchaine, Neuhaus, Zalewski, Crowell, & Potapova, in press).

Social anxiety, often combined with depression, was the most likely diagnosis for high reactives in our cultural setting because strangers and new places are common events and social acceptance is an important motive. The Saulteaux Indians of Manitoba worry about contracting a serious disease because illness is a sign that they violated an ethical norm on sexual, aggressive, or sharing behavior with others (Hallowell, 1941). A temperamental bias renders individuals vulnerable to some form of anxiety; their history and culture supply the specific target of this emotional family. Some U.S. males, but few Asian males, worry that their body is insufficiently muscular because physical strength has been a traditional value in Western but not Asian cultures (Kanayama & Pope, 2011). In contemporary United States, social failure has been added to the seven traditional sins of pride, anger, envy, avarice, sloth, gluttony, and lust as bases for anxiety, shame, and guilt.

Although high reactives are more likely than others to become shy, socially anxious, introverted adults, most will not meet criteria for a psychiatric diagnosis of social phobia and many will not be unusually shy. Only 1 of every 2 adults who score in the 90th percentile or above on a scale for self-reported shyness receive a diagnosis of social phobia (Chavira, Stein, & Malcarne, 2002). Furthermore, fewer than 15% of chronically shy children develop social anxiety disorder (Biederman et al., 2001; Prior, Smart, Sanson, & Oberklaid, 2000), and about half of adults with social phobia do not remember being excessively shy as young children, although they may distort their recollections of their childhood personality (Cox, McPherson, & Ens, 2005). Thus, the probability that an infant with a high-reactive temperament will become an intensely anxious or depressed adolescent is not high. However, the probability that such children will *not* be ebullient, relaxed, bold risk takers is greater than 90%. The power of a temperamental bias lies in its ability to restrict the development of certain future profiles rather than determine a particular personality trait. The same is true for experiences. The probability that children reared by wealthy, well-educated parents will not become prostitutes or homeless drug addicts is very high but the probability that they will occupy a specific vocational niche, say professional musicians in a symphony orchestra or research scientists, is much lower.

*Anhedonia.* The neurochemistry of high reactives could interfere with the intensity or frequency of the subjective feeling of pleasure that often occurs when a person is the recipient of an unexpected or larger-than-anticipated desirable experience. This state is mediated in part by the discharge of dopamine (DA)-producing neurons that accompany the anticipation of a desired event (Schultz, 2006; Chapter 6). Furthermore, *corticotropin-releasing hormone* (CRH), usually activated by the anticipation of threat and present in DA-producing brain sites, can suppress the release of DA to imminent reward (Austin, Rhodes, & Lewis, 1997). There also appears to be an association between an introverted personality and polymorphisms of the catechol-O-methyltransferase (COMT) gene, which affects the efficiency of DA degradation in the synapse (Golimbet, Gritsenko, Alfimova, & Ebstein, 2005; Stein, Fallin, Schork, & Gelernter, 2005).

Perhaps one reason why high-reactive adolescents do not like new activities (whether risky or not), even though they promise excitement, is that these youth fail to experience a great deal of pleasure when they anticipate visiting a new city, meeting a new person, or engaging in a novel activity (Netter, 2006). This argument is supported by a study of 111 college students who initially filled out a questionnaire measuring social anxiety and then rated their mood on each of 21 consecutive days. The students with high scores on the social anxiety scale were least likely to report pleasurable experiences and more likely to confess to a melancholic mood across the 3 weeks (Kashdan & Steger, 2006).

## Some Caveats

Verbal reports of moods and actions, usually without any direct behavioral observations or biological evidence, represent the usual information clinicians use in arriving at diagnoses of mental illness. But, as noted earlier, the meaning and therefore validity of every conclusion is dependent on the quality of evidence used to arrive at the inference. The same is true of single variables in a research study. A single measure, whether self-report, behavioral, or biological, rarely has an unequivocal meaning. Verbal replies to a question as simple as "Are you happy most of the time?" are ambiguous because this self-report has different correlates in adolescents with high compared with low reactive temperaments. It is likely that the self-reports of more complex psychological states are equally ambiguous because they can result from different histories and psychological states.

Accordingly, investigators should not treat similar answers to a questionnaire or interview as having an equivalent and transparent meaning (Schienle et al., 2006). Adults instructed to worry about issues they had previously told an investigator were serious sources of concern showed activation of frontal sites (measured by PET), but less activity in the amygdala and insula, and no change in heart rate or skin conductance. This suggests that some self-reports of anxiety are purely cognitive judgments unaccompanied by any somatic component of feelings (Hoehn-Saric,

Lee, McLeod, & Wong, 2005). Investigators should not assume that a verbal report of an emotional state reflects the same biological or psychological condition in all respondents offering identical descriptions.

Many popular psychopathological constructs, including anxiety, can be created by more than one pattern of conditions. There is, most of the time, more than one pathway to any psychiatric disorder, exemplifying the construct of equifinality (Chapter 1). A person could be classified as impulsive because of a life history that led to minimal concern with quality of performance or because of a biology that compromised frontal lobe function. Two photographs of the Washington monument, one made with a traditional camera and the other with a digital camera, appear similar despite the distinctly different mechanisms that produced the two pictures. Mice can develop the same phenotype of light-color fur as a function of two different polymorphisms (Hoekstra, Hirschmann, Bundey, Insel, & Crossland, 2006).

## Hyping Biology

Although almost all psychopathological profiles are a joint function of a biologically based vulnerability and a history of environmental experiences (Chapter 3), there is currently more enthusiasm and more adequate financial support for research that probes the biological rather than the environmental contributions to these profiles. This situation was reversed a half-century earlier. I end this chapter by addressing some reasons for the current bias.

First, U.S. and European scientists prefer materialistic explanations of all natural phenomena. Genes, neurons, transmitters, and circuits are material entities whose forms can be observed or imagined. Neither feelings nor thoughts, which the Greeks assigned to the soul, possess this quality. This perspective tempts investigators to ignore the child's private interpretation of a potentially stressful experience and assume, incorrectly, that harsh parental practices have the same consequences for all children and, therefore, are synonymous with abuse. If this were true, a majority of children raised by 17th-century New England Puritan parents would have to be classified as abused.

Second, anxiety, depression, criminality, and alcohol or drug dependence are more prevalent among those who are poor and/or belong to a disadvantaged ethnic minority. Investigators who claimed that the child-rearing practices of these parents made a contribution to the symptoms of their child would be accused of harboring prejudicial attitudes toward the socially disadvantaged. It has become politically incorrect to blame the victim.

Third, theoretical advances in every discipline often follow the introduction of new, more powerful methods. Investigators studying the importance of the social environment continue to use the traditional methods of questionnaires, interviews, and only occasionally, behavioral observations. These social scientists have not invented more sensitive ways to measure the private psychological consequences of experience. In contrast, geneticists, molecular biologists, and neuroscientists enjoy many new technologies, but many of these procedures are more easily implemented with rats and mice than with humans. As a result, scientists seeking research funds and acceptance from respected colleagues rationalize the use of rodents as a useful model for many forms of human mental illness.

One problem with this strategy is that there is no experimental manipulation with mice that could simulate the effects of being an economically disadvantaged member of an ethnic minority who is rejected by peers, a child with illiterate parents, or a parent who believes she was responsible for her child's current difficulties.

Fourth, investigators tend to ignore the transitions that occur between the presence of a particular genome and a specific symptom profile. There is a transition between the genome and the usual brain state it creates, between that tonic state and the brain state created by an incentive, between the induced brain state and a conscious feeling, between the feeling and a private interpretation, and between the interpretation and a behavioral symptom. Because a certain level of indeterminism is added at each transition, due to local conditions, the probability that a particular symptom will accompany a specific genome is quite low. The proportion of women possessing the risk genes for breast cancer is far larger than the proportion who develop a breast tumor. Most low-pressure regions that form off the east coast of Africa do not develop into hurricanes that strike the Gulf coast of the United States. Thus, materialism, a reluctance to blame the victim, powerful biological techniques that can be used more effectively with animals than with humans, and denying the transitions between genes and psychological states over the course of development all tend to create the current imbalance in the study of the causes of and cures for human psychopathology.

Obviously, the current emphasis on the biological contribution has considerable value. But it has two serious disadvantages. It fails to raise public consciousness over the contributions of the many adults and peers whose interactions with a particular child can place that youth at risk for pathology. Second, this frame of mind motivates a single-minded approach to finding risk genes and drug cures for all disorders and fails to motivate clinicians to consider combining medicines with strategies that might alter the child's circumstances. Every river is capable of becoming polluted and losing its capacity to sustain life. However, ecologists do not attribute an inherent flaw to a river that has become polluted. Rather, they urge changes in the practices of industry and agriculture that are the root causes of the pollution. Psychiatrists and psychologists should adopt a similar strategy with mood and character disorders.

The current Zeitgeist among molecular biologists and like-minded psychiatrists and psychologists is too friendly to a view of causality, reminiscent of Leibniz, which assumes that certain genetically mediated brain states automatically provoke particular mental states. Clinicians and scientists should be more receptive to Newton's argument that an apple falls from a tree when the gravitational force on the apple exceeds that of the force that holds the fruit to the branch on which it rests (Hall, 1980). It is useful to reflect on the fact that the civilizations of the Near and Far East had, during the 17th century, access to the first telescopes and were aware of Galileo's discoveries. But because Galileo's conclusions and views of nature were inconsistent with the varied philosophical premises held by these societies, their scholars did not take advantage of this new technology and the natural sciences failed to progress in these cultures. Similarly, as late as 1936 many eminent neurophysiologists were so committed to an electrical basis for all neuronal activity they resisted acknowledging that chemicals could mediate synaptic transmission in the brain, even though Otto Loewi had demonstrated that fact in the 1920s (Valenstein, 2005). An unquestioned loyalty to dogma exacts a stiff price.

## REFERENCES

Adamec, R. E., Blundell, J., & Burton, P. (2005). Neural circuit changes mediating a lasting bias and behavioral response to predator stress. *Neuroscience and Biobehavioral Reviews, 29,* 1225–1241.

Arbelle, S., Benjamin, J., Golin, M., Kremer, I., Belmaker, R. H., & Ebstein, R. P. (2003). Relation of shyness in grade school children to the genotype for the long form of the serotonin transporter promoter region polymorphism. *American Journal of Psychiatry, 160,* 671–676.

Arcus, D., & Kagan, J. (1995). Temperament and craniofacial variation in the first two years. *Child Development, 66,* 1529–1540.

Asendorpf, J. B. (1989). Shyness as a final pathway for two different kinds of inhibition. *Journal of Personality and Social Psychology, 57,* 481–492.

Asendorpf, J. B. (1991). Development of inhibited children's coping with unfamiliarity. *Child Development, 62,* 1460–1474.

Austin, M. C., Rhodes, J. L., & Lewis, D. A. (1997). Differential distribution of corticotropin-releasing hormone immunoreactive axons in monoaminergic nuclei of the human brainstem. *Neuropsychopharmacology, 17,* 326–341.

Baas, M. P., Milstein, J., Donlevy, M., & Grillon, C. (2006). Brainstem correlates of defensive states in humans. *Biological Psychiatry, 59,* 588–593.

Bartels, M., van den Oord, E. J., Hudziak, J. J., Rietveld, M. J., van Beijsterveldt, C. E., & Boomsa, D. I. (2004). Genetic and environmental mechanisms underlying stability and change in problem behaviors at ages 3, 7, 10 and 12. *Developmental Psychology, 40,* 852–867.

Bates, J. E. (1989). Concepts and measures of temperament. In J. A. Kohnstamm, J. E. Bates, & M. K. Rothbart (Eds.), *Temperament and childhood* (pp. 3–26). New York, NY: Wiley.

Battaglia, M., Ogliari, A., Zanoni, A., Citterio, A., Pozzoli, U., Giorda, R., et al. (2005). Influence of the serotonin transporter promoter gene and shyness on children's cerebral responses to facial expressions. *Archives of General Psychiatry, 62,* 85–94.

Beauchaine, T. P., Neuhaus, E., Brenner, S. L., & Gatzke-Kopp, L. (2008). Ten good reasons to consider biological processes in prevention and intervention research. *Development and Psychopathology, 20,* 745–774.

Beauchaine, T. P., Neuhaus, E., Zalewski, M., Crowell, S. E., & Potapova, N. (in press). The effects of allostatic load on neural systems subserving motivation, mood regulation, and social affiliation. *Development and Psychopathology.*

Bethea, C. L., Streicher, J. M., Coleman, K., Pau, F. K., Moessner, R., & Cameron, J. L. (2004). Anxious behavior and fenfluramine-induced prolactin secretion in young rhesus macaques with different alleles of the serotonin reuptake transporter polymorphism (5HTTLPR). *Behavior Genetics, 34,* 295–307.

Biederman, J., Hirshfeld-Becker, D. R., Rosenbaum, J. F., Herot, C., Friedman, D., Snidman, N., et al. (2001). Further evidence of association between behavioral inhibition and social anxiety in children. *American Journal of Psychiatry, 158,* 1673–1679.

Blackford, J. U., Allen, A., Cowan, R. L., & Avery, S. N. (2010). *Failure of amygdala and hippocampus to habituate to novel faces is associated with inhibited temperament in young adults.* Unpublished manuscript, Vanderbilt University.

Blackhart, G. C., Minnix, J. A., & Kline, J. P. (2006). Can EEG asymmetry patterns predict future development of anxiety and depression? *Biological Psychology, 72,* 46–60.

Bowlby, J. (1969). *Attachment* (Vol. I of Attachment and loss). New York, NY: Basic Books.

Bowlby, J. (1973). *Separation-anxiety and anger* (Vol. II of Attachment and Loss). New York, NY: Basic Books.

Bowlby, J. (1980). *Loss: Sadness and depression* (Vol. III of Attachment and loss). New York, NY: Basic Books.

Brandao, M. L., Coimbra, N. C., & Osaki, M. Y. (2001). Changes in the auditory-evoked potentials induced by fear-evoking stimulation. *Physiology and Behavior, 72,* 365–372.

Brendgen, M., Wanner, B., Morin, A. J. S., & Vitaro, F. (2005). Relations with parents and with peers, temperament, and trajectories of depressed mood during early adolescence. *Journal of Abnormal Child Psychology, 33,* 579–594.

Buss, K. A. (2011). Which fearful toddlers should we worry about? *Developmental Psychology, 47,* 804–819.

Cameron, O. G. (2002). *Visceral sensory neuroscience.* New York, NY: Oxford University Press.

Caspi, A., Sugden, K., Moffitt, T. E., Taylor, A., Craig, I. W., Harrington, H., et al. (2003). Influence of life stress on depression: moderation by a polymorphism in the 5-HTT gene. *Science, 301,* 386–389.

Chavira, D. A., Stein, M. B., & Malcarne, V., L. (2002). Scrutinizing the relationship between shyness and social phobia. *Journal of Anxiety Disorders, 16,* 585–598.

Colman, I., Wadsworth, M. E. J., Croudace, T. J., & Jones, P. B. (2007). Forty-year psychiatric outcomes following assessment for internalizing disorder in adolescence. *American Journal of Psychiatry, 164,* 126–133.

Cox, B. J., MacPherson, P. S., & Enns, M. W. (2005). Psychiatric correlates of childhood shyness in a nationally representative sample. *Behavior Research and Therapy, 43,* 1019–1027.

Davey, G. C., McDonald, A. S., Hirisave, U., Prabhu, G. G., Iwawaki, S., Jim, C. I., et al., (1998). A cross-cultural study of animal fears. *Behaviour Research and Therapy, 36,* 735–50.

Davidson, R. J. (2003). Right frontal brain activity, cortisol, and withdrawal behavior in 6-month-old infants. *Behavioral Neuroscience, 117,* 11–20.

Davidson, R. J., Jackson, D. L., & Kalin, N. H. (2000). Emotion, plasticity, context, and regulation. *Psychological Bulletin, 126,* 890–909.

Degnan, K. A., Hane, A. A., Henderson, H. A., Moas, O. L., Reeb-Sutherland, B. C., & Fox, N. A. (2011). Longitudinal stability of temperamental exuberance and social-emotional outcomes in early childhood. *Developmental Psychology, 47,* 765–780.

Diekelmann, S., Wilhelm, I., Wagner, U., & Born, J. (2011). Elevated cortisol at retrieval suppresses false memories in parallel with correct memories. *Journal of Cognitive Neuroscience, 23,* 772–781.

Eley, T. C. (2011). The interplay between genes and environment in the development of anxiety and depression. In K. S. Kendler, S. R. Jaffee, & D. Romer (Eds.), *The dynamic genome and mental health* (pp. 229–254). New York, NY: Oxford University Press.

Eley, T. C., Sugden, K., Corsico, A., Gregory, A. M., Shaw, P., McGuffin, P., et al. (2004). Gene-environment interaction analysis of serotonin system markers with adolescent depression. *Molecular Psychiatry, 9,* 908–915.

Fitzgerald, D. A., Angstadt, M., Jelsone, L. M., Nathan, P. J., & Phan, K. L. (2006). Beyond threat. *Neuroimage, 30,* 1441–1448.

Foland-Ross, L. C., Altshuler, L. L., Bookheimer, S. Y., Lieberman, M. D., Townsend, J., Penfield, C., et al. (2010). Amygdala responsivity in healthy adults is correlated with prefrontal cortical thickness. *Journal of Neuroscience, 30,* 16673–16678.

Fox, N. A., Calkins, S. D., & Bell, M. A. (1994). Neural plasticity and development in the first two years of life. *Development and Psychopathology, 6,* 677–696.

Fox, N. A., Henderson, H. A., Marshall, T. J., Nichols, K. E., & Ghera, M. N. (2005). Behavioral inhibition: Linking biology and behavior within a developmental framework. In S. Fiske, A. Kazdin, & D. Schacter (Eds.), *Annual Review of Psychology, 56,* 235–262.

Gladstone, G. L., & Parker, G. B. (2006). Is behavioral inhibition a risk factor for depression? *Journal of Affective Disorders, 95,* 85–94.

Golimbet, V. E., Gritsenko, I. K., Alfimova, M. V., & Ebstein, R. P. (2005). Polymorphic markers of the dopamine D4 receptor gene promoter region and personality traits in mentally healthy individuals from the Russian population. *Genetika, 41,* 966–972.

Hall, A. R. (1980). *Philosophers at war.* New York, NY: Cambridge University Press.

Hallowell, A. I. (1941). The social function of anxiety in a primitive society. *American Sociological Review, 6,* 869–891.

Hartl, D., & Jones, E. W. (2005). *Genetics* (6th ed.). Sudbury, MA: Jones & Bartlett.

Hill, S. Y., Tessner, K., Wang, S., Carter, H., & McDermott, M. (2010). Temperament at 5 years of age predicts amygdale and orbitofrontal volume in the right hemisphere in adolescence. *Psychiatry Research: Neuroimaging, 182,* 14–21.

Hinton, D. E., Pich, V., Safren, S. A., Pollack, M. H., & McNally, R. J. (2005a). Anxiety sensitivity in traumatized Cambodian refugees. *Behavioral Research and Therapy, 43,* 1631–1643.

Hinton, D. E., Pich, V., Chhean, D., Pollack, M. H., & McNally, R. J. (2005b). Sleep paralysis among Cambodian refugees: Association with PTSD diagnosis and severity. *Depression and Anxiety, 22,* 47–51.

Hoehn-Saric, R., Lee, J., McLeod, D., & Wong, D. (2005). Effect of worry on regional cerebral blood flow in nonanxious subjects. *Psychiatry Research: Neuroimaging, 140,* 259–269.

Hoekstra, H. E., Hirschmann, R. J., Bundey, R., Insel, P., & Crossland, J. (2006). A single amino acid mutation contributes to adaptive beach mouse color pattern. *Science, 313*, 101–104.

Irizarry, Y., & Galbraith, S. J. (2004). Complex disorders reloaded: Causality, action, reaction, cause and effect. *Molecular Psychiatry, 9*, 431–432.

Kagan, J. (1994). *Galen's prophecy.* New York, NY: Basic Books.

Kagan, J. (2011). Three lessons learned. *Perspectives on Psychological Science, 6*, 107–113.

Kagan, J. (2012). *Recalcitrant ghosts.* New Haven, CT: Yale University Press.

Kagan, J., & Saudino, K. J. (2001). Behavioral inhibition and related temperaments. In R. N. Emde & J. K. Hewitt (Eds.), *Infancy and early childhood* (pp. 111–122). New York, NY: Oxford University Press.

Kagan, J., & Snidman, N. (2004). *The long shadow of temperament.* Cambridge, MA: Harvard University Press.

Kagan, J., Snidman, N., Kahn, V., & Towsley, S. (2007). The preservation of two infant temperaments into adolescence. *Monographs of the Society for Research in Child Development, 72*, 1–75.

Kanayama, G., & Pope, H. G. (2011). Gods, men, and muscle dysmorphia. *Harvard Review of Psychiatry, 19*, 95–98.

Karg, K., Burmeister, M., Shedden, K., & Sen. S. (2011). The serotonin transporter promoter variant (5-HTTLPR), stress, and depression. *Archives of General Psychiatry, 68*, 444–454.

Kashdan, T. B., & Steger, M. F. (2006). Expanding the topography of social anxiety. *Psychological Science, 17*, 120–128.

Kaufman, J., Yang, B. Z., Douglas-Palumberi, H., Houssyar, S., Lipschitz, D., Krystal, J. H., et al. (2004). Social supports and serotonin transporter gene modulate depression in maltreated children. *Proceedings of the National Academy of Sciences, 101*, 17316–17321.

Kaufman, J., Yang, B. Z., Douglas-Palumberi, H., Grasso, D., Lipschitz, D., Houshyar, S., et al., (2006). Brain-derived neurotrophic factor-5HTTLPR gene interactions and environmental modifiers of depression in children. *Biological Psychiatry, 59*, 673–680.

Kelly, O., McIntosh, J., McIntyre, D., Merali, Z., & Anisman, H. (2003). Anxiety in rats selectively bred for fast and slow kindling rates: Situation-specific outcomes. *Stress, 6*, 289–295.

Kirsch, P. Esslinger, C., Chen, Q., Mier, D., Lis, S., Siddhanti, S., et al. (2005). Oxytocin modulates neural circuitry for social cognition and fear to humans. *Journal of Neuroscience, 49*, 11489–11493.

LaGasse, L., Gruber, C., & Lipsitt, L. P. (1989). The infantile expression of avidity in relation to later assessments. In J. S. Reznick (Ed.), *Perspectives on behavioral inhibition* (pp. 159–176). Chicago, IL: University of Chicago Press.

Lahti, J., Raikkonen, K., Ekelund, J., Peltonen, Raitakari, O. T., & Keltikangas-Jarvinen, L. (2006). Socio-demographic characteristics moderate the association between DRD4 and novelty seeking. *Personality and Individual Differences, 40*, 533–543.

Lakatos, K., Nemoda, Z., Birkas, E., Ronai, Z., Kovacs, E., Ney, K., et al. (2003). Association of D4 dopamine receptor gene and serotonin transporter promoter polymorphism with infants' response to novelty. *Molecular Psychiatry, 8,* 90–98.

Larsen, M. B., Sonders, M. S., Mortensen, O. V., Larson, G. A., Zahniser, N. R., & Amara, S. G. (2011). Dopamine transport by the serotonin transporter. *Journal of Neuroscience, 31,* 6605–6615.

McDougall, W. (1908). *Introduction to social psychology.* London, United Kingdom: Methuen.

McHugh, P. R. (2008). *Try to remember.* Washington, DC: Dana Press.

Mian, N. D., Wainwright, L., Briggs-Gowan, M. J., & Carter, A. S. (2011). An ecological risk model for early childhood anxiety. *Journal of Abnormal Child Psychology, 39,* 501–512.

Mick, M. A., & Telch, M. J. (1998). Social anxiety and history of behavioral inhibition in young adults. *Journal of Anxiety Disorders, 12,* 1–20.

Moretto, G., Ladavas, E., Mattioli, F., & di Pellegrino, G. (2010). A psychophysiological investigation of moral judgment after ventromedial prefrontal damage. *Journal of Cognitive Neuroscience, 22,* 1888–1899.

Netter, P. (2006). Dopamine challenge tests as an indicator of psychological traits. *Human Psychopharmacology, 21,* 91–99.

Pape, H. C., & Stork, O. (2003). Genes and mechanisms in the amygdala involved in the formation of fear memory. *Annals of the New York Academy of Sciences, 985,* 92–105.

Pickett, K. E., & Wilkinson, R. G. (2010). Inequality: An underacknowledged source of mental illness and disorder. *British Journal of Psychiatry, 197,* 426–428.

Pitkanen, A. (2000). Connectivity of the rat amygdaloid complex. In J. P. Aggleton (Ed.), *The amygdala* (2nd ed.). New York, NY: Oxford University Press.

Prior, M., Smart, D., Sanson, A., & Oberklaid, F. (2000). Does shy-inhibited temperament in childhood lead to anxiety problems in adolescence? *Journal of the American Academy of Child and Adolescent Psychiatry, 39,* 461–468.

Raczka, K. A., Gartmann, N., Mechias, M., Reif, A., Buchel, C., Deckert, J., et al. (2010). A neuropeptide S receptor variant associated with over-interpretation of fear. *Molecular Psychiatry, 15,* 1067–1074.

Rich, G. J. (1928). A biochemical approach to the study of personality. *Journal of Abnormal and Social Psychology, 23,* 158–179.

Rotge, J. Y., Grabot, D., Aouizerate, B., Pelissolo, A., Lepine, J. P., & Tignol, J. (2011). Childhood history of behavioral inhibition and comorbidity status in 256 adults with social phobia. *Journal of Affective Disorders, 129,* 338–341.

Rothbart, M. K. (1989). Temperament in childhood. In J. A. Kohnstamm, J. E. Bates, & M. K. Rothbart (Eds.), *Temperament in childhood* (pp. 59–76). New York, NY: Wiley.

Schienle, A., Schafer, A., Hermann, A., Walter, B., Stark, R., & Vaitl, D. (2006). fMRI responses to pictures of mutilation and contamination. *Neuroscience Letters, 393,* 174–178.

Schmidt, L. A. (2008). Patterns of second-by-second resting frontal brain (EEG) asymmetry and their relation to heart rate and temperament in 9-month-old human infants. *Personality and Individual Differences, 44,* 216–225.

Schmidt, L. A., Fox, N. A., Schulkin, J., & Gold, P. W. (1999). Behavioral and psychophysiological correlates of self-presentation in temperamentally shy children. *Developmental Psychobiology, 35*, 119–135.

Schneirla, T. C. (1959). An evolutionary and developmental theory of biphasic processes approach and withdrawal. In M. R. Jones (Ed.), *Nebraska symposium on motivation* (pp. 1–44). Lincoln, NE: University of Nebraska Press.

Schultz, W. (2006). Reward and addiction. In S. T. Fiske, A. E. Kazdin, & D. L. Schacter (Eds.), *Annual Review of Psychology, 57*, 87–116.

Schwartz, C. E., Kunwar, P. S., Greve, D. N., Moran, L. R., Viner, J. C., Covino, J. C., et al. (2010). Structural differences in adult orbital and ventromedial prefrontal cortex predicted by infant temperament at 4 months of age. *Archives of General Psychiatry, 67*, 1–9.

Schwartz, C. E., Kunwar, P. S., Greve, D. N., Kagan, J., & Snidman, N. C. (in press). A phenotype of early infancy predicts reactivity of the amygdale in male adults. *Molecular Psychiatry.*

Scott, J. P., & Fuller, J. (1965). *Genetics and the social behavior of the dog*. Chicago, IL: University of Chicago Press.

Segalowitz, S. J., Santesso, D. L., Willoughby, T., Relker, D. L., Campbell, K., Chalmers, H., et al. (2011). Adolescent peer interaction and trait surgency weaken medial prefrontal cortex response to failure. *Social Cognitive and Affective Neuroscience.*

Stefanacci, L., & Amaral, D. G. (2002). Some observations on cortical input for the macaque amygdala. *Journal of Comparative Neurology, 451*, 301–323.

Stein, M. B., Fallin, M. D., Schork, N. J., & Gelernter, J. (2005). COMT polymorphisms and anxiety-related personality traits. *Neuropsychopharmacology, 30*, 2092–2102.

Sundet, J. M., Skre, I., Okkenhaug, J. J., & Tambs, K. (2003). Genetic and environmental causes of the interrelationships between self-reported fears. A study of a non-clinical sample of Norwegian identical twins and their families. *Scandinavian Journal of Psychology, 44*, 97–106.

Sussman, A., & Ha, J. (2011). Developmental and cross-situational stability in infant pigtailed macaque temperament. *Developmental Psychology, 47*, 781–791.

Uher, R., Caspi, A., Houts, R., Sugden, K., Williams, B., Poulton, R., et al. (2011). Serotonin transporter gene moderates childhood maltreatment's effect on persistent but not single episode depression. *Journal of Affective Disorders, 132*, 112–120.

Valenstein, E. S. (2005). *The war between the soups and the sparks*. New York, NY: Columbia University Press.

Volbrecht, M. M., & Goldsmith, H. H. (2010). Early temperament and family predictors of shyness and anxiety. *Developmental Psychology, 46*, 1192–1205.

Welborn, B. L., Papademetris, X., Reis, D. L., Rajeevan, N., Bloise, S. M., & Gray, J. R. (2009). Variation in orbitofrontal cortex volume. *Social, Cognitive and Affective Neuroscience, 4*, 328–339.

Werner, E., & Smith, R. S. (1982). *Vulnerable but invincible*. New York, NY: McGraw-Hill.

Wirtschafter, D. (2005). Cholinergic involvement in the cortical and hippocampal Fos expression induced in the rat by placement in a novel environment. *Brain Research, 1051*, 57–65.

Xin, Z., Zhang, L., & Liu, D. (2010). Birth cohort changes of Chinese adolescents' anxiety. *Personality and Individual Differences, 48,* 208–212.

Yeh, T. L., Lee, I. H., & Chen, K. L. (2009). The relationships between life events and the availability of serotonin transporters and dopamine transporters in healthy volunteers. *Neuroimage, 45,* 275–279.

Young, L., Bechara, A., Tranel, D., Damasio, H., Hauser, M., & Damasio, A. (2010). Damage to ventromedial prefrontal cortex impairs judgment of harmful intent. *Neuron, 25,* 845–851.

# CHAPTER 8

# Beyond Allostatic Load

## The Stress Response System as a Mechanism of Conditional Adaptation

BRUCE J. ELLIS, MARCO DEL GIUDICE, AND ELIZABETH A. SHIRTCLIFF

## HISTORICAL CONTEXT

THE STRESS RESPONSE SYSTEM (SRS) has a central role in orchestrating physical and psychosocial development of both human and nonhuman species (Ellis, Jackson, & Boyce, 2006; Korte, Koolhaas, Wingfield, & McEwen, 2005). For many organisms, the SRS contributes crucially to responding flexibly to environmental opportunities and challenges. One of the most remarkable features of the SRS is the wide range of individual variation in physiological parameters. Some respond quickly and strongly even to minor events, whereas others show flat response profiles across situations. Furthermore, the balance of activation among primary SRS subsystems—the sympathetic nervous system (SNS), the parasympathetic nervous system (PNS), and limbic-hypothalamic-pituitary-adrenal (LHPA) axis—can vary considerably across individuals.

It is difficult to overstate the real-world relevance of such individual variability. Decades of research demonstrate not only that physiological patterns of stress responsivity constitute a primary integrative pathway through which *psychosocial environmental factors* are transmuted into the behavioral, autonomic, and immunologic manifestations of human pathology (reviewed in Boyce & Ellis, 2005), but also that patterns of stress responsivity regulate variation in a wide range of adaptive processes and behaviors including (but not limited to) growth and metabolism, reproductive status and fertility, aggression and risk taking, pair bonding and caregiving, and memory and learning (reviewed in Del Giudice, Ellis, & Shirtcliff, 2011). Clearly, understanding the causes of such individual differences and their development over the life course has important implications for medicine, psychology, and psychiatry, among other disciplines.

One approach has been to view individual differences in stress reactivity through a pathology lens. Indeed, a common assumption in the stress literature is that there is an optimal level of stress responsivity and that overly heightened or dampened SRS reactivity is dysfunctional and tends to undermine emotional and behavioral regulation (e.g., Evans & English, 2002). This purported biological dysregulation of the SRS is typically interpreted in an allostatic load framework (e.g., Juster, McEwen, & Lupien, 2010), whereby wear and tear of chronic stress is presumed to impair SRS functioning (see extended discussion below).

This allostatic load model (ALM) has recently been promoted in a double Special Issue of *Development and Psychopathology* (Cicchetti, 2011). In this chapter, however, we argue that enthusiasm for the ALM may have been overstated. Specifically, we contend that the ALM has strengths, but also serious limitations when evaluated from the vantage point of evolutionary biology; that the ALM does not address the role of allostasis in regulating adaptive developmental plasticity; that, in most instances, the core metaphor of "stress dysregulation" could usefully be replaced by "adaptive calibration" of SRS parameters; and that explicit modeling of biological fitness trade-offs, as instantiated in life history theory (LHT), is needed to more fully explain the complex relations between developmental exposures to stress, stress responsivity, behavioral strategies, and health. As an alternative to the ALM, we present the adaptive calibration model of stress responsivity (ACM; Del Giudice et al., 2011). We begin by reviewing the concepts of adaptive calibration and miscalibration more generally. We then summarize key ACM concepts and discuss their implications for developmental psychopathology. We conclude by comparing the ALM and ACM explicitly and suggest that it is time for the field to move beyond the ALM perspective.

## CONDITIONAL ADAPTATION AND MALADAPTATION

A large body of scientific work has sought to explain the relations between developmental exposures to stress, stress responsivity, behavioral strategies, and health. Unfortunately, this work has been hampered by patchy, inconsistent, and sometimes confusing usage of the concepts of adaptation and maladaptation. Here we attempt to define and explain these concepts from an evolutionary–developmental perspective.

### CONDITIONAL ADAPTATION

Developmental exposures to stress have always been part of the human experience. For example, almost half of children in hunter-gatherer societies—the best model for human demographics before the agricultural revolution—die before reaching adulthood (Kaplan & Lancaster, 2003). Thus, from an evolutionary–developmental perspective, stressful rearing conditions, even if those conditions engender sustained stress responses that must be maintained over time, should not so much impair SRS functioning ("dysregulation" in the ALM) as direct or regulate it toward response patterns that are adaptive under stressful conditions, even if those patterns are harmful in terms of the long-term welfare of the individual or society as a whole (e.g., Ellis, Boyce, Belsky, Bakermans-Kranenburg, & van Ijzendoorn, 2011; Mead,

Beauchaine, & Shannon, 2010). From an evolutionary perspective, there is no optimal level of stress responsivity; adaptation is context-specific.

Consider the extensive experimental work conducted by Michael Meaney and colleagues showing that putatively low quality maternal care in the rat (i.e., low levels of maternal licking and grooming) alters pups' stress physiology and brain morphology. Although such changes seem disadvantageous (i.e., higher corticosterone levels, shorter dendritic branch lengths, and lower spine density in hippocampal neurons), they actually enhance learning and memory processes under stressful conditions (e.g., Champagne et al., 2008). Moreover, such physiological and morphological changes mediate the effects of maternal behavior on central features of defensive and reproductive strategies: behavior under threat, open-field exploration, pubertal development, sexual behavior, and parenting (Cameron et al., 2005, 2008).

In total, enhanced learning under stressful conditions, increased fearful and defensive behaviors, accelerated sexual maturation, increased sexual behavior, and reduced parental investment in offspring apparently represent strategic—that is, functional—ways of developing when the young organism is relatively neglected. In such contexts, neglect itself can be regarded as a behavioral mechanism through which rat parents guide their offspring's development toward optimal survival and reproductive strategies under conditions of adversity. It would seem mistaken, therefore, to view diminished licking and grooming as "poor maternal care" or the development induced by such care as "disturbed," even though this is how they are often characterized. From an evolutionary perspective, altered care provided by parents may be appropriate preparation of their offspring for expected ecological conditions.

Accordingly, the evolutionary perspective emphasizes *conditional adaptation*: "evolved mechanisms that detect and respond to specific features of childhood environments, features that have proven reliable over evolutionary time in predicting the nature of the social and physical world into which children will mature, and entrain developmental pathways that reliably matched those features during a species' natural selective history" (Boyce & Ellis, 2005, p. 290; for a comprehensive treatment of conditional adaptation, see West-Eberhard, 2003). From this perspective, variation in SRS functioning results largely from individuals tracking different environmental conditions and altering their SRS profiles to match those conditions. Presumably, this matching process promoted fitness—survival and ultimately reproduction—across heterogeneous environmental contexts over human evolution.

However, an evolutionary history of exposure to such heterogeneous contexts, in which the fitness of different phenotypes varied across time and/or space, is a necessary but not sufficient condition for the evolution of conditional adaptations. The fitness of the alternative phenotypes must also be predictable on the basis of reliable cues that can be observed by the individual (Pigliucci, 2001). For example, tadpoles (*rana sylvatica*) alter their size and shape based on the presence of dragonfly larvae in their rearing environment (Van Buskirk & Relyea, 1998). These alterations involve development of smaller and shorter bodies and deep tail fins. Although tadpoles that do not undergo these morphological changes are highly vulnerable to predation by dragonflies, those that do but end up inhabiting environments that are not shared with dragonflies have relatively poor developmental and survival outcomes. In short, the predator-induced phenotype is only conditionally adaptive. This process highlights that in many cases, natural selection favors a primary phenotype that yields high payoffs under favorable circumstances and a secondary phenotype that "makes the best of a bad situation" (West-Eberhard, 2003).

## THE MEANING OF ADAPTIVE

The foregoing discussion highlights that the term *adaptive* has different meaning when viewed from evolutionary and mental health perspectives (see also Ellis et al., 2012; Mead et al., 2010). Because evolution by natural selection is driven by differences among individuals in reproductive success, the evolutionary significance of any behavior, or its "adaptive value," depends ultimately on its costs and benefits with respect to the organism's fitness (i.e., the contribution of offspring to future generations by an individual and its relatives). Even high-risk behaviors that result in net harm in terms of a person's own phenomenology and well-being (e.g., producing miserable feelings or a shortened life), the welfare of others around them, or the society as a whole, can still be *adaptive* in an evolutionary sense. Consider, for example, risky behaviors that expose adolescents to danger and/or inflict harm on others but increase dominance in social hierarchies and leverage access to mates (Ellis et al., 2012). On the other hand, from a mental health perspective, different patterns of behavior are regarded as "adaptive versus maladaptive" depending on the extent to which they promote versus threaten people's health, development, and safety. Adaptive developmental outcomes are thus equated with "desirable" outcomes (as defined by dominant Western values; e.g., health, happiness, secure attachment, high self-esteem, emotion regulation, educational and professional success, stable marriage), whereas maladaptive developmental outcomes are equated with "undesirable" outcomes constituting the opposite poles of these traits and variables. For the remainder of this paper, we use "adaptive" only in the evolutionary sense of the term. In contrast, the word *desirable* is used to connote adaptiveness from a mental health perspective.

## MALADAPTATION

The converse of adaptation is maladaptation. Biological maladaptation can occur for many reasons. Sometimes, an evolved mechanism ceases to perform its intended function because of, for example, harmful genetic mutations, accidents, or manipulation by other organisms (e.g., pathogens). Even when biological mechanisms perform normally, an organism may develop a phenotype that is poorly suited for its environment and as a consequence experiences a diminution in fitness (often accompanied by other "undesirable" outcomes). Thus, maladaptation is closely connected to the concept of developmental miscalibration or mismatch (see Frankenhuis & Del Giudice, 2012, for an extended discussion). There are a number of causes of such developmental miscalibration or mismatch. First, an individual may experience novel environments that are outside the range recurrently encountered over evolutionary history. In this case, all developmental bets are off and the person may experience abnormal outcomes. For example, Romanian or Ukrainian orphanages (Dobrova-Krol, Van IJzendoorn, Bakermans-Kranenburg, & Juffer, 2010; Nelson et al., 2007) constitute genuinely substandard, novel environments that are beyond the normative range of conditions encountered over human evolution. Children's brains and bodies simply could not have responded adaptively to collective rearing by paid, custodial, nonkin caregivers with minimal human contact (Hrdy, 1999). Exposures to such challenging and (evolutionarily) unprecedented conditions are likely to induce pathological development, not evolutionarily adaptive strategies.

Second, individuals may become maladapted to their environments because of a lack of behavioral plasticity. As discussed later, one of the responsivity profiles highlighted by the ACM is the unemotional pattern, which is characterized by low susceptibility to environmental influence (i.e., dampened physiological stress reactivity), which generally inhibits social learning and sensitivity to social feedback. One hypothesized pathway here is a genetic disposition toward hypoarousal of stress systems. Such a disposition could translate into a wide distribution of unemotional phenotypes across a range of familial and ecological conditions, including supportive and well-resourced rearing environments. Maladaptation may occur in this context because unemotional phenotypes are not susceptible to environmental influence and thus may not adjust their behavioral strategies to match the high levels of support and resources available to them (e.g., they may not adequately detect positive opportunities and learn to capitalize on them, such as seeing a teacher as a prospective mentor or taking advice from a loving parent; and/or they may develop a manipulative, antagonistic social strategy when trust and cooperation would better fit their social context). In total, increased probability of mismatch is a clear cost of low developmental plasticity.

Third, mismatch can occur because the validity of environmental cues that guide conditional adaptation is limited spatially, so such cues become invalid in other contexts. For example, according to LHT, children's brains and bodies tend to respond to dangerous or unpredictable environments by growing up fast and "living for the here and now" (e.g., Belsky, Steinberg, & Draper, 1991; Ellis, Schlomer, Figueredo, & Brumbach, 2009). This "get it while you can" strategy often translates into high-risk activities such as early initiation of sexual behavior, greater numbers of sexual partners, infrequent contraceptive use, delinquency, substance use, violence, and risky driving. These high-risk behaviors may only be locally adaptive, however. The research of Gibbons et al. (2012) on African American males is instructive in this context. Youth who were exposed to greater stress while growing up (e.g., more dangerous neighborhoods, lower quality parental investment, greater racial discrimination) developed "fast" life history strategies that may have been adaptive in their local context (e.g., participation in risky behaviors that leveraged positions in dominance hierarchies, increased access to mates) but clearly undesirable—and probably biologically maladaptive—in the wider U.S. society (e.g., dropping out of school, high rates of arrest and incarceration).

Fourth, mismatch can occur because the validity of environmental cues that guide conditional adaptation is temporally limited, so that those cues may become invalid at later times. One hypothesis is that individuals calibrate to environmental parameters early in life, even prenatally. When these values differ from those experienced later in life, normative processes of developmental plasticity can become maladaptive, resulting in a mismatched phenotype with increased likelihood of physical health problems (e.g., Gluckman, Low, Buklijas, Hanson, & Beedle, 2011). For instance, prenatal exposure to undernutrition may result in the development of metabolic processes designed to retain and store insulin and fatty acids (Barker, 1994). However, if resources are plentiful in the postnatal environment, the individual may be at increased risk for obesity and metabolic syndrome throughout life. This hypothesis is supported by data showing that detrimental effects seem absent when the postnatal environment continues to be lacking in resources (Stanner & Yudkin, 2001), suggesting that mismatch (rather than undernutrition) may be the root cause.

Finally, mismatch can occur due to a restricted range of niches that undermine the ability of organisms to choose environments that match their phenotypes. For example, in a study of semi-free ranging rhesus macaques (Boyce, O'Neill-Wagner, Price, Haines, & Suomi, 1998), the troop lived in a 5-acre wooded habitat in rural Maryland, on the grounds of the National Institutes of Health Primate Center. In 1993, the troop encountered a 6-month period of protective confinement to a small, 1,000-square-foot building, during a construction project on the habitat grounds. The confinement proved highly stressful, however, and the incidence of violent injuries increased fivefold during the 6-month period. During this period, when behavioral strategies available to troop members were severely curtailed, monkeys who had been previously characterized as high in biobehavioral reactivity to stress suffered dramatically higher rates of violent injuries than their less reactive peers. In the free-ranging wooded habitat, however, where a wide range of behavioral strategies could be employed, including escape from conflict, highly reactive monkeys suffered comparatively low rates of violent injury.

In summary, processes of conditional adaptation and phenotype-environment matching are fallible, and a number of circumstances can lead to maladaptation. Understanding this set of circumstances is critical to understanding the developmental origins of psychopathology.

## FUNCTIONS OF THE STRESS-RESPONSE SYSTEM

Environmental events signaling threats to survival or well-being produce a set of complex, highly orchestrated responses within the neural circuitry of the brain and peripheral neuroendocrine pathways regulating metabolic, immunologic, and other physiological functions. The SRS comprises primarily three anatomically distinct neuroendocrine circuits: the sympathetic (SNS) and parasympathetic (PNS) branches of the autonomic nervous system and the LHPA axis. Activity of these circuits is integrated and cross-regulated, so that they can be considered as partially independent yet interrelated components of a single functional system despite their anatomical and physiological diversity (e.g., Boyce & Ellis, 2005; Porges, 1995; Schlotz et al., 2008).

The general function of the PNS is to promote vegetative functions and reduce physiological arousal (see Del Giudice et al., 2011; Porges, 2007). However, when a stressor is encountered, the PNS responds quickly by withdrawing this inhibitory influence (Lovallo & Sollers, 2007), allowing the SNS to operate unopposed, thereby causing rapid increases in physiological arousal. More extreme defense reactions associated with "freeze/hide" behaviors also involve PNS activation, albeit via different efferent fibers (Porges, 2007). If parasympathetic deactivation is not sufficient to cope with the present challenge, activation of the SNS occurs within 20 to 30 seconds, providing a second layer of response in this hierarchy. Sympathetic activation mediates fight/flight responses and is coordinated by the locus coeruleus-norepinephrine (LCNE) system. SNS activation follows a fast, direct pathway via the noradrenergic innervation of visceral organs and a slower, hormonal pathway through innervation of the adrenal medulla (see, e.g., Goldstein & Kopin, 2008; Gunnar & Vazquez, 2006). Following SNS activation, the adrenal medulla secretes epinephrine (E) and smaller quantities of norepinephrine (NE) to increase heart rate, respiration, blood supply to skeletal muscles, and glucose release in the bloodstream.

The third component of the SRS is the LHPA axis, which mounts a delayed, long-term response to environmental challenges. The end point of the LHPA response is cortisol release by the adrenal cortex, typically within 5 minutes after the triggering event, with a cortisol peak between 10 and 30 minutes. The effects of cortisol secretion may be observed for several hours or more (Sapolsky, Romero, & Munck, 2000). Cortisol binds to nuclear receptors and regulates gene transcription. Its main effects are to (1) mobilize physiological and psychological resources (e.g., energy release, alertness and vigilance, memory sensitization; e.g., Flinn, 2006; Van Marle, Hermans, Qin, & Fernández, 2009), and (2) counter-regulate physiological effects of SNS activation, facilitating stress recovery (Munck, Guyre, & Holbrook, 1984). The joint effects of the SNS and LHPA axis are complex (Hastings et al., 2011), and can be synergistic (especially in the short term) or antagonistic (especially at later phases of responding).

## BIOLOGICAL SENSITIVITY TO CONTEXT

The foregoing summary of the SRS is a widely accepted description of how peripheral neuroendocrine responses prepare the organism for challenge or threat. However, according to the theory of Biological Sensitivity to Context (BSC; Boyce & Ellis, 2005), these "stress response" systems also function to increase susceptibility to resources and support in the ambient environment (e.g., positive social opportunities, cooperative information; see also Porges, 1995, 2007). This dual function signified the need to conceptualize stress reactivity more broadly as biological sensitivity to context, which Boyce and Ellis (2005) defined as neurobiological susceptibility to both cost-inflicting and benefit-conferring features of the environment and operationalized as a biological property indexed by heightened reactivity in one or more of the stress response systems (PNS, SNS, LHPA). Depending on levels of nurturance and support versus harshness and unpredictability in their developmental environments, highly reactive children experience either the best or the worst of psychiatric and biomedical outcomes within the populations from which they are drawn (reviewed in Ellis et al., 2011). BSC theory therefore posits that individual differences in the magnitude of biological stress responses function to regulate openness or susceptibility to environmental influences, ranging from harmful to protective (see Sijtsema et al., in press, for a review and critical analysis of BSC assumptions).

Given past evidence that early trauma increases stress reactivity and newer evidence that high reactivity may enhance developmental functioning in highly supportive settings, Boyce and Ellis (2005) postulated a curvilinear, U-shape relation between levels of early support-adversity and the magnitude of biological response dispositions. Specifically, we hypothesized that (1) exposure to acutely stressful childhood environments up-regulates BSC, increasing the capacity and tendency of individuals to detect and respond to environmental dangers and threats; (2) exposure to especially supportive childhood environments also up-regulates BSC, increasing susceptibility to social resources and support; and (3) by contrast, and typical of the majority of children, exposure to childhood environments that are not extreme in either direction down-regulates BSC, buffering individuals against the chronic stressors encountered in a world that is neither highly threatening nor consistently safe. Exploratory analyses in two studies offered confirmatory evidence that the lowest rates of high reactivity phenotypes were found in conditions of moderate stress and that both tails of the support-adversity distribution were associated with higher proportions of reactive children (Ellis, Essex, & Boyce, 2005; see also Bush, Obradovic, Adler, & Boyce, 2011; Gunnar, Frenn, Wewerka, & Van Ryzin, 2009).

Although BSC theory has moved the field toward a new conceptualization of stress responsivity, it has a number of significant limitations. First, BSC theory does not systematically link the different stress reactivity patterns to functional variation in behavior, such as individual differences in social and reproductive behaviors that are specified by LHT. Second, although BSC theory advances a general developmental prediction (the U-shape curve), it does not model the developmental trajectories leading to individual differences in a more fine-grained way (e.g., by discussing the development of stress responsivity at different life stages and identifying "switch points" when plasticity is preferentially expressed). Third, BSC does not address the adaptive meaning and developmental origins of sex differences in responsivity. Fourth, BSC focuses on explaining heightened reactivity to stress and does not afford a theory of hypoarousal (or dampened reactivity), in terms of its development or functional significance. Fifth, BSC does not address the development or functions of basal (tonic) levels of activity of the SRS. Finally, BSC theory does not advance discriminative predictions regarding PNS, SNS, and LHPA. The ACM, an extension and refinement of BSC, was formulated to address these issues.

## The Adaptive Calibration Model of Stress Responsivity

Goals of the ACM are to provide (1) a coherent, systematic account of the biological functions of the SRS; (2) an evolutionary-developmental theory of individual differences capable of explaining adaptation—and maladaptation—of stress physiology and behavior to local environmental conditions; and (3) a functionally valid taxonomy of stress response profiles, including neurobiological correlates (e.g., serotonergic function), behavioral correlates (e.g., aggression, self-regulation), and developmental trajectories, which integrates across baseline activity and responsivity measures of the SRS (Del Giudice et al., 2011). Achieving these goals would enable scientists to move beyond the purely inductive theory-building that now dominates the field and increase their ability to advance targeted hypotheses about individual differences and their development. The ACM has its main theoretical foundations in LHT, an evolutionary biological framework for describing the developmental "decisions" of organisms and their allocation of resources over the life course (Ellis et al., 2009; Kaplan & Gangestad, 2005), and the theory of adaptive developmental plasticity (West-Eberhard, 2003). In the ACM, individual differences in the functioning of the SRS are thought to result largely (though not exclusively) from the operation of evolved mechanisms that match the individual's physiology and behavior to local environmental conditions (i.e., calibration to the environment). Thus, patterns of stress responsivity are seen as *adaptive* in the biological sense, as they function in a way that ultimately tends to maximize the individual's survival and reproduction.

The ACM can be summarized in seven points (see Del Giudice et al., 2011, for complete explication of the model):

1. The SRS has three main biological functions: to coordinate the organism's allostatic response to physical and psychosocial challenges; to encode and filter information from the environment, thus mediating the organism's openness to environmental inputs; and to regulate a range of life history-relevant traits and behaviors.

2. The SRS works as a mechanism of conditional adaptation, regulating the development of alternative life history strategies (i.e., suites of reproductively relevant traits such as sexual maturation, intrasexual competitive behaviors and risk taking, and patterns of mating and parenting). Different patterns of baseline activity and responsivity in early development modulate differential susceptibility to environmental influence and shift susceptible children on alternative pathways, leading to individual differences in life history strategies.

3. Activation of the SRS during the first years of life provides crucial information about life history-relevant dimensions of the child's environment, namely, danger and unpredictability (see Ellis et al., 2009). This information is used to adaptively regulate stress responsivity and associated development of life history strategies.

4. At a general level, a nonlinear relation exists between exposures to environmental stress during development and optimal levels of stress responsivity (see Figure 8.1). This nonlinear relation can be characterized by a taxonomy of four prototypical responsivity patterns (labeled sensitive [I], buffered [II], vigilant [III], and unemotional [IV]). The four patterns constitute combinations of physiological parameters indexing functioning of the PNS, SNS, and LHPA axis (see Figure 8.1 and Table 8.1) and include neurobiological indicators,

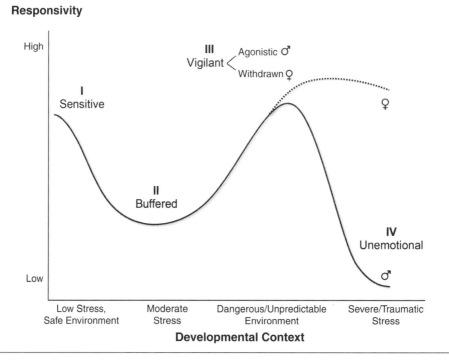

**Figure 8.1** The Adaptive Calibration Model of individual differences in development of stress responsivity.

At a general level, a nonlinear relation exists between exposures to environmental stress and support during development and optimal levels of stress responsivity. Although this nonlinear relation is specified for the stress response system (SRS; see Table 8.1), it may apply to other neurobiological systems as well. The figure does not imply that all components of the SRS will show identical responsivity profiles, nor that they will activate at the same time or over the same time course. Male/female symbols indicate sex-typical patterns of responsivity, but substantial within-sex differences in responsivity are expected as well. From Del Giudice et al. (2011).

**Table 8.1**
Predicted Physiological Profiles of the Four Responsivity Patterns

| | | Responsivity patterns | | | |
|---|---|---|---|---|---|
| | | I | II | III | IV |
| Physiological profile | | **Sensitive** | **Buffered** | **Vigilant** | **Unemotional** |
| PNS | responsivity | High | Moderate | Low/moderate | Low* |
| | basal | High | Moderate | Low | Low |
| SNS | responsivity | High/moderate | Low/moderate | High | Low* |
| | basal | Moderate | Low/moderate | High | Low |
| HPA | responsivity | High | Moderate | High | Low |
| | basal | Moderate | Moderate | High/moderate | Low |

*Unemotional individuals may display autonomic activation when faced with immediate physical threats and during agonistic confrontations, in contrast with their general pattern of unresponsivity to nonagonistic stressors.

From Del Giudice et al. (2011).

behavioral outcomes, and developmental trajectories. Note that environment-responsivity relations need not be the same for all the components of the SRS (see Table 8.1 for detailed predictions).

5. Sensitive and vigilant individuals display relatively high responsivity to the environment, whereas buffered and unemotional individuals display relatively low responsivity. Although comparisons between the two patterns of high responsivity (sensitive vs. vigilant) and the two patterns of low responsivity (buffered vs. unemotional) show substantial *convergence* in SRS baseline activity and responsivity (Table 8.1 and Figure 8.1), there is marked *divergence* in both antecedent environmental conditions and behavioral outcomes.

6. Because of sex differences in optimal life history strategies, sex differences are expected in the distribution of responsivity patterns and in their specific behavioral correlates. Sex differences should become more pronounced at increasing levels of environmental stress; in particular, contexts characterized by severe/traumatic stress should favor the emergence of a male-biased pattern of low responsivity (the unemotional pattern) and a female-biased pattern of high responsivity (the vigilant-withdrawn pattern).

7. Pre- and early postnatal development, the transition from early to middle childhood, and puberty are likely "switch points" for the calibration of stress responsivity. Individual and sex differences in the functioning of the SRS are predicted to emerge according to the evolutionary function of each developmental stage.

## ENVIRONMENTAL INFORMATION

One of the crucial functions of the SRS is to collect and integrate information about changing states in the environment (including the presence of threats, dangers, and opportunities) to adjust the state of the whole organism accordingly. This information can be encoded by the SRS and, in the long run, provides the organism with a statistical "summary" of key dimensions of the environment. In the ongoing process of physiological adjustment, the system's level of responsivity acts as an amplifier (when highly responsive) or filter (when unresponsive) of various types of contextual information. In this section we consider this function of the SRS in more detail, and take a closer look to the ecological information that can be encoded through repeated SRS activation.

### KEY DIMENSIONS OF THE ENVIRONMENT

Life history theory is a general framework for understanding biological trade-offs involved in development, such as those between growth and reproduction, current and future reproduction, and quality and quantity of one's offspring. According to LHT (Charnov, 1993; Stearns, 1992), variation in life history traits results from trade-offs in distribution of resources to competing life functions: bodily maintenance, growth, and reproduction. Due to structural and resource limitations, organisms cannot maximize all components of fitness simultaneously and instead are selected to make trade-offs that prioritize resource expenditures, so that greater investment in one domain occurs at the expense of investment in competing domains. For example, resources spent on an inflammatory host response to fight infection cannot be spent on reproduction. Thus, the benefits of an inflammatory host response are traded off against the costs of lower fertility. Each trade-off constitutes a decision node in allocation of resources, and each decision node influences the next decision node (opening up some options, foreclosing others) in an unending chain over the life course (Ellis et al., 2009).

Most important for the present discussion, LHT can be used to predict how organisms adjust their developmental trajectories according to variable ecological conditions. The key dimensions of the environment relevant to life history development are availability of resources, level of unavoidable danger (or, more precisely, extrinsic morbidity-mortality rate), and predictability of environmental change. Energetic resources—caloric intake, energy expenditures, and related health conditions—set the baseline for development, slowing growth and delaying sexual maturation and reproduction under energetic stress (i.e., favoring a "slow" life history strategy). When energetic resources are adequate, cues of extrinsic morbidity-mortality and unpredictability gain importance (Ellis et al., 2009). Given adequate bioenergetic resources to support growth and development, individuals should detect and respond to proximal cues of danger (e.g., exposures to violence, harsh childrearing practices) and unpredictability (e.g., stochastic changes in ecological context, economic conditions, family composition, parental behavior) by entraining faster life history strategies (see Belsky, Schlomer, & Ellis, 2012; Simpson, Griskevicius, Kuo, Sung, & Collins, 2012, for supporting longitudinal data). Fast life history strategies are comparatively high risk (taking benefits opportunistically with little regard for long-term consequences), focusing on mating opportunities (e.g., competitive risk taking, aggression), reproducing at younger ages, and producing a greater number of offspring with more variable outcomes. As discussed later, trade-offs incurred by the fast strategy include reduced health, vitality, and longevity—of self and offspring.

The SRS is attuned exquisitely to the life history-relevant features of the environment. Of particular interest, the level of extrinsic morbidity-mortality is conveyed both by frequent SNS activation (signaling a potentially dangerous ecology) and by repeated LHPA activation. Because it responds strongly to uncontrollable challenges and novel situations, the LHPA axis also encodes information about environmental unpredictability/uncontrollability, thus giving LHPA functioning a central role in the regulation of life history strategies (see Del Giudice et al., 2011). Across development, environmental information collected by the SRS (in interaction with the child's genotype) canalizes physiological and behavioral phenotypes to match local ecological contexts.

## The SRS as an Information Filter/Amplifier

If the SRS encodes environmental information as a statistical aggregation of repeated responses to challenge, it follows that SRS responsivity can function as an information filter. Low SRS responsivity results in a number of potential costs (e.g., reduced alertness, reduced sensitivity to social feedback) and potential benefits (e.g., resource economization, avoidance of immune suppression). A highly responsive SRS, by contrast, amplifies the signal coming from the environment and maximizes the chances that the organism will be modified by current experience. Potential costs of a highly responsive system include adverse physiological events, hypersensitivity to social feedback, and exposure to psychological manipulation. In addition, the organism's action plans can get interrupted easily by minor challenging events, and the ability to deal with future events may be reduced if physiological resources are already overwhelmed. On the other hand, a highly responsive system facilitates social learning and social bonding, enhances mental activities in localized domains, focuses attention, and primes memory storage, thus tuning cognitive processes to opportunities and threats in the environment.

Empirical studies (e.g., Pruessner et al., 2010) illustrate how SRS thresholds for responding to environmental stimuli differ dramatically from one person to another. It is also intriguing that such thresholds may show domain-specificity, as when challenges related to competition or achievement are more salient for males, but challenges related to social exclusion or rejection are more salient for females (Stroud et al., 2009; Stroud, Salavey, & Epel, 2002). Individual differences in the functional parameters of the SRS depend on complex causal chains across genetic, epigenetic, and neuroendocrine levels. Close social relationships can also filter/amplify more distal environmental factors, such as when cortisol reactivity is suppressed in the presence of a warm, supportive caregiver (e.g., Fries, Shirtcliff, & Pollak, 2008).

Although ACM terminology tends to emphasize the role of responsivity, components of the SRS operate at both state (situation-specific) and trait (basal) levels. Basal functioning indicates a level of physiological preparedness or anticipation of the individual's context (Pruessner et al., 2010), exerting a permissive effect on the individual's ability to respond to novel events and encode environmental information (e.g., Gunnar & Quevedo, 2007). It may also provide a rough index of the physiological accumulation of prior stressful events. High basal SRS activity is expected when the individual anticipates or needs to be engaged, aroused, or active in that context. High basal activation of the PNS promotes calm, concentration, and self-regulation (e.g., Fabes & Eisenberg, 1997; Porges, 2007), whereas high SNS baseline relates to anxiety (El-Sheikh, Erath, Buckhalt, Granger, & Mize, 2008), and baseline cortisol secretion regulates energy mobilization and engagement with the physical and social environment (Booth, Granger, & Shirtcliff, 2008). This role of the SRS in relation to anticipation is emphasized, for example, in an extensive literature demonstrating high cortisol in contexts characterized by unpredictability (Dickerson & Kemeny, 2004). Empirical findings that cortisol levels elevate prior to laboratory arrival (e.g., Ellis et al., 2005; Hastings et al., 2011) or in anticipation of challenges of the day (e.g., Fries, Dettenborn, & Kirschbaum, 2009; Schmidt-Reinwald et al., 1999) further bolster the interpretation that basal SRS activity serves an anticipatory or preparatory function.

Over time, repeated SRS responses to environmental challenges may accumulate so that state-specific activity patterns become part of the individual's trait-like functional parameters (Shirtcliff, Granger, Booth, & Johnson, 2005). Basal functioning of the SRS achieves set-points that calibrate the individual's physiology with the expected environmental demands, but as the environment changes, so, too, may the optimal set-point (McEwen & Wingfield, 2003). This implicates one of the most important functions of the SRS: to change according to anticipated or current context, using those changes to optimize physiological functioning for the expected future conditions.

## IMPLICATIONS FOR DEVELOPMENTAL PSYCHOPATHOLOGY

Looking at the SRS through the lens of information filtering and encoding provides useful insights into the developmental processes that ultimately lead to psychopathological outcomes. First, and foremost, this reconceptualization of the functioning of the SRS as a mechanism of susceptibility to environment influence (Boyce & Ellis, 2005) helps to explain the bivalent effects of stress responsivity on mental and physical health, whereby highly reactive children experience either the best or the worst of psychiatric and biomedical outcomes depending on levels of stress and support encountered over development (see earlier, BSC). A radical implication of this theory is that the very children whose heightened responsivity appears to make them vulnerable to developing psychopathology may also be most able to benefit from positive, supportive environments and interventions. For example, consider the results of two studies of naturally occurring environmental adversities and stress reactivity as predictors of respiratory illnesses in 3- to 5-year-old children (Boyce et al., 1995). Results revealed, first, that children showing low cardiovascular or immune reactivity to stressors had approximately equal rates of respiratory illnesses in both low and high adversity settings. Second, and consistent with the prevailing ALM of developmental psychopathology, highly biologically reactive children exposed to high adversity child care settings or home environments had substantially higher illness incidences than all other groups of children. The third finding, however, was that highly reactive children living in lower adversity conditions—that is, more supportive child care or family settings—had the *lowest* illness rates, significantly lower than even low reactivity children in comparable settings, supporting a BSC interpretation. Thus, the very qualities that appear to increase children's frailties may also be their strength, given supportive contexts, thus inspiring the metaphor of "orchid children" (Boyce & Ellis, 2005).

In addition, LHT delineates basic dimensions of environmental stress and support—underscoring resource availability, morbidity-mortality risk, and unpredictability as key dimensions of the environment that regulate development of SRS responsivity patterns and their behavioral correlates (see the next section). This has already proven to be a valuable tool in empirical research (e.g., Belsky et al., 2012; Simpson et al., 2012), given the confusing abundance of environmental/contextual variables that might be measured and correlated with developmental outcomes. Furthermore, LHT provides organizing principles needed to understand the broad network of interactions between the SRS and other physiological response systems, such as the immune system (see Miller, Chen, & Parker, 2011).

Another important implication of the concepts reviewed in this section is that both high- and low SRS responsivity can be adaptive precisely because they modulate the organism's openness to environmental information. As discussed earlier, there is no optimal level of responsivity; rather, the value of high versus low informational openness varies depending on the local ecology, and in some cases an unresponsive system can be highly functional in the context of an individual's life history strategy. This idea is developed in the next section.

## PATTERNS OF RESPONSIVITY

The ACM builds on the theoretical principles outlined in the previous sections to derive a taxonomy of four prototypical responsivity patterns. Each pattern describes an integrated mode of SRS functioning, life history-relevant behavioral tendencies, and plausible neurobiological correlates. Three of the patterns correspond to regions on the U-shape curve of the BSC theory; the fourth pattern is a novel addition, and accounts for the development of hypoarousal in severely stressful conditions.

### THE LOGIC OF HYPOAROUSAL

Some individuals show a persistent pattern of markedly reduced SRS basal activity and responsivity, even following stimuli that elicit strong physiological reactions in most people. So-called hypoarousal or hyporesponsivity is reliably associated with externalizing behaviors, conduct disorders, and psychopathic traits (especially from middle childhood on; e.g., Ortiz, & Raine, 2004), which makes it especially interesting from the perspective of developmental psychopathology. Hypoarousal is usually treated as a sign of physiological dysregulation (e.g., Lupien et al., 2006); interestingly, chronic early adversity can lead to both hyper- and hyporesponsivity of the SRS (e.g., De Bellis et al., 1999; Gustafsson et al., 2010; Tarullo & Gunnar, 2006; Yehuda, 2002). The ACM suggests that dampened responsivity may actually follow an adaptive logic, as a way to maximize the fitness benefit/cost ratio in severely dangerous and unpredictable environments (see Gatzke-Kopp, 2011, for a similar account regarding dopaminergic responsivity). In moderately dangerous contexts, a responsive SRS enhances the individual's ability to react appropriately to dangers and threats while maintaining a high level of engagement with the social and physical environment. Moreover, engaging in fast life history strategies should lead the individual to allocate resources in a manner that discounts the long-term physiological costs of the stress response in favor of more immediate advantages. In this context, the benefits of successful defensive strategies outweigh the costs of frequent, sustained LHPA and SNS activation.

When danger becomes severe, however, engaging in high levels of risk taking (e.g., antagonistic competition, impulsivity, and extreme discounting of the future) can become the optimal response from an evolutionary perspective (see Ellis et al., 2012). Note that such strategies require outright *insensitivity* to threats, dangers, and social feedback. An unresponsive SRS has a higher threshold for letting environmental signals in: Many potential threats will not be encoded as such, and many potentially relevant events will fail to affect physiology to a significant degree. For an extreme risk taker, however, informational insulation from environmental signals of threat is an asset, not a weakness (see also Korte et al., 2005). In particular, adopting an exploitative/antisocial interpersonal style requires one to be shielded from social rejection, disapproval, and feelings of shame (all amplified by heightened LHPA responsivity). In summary, generalized low responsivity can be evolutionarily adaptive (i.e., fitness-maximizing) at the high-risk end of the environmental spectrum, despite the possible negative consequences for the social group and for the individual's subjective well-being. This type of chronic low responsivity should be carefully distinguished from temporary "exhaustion" periods, usually arising after prolonged SRS activation in highly responsive individuals exposed to enduring stressors (Miller, Chen, & Zhou, 2007).

## THE LOGIC OF SEX DIFFERENCES

In sexually reproducing species, the two sexes differ predictably on life history–related dimensions. They are thus expected to employ different strategies in response to the same environmental cues (e.g., Geary, 2002; James, Ellis, Schlomer, & Garber, 2012). In mammals, including humans, males tend to engage in higher mating effort and lower parental effort than females (Geary, 2002; Kokko & Jennions, 2008; Trivers, 1972). In addition, males usually undergo stronger sexual selection; that is, their reproductive success is more variable than that of females, leading to higher risk propensity (Trivers, 1972; see also Frankenhuis & Del Giudice, 2012). The extent of sex differences in life history–related behavior, however, is not fixed but depends in part on the local environment.

At the slow end of the life history continuum, both sexes tend to engage in high parental investment, and male and female interests largely converge on long-term, committed pair bonds; sex differences in behavior are thus expected to be relatively small. As environmental danger and unpredictability increase, males benefit by shifting to low-investment, high-mating strategies; females, however, do not have the same flexibility since they benefit much less from mating with multiple partners and incur higher fixed costs through childbearing. Thus, male and female strategies should diverge increasingly at moderate to high levels of danger/unpredictability. In addition, sexual competition takes different forms in males and females, with males engaging in more physical aggression and substantially higher levels of risk-taking behavior. As life history strategies become faster, sexual competition becomes stronger, and sex differences in competitive strategies become more apparent.

For these reasons, sex differences in responsivity patterns and in the associated behavioral phenotypes should be relatively small at low to moderate levels of environmental stress, and increase as the environment becomes more dangerous and unpredictable. In particular, males should be more likely to develop unresponsive phenotypes in highly stressful contexts. Also, the behavioral correlates of both high and low responsivity in dangerous environments can be expected to differ between the sexes. As we discuss later, we do not expect sex differences in responsivity to be present from birth, but rather to emerge gradually during development.

267 Beyond Allostatic Load 267

## THE FOUR ACM PATTERNS

It is now possible to present a brief outline of the four ACM patterns (see Del Giudice et al., 2011, for a detailed description). Each pattern represents a stable configuration of SRS activity. Later, we discuss developmental pathways leading to establishment of these configurations.

*Sensitive pattern (Type I).* Sensitive patterns are hypothesized to develop in safe, predictable conditions and warm, family environments. High stress responsivity in sensitive individuals increases their openness to social and physical environments. Physiological profiles of those with this pattern (high LHPA and PNS responsivity, moderate SNS responsivity) favor sustained but flexible attention and sensitivity to social feedback. Sensitive individuals are reflective, self- and other-conscious, and engaged with the environment. They are high in inhibitory control, delay of gratification, and executive function. These traits promote sustained learning and cooperation. Other plausible correlates are high serotonergic function and slow sexual maturation.

*Buffered pattern (Type II).* Buffered patterns are predicted to develop preferentially in conditions of moderate environmental stress, where they strike a balance between costs and benefits of responsivity. Compared to Type III and IV patterns, buffered individuals should be lower in anxiety, aggression, and risk taking.

*Vigilant pattern (Type III).* Vigilant patterns develop in stressful contexts, where they enable people to cope effectively with dangers and threats in the physical and social environment. Their SNS-dominated physiological profile mediates heightened attention to threats and high trait anxiety. Increased SRS responsivity in dangerous environments can be expected to go together with increased responsivity in other neurobiological systems. For example, hyperdopaminergic function may contribute to the vigilant phenotype by boosting attention to threat-related cues and fast associative learning (Gatzke-Kopp, 2011). In the ACM, vigilance is not associated with a single behavioral pattern, but rather with a *distribution* of patterns involving different mixtures of aggressive/externalizing ("fight") and withdrawn/internalizing ("flight") behaviors. In males, vigilant responsivity should be associated more often with increased risk taking, impulsivity, agonistic social competition, and reactive aggression (the vigilant-agonistic subtype). In females, the typical pattern should involve social anxiety and fearful/withdrawn behavior (the vigilant-withdrawn subtype). Vigilant children who display high levels of both agonistic and withdrawn behaviors (typically females; Zahn-Waxler et al., 2006) may be best described as belonging to a third subtype, the vigilant-agonistic/withdrawn pattern.

*Unemotional pattern (Type IV).* Unemotional patterns are marked by a profile of low stress responsivity, with the possible exception of strong autonomic responses when facing immediate physical threats. Generalized unresponsivity inhibits social learning and sensitivity to social feedback; it can also increase risk taking by blocking information about dangers and threats in the environments. Predicted correlates of this pattern are low empathy and cooperation, impulsivity, competitive risk taking, and antisocial behavior, including high levels of proactive/instrumental aggression, especially in males. Based on LHT, the distribution of Type IV is expected to be male-biased, and its behavioral correlates are expected to differ between sexes.

For example, one key feature of unemotional responsivity in females may be a generalized pattern of aloof social relationships with parents, siblings, and peers. Low serotonergic and dopaminergic activity are likely neurobiological correlates of Type IV.

Preliminary empirical evidence supports the ACM taxonomy in children aged 8 to 10 years (Del Giudice, Hinnant, Ellis, & El-Sheikh, 2012), showing the presence of four major classes that provide a satisfactory match to the patterns described here. However, the sample size of this initial study is comparatively small; larger samples spanning a wider age range are needed to fully evaluate the ACM taxonomy, especially in view of the gradual emergence and consolidation of responsivity patterns and their distribution by sex (see next section).

## IMPLICATIONS FOR DEVELOPMENTAL PSYCHOPATHOLOGY

The logic sketched in this section has several implications for developmental psychopathology. First, it provides a functional account of hypoarousal that goes beyond "dysregulation," begins to explain why early adversity can have divergent outcomes (hyper- versus hypoarousal), and suggests that sex-related factors (such as sex hormones) may play an important role in determining the behavioral and physiological outcomes of early stress. Second, an evolutionary focus permits a better understanding of comorbidity patterns. For example, many superficially different traits and behaviors (e.g., aggression, early and promiscuous sexuality, substance abuse, reduced empathy) can be seen as manifestations of high-risk life history strategies that discount the future and increase mating effort. Consistent with this perspective, externalizing problems and precocious sexual behaviors in children not only covary, but also share many etiological factors (see Lévesque, Bigras, & Pauzé, 2010). Similarly, sex differences in the development of vigilant versus unemotional phenotypes may help to explain why girls show higher comorbidity between aggression and anxiety/depression: when exposed to highly stressful conditions, boys more than girls tend to develop an unemotional phenotype, characterized by high externalizing and low internalizing behaviors.

Finally, the ACM helps clarify complex relations between psychosocial environmental factors and stress responsivity patterns. Psychosocial stress and adversity over development can either up-regulate or down-regulate levels of SNS, PNS, and LHPA responsivity. The empirical literature on this topic remains highly conflicted: For every study linking stressful rearing experiences to hyperarousal (e.g., De Bellis et al., 1999; Essex, Klein, Cho, & Kalin, 2002; Yehuda, 2002), another study links such experiences to hypoarousal (e.g., Gunnar & Vazquez, 2006; Gustafsson et al., 2010; Tarullo & Gunnar, 2006). The ACM potentially explains both hyperarousal and hypoarousal by specifying nonlinear relations between environmental conditions and development of stress responsivity (Figure 8.1). According to the theory, developmental exposures to low- to moderate levels of stress either up-regulate (in the sensitive pattern) or down-regulate (in the buffered pattern) responsivity. Likewise, developmental exposures to high levels of stress either up-regulate (in the vigilant pattern) or down-regulate (in the unemotional pattern) responsivity.

Thus, if one considers the environment-responsivity curves shown in Figure 8.1, it is apparent that the results of any single study looking at linear statistical relationships can range from positive to null to negative, depending on the portion of the curve sampled in each case (Boyce & Ellis, 2005; Ellis et al., 2005). The many inconsistent results in the stress literature may depend, at least in part, on the failure to consider nonlinear relationships between environmental factors and SRS parameters, or the failure to assess the full range of environmental variance necessary to capture all four patterns of responsivity and associated behavioral strategies specified by the ACM.

## DEVELOPMENTAL PATHWAYS AND TRANSITIONS

Individual differences in stress responsivity are likely present prenatally, but patterns we described in the previous sections emerge as outcomes of long-term developmental processes. In these processes, the SRS collects environmental information and is shaped by that information, in a dynamic interplay with other key neurobiological systems. Developmental pathways are thus an integral aspect of the ACM, and they connect our model to a broader evolutionary theory of human development. Central to our discussion is the concept of a *developmental switch point*, the elementary unit in the development of plastic organisms.

### DEVELOPMENTAL SWITCH POINTS

West-Eberhard (2003) proposed that developmental change is coordinated by regulatory switch mechanisms, which serve as transducers (mediators) of genetic, environmental, and structural influences on phenotypic variation. These switch mechanisms control *developmental switch points*: "a point in time when some element of phenotype changes from a default state, action, or pathway to an alternative one—it is activated, deactivated, altered, or moved" (West-Eberhard, 2003, p. 67). This can involve a discrete structural change or a change in the rate of a process. Genetic and environmental inputs interact with phenotypic qualities to determine the functioning of regulatory switch mechanisms and influence their thresholds. Once a threshold is passed (i.e., the switch occurs), the regulatory mechanism coordinates expression and use of gene products and environmental elements that mediate the species-typical transition to the new phenotypic stage, as well as individually differentiated pathways within that stage. A concrete example of a switch-point in human development is puberty (see Ellis, 2011, for more details).

Critically, regulatory switch mechanisms provide a common locus of operations for genetic and environmental influences on phenotypic development; that is, these mechanisms are the vehicle through which gene-gene, environment-environment, and gene-environment interactions occur (see Chapter 3). These inputs structure the operation of regulatory switch mechanisms and may affect thresholds necessary for a developmental switch to occur and/or the organism's ability to cross that threshold (West-Eberhard, 2003). This is also the most crucial difference between a developmental switch point and a *sensitive* or *critical period*. A sensitive period is defined by increased susceptibility to environmental input, whereas a developmental switch point is marked by increased susceptibility to both environmental *and* genetic effects. For example, the activation of sex hormone-related biochemical pathways at puberty induces expression of genetic variation that was previously silent. This, in turn, creates new opportunities for gene-environment interactions, which may alter the direction of individual developmental trajectories.

## Stages and Transitions in Human Life History

Human life history can be described as a sequence of stages and transitions (Bogin, 1999). Life history strategies unfold progressively, according to the evolutionary function of each life stage. Del Giudice and Belsky (2011) proposed that the major switch points in human life history strategies occur during (a) pre- and early postnatal development, (b) the transition from early to middle childhood or *juvenile transition*, and (c) puberty. The juvenile transition (Del Giudice, Angeleri, & Manera, 2009) takes place at around 6 to 8 years in Western societies, and is marked by "adrenal puberty" or *adrenarche*, whereby the cortex of the adrenal glands begins to secrete increasing quantities of androgens, mainly dehydroepiandrosterone (DHEA) and its sulfate (DHEAS).

The onset of human juvenility (i.e., middle childhood) witnesses massive changes in children's social behavior, cognitive abilities, and the emergence or intensification of sex differences in aggression, attachment, play, language use, and so forth (reviewed in Del Giudice et al., 2009). In an evolutionary perspective, the main functions of juvenility are learning (including social and practical skills) and competition for status and social resources in the peer group. With the onset of puberty, sexual behavior and romantic attachment come to the forefront, and social competition further intensifies. Puberty affords another opportunity to revise one's life history strategy, depending for example on the success enjoyed—or the level of competition experienced—during juvenility.

## Developmental Pathways in the ACM

The development of stress responsivity begins prenatally, with interactions between fetal genes and maternal hormones (see Pluess & Belsky, 2011). The first years of life are also important because they provide the child with information about their local environment, both directly and indirectly through their parents' behavior. In this phase, high levels of stress are expected mainly to increase SRS responsivity (vigilant phenotypes), whereas moderate, repeated activation of the SRS leads to the development of buffered responsivity.

In the ACM, we argue that the juvenile transition is the first critical turning point in the development of stress responsivity. We predict that sex differences in responsivity patterns and their behavioral correlates should emerge from the beginning of middle childhood, with a further increase at puberty. Second, we expect individual changes in responsivity to be especially frequent in the transition from early to middle childhood, possibly driven by adrenal androgens. Some children (especially males) who grow up under conditions of severe stress may display a highly responsive profile in early childhood, then shift to low responsivity as social competition becomes a central developmental task. Thus, we expect a number of individuals—likely the most aggressive ones—to display a transition from Type III to Type IV during juvenility or adolescence. The development of unemotional responsivity may also follow a different pathway, dependent on strong genetic dispositions. In this pathway, unemotional traits may appear in childhood, even in low-stress environments (Del Giudice et al., 2011; see discussion earlier).

Finally, it is noteworthy that we predict sensitive patterns to develop in infants and young children who are emotionally labile initially and characterized by difficult or inhibited temperament. As they grow up in a protective environment, however, they may become less anxious, more stable emotionally, and more confident socially, possibly even more so than their temperamentally stable peers (reviewed in Ellis et al., 2011). At the physiological level, this shift is likely to be marked by increased PNS tone and responsivity (see Del Giudice et al., 2011).

## IMPLICATIONS FOR DEVELOPMENTAL PSYCHOPATHOLOGY

Much work needs to be done before we will achieve a principled, comprehensive description of developmental pathways, and many important details (for example, the mechanics of gene-environment interactions and epigenetic regulation) are yet to be filled in. However, we feel that our approach to human development has important heuristic advantages. At a general level, the life history perspective, with its emphasis on underlying trade-offs as explanations for manifest traits, is a natural framework for understanding equifinality and multifinality in development (Pickles & Hill, 2006), as well as the related issue of homotopic and heterotopic continuity (Costello & Angold, 2006). In a nutshell, the three main insights are that superficially similar behaviors may actually be serving different strategies (and reflect different patterns of responsivity); that the same strategy may require different behaviors at different times; and that the same feature of the environment may have very different biobehavioral implications for individuals engaging in different strategies with different cost-benefit balances.

Just as important, a biologically informed view of developmental stages and transitions provides content and specificity to the study of how stress exposure can have different effects according to its developmental timing (e.g., Ganzel & Morris, 2011). Also, empirical findings from developmental epidemiology (Costello & Angold, 2006) acquire more meaning when put in a proper evolutionary-developmental framework (see Del Giudice et al., 2009). As a specific example, the hypothesized transition from vigilant to unemotional patterns under the influence of adrenal androgens may explain the puzzling finding that externalizing and aggressive behavior are associated with high cortisol levels in preschoolers, but low cortisol levels from middle childhood on (Alink et al., 2008; Shirtcliff et al., 2005).

## ADAPTIVE CALIBRATION AND THE ALLOSTATIC LOAD MODEL

With the ACM we are seeking an integrative theoretical framework for the study of stress and stress responsivity across development. Presently, the main contender for this role is the allostatic load model (ALM; McEwen & Stellar, 1993). The ALM has become quite popular in developmental psychopathology (e.g., Beauchaine et al., 2011; Lupien et al., 2006), and in recent years researchers have started adopting it as a foundation for interdisciplinary integration (e.g., Ganzel, Morris, & Wethington, 2010; Juster et al., 2011). In this section, we review key points of convergence and divergence between the two models and explain why we consider the ACM to have many advantages and to be a more viable alternative in some important domains of inquiry.

### The Allostatic Load Model

The key concept of the ALM is that of allostasis, or "stability through change." Allostasis comprises processes through which an organism adapts to environmental challenges by modifying its regulatory parameters (e.g., by increasing or decreasing the set point of a homeostatic physiological mechanism). The term is typically used to describe the "moment to moment process of establishing a new homeostatic equilibrium in the face of challenge" (Ganzel & Morris, 2011, p. 956) or, stated differently, "how continuous reevaluation and readjustments create new set points that maximize the organism's resources (e.g., increased cardiac output when running)" (Juster et al., 2011, p. 727). Here allostasis enables accommodation to current stressors (Lupien et al., 2006). However, some authors (e.g., Beauchaine et al., 2011) restrict the meaning of allostasis to long-term, potentially permanent changes in the system's parameters in contexts of protracted stress—what McEwen and Wingfield (2003) labeled "allostatic states." The SRS is a crucial mediator of allostasis, though many other central and peripheral structures initiate and sustain allostatic responses (see Ganzel et al., 2010).

Allostatic load is a label for the costs of allostasis and is often described as the "wear and tear" that results from repeated allostatic adjustments, exposing the organism to adverse health consequences. The central tenet of the ALM is that the stress response is usually adaptive in the short term (i.e., acute stress responses mobilize biological resources that permit fight or flight responses that are normally protective against danger), but maladaptive and damaging in the long term (see Lupien et al., 2006; McEwen & Stellar, 1993). As eloquently stated by Juster et al. (2011, p. 725):

> Central to this biological damage is altered stress hormone functioning that inexorably strains interconnected biomarkers that eventually collapse like domino pieces trailing toward stress-related endpoints.

Among other adverse outcomes, allostatic load is thought to cause SRS dysregulation, resulting, for example, in excessive or insufficient responses to stressors and increasing the risk for psychopathology. The idea of physiological dysregulation is integral to the ALM, and both "hyperarousal" and "hypoarousal" are routinely described as dysfunctional deviations from the norm (e.g., Beauchaine et al., 2011; Juster et al., 2011; Lupien et al., 2006), usually caused by a combination of excessive stress exposure and genetic or epigenetic vulnerability.

## ACM VERSUS ALM

It should be noted at the outset that there are significant points of convergence between the ACM and the ALM. First, the ACM explicitly embraces the concept of allostasis and describes the coordination of allostatic responses as one of the main biological functions of the SRS. The ACM also acknowledges that chronic SRS activation does carry substantial costs, in terms of biological fitness as well as subjective well-being. Finally, whereas the ACM focuses on conditional adaptation, it leaves open the possibility that—for a number of reasons—some developmental outcomes are biologically maladaptive (see earlier discussion).

From an evolutionary standpoint, the biggest limitation of the ALM is that no distinction is made between the two meanings of "adaptive" (and maladaptive) described above: positive versus negative biological fitness outcomes, on the one hand, and desirable versus undesirable mental and physical health outcomes, on the other. Maladaptation is inferred whenever there are costs for the organism. For example, if elevated cortisol levels in children are associated with a negative outcome, such as reduced working memory, then elevated cortisol is classified as a marker of allostatic load (Juster et al., 2011). This reasoning ignores the crucial fact that biological processes are adaptive when their fitness benefits outweigh the costs, *not* when they are cost-free. As discussed earlier, even large costs can be offset by large enough expected benefits. For example, in dangerous and unpredictable environments, organisms often accept the risk of severe damage in exchange for a chance of improving their condition (see Ellis et al., 2012; Frankenhuis & Del Giudice, 2012). Similarly, when health and reproductive success conflict, natural selection favors the latter at the expense of the former (see Nesse, 2001).

Because of the failure to distinguish between (mal)adaptive and (un)desirable outcomes, most applications of the ALM do not address the trade-offs involved in the development of physiological and behavioral phenotypes; as a consequence, the ALM literature often lacks a theory of adaptive individual variation in stress responsivity (but see Korte et al., 2005, for a notable exception). Although the ALM is sophisticated in explaining the costs of allostasis, it only captures the short-term benefits of allostasis and does not consider the long-term benefits in terms of regulating conditional adaptation to varying environmental conditions. As a result, the development of enduring individual differences is usually traced to pathogenic processes.

In contrast, the ACM is built on life history theory, which is a theory of inherent trade-offs in the life cycle of organisms, and explicit consideration of these trade-offs is at the heart of the ACM taxonomy of responsivity patterns. For example, consider heightened SRS responsivity in vigilant patterns (Type III). In the ACM, it is hypothesized that the costs of repeated SRS activation are offset by improved management of danger. Although the system is on a hair trigger, with the resulting burden of anxiety and/or aggression, few instances of actual danger will be missed. In addition, engaging in a "fast," present-oriented life history strategy makes it optimal to discount the long-term health costs of chronic SRS activation if the immediate benefits are large enough (for in-depth discussion, see Del Giudice et al., 2011). In the ALM framework, the same pattern of responsivity would be treated as dysfunctional because the stress response is deployed even in absence of true dangers ("excessive" response, "unnecessary" triggering; see Beauchaine et al., 2011; Lupien et al., 2006) and because of the associated unpleasant states and health risks. This approach, however, fails to consider that natural defenses are usually designed by natural selection to accept a high rate of false positives (the so-called smoke detector principle; Nesse, 2005). Moreover, adaptive defenses, from environmentally triggered surges in catecholamines and glucocorticoids to development of fever in response to an infection, are often aversive, disabling, and occasionally harmful (or even fatal); but mistaking them for diseases because of these superficial features is a fallacy, though one that is exceedingly common in the psychopathology literature (see Nesse & Jackson, 2006).

A related point of divergence between the ACM and the ALM concerns responses to acute versus chronic stress. In the ALM, adaptive responses to acute stress are contrasted with the biological "wear and tear" caused by chronic stress and the resulting long-term modifications of SRS regulatory parameters. In the ACM, responses to both acute and chronic stress can be adaptive (though not cost-free); and, as a rule, the long-term adjustment of SRS parameters is seen as adaptive calibration rather than maladaptive dysregulation. Indeed, we anticipate that many of the allegedly "toxic" effects of chronic stress (e.g., its effects on immune function, brain physiology, memory, learning, and so forth) will ultimately find a better explanation as mediators of biological fitness trade-offs. In total, the ALM, relative to the ACM, overemphasizes the costs of allostasis and underappreciates its benefits.

For example, the ALM and ACM both recognize that childhood exposures to stress and adversity often result in physiological, cognitive, behavioral, and maturational changes in the developing organism (e.g., new SRS set points, elevated sensitivity to threat cues, attenuated delay of gratification, early puberty), and that over time these changes may mediate undesirable mental and physical health outcomes. From an evolutionary perspective, however, these outcomes reflect the costs of life history strategies—strategies instantiated in a chain of resource allocation decisions over the life course—that "make the best of a bad situation" by trading off survival for reproduction. According to the ACM, the SRS collects environmental information, is shaped by that information (allostasis), and uses it to adaptively match development of life history strategies to local conditions. Physiological, cognitive, behavioral, and maturational changes in response to environmental harshness and unpredictability function to accelerate life history strategies, shifting resource allocations toward more risky and aggressive behavior, earlier pubertal timing and sexual debut, less stable pair bonding, more children, and less parental investment per child (e.g., Ellis et al., 2009)—at the price of reduced health and longevity (i.e., allostatic load; see especially Allsworth, Weitzen, & Boardman, 2005). These biological fitness trade-offs are discussed further below.

## Implications for Developmental Psychopathology

The ALM and the concept of allostatic load have become remarkably popular in developmental psychopathology. Here we argue that the ALM has a number of limitations, and that the ACM provides researchers with a theory of stress responsivity that is broader and more consistent with the principles of evolutionary biology. We recognize that the ALM may be especially attractive because it conforms to the implicit assumptions of the standard mental health approach, particularly regarding stress-disease relationships, and therefore does not require any fundamental shift in thinking and logic. However, it also fails to deliver the insight and heuristic power of a modern evolutionary-developmental framework. In the long run, the field of developmental psychopathology may be better served by a model informed by life history theory, modeling of strategic trade-offs, and a more sophisticated consideration of the relations between adaptation, health, and well-being.

We believe that the ACM embodies the main insights of the ALM without sharing its limitations. Even more importantly, most of the work that is presently carried out under the ALM umbrella could be easily reframed in the perspective of the ACM. For example, the ACM taxonomy of responsivity patterns already contains predictions on likely neurobiological correlates such as dopaminergic, serotonergic, and noradrenergic function (Del Giudice et al., 2011). This makes the ACM a natural catalyst for the integrative work initiated by Beauchaine and colleagues (2011) and Ganzel and colleagues (2010). Similarly, the theory of developmental stages and switch points embodied in the ACM might serve as a detailed, biologically-grounded foundation for the analysis of the effects of stress exposure at different points in the life cycle (Ganzel et al., 2011).

Finally, the ACM addresses major anomalies in the field regarding complex relations between psychosocial environmental factors, stress responsivity, life history relevant traits and behaviors, and health. In the ALM, both hyperarousal and hypoarousal are considered indicators of stress dysregulation resulting from allostatic load, and the developmental pathways leading to systematic up-regulation versus down-regulation of SRS parameters are not theoretically modeled (rather, hyperarousal and hypoarousal are grouped together as dysfunctional deviations). We believe that this is a substantial limitation of the ALM. Valid explanatory models of the developmental pathways leading to both hyper- and hyporesponsivity are critical to explaining the development of psychopathology because both heightened and dampened responsivity can look either good or bad in terms of behavioral adjustment and health. Such bivalent effects of the SRS have been documented in SNS, PNS, and LHPA studies focusing on both baseline arousal and responsivity (e.g., Bauer, Quas, & Boyce, 2002; Burke, Davis, Otte, & Mohr, 2005; Evans & English, 2002).

A vast body of research has shown that children exposed to higher levels of psychosocial stress and adversity tend to develop more mental and physical health problems, and that these relations are often moderated by variation in stress responsivity. However, for every study showing that heightened stress reactivity operates as a *risk factor* that increases children's vulnerability to psychosocial stress (e.g., Boyce et al., 2006; Obradovic, Bush, & Boyce, 2011; Obradovic, Bush, Stamperdahl, Adler, & Boyce, 2010), another study shows that heightened stress reactivity operates as a *protective factor* that reduces children's vulnerability to psychosocial stress (e.g., Calkins & Keane, 2009; Degnan, Calkins, Keane, & Soderlund, 2008; El-Sheikh, Harger, & Whitson, 2001). The ACM potentially explains these anomalous findings by specifying two patterns of heightened stress reactivity (sensitive and vigilant phenotypes) and two patterns of dampened stress reactivity (buffered and unemotional phenotypes). Most importantly, each phenotype is characterized by different developmental histories and behavioral and health trajectories. Accordingly, *heightened* reactivity may look like a protective factor in sensitive phenotypes and a risk factor in vigilant phenotypes, while *dampened* reactivity may look like a protective factor in buffered phenotypes and a risk factor in unemotional phenotypes.

As discussed earlier, some people develop slower life history strategies characterized by later reproductive development and behavior. The slower strategy also involves greater allocation of resources toward enhancing growth, vitality, and long-term survival. By contrast, others develop faster strategies characterized by the opposite pattern. Because slower life history strategists, by definition, allocate more bioenergetic resources to somatic effort, meaning growth and maintenance of one's body (*soma* in Greek), life history theory predicts that they will generally experience better physical and mental health than will faster life history strategists, and more so as the life course progresses. This prediction has been supported by empirical research, both cross-sectional and longitudinal, showing that individuals who pursue faster life history strategies suffer from more mental health problems, medical ailments (e.g., thyroid disease, high blood pressure or hypertension, ulcers), and physical health symptoms (e.g., sore throat or cough, dizziness) (Brumbach, Figueredo, & Ellis, 2009; Figueredo, Vasquez, Brumbach, & Schneider, 2004; Sefcek & Figueredo, 2010). Furthermore, exposures to higher levels of psychosocial stress during childhood reliably predict the development of faster life history strategies in adolescence and beyond (reviewed in Ellis et al., 2009).

When viewed in the context of the ACM, these links between psychosocial stress, life history strategy, and health potentially explain why both heightened and dampened stress reactivity can either act as risk factors for or protective factors against psychiatric and biomedical disorder. Both sensitive phenotypes (↑ responsivity) and buffered phenotypes (↓ responsivity) are associated with lower levels of psychosocial stress and concomitant development of slower life history strategies (and thus better mental and physical health outcomes), whereas both vigilant phenotypes (↑ responsivity) and unemotional phenotypes (↓ responsivity) are associated with higher levels of psychosocial stress and concomitant development of faster life history strategies (and thus worse mental and physical health outcomes, especially in the long run).

# CONCLUSION

In this chapter we presented and elaborated an evolutionary-developmental theory of individual differences in stress responsivity—the ACM—that reorganizes many empirical findings from different research fields, weaves them together in a theoretically coherent manner, and advances novel and testable predictions about behavior, development, and neurobiology. Built explicitly on the foundation of modern evolutionary biology, the ACM provides a framework for research on stress and development that takes us beyond the ALM. We are not arguing that the ALM is *wrong* per se, nor that the extensive body of research documenting the negative effects of allostatic load on health is incorrect, but rather that the overemphasis of the ALM on the costs of allostasis weakens its conceptual power. The ALM does not address the adaptive role of allostasis in regulating developmental plasticity, which is the main objective—and strength—of the ACM. Because of their divergent focus and underlying assumptions, especially regarding adaptive calibration versus stress dysregulation, the ACM and ALM are only partially complementary. Nonetheless, conceptual differences between the two models should not be irreconcilable, and greater integration of the ACM and ALM in the future could potentially strengthen both approaches. Most relevant to the current volume, the ACM and ALM have rather different implications for understanding the development of psychopathology and, consequently, may support different intervention strategies.

# REFERENCES

Alink, L. R. A., van IJzendoorn, M. H., Bakermans-Kranenburg, M. J., Mesman, J., Juffer, F., & Koot, H. M. (2008). Cortisol and externalizing behavior in children and adolescents: Mixed meta-analytic evidence for the inverse relation of basal cortisol and cortisol reactivity with externalizing behavior. *Developmental Psychobiology, 50,* 427–450.

Allsworth, J. E., Weitzen, S., & Boardman, L. A. (2005). Early age at menarche and allostatic load: Data from the third national health and nutrition examination survey. *Annals of Epidemiology, 15,* 438–444.

Barker, D. (1994). *Mothers, babies, and disease in later life.* London, United Kingdom: BMJ.

Bauer, A. M., Quas, J. A., & Boyce, W. T. (2002). Associations between physiological reactivity and children's behavior: Advantages of a multisystem approach. *Journal of Developmental and Behavioral Pediatrics, 23,* 102–113.

Beauchaine, T. P., Neuhaus, E., Zalewski, M., Crowell, S. E., & Potapova, N. (2011). The effects of allostatic load on neural systems subserving motivation, mood regulation, and social affiliation. *Development and Psychopathology, 23,* 975–999.

Belsky, J., Schlomer, G. L., & Ellis, B. J. (2012). Beyond cumulative risk: Distinguishing harshness and unpredictability as determinants of parenting and early life history strategy. *Developmental Psychology, 48,* 662–673.

Belsky, J., Steinberg, L., & Draper, P. (1991). Childhood experience, interpersonal development and reproductive strategy: An evolutionary theory of socialization. *Child Development, 62,* 647–670.

Bogin, B. (1999). Evolutionary perspective on human growth. *Annual Review of Anthropology, 28,* 109–153.

Booth, A., Granger, D. A., & Shirtcliff, E. A. (2008). Gender- and age-related differences in the association between social relationship quality and trait levels of salivary cortisol. *Journal of Research on Adolescence, 18,* 239–260.

Boyce, W. T., Chesney, M., Alkon, A., Tschann, J. M., Adams, S., Chesterman, B., et al. (1995). Psychobiologic reactivity to stress and childhood respiratory illnesses: Results of two prospective studies. *Psychosomatic Medicine, 57,* 411–422.

Boyce, W. T., & Ellis, B. J. (2005). Biological sensitivity to context: I. An evolutionary-developmental theory of the origins and functions of stress reactivity. *Development and Psychopathology, 17,* 271–301.

Boyce, W. T., Essex, M. J., Alkon, A., Goldsmith, H. H., Kraemer, H. C., & Kupfer, D. J. (2006). Early father involvement moderates biobehavioral susceptibility to mental health problems in middle childhood. *Journal of the American Academy of Child and Adolescent Psychiatry, 45,* 1510–1520.

Boyce, W. T., O'Neill-Wagner, P., Price, C. S., Haines, M., & Suomi, S. J. (1998). Crowding stress and violent injuries among behaviorally inhibited rhesus macaques. *Health Psychology, 17,* 285–289.

Brumbach, B. H., Figueredo A. J., & Ellis, B. J. (2009). Effects of harsh and unpredictable environments in adolescence on development of life history strategies. *Human Nature, 20,* 25–51.

Burke, H. M., Davis, M. C., Otte, C., & Mohr, D. C. (2005). Depression and cortisol responses to psychological stress: A meta-analysis. *Psychoneuroendocrinology, 30,* 846–856.

Bush, N. R., Obradovic, J., Adler, N., & Boyce, W. T. (2011). Kindergarten stressors and cumulative adrenocortical activation: The "first straws" of allostatic load? *Development and Psychopathology, 23,* 1089–1106.

Calkins, S. D., & Keane, S. P. (2009). Developmental origins of early antisocial behavior. *Development and Psychopathology, 21,* 1095–1109.

Cameron, N. M., Champagne, F. A., Parent, C., Fish, E. W., Osaki-Kuroda, K., & Meaney, M. J. (2005). The programming of individual differences in defensive responses and reproductive strategies in the rat through variations in maternal care. *Neuroscience and Biobehavioral Review, 29,* 843–865.

Cameron, N. M., Del Corpo, A., Diorio, J., Mackallister, K., Sharma, S., & Meaney, M. J. (2008). Maternal programming of sexual behavior and hypothalamic-pituitary gonadal function in the female rat. *PLoS ONE, 3,* 1–12.

Champagne, D. L., Bagot, R. C., van Hasselt, F., Ramakers, G., Meaney, M. J., de Kloet, R. E., & Krugers, H. (2008). Maternal care and hippocampal plasticity: Evidence for experience-dependent structural plasticity, altered synaptic functioning, and differential responsiveness to glucocorticoids and stress. *Journal of Neuroscience, 28,* 6037–6045.

Charnov, E. L. (1993). *Life history invariants*. Oxford, England: Oxford University Press.

Cicchetti, D. (Ed.). (2011). Allostatic load. *Development and Psychopathology, 23,* 723–724.

Costello, E. J., & Angold, A. (2006). Developmental epidemiology. In D. Cicchetti & D. J. Cohen (Eds.), *Developmental psychopathology: Vol. 1. Theory and methods* (2nd ed., pp. 41–75). Hoboken, NJ: Wiley.

De Bellis, M. D., Baum, A. S., Birmaher, B., Keshavan, M. S., Eccard, C. H., Boring, A. M., & Ryan, N. D. (1999). Developmental traumatology. Part I: Biological stress systems. *Biological Psychiatry, 45,* 1259–1270.

Degnan, K. A., Calkins, S. D., Keane, S. P., & Hill-Soderlund, A. L. (2008). Profiles of disruptive behavior across early childhood: Contributions of frustration reactivity, physiological regulation, and maternal behavior. *Child Development, 79,* 1357–1376.

Del Giudice, M., Angeleri, R., & Manera, V. (2009). The juvenile transition: A developmental switch point in human life history. *Developmental Review, 29,* 1–31.

Del Giudice, M., Ellis, B. J., & Shirtcliff, E. A. (2011). The adaptive calibration model of stress responsivity. *Neuroscience and Biobehavioral Reviews, 35,* 1562–1592.

Del Giudice, M., Hinnant, J. B., Ellis, B. J., & El-Sheikh, M. (2012). Adaptive patterns of stress responsivity: A preliminary investigation. *Developmental Psychology, 48,* 775–790.

Dickerson, S. S., & Kemeny, M. E. (2004). Acute stressors and cortisol responses: A theoretical integration and synthesis of laboratory research. *Psychological Bulletin, 130,* 355–391.

Dobrova-Krol, N. A., Van IJzendoorn, M. H., Bakermans-Kranenburg, M. J., & Juffer, F. (2010). Effects of perinatal HIV infection and early institutional rearing on physical and cognitive development of children in Ukraine. *Child Development, 81,* 237–251.

Ellis, B. J. (2011). Toward an evolutionary-developmental explanation of alternative reproductive strategies: The central role of switch-controlled modular systems. In D. M. Buss & P. H. Hawley (Eds.), *The evolution of personality and individual differences* (pp. 177–209). New York, NY: Oxford University Press.

Ellis, B. J., Boyce, W. T., Belsky, J., Bakermans-Kranenburg, M. J., & van IJzendoorn, M. H. (2011). Differential susceptibility to the environment: An evolutionary-neurodevelopmental theory. *Development and Psychopathology, 23,* 7–28.

Ellis, B. J., Del Giudice, M., Dishion, T. J., Figueredo, A. J., Gray, P., Griskevicius, V., & Wilson, D. S. (2012). The evolutionary basis of risky adolescent behavior: Implications for science, policy, and practice. *Developmental Psychology, 48,* 598–623.

Ellis, B. J., Essex, M. J., & Boyce, W. T. (2005). Biological sensitivity to context II: Empirical explorations of an evolutionary-developmental theory. *Development and Psychopathology, 17,* 303–328.

Ellis, B. J., Jackson, J. J., & Boyce, W. T. (2006). The stress response system: Universality and adaptive individual differences. *Developmental Review, 26,* 175–212.

Ellis, B. J., Schlomer, G. L., Figueredo, A. J., & Brumbach, B. H. (2009). Fundamental dimensions of environmental risk: The impact of harsh versus unpredictable environments on the evolution and development of life history strategies. *Human Nature, 20*, 204–268.

El-Sheikh, M., Erath, S. A., Buckhalt, J. A., Granger, D. A., & Mize, J. (2008). Cortisol and children's adjustment: The moderating role of sympathetic nervous system activity. *Journal of Abnormal Child Psychology, 36*, 601–611.

El-Sheikh, M., Harger, J., & Whitson, S. M. (2001). Exposure to interparental conflict and children's adjustment and physical health: The moderating role of vagal tone. *Child Development, 72*, 1617–1636.

Essex, M. J., Klein, M. H., Cho, E., & Kalin, N. H. (2002). Maternal stress beginning in infancy may sensitize children to later stress exposure: Effects on cortisol and behavior. *Biological Psychiatry, 52*, 776–784.

Evans, G. W., & English, K. (2002). The environment of poverty: Multiple stressor exposure, psychophysiological stress, and socioemotional adjustment. *Child Development, 73*, 1238–1248.

Fabes, R. A., & Eisenberg, N. (1997). Regulatory control and adults' stress-related responses to daily life events. *Journal of Personality and Social Psychology, 73*, 1107–1117.

Figueredo, A. J., Vasquez, G., Brumbach, B. H., & Schneider, S. M. R. (2004). The heritability of life history strategy: The K-factor, covitality, and personality. *Social Biology, 51*, 121–143.

Flinn, M. V. (2006). Evolution and ontogeny of the stress response to social challenges in the human child. *Developmental Review, 26*, 138–174.

Frankenhuis, W. E., & Del Giudice, M. (2012). When do adaptive developmental mechanisms yield maladaptive outcomes? *Developmental Psychology, 48*, 628–642.

Fries, E., Dettenborn, L., & Kirschbaum, C. (2009). The cortisol awakening response (CAR): Facts and future directions. *International Journal of Psychophysiology, 72*, 67–73.

Fries, A. B., Shirtcliff, E. A., & Pollak, S. D. (2008). Neuroendocrine dysregulation following early social deprivation in children. *Developmental Psychobiology, 50*, 588–599.

Ganzel, B. L., Morris, P. A., & Wethington, E. (2010). Allostasis and the human brain: Integrating models of stress from the social and life sciences. *Psychological Review, 117*, 134–174.

Ganzel, B. L., & Morris, P. A. (2011). Allostasis and the developing human brain: Explicit consideration of implicit models. *Development and Psychopathology, 23*, 955–974.

Gatzke-Kopp, L. M. (2011). The canary in the coalmine: The sensitivity of mesolimbic dopamine to environmental adversity during development. *Neuroscience and Biobehavioral Reviews, 35*, 794–803.

Geary, D. C. (2002). Sexual selection and human life history. *Advances in Child Development and Behavior, 30*, 41–101.

Gibbons, F. X., Roberts, M. E., Gerrard, M., Li, Z., Beach, S. R., Simons, R. L., & Philibert, R. A. (2012). The impact of stress on the life history strategies of

African American adolescents: Cognitions, genetic moderation, and the role of discrimination. *Developmental Psychology, 48,* 772–739.

Gluckman, P. D., Low, F. M., Buklijas, T., Hanson, M. A., & Beedle, A. S. (2011). How evolutionary principles improve the understanding of human health and disease. *Evolutionary Applications, 4,* 249–263.

Goldstein, D. S., & Kopin, I. J. (2008). Adrenomedullary, adrenocortical, and sympathoneural responses to stressors: A meta-analysis. *Endocrine Regulations, 42,* 111–119.

Gunnar, M. R., Frenn, K., Wewerka, S. S., & Van Ryzin, M. J. (2009). Moderate versus severe early life stress: Associations with stress reactivity and regulation in 10–12-year-old children. *Psychoneuroendocrinology, 34,* 62–75.

Gunnar, M., & Quevedo, K. (2007). The neurobiology of stress and development. *Annual Review of Psychology, 58,* 145–173.

Gunnar, M. R., & Vazquez, D. (2006). Stress neurobiology and developmental psychopathology. In D. Cicchetti & D. J. Cohen (Eds.), *Developmental psychopathology: Vol. 2. Developmental neuroscience* (2nd ed., pp. 553–568). Hoboken, NJ: Wiley.

Gustafsson, P. E., Anckarsäter, H., Lichtenstein, P., Nelson, N., & Gustafsson, P. A. (2010). Does quantity have a quality all its own? Cumulative adversity and up- and down-regulation of circadian salivary cortisol levels in healthy children. *Psychoneuroendocrinology, 35,* 1410–1415.

Hastings, P. D., Shirtcliff, E. A., Klimes-Dougan, B., Allison, A. L., Derose, L., Kendziora, K. T., & Zahn-Waxler, C. (2011). Allostasis and the development of internalizing and externalizing problems: Changing relations with physiological systems across adolescence. *Development and Psychopathology, 23,* 1149–1165.

Hrdy, S. B. (1999). *Mother nature: A history of mothers, infants and natural selection.* New York, NY: Pantheon.

James, J., Ellis, B. J., Schlomer, G. L., & Garber, J. (2012). Sex-specific pathways to early puberty, sexual debut and sexual risk-taking: Tests of an integrated evolutionary-developmental model. *Developmental Psychology, 48,* 687–702.

Juster, R. P., Bizik, G., Picard, M., Arsenault-lapierre, G., Sindi, S., Trepanier, L., Lupien, S. J. (2011). A transdisciplinary perspective of chronic stress in relation to psychopathology throughout life span development. *Development and Psychopathology, 23,* 725–776.

Juster, R. P., McEwen, B. S., & Lupien, S. J. (2010). Allostatic load biomarkers of chronic stress and impact on health and cognition. *Neuroscience and Biobehavioral Reviews, 35,* 2–16.

Kaplan, H. S., & Gangestad, S. W. (2005). Life history theory and evolutionary psychology. In D. M. Buss (Ed.), *The handbook of evolutionary psychology* (pp. 68–95). Hoboken, NJ: Wiley.

Kaplan, H. S., & Lancaster, J. B. (2003). An evolutionary and ecological analysis of human fertility, mating patterns, and parental investment. In K. W. Wachter & R. A. Bulatao (Eds.), *Offspring: Human fertility behavior in biodemographic perspective* (pp. 170–223). Washington, DC: National Academies Press.

Kokko, H., & Jennions, M. (2008). Parental investment, sexual selection and sex ratios. *Journal of Evolutionary Biology, 21,* 919–948.

Korte, S. M., Koolhaas, J. M., Wingfield, J. C., & McEwen, B. S. (2005). The Darwinian concept of stress: Benefits of allostasis and costs of allostatic load and the trade-offs in health and disease. *Neuroscience and Biobehavioral Reviews, 29,* 3–38.

Lévesque, M., Bigras, M., & Pauzé, R. (2010). Externalizing problems and problematic sexual behaviors: Same etiology? *Aggressive Behavior, 36,* 358–370.

Lovallo, W. R., & Sollers III,, J. J. (2007). Autonomic nervous system. In J. Fink (Ed.), *Encyclopedia of stress* (2nd ed., pp. 282–289). San Diego, CA: Academic Press.

Lupien, S. J., Ouellet-Morin, I., Hupbach, A., Tu, M. T., Buss, C., Walker, D., & McEwen, B. S. (2006). Beyond the stress concept: Allostatic load: A developmental biological and cognitive perspective. In D. Cicchetti & D. J. Cohen (Eds.), *Developmental psychopathology: Vol. 2. Developmental neuroscience* (2nd ed., pp. 578–628). Hoboken, NJ: Wiley.

McEwen, B. S., & Stellar, E. (1993). Stress and the individual: Mechanisms leading to disease. *Archives of Internal Medicine, 153,* 2093–2101.

McEwen, B. S., & Wingfield, J. C. (2003). The concept of allostasis in biology and biomedicine. *Hormones and Behavior, 43,* 2–15.

Mead, H. K., Beauchaine, T. P., & Shannon, K. E. (2010). Neurobiological adaptations to violence across development. *Development and Psychopathology, 22,* 1–22.

Miller, G. E., Chen, E., & Zhou, E. S. (2007). If it goes up, must it come down? Chronic stress and the hypothalamic-pituitary-adrenocortical axis in humans. *Psychological Bulletin, 133,* 25–45.

Miller, G. E., Chen, E., & Parker, K. J. (2011). Psychological stress in childhood and susceptibility to the chronic diseases of aging: Moving toward a model of behavioral and biological mechanisms. *Psychological Bulletin, 137,* 959–997.

Munck, A., Guyre, P. M., & Holbrook, N. J. (1984). Physiological functions of glucocorticoids in stress and their relation to pharmacological actions. *Endocrinology Review, 5,* 25–43.

Nelson, C. A., Zeanah, C. H., Fox, N. A., Marshall, P. J., Smyke, A., & Guthrie, D. (2007). Cognitive recovery in socially deprived young children: The Bucharest early intervention project. *Science, 318,* 1937–1940.

Nesse, R. M. (2001). On the difficulty of defining disease: A Darwinian perspective. *Medicine, Health Care and Philosophy, 4,* 37–46.

Nesse, R. M. (2005). Natural selection and the regulation of defenses: A signal detection analysis of the smoke detector principle. *Evolution and Human Behavior, 26,* 88–105.

Nesse, R. M., & Jackson, E. D. (2006). Evolution: psychiatric nosology's missing biological foundation. *Clinical Neuropsychiatry, 3,* 121–131.

Obradovic, J., Bush, N. R., & Boyce, W. T. (2011). The interactive effect of marital conflict and stress reactivity on externalizing and internalizing symptoms: The role of laboratory stressors. *Development & Psychopathology, 23,* 101–114.

Obradovic, J., Bush, N. R., Stamperdahl, J., Adler, N. E., & Boyce, W. T. (2010). Biological sensitivity to context: The interactive effects of stress reactivity and family adversity on socioemotional behavior and school readiness. *Child Development, 81*, 270–289.

Ortiz, J., & Raine, A. (2004). Heart rate level and antisocial behavior in children and adolescents: A meta-analysis. *Journal of the American Academy of Child and Adolescent Psychiatry, 43*, 154–162.

Pickles, A., & Hill, J. (2006). Developmental pathways. In D. Cicchetti & D. J. Cohen (Eds.), *Developmental psychopathology: Vol. 1. Theory and method* (2nd ed., pp. 211–243). Hoboken, NJ: Wiley.

Pigliucci, M. (2001). *Phenotypic plasticity: Beyond nature and nurture.* Baltimore, MD: Johns Hopkins University Press.

Pluess, M., & Belsky, J. (2011). Prenatal programming of postnatal plasticity? *Development and Psychopathology, 23*, 29–38.

Porges, S. W. (1995). Orienting in a defensive world: Mammalian modifications of our evolutionary heritage. A polyvagal theory. *Psychophysiology, 32*, 301–318.

Porges, S. W. (2007). The polyvagal perspective. *Biological Psychology, 74*, 116–143.

Pruessner, J. C., Dedovic, K., Pruessner, M., Lord, C., Buss, C., Collins, L., & Lupien, S. J. (2010). Stress regulation in the central nervous system: Evidence from structural and functional neuroimaging studies in human populations. *Psychoneuroendocrinology, 35*, 179–191.

Sapolsky, R. M., Romero, L. M., & Munck, A. U. (2000). How do glucocorticoids influence stress responses? Integrating permissive, suppressive, stimulatory, and preparative actions. *Endocrine Reviews, 21*, 55–89.

Schlotz, W., Kumsta, R., Layes, I., Entringer, S., Jones, A., & Wust, S. (2008). Covariance between psychological and endocrine responses to pharmacological challenge and psychosocial stress: A question of timing. *Psychosomatic Medicine, 70*, 787–796.

Schmidt-Reinwald, A., Pruessner, J. C., Hellhammer, D. H., Federenko, I., Rohleder, N., Schurmeyer, T. H., & Kirschbaum, C. (1999). The cortisol response to awakening in relation to different challenge tests and a 12-hour cortisol rhythm. *Life Sciences, 64*, 1653–1660.

Sefcek, J. A., & Figueredo, A. J. (2010). A life history model of human fitness indicators. *Biodemography and Social Biology, 56*, 42–66.

Shirtcliff, E. A., Granger, D. A., Booth, A., & Johnson, D. (2005). Low salivary cortisol levels and externalizing behavior problems in youth. *Development and Psychopathology, 17*, 167–184.

Sijtsema, J. J., Nederhof, E., Veenstra, R., Ormel, J., Oldehinkel, A. J., & Ellis, B. J. (in press). Family cohesion, prosocial behavior, and antisocial behavior in adolescence: Moderating effects of biological sensitivity to context. The TRAILS study. *Development and Psychopathology.*

Simpson, J. A., Griskevicius, V., Kuo, S. I., Sung, S., & Collins, W. A. (2012). Evolution, stress, and sensitive periods: The influence of unpredictability in early versus late childhood on sex and risky behavior. *Developmental Psychology, 48*, 674–686.

Stanner, S. A., & Yudkin, J. S. (2001). Fetal programming and the Leningrad siege study. *Twin Research, 4*, 287–292.

Stearns, S. (1992). *The evolution of life histories*. Oxford, England: Oxford University Press.

Stroud, L., Salavey, P., & Epel, E. (2002). Sex differences in stress responses: Social rejection versus achievement stress. *Biological Psychiatry, 52,* 318–328.

Stroud, L. R., Foster, E., Papandonatos, G. D., Handwerger, K., Granger, D. A., Kivlighan, K. T., & Niaura, R. (2009). Stress response and the adolescent transition: Performance versus peer rejection stressors. *Development and Psychopathology, 21,* 47–68.

Tarullo, A. R., & Gunnar, M. R. (2006). Child maltreatment and the developing HPA axis. *Hormones and Behavior, 50,* 632–639.

Trivers, R. L. (1972). Parental investment and sexual selection. In B. Campbell (Ed.), *Sexual selection and the descent of man 1871–1971* (pp. 136–179). Chicago, IL: Aldine.

Van Buskirk, J., & Relyea, R. A. (1998). Selection for phenotypic plasticity in *Rana sylvatica* tadpoles. *Biological Journal of the Linnean Society, 65,* 301–328.

Van Marle, H. J. F., Hermans, E. J., Qin, S., & Fernández, G. (2009). From specificity to sensitivity: How acute stress affects amygdala processing of biologically salient stimuli. *Biological Psychiatry, 66,* 649–655.

West-Eberhard, M. J. (2003). *Developmental plasticity and evolution*. New York, NY: Oxford University Press.

Yehuda, R. (2002). Post-traumatic stress disorder. *New England Journal of Medicine, 346,* 108–114.

Zahn-Waxler, C., Crick, N. R., Shirtcliff, E. A., & Woods, K. E. (2006). The origins and development of psychopathology in females and males. In D. Cicchetti & D. J. Cohen (Eds.). *Developmental Psychopathology, 2nd ed., Vol. 1.* (pp. 76–138). Hoboken, NJ: Wiley.

# CHAPTER 9

# Exposure to Teratogens as a Risk Factor for Psychopathology

NICOLE A. CROCKER, SUSANNA L. FRYER, AND SARAH N. MATTSON

## INTRODUCTION AND ETIOLOGICAL FORMULATIONS

A TERATOGEN IS AN agent that causes birth defects by altering the course of typical development. Examples of human teratogens exist in several classes of substances including drugs of abuse (e.g., alcohol, cocaine, nicotine), prescription medications (e.g., retinoic acid, valproic acid, thalidomide), environmental contaminants (e.g., pesticides, lead, methylmercury), and diseases (e.g., varicella, herpes simplex virus, rubella). Pregnant women are exposed to teratogens for a variety of reasons. Some women may be unaware of the teratogenic nature of certain substances. Or, in the case of viruses such as varicella, even if awareness exists, prevention of exposure may not be possible. Similarly, with medical conditions such as seizure disorder or severe depression, termination of pharmacologic treatment during pregnancy may not be advisable. Furthermore, given that about half of pregnancies in the United States are unplanned, and given that pregnancy detection may not occur until fetal development is well underway, many teratogenic exposures occur prior to pregnancy recognition (Henshaw, 1998). As an example, more than 130,000 pregnant women per year in the United States consume alcoholic beverages at levels believed to pose teratogenic risk to their fetuses (Lupton, Burd, & Harwood, 2004), and 10% of women who know they are pregnant report drinking alcohol during pregnancy (Centers for Disease Control and Prevention, 2004). These rates exist despite more than three decades of research on the effects of alcohol-induced birth defects and the presence of government-mandated labels on alcoholic beverages that warn of the association between drinking during

Acknowledgments: Preparation of this chapter was supported in part by National Institute on Alcohol Abuse and Alcoholism Grant numbers U01 AA014834, R01 AA019605, R01 AA010417, and F31 AA020142. We gratefully acknowledge the assistance and support of the Center for Behavioral Teratology, San Diego State University.

pregnancy and harmful fetal effects. Thus, teratogenic exposures are common, and birth defects that can result from prenatal exposures constitute a major public health concern.

Behavioral teratogens are agents that cause changes in central nervous system function (e.g., cognitive, affective, sensorimotor, or social) when individuals are exposed during gestation (Vorhees, 1986). Behavioral teratogens can cause damage to the fetus even in the absence of gross physical or structural abnormalities that may occur with physical teratogens. The effects of behavioral teratogens may be subtle and are not necessarily easily recognizable at birth. The purpose of research aimed at identifying and characterizing the effects of behavioral teratogens is to determine the degree and nature of behavioral dysfunction attributable to fetal exposure to drugs or other agents capable of causing birth defects. The hope is that identifying substances that can act as behavioral teratogens and increasing public awareness of teratogenic effects can reduce exposure to teratogens and resulting fetal damage.

As noted earlier, the effects of behavioral teratogenic exposures are diverse and may include structural damage to the developing brain, cognitive impairments, and emotional dysfunction. In this chapter, we focus on associations between teratogenic exposures and the development of mental illnesses. The etiology of psychopathology is complicated by gene-environment interactions (including epigenetic effects) through which only certain genotypes may be activated by certain environmental risks (cf. Rutter, 2005; see Chapter 3). Gene-environment correlation is also possible. For example, genes predisposing to maternal substance abuse may co-occur with maladaptive childrearing environments. In short, it is difficult to pinpoint the multifaceted etiology of psychopathology to single genetic or environmental causes. Rather, the complex behaviors that comprise psychopathology manifest in an emergent fashion from a continuous interplay between an individual's genetic expression patterns and his or her environment. Certain individuals may be genetically predisposed to development of mental illness, yet nongenetic factors, such as perinatal complications, early childhood experiences, and socioeconomic factors may also be involved. Factors such as family placement (e.g., being raised in a biological, foster, or adoptive home; Viner & Taylor, 2005), socioeconomic status (SES; Rutter, 2003), and general intelligence (Dykens, 2000) are potential sources of variance in mental health outcomes that may be of particular concern in evaluating the mental health status in individuals with teratogenic exposures.

Alcohol is the main focus of this chapter, as it is both an archetypal and widely studied behavioral teratogen. The association between psychopathology and fetal exposure to nicotine, stimulant drugs, methylmercury, and lead is discussed briefly, as the effects of these exposures on mental health outcomes are less well studied.

## HISTORICAL CONTEXT

Knowledge of birth defects and their associations with teratogenic exposures has evolved over the course of history. Early depictions, including carvings and drawings, indicate knowledge of birth defects as early as 6500 B.C., and early written records indicate beliefs that birth defects were caused by various factors including witchcraft. Birth defects were also thought to portend adverse events. Moving into the 20th century, it was thought that the fetus was afforded significant protection by the uterus, and it was not until 1941 that an association between prenatal exposure to the rubella virus and subsequent birth defects was reported in the scientific literature. Even so, it took the experience with thalidomide in the late 1950s to confirm the association between teratogens and resulting birth defects (Vorhees, 1986).

Similarly, an association between gestational alcohol exposure and deleterious fetal effects was described anecdotally for centuries. Some contend that the association was documented in Greek and Roman mythology and in the Bible. Yet throughout the majority of the 20th century, alcohol was not recognized as a human teratogen. In fact, for much of the century, alcohol was used by physicians to treat premature labor, in a procedure referred to as an *ethanol drip*. Perhaps in part due to this medical usage, the first descriptions in the scientific literature of alcohol as a human teratogen were met with considerable resistance. Instead, it was posed that the constellation of symptoms identified as the fetal alcohol syndrome (FAS) were due to other factors such as inadequate prenatal nutrition or genetics ("Effect of alcoholism at time of conception," 1946). Because of their ability to control confounding factors, preclinical animal models were crucial in establishing the causal role of alcohol in bringing about the effects now recognized as fetal alcohol spectrum disorders (FASD). After more than 30 years of research on alcohol teratogenesis, prenatal alcohol exposure is now recognized as a major public health concern (e.g., Streissguth, 2007). As an example of this increased public awareness, in 1989 the United States Government passed the Alcoholic Beverage Warning Label Act, which mandates that alcoholic beverages contain labels that warn of alcohol's capability to cause harmful effects on the developing fetus. In addition, in February 2005, the U.S. Surgeon General issued an updated "Advisory on Alcohol Use and Pregnancy." This advisory recommended that (1) pregnant women should not drink alcohol, (2) pregnant women who have already consumed alcohol during pregnancy should stop drinking to minimize further risk, and (3) women who are considering pregnancy or who might become pregnant should also abstain from alcohol (http://www.hhs.gov/surgeongeneral/pressreleases/sg02222005.html). Despite this progress, women continue to drink in pregnancy.

## TERMINOLOGICAL AND CONCEPTUAL ISSUES

Since the first descriptions of FAS appeared in the scientific literature (Jones & Smith, 1973; Jones, Smith, Ulleland, & Streissguth, 1973; Lemoine, Harousseau, Borteyru, & Menuet, 1968), the pattern of birth defects associated with maternal alcohol consumption has been studied extensively. FAS is characterized by a triad of presenting symptoms: (1) pre- and/or postnatal growth deficiency, (2) dysmorphic facial features (short palpebral fissures, indistinct philtrum, and a thin upper lip), and (3) central nervous system (CNS) dysfunction. Although CNS dysfunction is required for the diagnosis of FAS, cognitive deficits and behavioral abnormalities are commonly observed following prenatal alcohol exposure even in the absence of the growth deficiency and facial stigmata required for clinical recognition of FAS (e.g., Mattson, Riley, Gramling, Delis, & Jones, 1997, 1998).

Given the variable clinical presentation of individuals with histories of gestational alcohol exposure, the term FASD is now used to describe the range of effects attributable to prenatal alcohol exposure (Bertrand, Floyd, & Weber, 2005). These effects may range from the complete manifestation of FAS (i.e., meeting all diagnostic criteria) to subtle neurobehavioral or physical defects. The umbrella term FASD includes both dysmorphic (i.e., FAS) and nondysmorphic cases of prenatal alcohol exposure, and is designed to encompass historical terms such as fetal alcohol effects (FAE) and current diagnoses of partial FAS (PFAS), alcohol-related birth defects (ARBD), and alcohol-related neurodevelopmental disorder (ARND).

Birth defects caused by maternal alcohol consumption constitute a serious public health concern, both in the United States and internationally. Incidence rates of FAS average about 1 case per 1,000 live births (Bertrand et al., 2005), making FAS the leading preventable cause of mental retardation (Pulsifer, 1996). Moreover, more subtle birth defects due to prenatal alcohol exposure occur more frequently, as the combined rate for dysmorphic (i.e., FAS) and nondysmorphic FASD cases has been conservatively estimated at 9.1 cases per 1,000 live births (May et al., 2009; Sampson et al., 1997). The costs of fetal alcohol effects pose a heavy burden on society, ranging from $4 billion to $9.7 billion annually (Lupton et al., 2004; Thanh, Jonsson, Dennett, & Jacobs, 2011). Costs related to FASD are bound to be considerably higher.

## MENTAL HEALTH OUTCOMES IN FASD

Although not as well studied as the cognitive deficits associated with prenatal alcohol exposure, there is a sizeable literature focused on mental health outcomes in FASD. Studies of affected individuals consistently demonstrate deficits in parent and self-reported behavior (Coles, Platzman, Brown, Smith, & Falek, 1997; Coles, Platzman, & Lynch, 1999; Mattson & Riley, 2000; Nash et al., 2006; O'Leary et al., 2009; Sayal et al., 2009; Sayal, Heron, Golding, & Emond, 2007; Steinhausen, Willms, Metzke, & Spohr, 2003). In one early longitudinal investigation, behavior associated with psychopathology was rated in children with FAS, a large portion of whom were mentally retarded (Steinhausen, Nestler, & Spohr, 1982; Steinhausen, Willms, & Spohr, 1993, 1994). Increased rates of many maladaptive behaviors were observed, including stereotypies, sleeping problems, tics, head and body rocking, peer relationship difficulties, and phobic behaviors. Moreover, an index of psychopathological behavior, created from the sum of symptom scores, correlated with degree of dysmorphology (Steinhausen et al., 1982). A follow-up report demonstrated persistence of psychopathological symptoms through late childhood, including hyperkinetic behaviors, sleep disturbances, abnormal habits, stereotyped behaviors, and emotional disorders (Steinhausen & Spohr, 1998). In another investigation that used IQ-matched controls, alcohol-exposed children had significantly more parent-reported behavioral and emotional disturbances than controls on 5 of 8 subscales on the Child Behavior Checklist (Mattson & Riley, 2000). As a group, children with prenatal alcohol exposure had clinically significant scores on several externalizing behavior domains including social problems, attention problems, and aggressive behavior. Children with FASD also demonstrated elevated internalizing difficulties, but differences on these scales were not as large as on externalizing behavior domains.

Other studies that have used *Diagnostic and Statistical Manual of Mental Disorders-IV* (*DSM-IV*, American Psychiatric Association, 1994, 2000) criteria to evaluate psychopathology demonstrate that rates of clinical diagnoses are also elevated in children with FASD. In one sample of 23 children with histories of heavy prenatal alcohol exposure, ages 5 to 13 (O'Connor et al., 2002), 87% (20 out of 23) met criteria for at least one of the psychiatric disorders examined based on psychiatric interview, with mood disorders being the most common (including both major depressive and bipolar disorders). These data also suggested comparable mental health outcomes regardless of the severity of fetal alcohol effects; nondysmorphic individuals were as likely to have clinically significant psychopathology as children with hallmark facial features of FAS. In an effort to focus on the development of psychiatric illness in children with FASD independent of mental retardation, children with an intelligence quotient (IQ) below 70 were excluded from this study. In addition, the authors noted that because the sample was clinically referred, the high rates of observed psychopathology may not generalize to the entire alcohol-exposed population (O'Connor et al., 2002). In a later study conducted by Fryer, McGee, Matt, Riley, and Mattson (2007), also of a clinically referred FASD sample, 97% of alcohol-exposed children met criteria for at least one Axis I disorder based on *DSM-IV* interview compared with only 40% of control children. Of the children with FASD, 28% met criteria for a mood or anxiety disorder and 59% met criteria for externalizing disorders such as attention-deficit/hyperactivity disorder (ADHD), conduct disorder, and/or oppositional defiant disorder. These rates were higher than rates demonstrated by both children in the control group and the general population.

Because these studies involve participants who were identified on the basis of clinically significant behavioral problems or recognition of fetal alcohol effects, mental health outcome results may not generalize to the entire alcohol-exposed population. That is, these studies select against individuals who were exposed to alcohol prenatally but experience few or no psychiatric or behavioral symptoms. Although retrospective studies are important in characterizing individuals most in need of clinical services, studies that identify participants prospectively (i.e., at or near the time of teratogenic exposure) can increase the external validity of research findings. Also, prospective studies typically enable better control of confounding factors, because environmental and demographic information can be collected more accurately closer to the time of exposure.

The Seattle Study on Alcohol and Pregnancy, a large-scale population-based study of alcohol's behavioral teratogenicity, used a prospective design. Streissguth and colleagues identified 1,529 pregnant women in the mid-1970s and collected information about their use of alcohol, cigarettes, caffeine, and other recreational and prescription drugs (Barr et al., 2006). Importantly, these pregnancies were not considered high risk, and all women received prenatal care. A cohort of 500 mother-infant pairs was selected—oversampling for alcohol use—and followed through adulthood. Of this birth cohort, 400 young adults, including individuals with and without prenatal alcohol exposure, were interviewed at about age 25 using Structured Clinical Interviews for *DSM-IV* (both the Axis I and Axis II versions were administered). The purpose of this study was to determine whether high rates of psychiatric illness observed in clinical samples of individuals with FASD would replicate in a nonclinical, community sample.

The odds of developing Axis I somatoform and substance use disorders and Axis II paranoid, passive-aggressive, and antisocial traits were at least doubled in individuals who had been exposed to one or more binge drinking episodes versus those who had not. Substance use disorders and Axis II passive-aggressive and antisocial personality traits remained at least a twofold risk in alcohol-exposed individuals, even after controlling for confounding factors including prenatal nicotine or marijuana exposure, family placement, low SES, poor maternal nutrition, breast-feeding, and family history of psychiatric problems and alcoholism. The authors noted that given the epidemiological focus of their study, including thorough control of many other factors that predict mental health, prenatal alcohol exposure is likely to play a causal role in increased rates of the disorders noted.

The consensus from these global mental health outcome studies suggests that individuals with fetal alcohol exposure histories suffer from substantial psychiatric illness. Moreover, the diversity of study methodologies (e.g., both prospective and retrospective subject ascertainment, longitudinal versus cross-sectional design, different portions of the age span) supports the generalizability of the association between FASD and increased psychopathology.

## DISRUPTIVE BEHAVIOR DISORDERS

A review of available literature suggests that certain types of psychopathology may be more likely than others to follow gestational alcohol exposure. Among these are disorders on the disruptive behavior spectrum (e.g., ADHD, oppositional defiant disorder, conduct disorder). As stated earlier, findings from the Fryer et al. (2007) study indicated group differences between alcohol-exposed and typically developing peers in rates of ADHD, oppositional defiant disorder, conduct disorder, depressive disorders, and specific phobias, with the group difference in the ADHD category the largest effect observed by far. This finding is consistent with other research suggesting that increased attention difficulties and ADHD are among the most notable psychopathological outcomes within the FASD population (Burd, Klug, Martsolf, & Kerbeshian, 2003; Coles, Platzman, Lynch, & Freides, 2002; Mattson & Riley, 1998; Steinhausen et al., 1993; Streissguth, Barr, Kogan, & Bookstein, 1996; Steinhausen & Spohr, 1998). Given the high rates of ADHD in FASD, an entire body of research comparing these two clinical groups has formed with the goal of differentiating their cognitive and behavioral function to aid in better identification of alcohol exposed individuals (Burden et al., 2010; Coffin, Baroody, Schneider, & O'Neill, 2005; Coles, Platzman, Raskind-Hood, et al., 1997; Crocker, Vaurio, Riley,

& Mattson, 2009, 2011; Greenbaum, Stevens, Nash, Koren, & Rovet, 2009; Jacobson, Dodge, Burden, Klorman, & Jacobson, 2011; Kooistra, Crawford, Gibbard, Kaplan, & Fan, 2011; Kooistra, Crawford, Gibbard, Ramage, & Kaplan, 2010; Kooistra et al., 2009; Nanson & Hiscock, 1990; Nash et al., 2006; Vaurio, Riley, & Mattson, 2008). In one such investigation, parent-report items reflecting hyperactivity, inattention, lying and cheating, lack of guilt, and disobedience were particularly useful at discriminating children with FASD from children with ADHD (Nash et al., 2006), with 6 or more reported symptoms being indicative of FASD.

Several recent studies have examined the interaction between prenatal alcohol exposure and ADHD on behavioral and psychiatric outcomes. These studies suggest a possible synergistic effect of these two factors where children with both alcohol exposure and ADHD have worse outcomes than children with either condition alone (Graham et al., 2011; Ware et al., 2011; Ware et al., 2012). Interestingly, the same does not appear to be true for neuropsychological abilities; alcohol-exposed children with and without ADHD appear to have similar neuropsychological profiles (Glass et al., 2012).

Increased delinquent behavior and deficient moral decision making have also been reported in alcohol-exposed youth (Roebuck, Mattson, & Riley, 1999; Schonfeld, Mattson, & Riley, 2005; Streissguth et al., 1996), and subsequently, rates of conduct disorder and oppositional defiant disorder are increased in these individuals (Disney, Iacono, McGue, Tully, & Legrand, 2008; Fryer et al., 2007; Hill, Lowers, Locke-Wellman, & Shen, 2000). In one population study of 626 adolescent twin pairs, prenatal alcohol exposure was associated with higher rates of conduct disorder symptoms even after controlling statistically for parental externalizing disorders, prenatal nicotine exposure, monozygosity, gestational age, and birth weight (Disney et al., 2008). In another study, low IQ of children with prenatal alcohol exposure predicted lowered moral maturity relative to typically developing children. In addition, children with FASD displayed a specific deficit in moral value judgments in their relationships with others (Schonfeld et al., 2005). Other studies have demonstrated that children with prenatal alcohol exposure are more likely to lie about their behavior and are more skilled lie tellers at younger ages than their nonexposed peers (Rasmussen, Talwar, Loomes, & Andrew, 2008).

Given the increase in delinquent behavior demonstrated by individuals with prenatal alcohol exposure, it is not surprising that alcohol-exposed youth are significantly overrepresented in the criminal justice system (Boland, Burrill, Duwyn, & Karp, 1998; Fast & Conry, 2004, 2009). Interestingly, corrections staff are largely unaware of this phenomenon (Burd, Selfridge, Klug, & Bakko, 2004). One of the few systematic FASD screens of a delinquent group undertaken by a forensic psychiatric facility in Canada revealed that 23% of juvenile detainees were exposed to significant amounts of alcohol prenatally (Fast, Conry, & Loock, 1999). Of the 67 individuals who were identified as having birth defects related to alcohol exposure, only 3 had been given an alcohol-related diagnosis prior to the screen. Overall, the association between prenatal alcohol exposure and disruptive behavior appears to be reliable and persistent, and it is evident at relatively low exposure levels. For example, when researchers in the Seattle project conducted psychosocial assessments of 14-year-old exposed offspring, misbehaviors were among the outcomes most strongly associated with alcohol exposure (Carmichael Olson et al., 1997). However, whether this association between prenatal alcohol exposure and delinquency is direct—or is mediated by a more proximal linkage between FASD and early-appearing attention/impulse control problems and/or learning difficulties, which themselves predict later conduct problems—is indeterminate (e.g., Hinshaw, 1992).

## Mood Disorders

Psychopathology associated with alcohol teratogenesis is not limited to the disruptive behaviors. Elevated rates of depressive disorders have also been noted in children with FASD, based on parent interviews (Fryer et al., 2007; O'Connor et al., 2002). Also, depressive features are noted on parent questionnaires (Mattson & Riley, 2000; Roebuck et al., 1999). The potential link between fetal alcohol exposure and depression has been less frequently investigated than relations with disruptive psychopathology, although research is increasingly focusing on this important topic. Moreover, data examining child and adolescent psychopathology rates indicate that the comorbidities among disruptive behavior disorders and mood disorders are high in the general population (Angold, Costello, & Erkanli, 1999) and similarly, psychiatric comorbidities are common among children with FASD. Thus, some degree of overlap among those needing services for problems such as mood and disruptive disorders is to be expected.

One longitudinal study examined the relation between prenatal alcohol exposure, negative infant affect, and subsequent symptoms of childhood depression (O'Connor, 2001). Results indicated that gestational alcohol exposure was a significant risk factor for developing depressive features at age 6 years, both as a direct effect and as an indirect effect, mediated through negative infant affect. Interestingly, the authors note that the association between alcohol exposure and depressive symptoms may be moderated by factors such as sex and maternal depression status, as girls whose mothers had high levels of depression were among those most affected in the sample (O'Connor & Kasari, 2000). More recent work used structural equation modeling to evaluate the relationship between prenatal alcohol exposure and childhood depression (O'Connor & Paley, 2006). This model consisted of both pre- and postnatal factors, indicating that prenatal alcohol exposure is a possible etiological factor in increased negative affect and depressive symptoms. However, this association appeared to also be mediated by the quality and nature of mother-child interactions.

## Potential Mediating and Moderating Factors

As discussed previously, factors such as general intelligence, SES, and family placement are important sources of variance in mental health outcomes, and several authors have attempted to tease apart the effects of environmental risk factors from prenatal alcohol exposure when evaluating behavioral difficulties in affected children (D'Onofrio et al., 2007; Hill et al., 2000; Rodriguez et al., 2009; Staroselsky et al., 2009). Some findings suggest that maternal psychopathology may be a better predictor of internalizing problems in children with FASD but that alcohol exposure is more directly related to externalizing problems (Staroselsky et al., 2009). However, other studies fail to find strong associations between prenatal alcohol exposure and externalizing difficulties once environmental factors are taken into account (D'Onofrio et al., 2007). For example, in terms of delinquent behaviors noted in cases with FASD, factors such as amount of exposure (Lynch, Coles, Corley, & Falek, 2003) and home placement (biological, foster, or adoptive; Schonfeld et al., 2005) are likely to exacerbate the relation between prenatal alcohol exposure and delinquency. In one investigation of a low-SES community sample, investigators did not find an increased rate of delinquency when alcohol-exposed youth were compared to either nonexposed peers (also low SES) or a special education comparison group (Lynch et al., 2003). Rather, within this sample, delinquency was related to environmental and behavioral variables such as low parental supervision, adolescent life stress, and self-reported drug use. In terms of family placement, higher rates of delinquent behavior were endorsed by alcohol-exposed adolescents in biological and foster homes versus those in adoptive homes (Schonfeld et al., 2005).

## ADAPTIVE DYSFUNCTION

As might be expected in a population characterized by cognitive impairments and increased rates of mental illness, adaptive dysfunction has been documented in individuals with prenatal alcohol exposure histories (Carr, Agnihotri, & Keightley, 2010; Crocker et al., 2009; Jirikowic, Carmichael Olson, & Kartin, 2008; Streissguth et al., 1991; Thomas, Kelly, Mattson, & Riley, 1998; Whaley, O'Connor, & Gunderson, 2001). The Seattle study found that as alcohol-exposed individuals reached adulthood, their overall adaptive abilities were equivalent to those of a typically developing 7-year-old, with social skills showing the most severe detriment (Streissguth et al., 1991). More recent studies confirm that socialization of children with FASD may be the most affected domain within adaptive function (Crocker et al., 2009; McGee, Bjorkquist, Price, Mattson, & Riley, 2009; McGee, Fryer, Bjorkquist, Mattson, & Riley, 2008; Thomas et al., 1998; Whaley et al., 2001) and that these abilities fail to improve with increasing age, suggesting an arrest in development of these skills (Crocker et al., 2009; Thomas et al., 1998; Whaley et al., 2001), rather than a delay. A similar arrest in development in communication skills was documented in an investigation comparing children with FASD to children with ADHD and controls on adaptive ability (Crocker et al., 2009). Thus, children with prenatal alcohol exposure are likely to have increasing difficulty meeting greater demands in social and communication function as they become teenagers and adults.

## PSYCHOPATHOLOGY IN ADULTS WITH FASD

Evidence suggests that behavioral difficulties and psychopathology of children with FASD persist into adulthood (Barr et al., 2006; Famy, Streissguth, & Unis, 1998; Spohr, Willms, & Steinhausen, 2007; Streissguth, 2007), often resulting in adverse life events such as substance abuse problems (Alati et al., 2006; Alati et al., 2008; Baer, Barr, Bookstein, Sampson, & Streissguth, 1998; Baer, Sampson, Barr, Connor, & Streissguth, 2003) and trouble with the law (Fast et al., 1999; Streissguth et al., 2004). In the Seattle cohort of prospectively identified participants, prenatal alcohol exposure was associated with alcohol problems at age 21, effects that remained after controlling for family history of alcohol use disorders, other prenatal exposures, and other environmental factors such as postnatal parental use of other drugs (Baer et al., 2003). These findings are supported by more recent studies (Alati et al., 2006; Alati et al., 2008) and demonstrate the persistent nature of the behavioral effects of prenatal alcohol exposure. Furthermore, the wide range of clinical difficulties associated with prenatal alcohol exposure, such as impulsivity, mood disorder, and substance abuse, place affected individuals at high risk for suicide. Indeed, individuals with FASD have an increase in lifetime suicide attempts relative to the general population (Baldwin, 2007; O'Malley & Huggins, 2005; Streissguth et al., 1996). In one account, 43% of adults with FASD reported suicide threats and 23% reported a history of suicide attempts throughout the lifetime (Streissguth et al., 1996).

## Possible Mechanisms of Action

Because of the infeasibility of controlling for confounding factors such as maternal nutrition and timing and dose of alcohol exposure in humans, research focused on identifying mechanisms of alcohol teratogenesis is typically derived from preclinical animal models of FASD and in vitro tissue culture studies. It is unlikely that the variable and wide-ranging effects associated with prenatal alcohol exposure are produced via a single process or pathway. Rather, a multitude of possible mechanisms for causing the pathology associated with FASD have been identified, including oxidative stress, changes in glucose metabolism, mitochondrial damage, abnormal growth factor activity, dysregulation of developmental gene expression, anomalous cell adhesion, and abnormalities in the development and regulation of neurotransmitter systems (e.g., excitotoxicity; Goodlett & Horn, 2001; Uban et al., 2011). The majority of these potential mechanisms may result in CNS damage by inducing either necrotic or apoptotic cell death, although disturbance to normal cell division and maturation could also be operative. Unfortunately, pinpointing the exact mechanisms through which alcohol exerts teratogenic effects in any given individual is complicated by a host of factors, including variations in timing, dose, and pattern of exposure, maternal characteristics, and fetal genetic factors. Further complicating matters, mechanisms of damage are likely to vary by brain region and cell type (Goodlett, Horn, & Zhou, 2005). Despite these complexities, mechanistic studies have been invaluable in clarifying alcohol's negative effects on the developing fetus and will continue to be of great utility in the future, particularly in the development of prevention and treatment efforts, which are lacking for this population. With regard to treating the psychopathology associated with FASD, preclinical studies can inform intervention efforts by refining our understanding of the structural and functional CNS deficits that may contribute to mental illness in this population. Such translational research is crucial to developing effective, evidence-based treatments.

In summary, prenatal alcohol exposure is associated with clinically significant psychopathology. Moreover, certain psychiatric sequelae, such as those occurring with disruptive behavior disorders, delinquency, substance use disorders, and depressive disorders appear to be more prevalent in individuals with FASD than in comparison populations. As discussed above, etiologic pathways are likely to be complex (i.e., equifinality, see Chapter 1). Indeed, it is not always possible to disentangle the direct effects of prenatal alcohol exposure from important correlates. Ultimately, this body of research suggests that alcohol teratogenesis should be considered as a possible etiological factor contributing to mental illness, and individuals with histories of prenatal alcohol exposure should be referred for psychiatric evaluation.

## PSYCHOPATHOLOGY RELATED TO OTHER PRENATAL EXPOSURES

In comparison to alcohol, much less is known about the effects of other potential teratogens on behavioral and psychopathological outcomes. This section describes research findings related to prenatal nicotine, stimulant drugs, methylmercury, and lead exposures.

### NICOTINE

Perhaps because of the high frequency at which fetuses are exposed to cigarette smoke, the effects of gestational nicotine exposure on resulting offspring have been studied fairly extensively, although less is known about behavioral and psychopathological outcomes. It is estimated that nearly a quarter of pregnant women in the United States continue to smoke during pregnancy (National Institute on Drug Abuse, 1996). The most commonly reported effects include increases in antisocial or delinquent behavior and ADHD.

Several studies have focused on the effects of nicotine exposure on antisocial and/or delinquent behavior. Converging data from criminal records (Brennan, Grekin, & Mednick, 1999; Gibson, Piquero, & Tibbetts, 2000; Piquero, Gibson, Tibbetts, Turner, & Katz, 2002; Rantakallio, Läärä, Isohanni, & Moilanen, 1992; Räsänen et al., 1999), parental reports of child behavior (Gatzke-Kopp & Beauchaine, 2007; Maughan, Taylor, Taylor, Butler, & Bynner, 2001; Ruckinger et al., 2010; Wasserman, Liu, Pine, & Graziano, 2001), and structured psychiatric clinical interviews (Langley, Holmans, van den Bree, & Thapar, 2007; Nigg & Breslau, 2007; Wakschlag et al., 1997; Wakschlag, Pickett, Cook, Benowitz, & Leventhal, 2002; Wakschlag, Pickett, Kasza, & Loeber, 2006; Weissman, Warner, Wickramaratne, & Kandel, 1999) support a relation between prenatal nicotine exposure and increased delinquency. Importantly, the relation between conduct problems in offspring and fetal nicotine exposure remains after controlling for potential confounds (Ruckinger et al., 2010), such as genetic factors (Maughan, Taylor, Caspi, & Moffitt, 2004), parental antisocial behavior (Gatzke-Kopp & Beauchaine, 2007; Maughan et al., 2004), income, prematurity, birth weight, and poor parenting practices (Gatzke-Kopp & Beauchaine, 2007).

The relation between prenatal nicotine exposure and the development of ADHD is also supported by several studies. Offspring exposed to nicotine during gestation are at increased risk for ADHD symptoms (Batstra, Hadders-Algra, & Neeleman, 2003; Fried, Watkinson, & Gray, 1992; Langley et al., 2007; Mick, Biederman, Faraone, Sayer, & Kleinman, 2002; Naeye & Peters, 1984; Rodriguez & Bohlin, 2005; Romano, Tremblay, Farhat, & Côté, 2006), and some research suggests that the effects of fetal nicotine exposure on attention are independent of those associated with antisocial behaviors (Button, Thapar, & McGuffin, 2005; Langley et al., 2007) and genetic transmission (Thapar et al., 2003). In a study comparing a large sample of boys with ADHD to their peers, increased rates of maternal smoking were documented retrospectively in the ADHD group (Milberger, Biederman, Faraone, Chen, & Jones, 1996). Importantly, the relation remained significant after controlling for SES, parental IQ, and parental ADHD diagnosis. Similarly, a case–control study estimated that maternal smoking was associated with a threefold increase in developing a hyperkinetic disorder, although other predictive factors such as SES and family psychiatric history partially weakened this association (Linnet et al., 2005). In spite of this evidence, the relation between nicotine exposure and disruptive psychopathology is not universally accepted, and some researchers have contested the degree of risk once confounding factors are controlled (D'Onofrio et al., 2010; Hill et al., 2000; Knopik et al., 2005; Nigg & Breslau, 2007; Roza et al., 2009; Silberg et al., 2003). In one study, researchers evaluated offspring of women who were conceived using assisted reproduction technologies in an attempt to remove the confound of inherited genetic risk for ADHD, as these children are genetically unrelated to the women who carry them during pregnancy. This study demonstrated that the association between prenatal smoking exposure and ADHD was significantly higher in genetically related mother-child pairs than in genetically unrelated pairs, suggesting ADHD is linked to inherited genetic effects rather than prenatal smoking exposure, per se (Thapar et al., 2009). This study and others highlight the need to test causal hypotheses regarding behavioral teratogenesis with careful consideration for confounding factors.

Prenatal nicotine exposure is also associated with other indicators of disruptive behavior, such as increases in dimensional measures of externalizing behavior, delinquency, and ADHD-like symptoms (Cornelius et al., 2011; Fergusson, 1999; Griesler, Kandel, & Davies, 1998; Indredavik, Brubakk, Romundstad, & Vik, 2007; Obel et al., 2009; Orlebeke, Knol, & Verhulst, 1997; Stene-Larsen, Borge, & Vollrath, 2009; Williams et al., 1998). In some samples, these effects survive statistical control of potentially confounding influences including child variables (e.g., sex, ethnicity), maternal variables (e.g., education, age, emotional responsiveness), SES, and parental histories of substance use and criminality (Cornelius et al., 2011; Fergusson, Horwood, & Lynskey, 1993; Indredavik et al., 2007; Obel et al., 2009). There is some evidence that teratogenic exposure may interact with genetic factors in producing psychological outcomes: a polymorphism of the dopamine transporter (DAT1) gene was associated with increases in hyperactive/impulsive and oppositional behaviors, but only in children who were prenatally exposed to nicotine (Kahn, Khoury, Nichols, & Lanphear, 2003). Another study demonstrated an interaction between prenatal exposure to smoking and variations in the DAT1 and DRD4 loci in children with ADHD. Children who inherited the DAT1 440 allele or the DRD 7-repeat allele and were exposed were almost 3 times more likely than nonexposed children to be diagnosed with ADHD (Neuman et al., 2007). Some research suggests that the interaction between DAT1 genotype and prenatal smoke exposure increases risk for hyperactivity and impulsivity only in males (Becker, El-Faddagh, Schmidt, Esser, & Laucht, 2008). Although the etiology of such behaviors is clearly multifaceted, these studies identify potential mechanisms through which gene-environment interactions increase psychopathological risk.

The association between disruptive, externalizing behavior and prenatal nicotine exposure appears to manifest in offspring at a young age. Assessments of toddlers whose mothers smoked during pregnancy reveal higher rates of negative conduct, including aggressive, oppositional behaviors, and/or hyperactive behaviors even after controlling for socioeconomic and child rearing variables (Brook, Brook, & Whiteman, 2000; Day, Richardson, Goldschmidt, & Cornelius, 2000; Linnet et al., 2006; Stene-Larsen et al., 2009). Poor peer relations and increased tantrums have also been described among toddlers exposed to nicotine, while covarying the effects of other drug exposures such as alcohol, marijuana, and cocaine (Faden & Graubard, 2000). Finally, maternal smoking during pregnancy was identified as a risk factor for persisting generalized behavioral problems, as measured by the Child Behavior Checklist Total Problems summary score, in a large sample of low weight, premature offspring assessed at 3, 5, and 8 years of age (Gray, Indurkhya, & McCormick, 2004). Although the disruptive disorders are the most commonly studied, a smaller body of literature suggests that higher rates of substance use problems, depression, and other internalizing symptoms are also associated with nicotine exposure (Ashford, van Lier, Timmermans, Cuijpers, & Koot, 2008; Brennan, Grekin, Mortensen, & Mednick, 2002; Ekblad, Gissler, Lehtonen, & Korkeila, 2010; Fergusson, Woodward, & Horwood, 1998; Indredavik et al., 2007; Weissman et al., 1999).

In summary, prenatal nicotine exposure appears to increase risk for psychiatric symptoms, although other important explanatory variables, such as concurrent prenatal exposures and family history, likely contribute to the association. Future research with greater control of confounding variables will be useful in further defining the role that prenatal nicotine exposure plays in the development of psychiatric symptoms.

## OTHER STIMULANT DRUGS

The teratogenic effects of other drugs of abuse are less studied than those of alcohol and nicotine, but there is some evidence that prenatal exposure to stimulants may be associated with subtle neurobehavioral alterations. Although early depictions of fetal cocaine exposure in the popular media were somewhat exaggerated, more recent research has attempted to clarify this issue. Regarding psychopathology, increased levels of aggressive behavior have been reported in cocaine-exposed children (Bada et al., 2007; Bada et al., 2011; Bendersky, Bennett, & Lewis, 2006; Griffith, Azuma, & Chasnoff, 1994; Linares et al., 2006; Minnes et al., 2010; Richardson, Goldschmidt,

Leech, & Willford, 2011; Sood et al., 2005), although the moderating effects of sex and comorbid alcohol exposure are important to consider (Nordstrom Bailey et al., 2005). Several studies have demonstrated that group differences remain even after controlling for potential confounds (Bada et al., 2007; Bada et al., 2011; Minnes et al., 2010; Richardson et al., 2011) and that behavior problems manifest in boys more than girls with prenatal cocaine exposure (Bendersky et al., 2006; Bennett, Bendersky, & Lewis, 2007; Delaney-Black et al., 2004; Dennis, Bendersky, Ramsay, & Lewis, 2006). However a few recent investigations have found the opposite, with cocaine-exposed girls being at greater risk for delinquent behaviors (McLaughlin et al., 2011; Minnes et al., 2010; Sood et al., 2005).

Prenatal cocaine exposure may also relate to increased infant and toddler irritability and mood lability (Behnke, Eyler, Garvan, Wobie, & Hou, 2002; Chaplin, Fahy, Sinha, & Mayes, 2009; Richardson, 1998; Richardson, Goldschmidt, & Willford, 2008). Still, it is not clear whether these behaviors observed in infancy correlate directly with increased psychopathology later in life. One follow-up study of 6-year-olds did not find effects of prenatal cocaine exposure on teacher ratings of child behavior after controlling for the influences of race, child IQ, school grade, and fetal exposure to alcohol, marijuana, and tobacco (Richardson, Conroy, & Day, 1996). However, in another investigation that evaluated prenatal cocaine exposure during the first trimester of pregnancy versus exposure throughout pregnancy demonstrated that school-aged children of mothers who used cocaine through the third trimester had increased externalizing behaviors after addressing confounding variables (Richardson et al., 2011). Furthermore, a recent study indicated that prenatal cocaine exposure was related to teen use of cocaine at age 14 (Delaney-Black et al., 2011). These findings suggest that the neurobehavioral effects of cocaine teratogenesis are subtle and may manifest differently as a factor of the exposed child's age and dose and timing of maternal cocaine use; they may also interact with a host of other risk factors. Interestingly, cognitive deficits, particularly deficits in attention, have been associated with prenatal cocaine exposure (Ackerman, Riggins, & Black, 2008; Bandstra, Morrow, Anthony, Accornero, & Fried, 2001; Heffelfinger, Craft, White, & Shyken, 2002; Noland et al., 2005; Savage, Brodsky, Malmud, Giannetta, & Hurt, 2005); however, the relation of these deficits to the development of ADHD remains unclear.

Despite the effects noted above, many studies have failed to find a sizeable association between prenatal cocaine exposure and the development of psychopathology such as behavior problems (Accornero, Morrow, Bandstra, Johnson, & Anthony, 2002; Azuma & Chasnoff, 1993; Bennett, Bendersky, & Lewis, 2002; Frank, Augustyn, Knight, Pell, & Zuckerman, 2001; Messinger et al., 2004; Nair, Black, Ackerman, Schuler, & Keane, 2008; Phelps, Wallace, & Bontrager, 1997; Warner et al., 2006), depressive symptoms (O'Leary et al., 2006), or poor impulse control (Bendersky & Lewis, 1998). Rather, research has suggested that postnatal variables such as the mother's continued drug use, level of mental functioning, and depressive symptoms may be better predictors of mental health status in cocaine-exposed children than exposure-related variables per se. In one previously discussed study that focused on alcohol exposure and development of depressive features in children, exposure to cocaine was associated with negative infant affect, but not with subsequent development of depressive features (O'Connor & Paley, 2006). Nicotine, marijuana, and caffeine were also examined in this sample. They were not associated with childhood depression, although it is unclear whether exposure to these other drugs occurred at rates high enough to afford adequate statistical power to detect effects, were they to exist.

## Possible Mechanisms of Action

As with the study of FASD, preclinical animal models of gestational stimulant drug exposure have been invaluable in elucidating the role of drugs of abuse on the developing CNS. In particular, monoaminergic systems have been implicated as targets of such exposure (cf. Mayes, 2002; Middaugh, 1989), although factors such as age and sex may be important moderators of outcome (Glatt, Bolaños, Trksak, & Jackson, 2000). Atypical development of monoamine transmission may help to explain the attention and arousal dysfunction observed in prenatal exposure cases to stimulants. For example, one possible causal model of arousal dysregulation following prenatal cocaine exposure is impairment in the ability to switch between executively versus automatically driven arousal (Mayes, 2002), functions subserved by the prefrontal cortex that rely on intact dopamine and norepinephrine transmission systems. Due to cocaine's effects on the developing monoaminergic system (e.g., uncoupling of the $D_1$ receptor), it is possible that the normal balance between dopaminergically mediated and noradrenergically mediated arousal regulatory systems is disrupted, leading to hyperarousal (Mayes, 2002). As with the case of alcohol, the mechanisms through which stimulant drugs affect prenatal development are likely to be multifaceted.

In summary, it appears that the behavioral effects of prenatal stimulant exposure are less pronounced than those associated with alcohol and nicotine teratogenesis and that environmental factors related to caregivers may be especially important to consider in stimulant exposure cases. Ultimately, more research is needed to clarify the extent to which exposure to stimulants increases the risk for developing psychopathology.

## Methylmercury and Lead

Methylmercury toxicity has also been associated with neurobehavioral deficits, as a result of both developmental and prenatal exposure (Debes, Budtz-Jorgensen, Weihe, White, & Grandjean, 2006; Julvez, Debes, Weihe, Choi, & Grandjean, 2010; Mendola, Selevan, Gutter, & Rice, 2002). However, there is little existing evidence that low-level exposures are associated with marked alterations of the course of typical behavioral development (Davidson et al., 2011; Davidson, Myers, Shamlaye, Cox, & Wilding, 2004; Myers et al., 2003). Much of the research on methylmercury derives from one longitudinal study of relatively low levels of exposure resulting from fish consumption (for review, see Davidson, Myers, Weiss, Shamlaye, & Cox, 2006). Findings do not indicate an association between prenatal methylmercury exposure and later adverse developmental outcomes in offspring. The most recent study evaluated the main cohort at age 17 years and found improved performance or no association between prenatal methylmercury exposure on 26 of 27 cognitive and behavioral measures (Davidson et al., 2011). However, in another cohort exposed to methylmercury through maternal consumption of whale meat, mercury-related cognitive deficits were found (Grandjean et al., 1997; Julvez et al., 2010). Although developmental outcome studies of prenatal exposure to methylmercury have revealed inconsistent findings (e.g., Spurgeon, 2006), only a few have examined behavior. Of the studies in which a behavioral measure was used, prenatal exposure to methylmercury was not related to negative outcomes (reviewed in Davidson et al., 2011; Myers & Davidson, 1998). Thus, although existing data do not suggest a link between methylmercury teratogenesis and psychopathology, more research is needed to confirm this preliminary conclusion, particularly in cases with higher exposure levels.

In considering teratogenic exposure to lead, it is often difficult to differentiate between prenatal and postnatal exposure, given the likelihood of continued environmental exposure after birth (Burns, Baghurst, Sawyer, McMichael, & Tong, 1999; Needleman, McFarland, Ness, Fienberg, & Tobin, 2002; Wasserman, Staghezza-Jaramillo, Shrout, Popovac, & Graziano, 1998). Research aimed at disambiguating the effects of timing of lead exposure suggests that postnatal lead exposure may be more influential than prenatal exposure (Bellinger, 1994; Leviton et al., 1993). However, there is some evidence for increased rates of delinquency in children exposed prenatally to lead. The Cincinnati Lead Study, which identified a cohort of pregnant women prospectively in order to examine the effects of lead toxicity on child development, found increased rates of both self- and parent-reported delinquency and antisocial behavior associated with prenatal lead exposure (Dietrich, Ris, Succop, Berger, & Bornschein, 2001). This relation was independent of birth weight, parental IQ, quality of home environment, and SES. In a later investigation conducted on the same cohort, prenatal lead exposure was related to high numbers of arrests in early adulthood (Wright et al., 2008). Thus, although developmental lead exposure has received the most attention regarding cognitive and behavioral outcomes in children, the potential importance of prenatal lead exposure should not be underestimated as there is some evidence that it can lead to deleterious consequences throughout the life span.

## Conclusions

Available data underscore the need for clinicians to take thorough prenatal exposure histories and consider the possible influence of teratogens when assessing psychiatric symptoms. The examples discussed in this chapter demonstrate that teratogenic exposure may increase risk for several common psychiatric disorders. However, the effects of potential mediating and moderating factors underscore a common theme: fetal exposures to teratogenic agents are not necessarily the sole or direct cause of mental illness. Rather, it seems teratogenic exposures act in concert with other risk factors, and a combination of interacting determinants is likely necessary to lead to the development of psychopathological behavior. Also, individuals with teratogenic exposures, such as alcohol, may not respond in the same manner as other mental health patients to psychotherapeutic and/or pharmacological treatments (Doig, McLennan, & Gibbard, 2008; O'Connor et al., 2002). Thus, taking an accurate prenatal history could be important for determining the most effective treatment.

## RISK AND PROTECTIVE FACTORS

Although complete prevention of teratogenic exposure is clearly ideal, this may not always be possible or practical. In addition, given the multifactorial nature of the etiology of psychiatric illness, it is important to identify factors that may prevent or limit the development of mental health problems in the face of teratogenic exposure. Such protective factors can form the cornerstone of effective mental health intervention and prevention efforts. An equally important task is to identify variables that increase the likelihood of developing psychopathology in cases of teratogenic exposures. Hopefully, once identified, exposure to such risk factors can be minimized. For example, in the case of alcohol, potential aspects that may protect individuals against a negative mental health outcome status include disability service eligibility; a nurturing, stable home (Streissguth et al., 1996); and early identification and treatment of children (Streissguth et al., 2004). Based on caregiver interviews, children who were reared in more stable home settings were three- to fourfold less likely to have experienced the majority of adverse life events examined (i.e., disrupted schooling, legal trouble, substance abuse, inappropriate sexual behaviors; Streissguth et al., 2004). In a more recent study, behavioral problems in alcohol-exposed children were related to the length of time spent in out-of-home placements (Fagerlund, Autti-Ramo, Hoyme, Mattson, & Korkman, 2011). This is an important point to underscore, as it highlights the interactive nature of biology-environment relationships that drive the development of psychopathology. Thus, a stable and nurturing home is one potential and salient environmentally-mediated pathway to protect children with prenatal alcohol exposure from developing psychopathological behavior.

## SYNTHESIS AND FUTURE DIRECTIONS

Insufficient data exist to determine conclusively whether there are associations between all known teratogens and psychopathology. Furthermore, the behavioral teratogenicity of many additional compounds, such as common prescription medications, remains virtually unknown. However, the effect of prenatal alcohol exposure on the development of psychiatric symptoms provides clear evidence that teratogenic exposure can increase the risk of developing psychopathology. More research is needed to provide pregnant women and their health care providers with adequate information to promote the health of both the mother and her child. In particular, future studies might focus on developing a profile of potential mental health problems for exposed individuals, while also distilling factors that may prevent development of mental health problems in these children. To promote factors that protect against mental illness and to deliver interventions effectively, valid early detection methods and increased awareness of teratogenic exposures, especially among pediatric healthcare providers, are necessary.

# REFERENCES

Accornero, V. H., Morrow, C. E., Bandstra, E. S., Johnson, A. L., & Anthony, J. C. (2002). Behavioral outcome of preschoolers exposed prenatally to cocaine: Role of maternal behavioral health. *Journal of Pediatric Psychology, 27,* 259–269.

Ackerman, J. P., Riggins, T., & Black, M. M. (2008). A review of the effects of prenatal cocaine exposure among school-aged children. *Pediatrics, 125,* 554–565.

Alati, R., Al Mamun, A., Williams, G. M., O'Callaghan, M., Najman, J. M., & Bor, W. (2006). In utero alcohol exposure and prediction of alcohol disorders in early adulthood: A birth cohort study. *Archives of General Psychiatry, 63,* 1009–1016.

Alati, R., Clavarino, A., Najman, J. M., O'Callaghan, M., Bor, W., Mamun, A. A., & Williams, G. M. (2008). The developmental origin of adolescent alcohol use: Findings from the Mater University Study of Pregnancy and its outcomes. *Drug and Alcohol Dependence,* 136–143.

American Psychiatric Association. (1994). *Diagnostic and statistical manual of mental disorders* (4th ed.). Washington, DC: American Psychiatric Association.

American Psychiatric Association. (2000). *Diagnostic and statistical manual of mental disorders,* (4th ed., text revision). Washington, DC: American Psychiatric Association.

Angold, A., Costello, E. J., & Erkanli, A. (1999). Comorbidity. *Journal of Child Psychology and Psychiatry and Allied Disciplines, 40,* 57–87.

Ashford, J., van Lier, P. A., Timmermans, M., Cuijpers, P., & Koot, H. M. (2008). Prenatal smoking and internalizing and externalizing problems in children studied from childhood to late adolescence. *Journal of the American Academy of Child & Adolescent Psychiatry, 47,* 779–787.

Azuma, S. D., & Chasnoff, I. J. (1993). Outcome of children prenatally exposed to cocaine and other drugs: A path analysis of three-year data. *Pediatrics, 92,* 396–402.

Bada, H. S., Bann, C. M., Bauer, C. R., Shankaran, S., Lester, B., LaGasse, L., . . . Higgins, R. (2011). Preadolescent behavior problems after prenatal cocaine exposure: Relationship between teacher and caretaker ratings (Maternal Lifestyle Study). *Neurotoxicology and Teratology, 33,* 78–87.

Bada, H. S., Das, A., Bauer, C. R., Shankaran, S., Lester, B., LaGasse, L., . . . Higgins, R. (2007). Impact of prenatal cocaine exposure on child behavior problems through school age. *Pediatrics, 119,* e348–359.

Baer, J. S., Barr, H. M., Bookstein, F. L., Sampson, P. D., & Streissguth, A. P. (1998). Prenatal alcohol exposure and family history of alcoholism in the etiology of adolescent alcohol problems. *Journal of Studies on Alcohol, 59,* 533–543.

Baer, J. S., Sampson, P. D., Barr, H. M., Connor, P. D., & Streissguth, A. P. (2003). 21-year longitudinal analysis of the effects of prenatal alcohol exposure on young adult drinking. *Archives of General Psychiatry, 60,* 377–385.

Baldwin, M. R. (2007). Fetal alcohol spectrum disorders and suicidality in a healthcare setting. *International Journal of Circumpolar Health, 66*, 54–60.

Bandstra, E. S., Morrow, C. E., Anthony, J. C., Accornero, V. H., & Fried, P. A. (2001). Longitudinal investigation of task persistence and sustained attention in children with prenatal cocaine exposure. *Neurotoxicology and Teratology, 23*, 545–559.

Barr, H. M., Bookstein, F. L., O'Malley, K. D., Connor, P. D., Huggins, J. E., & Streissguth, A. P. (2006). Binge drinking during pregnancy as a predictor of psychiatric disorders on the structured clinical interview for DSM-IV in young adult offspring. *American Journal of Psychiatry, 163*, 1061–1065.

Batstra, L., Hadders-Algra, M., & Neeleman, J. (2003). Effect of antenatal exposure to maternal smoking on behavioural problems and academic achievement in childhood: Prospective evidence from a Dutch birth cohort. *Early Human Development, 75*, 21–33.

Becker, K., El-Faddagh, M., Schmidt, M. H., Esser, G., & Laucht, M. (2008). Interaction of dopamine transporter genotype with prenatal smoke exposure on ADHD symptoms. *Journal of Pediatrics, 152*, 263–269.

Behnke, M., Eyler, F. D., Garvan, C. W., Wobie, K., & Hou, W. (2002). Cocaine exposure and developmental outcome from birth to 6 months. *Neurotoxicology and Teratology, 24*, 283–295.

Bellinger, D. (1994). Teratogen update: Lead. *Teratology, 50*, 367–373.

Bendersky, M., Bennett, D., & Lewis, M. (2006). Aggression at age 5 as a function of prenatal exposure to cocaine, gender, and environmental risk. *Journal of Pediatric Psychology, 31*, 71–84.

Bendersky, M., & Lewis, M. (1998). Prenatal cocaine exposure and impulse control at two years. *Annals of the New York Academy of Sciences, 846*(11 Suppl), 365–367.

Bennett, D. S., Bendersky, M., & Lewis, M. (2002). Children's intellectual and emotional-behavioral adjustment at 4 years as a function of cocaine exposure, maternal characteristics, and environmental risk. *Developmental Psychology, 38*, 648–658.

Bennett, D., Bendersky, M., & Lewis, M. (2007). Preadolescent health risk behavior as a function of prenatal cocaine exposure and gender. *Journal of Developmental & Behavioral Pediatrics, 28*, 467–472.

Bertrand, J., Floyd, R. L., & Weber, M. K. (2005). Guidelines for identifying and referring persons with fetal alcohol syndrome. *Morbidity and Mortality Weekly Report Recommendations and Reports, 54* (RR-11), 1–14.

Boland, F. J., Burrill, R., Duwyn, M., & Karp, J. (1998). *Fetal alcohol syndrome: Implications for correctional service*. Ottawa, Canada: Correctional Service of Canada.

Brennan, P. A., Grekin, E. R., & Mednick, S. A. (1999). Maternal smoking during pregnancy and adult male criminal outcomes. *Archives of General Psychiatry, 56*, 215–219.

Brennan, P. A., Grekin, E. R., Mortensen, E. L., & Mednick, S. A. (2002). Relationship of maternal smoking during pregnancy with criminal arrest and hospitalization for substance abuse in male and female adult offspring. *American Journal of Psychiatry, 159*, 48–54.

Brook, J. S., Brook, D. W., & Whiteman, M. (2000). The influence of maternal smoking during pregnancy on the toddler's negativity. *Archives of Pediatrics & Adolescent Medicine, 154,* 381–385.

Burd, L., Klug, M. G., Martsolf, J. T., & Kerbeshian, J. (2003). Fetal alcohol syndrome: Neuropsychiatric phenomics. *Neurotoxicology and Teratology, 25,* 697–705.

Burd, L., Selfridge, R. H., Klug, M. G., & Bakko, S. A. (2004). Fetal alcohol syndrome in the United States corrections system. *Addiction Biology, 9,* 169–176.

Burden, M. J., Jacobson, J. L., Westerlund, A., Lundahl, L. H., Morrison, A., Dodge, N. C., . . . Jacobson, S. W. (2010). An event-related potential study of response inhibition in ADHD with and without prenatal alcohol exposure. *Alcoholism: Clinical and Experimental Research, 34,* 617–627.

Burns, J. M., Baghurst, P. A., Sawyer, M. G., McMichael, A. J., & Tong, S.-l. (1999). Lifetime low-level exposure to environmental lead and children's emotional and behavioral development at ages 11–13 years. The Port Pirie cohort study. *American Journal of Epidemiology, 149,* 740–749.

Button, T. M. M., Thapar, A., & McGuffin, P. (2005). Relationship between anti-social behaviour, attention-deficit hyperactivity disorder and maternal prenatal smoking. *British Journal of Psychiatry, 187,* 155–160.

Carmichael Olson, H., Streissguth, A. P., Sampson, P. D., Barr, H. M., Bookstein, F. L., & Thiede, K. (1997). Association of prenatal alcohol exposure with behavioral and learning problems in early adolescence. *Journal of the American Academy of Child and Adolescent Psychiatry, 36,* 1187–1194.

Carr, J. L., Agnihotri, S., & Keightley, M. (2010). Sensory processing and adaptive behavior deficits of children across the fetal alcohol spectrum disorder continuum. *Alcoholism: Clinical and Experimental Research, 34,* 1022–1032.

Centers for Disease Control and Prevention. (2004). Alcohol consumption among women who are pregnant or who might become pregnant—United States, 2002. *Morbidity and Mortality Weekly Report, 53,* 1178–1181.

Chaplin, T. M., Fahy, T., Sinha, R., & Mayes, L. C. (2009). Emotional arousal in cocaine exposed toddlers: Prediction of behavior problems. *Neurotoxicology and Teratology, 31,* 275–282.

Coffin, J. M., Baroody, S., Schneider, K., & O'Neill, J. (2005). Impaired cerebellar learning in children with prenatal alcohol exposure: A comparative study of eyeblink conditioning in children with ADHD and dyslexia. *Cortex, 41,* 389–398.

Coles, C. D., Platzman, K. A., Brown, R. T., Smith, I. E., & Falek, A. (1997). Behavior and emotional problems at school age in alcohol-affected children. *Alcoholism: Clinical and Experimental Research, 21*(3 Suppl), 116A.

Coles, C. D., Platzman, K. A., & Lynch, M. E. (1999). Behavior problems reported by alcohol-affected adolescents and caregivers. *Alcoholism: Clinical and Experimental Research, 23*(5 Suppl), 107A.

Coles, C. D., Platzman, K. A., Lynch, M. E., & Freides, D. (2002). Auditory and visual sustained attention in adolescents prenatally exposed to alcohol. *Alcoholism: Clinical and Experimental Research, 26,* 263–271.

Coles, C. D., Platzman, K. A., Raskind-Hood, C. L., Brown, R. T., Falek, A., & Smith, I. E. (1997b). A comparison of children affected by prenatal alcohol exposure and attention deficit, hyperactivity disorder. *Alcoholism: Clinical and Experimental Research, 21*, 150–161.

Cornelius, M. D., De Genna, N. M., Leech, S. L., Willford, J. A., Goldschmidt, L., & Day, N. L. (2011). Effects of prenatal cigarette smoke exposure on neurobehavioral outcomes in 10-year-old children of adolescent mothers. *Neurotoxicology and Teratology, 33*, 137–144.

Crocker, N., Vaurio, L., Riley, E. P., & Mattson, S. N. (2009). Comparison of adaptive behavior in children with heavy prenatal alcohol exposure or attention-deficit/hyperactivity disorder. *Alcoholism: Clinical and Experimental Research, 33*, 2015–2023.

Crocker, N., Vaurio, L., Riley, E. P., & Mattson, S. N. (2011). Comparison of verbal learning and memory in children with heavy prenatal alcohol exposure or attention-deficit/ hyperactivity disorder. *Alcoholism: Clinical and Experimental Research, 35*, 1114–1121.

Davidson, P. W., Cory-Slechta, D. A., Thurston, S. W., Huang, L. S., Shamlaye, C. F., Gunzler, D., . . . Myers, G. J. (2011). Fish consumption and prenatal methylmercury exposure: Cognitive and behavioral outcomes in the main cohort at 17 years from the Seychelles child development study. *Neurotoxicology, 32*, 711–717.

Davidson, P. W., Myers, G. J., Shamlaye, C., Cox, C., & Wilding, G. E. (2004). Prenatal exposure to methylmercury and child development: Influence of social factors. *Neurotoxicology and Teratology, 26*, 553–559.

Davidson, P. W., Myers, G. J., Weiss, B., Shamlaye, C. F., & Cox, C. (2006). Prenatal methylmercury exposure from fish consumption and child development: A review of evidence and perspectives from the Seychelles child development study. *NeuroToxicology, 27*, 1106–1109.

Day, N. L., Richardson, G. A., Goldschmidt, L., & Cornelius, M. D. (2000). Effects of prenatal tobacco exposure on preschoolers' behavior. *Journal of Developmental and Behavioral Pediatrics, 21*, 180–188.

Debes, F., Budtz-Jorgensen, E., Weihe, P., White, R. F., & Grandjean, P. (2006). Impact of prenatal methylmercury exposure on neurobehavioral function at age 14 years. *Neurotoxicology and Teratology, 28*, 363–375.

Delaney-Black, V., Chiodo, L. M., Hannigan, J. H., Greenwald, M. K., Janisse, J., Patterson, G., . . . Sokol, R. J. (2011). Prenatal and postnatal cocaine exposure predict teen cocaine use. *Neurotoxicology and Teratology, 33*, 110–119.

Delaney-Black, V., Covington, C., Nordstrom, B., Ager, J., Janisse, J., Hannigan, J. H., . . . Sokol, R. J. (2004). Prenatal cocaine: Quantity of exposure and gender moderation. *Journal of Developmental and Behavioral Pediatrics, 25*, 254–263.

Dennis, T., Bendersky, M., Ramsay, D., & Lewis, M. (2006). Reactivity and regulation in children prenatally exposed to cocaine. *Developmental Psychology, 42*, 688–697.

Dietrich, K. N., Ris, M. D., Succop, P. A., Berger, O. G., & Bornschein, R. L. (2001). Early exposure to lead and juvenile delinquency. *Neurotoxicology and Teratology, 23*, 511–518.

Disney, E. R., Iacono, W., McGue, M., Tully, E., & Legrand, L. (2008). Strengthening the case: Prenatal alcohol exposure is associated with increased risk for conduct disorder. *Pediatrics, 122*, e1225–e1230.

Doig, J., McLennan, J. D., & Gibbard, W. B. (2008). Medication effects on symptoms of attention-deficit/hyperactivity disorder in children with fetal alcohol spectrum disorder. *Journal of Child and Adolescent Psychopharmacology, 18,* 365–371.

D'Onofrio, B. M., Singh, A. L., Iliadou, A., Lambe, M., Hultman, C. M., Grann, M.,...Lichtenstein, P. (2010). Familial confounding of the association between maternal smoking during pregnancy and offspring criminality: A population-based study in Sweden. *Archives of General Psychiatry, 67,* 529–538.

D'Onofrio, B. M., Van Hulle, C. A., Waldman, I. D., Rodgers, J. L., Rathouz, P. J., & Lahey, B. B. (2007). Causal inferences regarding prenatal alcohol exposure and childhood externalizing problems. *Archives of General Psychiatry, 64,* 1296–1304.

Dykens, E. M. (2000). Psychopathology in children with intellectual disability. *Journal of Child Psychology and Psychiatry and Allied Disciplines, 41,* 407–417.

Effect of alcoholism at time of conception. (1946). *Journal of the American Medical Association, 132,* 419.

Ekblad, M., Gissler, M., Lehtonen, L., & Korkeila, J. (2010). Prenatal smoking exposure and the risk of psychiatric morbidity into young adulthood. *Archives of General Psychiatry, 67,* 841–849.

Faden, V. B., & Graubard, B. I. (2000). Maternal substance use during pregnancy and developmental outcome at age three. *Journal of Substance Abuse, 12,* 329–340.

Fagerlund, A., Autti-Ramo, I., Hoyme, H. E., Mattson, S. N., & Korkman, M. (2011). Risk factors for behavioural problems in foetal alcohol spectrum disorders. *Acta Paediatrica, 100,* 1481–1488.

Famy, C., Streissguth, A. P., & Unis, A. S. (1998). Mental illness in adults with fetal alcohol syndrome or fetal alcohol effects. *American Journal of Psychiatry, 15,* 552–554.

Fast, D. K., & Conry, J. (2004). The challenge of fetal alcohol syndrome in the criminal legal system. *Addiction Biology, 9,* 161–166.

Fast, D. K., & Conry, J. (2009). Fetal alcohol spectrum disorders and the criminal justice system. *Developmental Disabilities Research Reviews, 15,* 250–257.

Fast, D. K., Conry, J., & Loock, C. A. (1999). Identifying fetal alcohol syndrome among youth in the criminal justice system. *Journal of Developmental and Behavioral Pediatrics, 20,* 370–372.

Fergusson, D. M. (1999). Prenatal smoking and antisocial behavior. *Archives of General Psychiatry, 56,* 223–224.

Fergusson, D. M., Horwood, L. J., & Lynskey, M. T. (1993). Maternal smoking before and after pregnancy: Effects on behavioral outcomes in middle childhood. *Pediatrics, 92,* 815–822.

Fergusson, D. M., Woodward, L. J., & Horwood, L. J. (1998). Maternal smoking during pregnancy and psychiatric adjustment in late adolescence. *Archives of General Psychiatry, 55,* 721–727.

Frank, D. A., Augustyn, M., Knight, W. G., Pell, T., & Zuckerman, B. (2001). Growth, development, and behavior in early childhood following prenatal cocaine exposure. *Journal of the American Medical Association, 285,* 1613–1625.

Fried, P. A., Watkinson, B., & Gray, R. (1992). A follow-up study of attentional behavior in 6-year-old children exposed prenatally to marijuana, cigarettes, and alcohol. *Neurotoxicology and Teratology, 14*, 299–311.

Fryer, S. L., McGee, C. L., Matt, G. E., Riley, E. P., & Mattson, S. N. (2007). Evaluation of psychopathological conditions in children with heavy prenatal alcohol exposure. *Pediatrics, 119*, e733–e741.

Gatzke-Kopp, L. M., & Beauchaine, T. P. (2007). Direct and passive prenatal nicotine exposure and the development of externalizing psychopathology. *Child Psychiatry and Human Development, 38*, 255–269.

Gibson, C. L., Piquero, A. R., & Tibbetts, S. G. (2000). Assessing the relationship between maternal cigarette smoking during pregnancy and age at first police contact. *Justice Quarterly, 17*, 519–542.

Glass, L., Ware, A. L., Crocker, N., Coles, C. D., Kable, J. A., May, P. A., . . . CIFASD. (2012). Prenatal alcohol exposure X ADHD: Interactive effects on neuropsychological performance. *Manuscript submitted for publication*.

Glatt, S. J., Bolaños, C. A., Trksak, G. H., & Jackson, D. (2000). Effects of prenatal cocaine exposure on dopamine system development: A meta-analysis. *Neurotoxicology and Teratology, 22*, 617–629.

Goodlett, C. R., & Horn, K. H. (2001). Mechanisms of alcohol-induced damage to the developing nervous system. *Alcohol Research and Health, 25*, 175–184.

Goodlett, C. R., Horn, K. H., & Zhou, F. C. (2005). Alcohol teratogenesis: Mechanisms of damage and strategies for intervention. *Experimental Biology and Medicine, 230*, 394–406.

Graham, D. M., Crocker, N., Deweese, B. N., Roesch, S. C., Coles, C. D., Kable, J. A., . . . CIFASD. (2011). Prenatal alcohol exposure, ADHD, and sluggish cognitive tempo. *Manuscript submitted for publication*.

Grandjean, P., Weihe, P., White, R. F., Debes, F., Araki, S., Yokoyama, K., . . . Jørgensen, P. J. (1997). Cognitive deficit in 7-year-old children with prenatal exposure to methylmercury. *Neurotoxicology and Teratology, 19*, 417–428.

Gray, R. F., Indurkhya, A., & McCormick, M. C. (2004). Prevalence, stability, and predictors of clinically significant behavior problems in low birth weight children at 3, 5, and 8 years of age. *Pediatrics, 114*, 736–743.

Greenbaum, R. L., Stevens, S. A., Nash, K., Koren, G., & Rovet, J. (2009). Social cognitive and emotion processing abilities of children with fetal alcohol spectrum disorders: A comparison with attention deficit hyperactivity disorder. *Alcoholism: Clinical and Experimental Research, 33*, 1656–1670.

Griesler, P. C., Kandel, D. B., & Davies, M. (1998). Maternal smoking in pregnancy, child behavior problems, and adolescent smoking. *Journal of Research on Adolescence, 8*, 159–185.

Griffith, D. R., Azuma, S. D., & Chasnoff, I. J. (1994). Three-year outcome of children exposed prenatally to drugs. *Journal of the American Academy of Child and Adolescent Psychiatry, 33*, 20–27.

Heffelfinger, A. K., Craft, S., White, D. A., & Shyken, J. (2002). Visual attention in preschool children prenatally exposed to cocaine: Implications for behavioral regulation. *Journal of the International Neuropsychological Society, 8*, 12–21.

Henshaw, S. K. (1998). Unintended pregnancy in the United States. *Family Planning Perspectives, 30*, 24–29, 46.

Hill, S. Y., Lowers, L., Locke-Wellman, J., & Shen, S. (2000). Maternal smoking and drinking during pregnancy and the risk for child and adolescent psychiatric disorders. *Journal of Studies on Alcohol, 61*, 661–668.

Hinshaw, S. P. (1992). Externalizing behavior problems and academic under-achievement in childhood and adolescence: Causal relationships and underlying mechanisms. *Psychological Bulletin, 111*, 127–155.

Indredavik, M. S., Brubakk, A. M., Romundstad, P., & Vik, T. (2007). Prenatal smoking exposure and psychiatric symptoms in adolescence. *Acta Paediatrica, 96*, 377–382.

Jacobson, J. L., Dodge, N. C., Burden, M. J., Klorman, R., & Jacobson, S. W. (2011). Number processing in adolescents with prenatal alcohol exposure and ADHD: Differences in the neurobehavioral phenotype. *Alcoholism: Clinical and Experimental Research, 35*, 431–442.

Jirikowic, T., Carmichael Olson, H., & Kartin, D. (2008). Sensory processing, school performance, and adaptive behavior of young school-age children with fetal alcohol spectrum disorders. *Physical and Occupational Therapy in Pediatrics, 28*, 117–136.

Jones, K. L., & Smith, D. W. (1973). Recognition of the fetal alcohol syndrome in early infancy. *Lancet, 2*(7836), 999–1001.

Jones, K. L., Smith, D. W., Ulleland, C. N., & Streissguth, A. P. (1973). Pattern of malformation in offspring of chronic alcoholic mothers. *Lancet, 1*(7815), 1267–1271.

Julvez, J., Debes, F., Weihe, P., Choi, A., & Grandjean, P. (2010). Sensitivity of continuous performance test (CPT) at age 14 years to developmental methylmercury exposure. *Neurotoxicology and Teratology, 32*, 627–632.

Kahn, R. S., Khoury, J., Nichols, W. C., & Lanphear, B. P. (2003). Role of dopamine transporter genotype and maternal prenatal smoking in childhood hyperactive-impulsive, inattentive, and oppositional behaviors. *Journal of Pediatrics, 143*, 104–110.

Knopik, V. S., Sparrow, E. P., Madden, P. A. F., Bucholz, K. K., Hudziak, J. J., Reich, W., . . . Heath, A. C. (2005). Contributions of parental alcoholism, prenatal substance exposure, and genetic transmission to child ADHD risk: A female twin study. *Psychological Medicine, 35*, 625–635.

Kooistra, L., Crawford, S., Gibbard, B., Kaplan, B. J., & Fan, J. (2011). Comparing attentional networks in fetal alcohol spectrum disorder and the inattentive and combined subtypes of attention deficit hyperactivity disorder. *Developmental Neuropsychology, 36*, 566–577.

Kooistra, L., Crawford, S., Gibbard, B., Ramage, B., & Kaplan, B. J. (2010). Differentiating attention deficits in children with fetal alcohol spectrum disorder or attention-deficit-hyperactivity disorder. *Developmental Medicine and Child Neurology, 52*, 205–211.

Kooistra, L., Ramage, B., Crawford, S., Cantell, M., Wormsbecker, S., Gibbard, B., & Kaplan, B. J. (2009). Can attention deficit hyperactivity disorder and fetal alcohol spectrum disorder be differentiated by motor and balance deficits? *Human Movement Science, 28*, 529–542.

Langley, K., Holmans, P. A., van den Bree, M. B., & Thapar, A. (2007). Effects of low birth weight, maternal smoking in pregnancy and social class on the phenotypic manifestation of Attention Deficit Hyperactivity Disorder and associated antisocial behaviour: Investigation in a clinical sample. *BMC Psychiatry, 7*, 1–8.

Lemoine, P., Harousseau, H., Borteyru, J.-P., & Menuet, J.-C. (1968). Les enfants de parents alcooliques. Anomalies observees. A propos de 127 cas [Children of alcoholic parents. Abnormalities observed in 127 cases]. *Ouest Medical, 21*, 476–482.

Leviton, A., Bellinger, D., Allred, E. N., Rabinowitz, M., Needleman, H., & Schoenbaum, S. (1993). Pre- and postnatal low-level lead exposure and children's dysfunction in school. *Environmental Research, 60*, 30–43.

Linares, T. J., Singer, L. T., Kirchner, H. L., Short, E. J., Min, M. O., Hussey, P., & Minnes, S. (2006). Mental health outcomes of cocaine-exposed children at 6 years of age. *Journal of Pediatric Psychology, 31*, 85–97.

Linnet, K. M., Obel, C., Bonde, E., Thomsen, P. H., Secher, N. J., Wisborg, K., & Henriksen, T. B. (2006). Cigarette smoking during pregnancy and hyperactive-distractible preschoolers: A follow-up study. *Acta Paediatrica, 95*, 694–700.

Linnet, K. M., Wisborg, K., Obel, C., Secher, N. J., Thomsen, P. H., Agerbo, E., & Henriksen, T. B. (2005). Smoking during pregnancy and the risk for hyperkinetic disorder in offspring. *Pediatrics, 116*, 462–467.

Lupton, C., Burd, L., & Harwood, R. (2004). Cost of fetal alcohol spectrum disorders. *American Journal of Medical Genetics Part C (Seminars in Medical Genetics), 127C*, 42–50.

Lynch, M. E., Coles, C. D., Corley, T., & Falek, A. (2003). Examining delinquency in adolescents differentially prenatally exposed to alcohol: The role of proximal and distal risk factors. *Journal of Studies on Alcohol, 64*, 678–686.

Mattson, S. N., & Riley, E. P. (1998). A review of the neurobehavioral deficits in children with fetal alcohol syndrome or prenatal exposure to alcohol. *Alcoholism: Clinical and Experimental Research, 22*, 279–294.

Mattson, S. N., & Riley, E. P. (2000). Parent ratings of behavior in children with heavy prenatal alcohol exposure and IQ-matched controls. *Alcoholism: Clinical and Experimental Research, 24*, 226–231.

Mattson, S. N., Riley, E. P., Gramling, L. J., Delis, D. C., & Jones, K. L. (1997). Heavy prenatal alcohol exposure with or without physical features of fetal alcohol syndrome leads to IQ deficits. *Journal of Pediatrics, 131*, 718–721.

Mattson, S. N., Riley, E. P., Gramling, L. J., Delis, D. C., & Jones, K. L. (1998). Neuropsychological comparison of alcohol-exposed children with or without physical features of fetal alcohol syndrome. *Neuropsychology, 12*, 146–153.

Maughan, B., Taylor, A., Caspi, A., & Moffitt, T. E. (2004). Prenatal smoking and early childhood conduct problems: Testing genetic and environmental explanations of the association. *Archives of General Psychiatry, 61*, 836–843.

Maughan, B., Taylor, C., Taylor, A., Butler, N., & Bynner, J. (2001). Pregnancy smoking and childhood conduct problems: A causal association? *Journal of Child Psychology and Psychiatry, 42,* 1021–1028.

May, P. A., Gossage, J. P., Kalberg, W. O., Robinson, L. K., Buckley, D., Manning, M., & Hoyme, H. E. (2009). Prevalence and epidemiologic characteristics of FASD from various research methods with an emphasis on recent in-school studies. *Developmental Disabilities Research Reviews, 15,* 176–192.

Mayes, L. C. (2002). A behavioral teratogenic model of the impact of prenatal cocaine exposure on arousal regulatory systems. *Neurotoxicology and Teratology, 24,* 385–395.

McGee, C. L., Bjorkquist, O. A., Price, J. M., Mattson, S. N., & Riley, E. P. (2009). Social information processing skills in children with histories of heavy prenatal alcohol exposure. *Journal of Abnormal Child Psychology, 37,* 817–830.

McGee, C. L., Fryer, S. L., Bjorkquist, O. A., Mattson, S. N., & Riley, E. P. (2008). Deficits in social problem solving in adolescents with prenatal exposure to alcohol. *American Journal of Drug and Alcohol Abuse, 34,* 423–431.

McLaughlin, A. A., Minnes, S., Singer, L. T., Min, M., Short, E. J., Scott, T. L., & Satayathum, S. (2011). Caregiver and self-report of mental health symptoms in 9-year old children with prenatal cocaine exposure. *Neurotoxicology and Teratology, 33,* 582–591.

Mendola, P., Selevan, S. G., Gutter, S., & Rice, D. (2002). Environmental factors associated with a spectrum of neurodevelopmental deficits. *Mental Retardation and Developmental Disabilities Research Reviews, 8,* 188–197.

Messinger, D. S., Bauer, C. R., Das, A., Seifer, R., Lester, B. M., Lagasse, L. L., . . . Poole, W. K. (2004). The maternal lifestyle study: Cognitive, motor, and behavioral outcomes of cocaine-exposed and opiate-exposed infants through three years of age. *Pediatrics, 113,* 1677–1685.

Mick, E., Biederman, J., Faraone, S. V., Sayer, J., & Kleinman, S. (2002). Case–control study of attention-deficit hyperactivity disorder and maternal smoking, alcohol use, and drug use during pregnancy. *Journal of the American Academy of Child and Adolescent Psychiatry, 41,* 378–385.

Middaugh, L. D. (1989). Prenatal amphetamine effects on behavior: Possible mediation by brain monoamines. *Annals of the New York Academy of Sciences, 562,* 308–318.

Milberger, S., Biederman, J., Faraone, S. V., Chen, L., & Jones, J. (1996). Is maternal smoking during pregnancy a risk factor for attention deficit hyperactivity disorder in children? *American Journal of Psychiatry, 153,* 1138–1142.

Minnes, S., Singer, L. T., Kirchner, H. L., Short, E., Lewis, B., Satayathum, S., & Queh, D. (2010). The effects of prenatal cocaine exposure on problem behavior in children 4–10 years. *Neurotoxicology and Teratology, 32,* 443–451.

Myers, G. J., & Davidson, P. W. (1998). Prenatal methylmercury exposure and children: Neurologic, developmental, and behavioral research. *Environmental Health Perspectives, 106*(Suppl 3), 841–847.

Myers, G. J., Davidson, P. W., Cox, C., Shamlaye, C. F., Palumbo, D., Cernichiari, E., . . . & Clarkson, T. W. (2003). Prenatal methylmercury exposure from ocean fish consumption in the Seychelles child development study. *Lancet, 361,* 1686–1692.

Naeye, R. L., & Peters, E. C. (1984). Mental development of children whose mothers smoked during pregnancy. *Obstetrics and Gynecology, 64,* 601–607.

Nair, P., Black, M. M., Ackerman, J. P., Schuler, M. E., & Keane, V. A. (2008). Children's cognitive-behavioral functioning at age 6 and 7: Prenatal drug exposure and caregiving environment. *Ambulatory Pediatrics, 8,* 154–162.

Nanson, J. L., & Hiscock, M. (1990). Attention deficits in children exposed to alcohol prenatally. *Alcoholism: Clinical and Experimental Research, 14,* 656–661.

Nash, K., Rovet, J., Greenbaum, R., Fantus, E., Nulman, I., & Koren, G. (2006). Identifying the behavioural phenotype in fetal alcohol spectrum disorder: Sensitivity, specificity and screening potential. *Archives of Women's Mental Health, 9,* 181–186.

National Institute on Drug Abuse. (1996). *National pregnancy and health survey: Drug use among women delivering livebirths, 1992* (Vol. Publication No. 96–3819). Rockville, MD: National Institutes of Health.

Needleman, H. L., McFarland, C., Ness, R. B., Fienberg, S. E., & Tobin, M. J. (2002). Bone lead levels in adjudicated delinquents. A case control study. *Neurotoxicology and Teratology, 24,* 711–717.

Neuman, R. J., Lobos, E., Reich, W., Henderson, C. A., Sun, L. W., & Todd, R. D. (2007). Prenatal smoking exposure and dopaminergic genotypes interact to cause a severe ADHD subtype. *Biological Psychiatry, 61,* 1320–1328.

Nigg, J. T., & Breslau, N. (2007). Prenatal smoking exposure, low birth weight, and disruptive behavior disorders. *Journal of the American Academy of Child and Adolescent Psychiatry, 46,* 362–369.

Noland, J. S., Singer, L. T., Short, E. J., Minnes, S., Arendt, R. E., Kirchner, H. L., & Bearer, C. (2005). Prenatal drug exposure and selective attention in preschoolers. *Neurotoxicology and Teratology, 27,* 429–438.

Nordstrom Bailey, B., Sood, B. G., Sokol, R. J., Ager, J., Janisse, J., Hannigan, J. H., . . . Delaney-Black, V. (2005). Gender and alcohol moderate prenatal cocaine effects on teacher-report of child behavior. *Neurotoxicology and Teratology, 27,* 181–189.

O'Connor, M. J. (2001). Prenatal alcohol exposure and infant negative affect as precursors of depressive features in children. *Infant Mental Health Journal, 22,* 291–299.

O'Connor, M. J., & Kasari, C. (2000). Prenatal alcohol exposure and depressive features in children. *Alcoholism: Clinical and Experimental Research, 24,* 1084–1092.

O'Connor, M. J., & Paley, B. (2006). The relationship of prenatal alcohol exposure and the post-natal environment to child depressive symptoms. *Journal of Pediatric Psychology, 31,* 50–64.

O'Connor, M. J., Shah, B., Whaley, S., Cronin, P., Gunderson, B., & Graham, J. (2002). Psychiatric illness in a clinical sample of children with prenatal alcohol exposure. *American Journal of Drug and Alcohol Abuse, 28,* 743–754.

O'Leary, C. C., Frank, D. A., Grant-Knight, W., Beeghly, M., Augustyn, M., Rose-Jacobs, R., . . . Gannon, K. (2006). Suicidal ideation among urban nine and ten year olds. *Journal of Developmental and Behavioral Pediatrics, 27,* 33–39.

O'Leary, C. M., Nassar, N., Zubrick, S. R., Kurinczuk, J. J., Stanley, F., & Bower, C. (2009). Evidence of a complex association between dose, pattern and timing of prenatal alcohol exposure and child behaviour problems. *Addiction, 105,* 74–86.

O'Malley, K., & Huggins, J. (2005). Suicidality in adolescents and adults with fetal alcohol spectrum disorders. *Canadian Journal of Psychiatry, 50,* 125.

Obel, C., Linnet, K. M., Henriksen, T. B., Rodriguez, A., Jarvelin, M. R., Kotimaa, A., . . . Olsen, J. (2009). Smoking during pregnancy and hyperactivity-inattention in the offspring—Comparing results from three Nordic cohorts. *International Journal of Epidemiology, 38,* 698–705.

Orlebeke, J. F., Knol, D. L., & Verhulst, F. C. (1997). Increase in child behavior problems resulting from maternal smoking during pregnancy. *Archives of Environmental Health, 52,* 317–321.

Phelps, L., Wallace, N. V., & Bontrager, A. (1997). Risk factors in early child development: Is prenatal cocaine/poly-drug exposure a key variable? *Psychology in the Schools, 34,* 245–252.

Piquero, A. R., Gibson, C. L., Tibbetts, S. G., Turner, M. G., & Katz, S. H. (2002). Maternal cigarette smoking during pregnancy and life-course-persistent offending. *International Journal of Offender Therapy and Comparative Criminology, 46,* 231–248.

Pulsifer, M. B. (1996). The neuropsychology of mental retardation. *Journal of the International Neuropsychological Society, 2,* 159–176.

Rantakallio, P., Läärä, E., Isohanni, M., & Moilanen, I. (1992). Maternal smoking during pregnancy and delinquency of the offspring: An association without causation? *International Journal of Epidemiology, 21,* 1106–1113.

Räsänen, P., Hakko, H., Isohanni, M., Hodgins, S., Järvelin, M.-R., & Tiihonen, J. (1999). Maternal smoking during pregnancy and risk of criminal behavior among adult male offspring in the northern Finland 1966 birth cohort. *American Journal of Psychiatry, 156,* 857–862.

Rasmussen, C., Talwar, V., Loomes, C., & Andrew, G. (2008). Brief report: Lie-telling in children with fetal alcohol spectrum disorder. *Journal of Pediatric Psychology, 33,* 220–226.

Richardson, G. A. (1998). Prenatal cocaine exposure. A longitudinal study of development. *Annals of the New York Academy of Sciences, 846,* 144–152.

Richardson, G. A., Conroy, M. L., & Day, N. L. (1996). Prenatal cocaine exposure: Effects on the development of school-age children. *Neurotoxicology and Teratology, 18,* 627–634.

Richardson, G. A., Goldschmidt, L., Leech, S., & Willford, J. (2011). Prenatal cocaine exposure: Effects on mother- and teacher-rated behavior problems and growth in school-age children. *Neurotoxicology and Teratology, 33,* 69–77.

Richardson, G. A., Goldschmidt, L., & Willford, J. (2008). The effects of prenatal cocaine use on infant development. *Neurotoxicology and Teratology, 30,* 96–106.

Rodriguez, A., & Bohlin, G. (2005). Are maternal smoking and stress during pregnancy related to ADHD symptoms in children? *Journal of Child Psychology and Psychiatry and Allied Disciplines, 46,* 246–254.

Rodriguez, A., Olsen, J., Kotimaa, A. J., Kaakinen, M., Moilanen, I., Henriksen, T. B., . . . Järvelin, M. R. (2009). Is prenatal alcohol exposure related to inattention and hyperactivity symptoms in children? Disentangling the effects of social adversity. *Journal of Child Psychology and Psychiatry, 5,* 1073–1083.

Roebuck, T. M., Mattson, S. N., & Riley, E. P. (1999). Behavioral and psychosocial profiles of alcohol-exposed children. *Alcoholism: Clinical and Experimental Research, 23,* 1070–1076.

Romano, E., Tremblay, R. E., Farhat, A., & Côté, S. (2006). Development and prediction of hyperactive symptoms from 2 to 7 years in a population-based sample. *Pediatrics, 117,* 2101–2110.

Roza, S. J., Verhulst, F. C., Jaddoe, V. W., Steegers, E. A., Mackenbach, J. P., Hofman, A., & Tiemeier, H. (2009). Maternal smoking during pregnancy and child behaviour problems: The Generation R Study. *International Journal of Epidemiology, 38,* 680–689.

Ruckinger, S., Rzehak, P., Chen, C. M., Sausenthaler, S., Koletzko, S., Bauer, C. P., . . . Heinrich, J. (2010). Prenatal and postnatal tobacco exposure and behavioral problems in 10-year-old children: Results from the GINI-plus prospective birth cohort study. *Environmental Health Perspectives, 118,* 150–154.

Rutter, M. (2003). Poverty and child mental health: Natural experiments and social causation. *Journal of the American Medical Association, 290,* 2063–2064.

Rutter, M. (2005). Environmentally mediated risks for psychopathology: Research strategies and findings. *Journal of the American Academy of Child and Adolescent Psychiatry, 44,* 3–18.

Sampson, P. D., Streissguth, A. P., Bookstein, F. L., Little, R. E., Clarren, S. K., Dehaene, P., . . . Graham, J. M. Jr. (1997). Incidence of fetal alcohol syndrome and prevalence of alcohol-related neurodevelopmental disorder. *Teratology, 56,* 317–326.

Savage, J., Brodsky, N. L., Malmud, E., Giannetta, J. M., & Hurt, H. (2005). Attentional functioning and impulse control in cocaine-exposed and control children at age ten years. *Journal of Developmental and Behavioral Pediatrics, 26,* 42–47.

Sayal, K., Heron, J., Golding, J., Alati, R., Smith, G. D., Gray, R., & Emond, A. (2009). Binge pattern of alcohol consumption during pregnancy and childhood mental health outcomes: Longitudinal population-based study. *Pediatrics, 123,* e289–e296.

Sayal, K., Heron, J., Golding, J., & Emond, A. (2007). Prenatal alcohol exposure and gender differences in childhood mental health problems: A longitudinal population-based study. *Pediatrics, 119,* e426–e434.

Schonfeld, A. M., Mattson, S. N., & Riley, E. P. (2005). Moral maturity and delinquency after prenatal alcohol exposure. *Journal of Studies on Alcohol, 66,* 545–554.

Silberg, J. L., Parr, T., Neale, M. C., Rutter, M., Angold, A., & Eaves, L. J. (2003). Maternal smoking during pregnancy and risk to boys' conduct disturbance: An examination of the causal hypothesis. *Biological Psychiatry, 53,* 130–135.

Sood, B. G., Nordstrom Bailey, B., Covington, C., Sokol, R. J., Ager, J., Janisse, J., . . . Delaney-Black, V. (2005). Gender and alcohol moderate caregiver reported child behavior after prenatal cocaine. *Neurotoxicology and Teratology, 27*, 191–201.

Spohr, H.-L., Willms, J., & Steinhausen, H.-C. (2007). Fetal alcohol spectrum disorders in young adulthood. *Journal of Pediatrics, 150*, 175–179.

Spurgeon, A. (2006). Prenatal methylmercury exposure and developmental outcomes: Review of the evidence and discussion of future directions. *Environmental Health Perspectives, 114*, 307–312.

Staroselsky, A., Fantus, E., Sussman, R., Sandor, P., Koren, G., & Nulman, I. (2009). Both parental psychopathology and prenatal maternal alcohol dependency can predict the behavioral phenotype in children. *Pediatric Drugs, 11*, 22–25.

Steinhausen, H.-C., Nestler, V., & Spohr, H.-L. (1982). Development and psychopathology of children with the fetal alcohol syndrome. *Journal of Developmental and Behavioral Pediatrics, 3*, 49–54.

Steinhausen, H.-C., & Spohr, H.-L. (1998). Long-term outcome of children with fetal alcohol syndrome: Psychopathology, behavior and intelligence. *Alcoholism: Clinical and Experimental Research, 22*, 334–338.

Steinhausen, H.-C., Willms, J., Metzke, C. W., & Spohr, H.-L. (2003). Behavioural phenotype in foetal alcohol syndrome and foetal alcohol effects. *Developmental Medicine and Child Neurology, 45*, 179–182.

Steinhausen, H.-C., Willms, J., & Spohr, H.-L. (1993). Long-term psychopathological and cognitive outcome of children with fetal alcohol syndrome. *Journal of the American Academy of Child and Adolescent Psychiatry, 32*, 990–994.

Steinhausen, H.-C., Willms, J., & Spohr, H.-L. (1994). Correlates of psychopathology and intelligence in children with fetal alcohol syndrome. *Journal of Child Psychology and Psychiatry and Allied Disciplines, 35*, 323–331.

Stene-Larsen, K., Borge, A. I., & Vollrath, M. E. (2009). Maternal smoking in pregnancy and externalizing behavior in 18-month-old children: Results from a population-based prospective study. *Journal of American Academy Child and Adolescent Psychiatry, 48*, 283–289.

Streissguth, A. (2007). Offspring effects of prenatal alcohol exposure from birth to 25 years: The Seattle prospective longitudinal study. *Journal of Clinical Psychology in Medical Settings, 14*, 81–101.

Streissguth, A. P., Aase, J. M., Clarren, S. K., Randels, S. P., LaDue, R. A., & Smith, D. F. (1991). Fetal alcohol syndrome in adolescents and adults. *Journal of the American Medical Association, 265*, 1961–1967.

Streissguth, A. P., Barr, H. M., Kogan, J., & Bookstein, F. L. (1996). *Final report: Understanding the occurrence of secondary disabilities in clients with fetal alcohol syndrome (FAS) and fetal alcohol effects (FAE)*. Seattle, WA: University of Washington.

Streissguth, A. P., Bookstein, F. L., Barr, H. M., Sampson, P. D., O'Malley, K., & Young, J. K. (2004). Risk factors for adverse life outcomes in fetal alcohol syndrome and fetal alcohol effects. *Journal of Developmental and Behavioral Pediatrics, 25*, 228–238.

Thanh, N. X., Jonsson, E., Dennett, L., & Jacobs, P. (2011). Costs of FASD. In E. P. Riley, S. Clarren, J. Weinberg, & E. Jonsson (Eds.), *Fetal alcohol spectrum disorder:*

*Management and policy perspectives of FASD* (pp. 45–69). Weinheim, Germany: Wiley-Blackwell.

Thapar, A., Fowler, T., Rice, F., Scourfield, J., van den Bree, M., Thomas, H., ... Hay, D. (2003). Maternal smoking during pregnancy and attention deficit hyperactivity disorder symptoms in offspring. *American Journal of Psychiatry, 160,* 1985–1989.

Thapar, A., Rice, F., Hay, D., Boivin, J., Langley, K., van den Bree, M., ... Harold, G. (2009). Prenatal smoking might not cause attention-deficit/hyperactivity disorder: Evidence from a novel design. *Biological Psychiatry, 66,* 722–727.

Thomas, S. E., Kelly, S. J., Mattson, S. N., & Riley, E. P. (1998). Comparison of social abilities of children with fetal alcohol syndrome to those of children with similar IQ scores and normal controls. *Alcoholism: Clinical and Experimental Research, 22,* 528–533.

Uban, K. A., Bodnar, T., Butts, K., Sliwowska, J. H., Comeau, W., & Weinberg, J. (2011). Direct and indirect mechanisms of alcohol teratogenesis: Implications for understanding alterations in brain and behavior in FASD. In E. P. Riley, S. Clarren, J. Weinberg, & E. Jonsson (Eds.), *Fetal alcohol spectrum disorder: Management and policy perspectives of FASD* (pp. 73–108). Weinheim, Germany: Wiley-Blackwell.

Vaurio, L., Riley, E. P., & Mattson, S. N. (2008). Differences in executive functioning in children with heavy prenatal alcohol exposure or attention-deficit/hyperactivity disorder. *Journal of the International Neuropsychological Society, 14,* 119–129.

Viner, R. M., & Taylor, B. (2005). Adult health and social outcomes of children who have been in public care: Population-based study. *Pediatrics, 115,* 894–899.

Vorhees, C. V. (1986). Principles of behavioral teratology. In E. P. Riley & C. V. Vorhees (Eds.), *Handbook of behavioral teratology* (pp. 23–48). New York, NY: Plenum Press.

Wakschlag, L. S., Lahey, B. B., Loeber, R., Green, S. M., Gordon, R. A., & Leventhal, B. L. (1997). Maternal smoking during pregnancy and the risk of conduct disorder in boys. *Archives of General Psychiatry, 54,* 670–676.

Wakschlag, L. S., Pickett, K. E., Cook, E. Jr., Benowitz, N. L., & Leventhal, B. L. (2002). Maternal smoking during pregnancy and severe antisocial behavior in offspring: A review. *American Journal of Public Health, 92,* 966–974.

Wakschlag, L. S., Pickett, K. E., Kasza, K. E., & Loeber, R. (2006). Is prenatal smoking associated with a developmental pattern of conduct problems in young boys? *Journal of the American Academy of Child and Adolescent Psychiatry, 45,* 461–467.

Ware, A. L., Crocker, N., O'Brien, J. W., Deweese, B. N., Roesch, S. C., Coles, C. D., ... CIFASD. (2012). Executive function predicts adaptive behavior in children with histories of heavy prenatal alcohol exposure and attention deficit/hyperactivity disorder. *Manuscript submitted for publication.*

Ware, A. L., O'Brien, J. W., Crocker, N., Deweese, B. N., Roesch, S. C., Coles, C. D., ... Mattson, S. M. (in press). The effects of prenatal alcohol exposure and ADHD on psychiatric comorbidity and behavior. *Alcoholism: Clinical and Experimental Research.*

Warner, T. D., Behnke, M., Hou, W., Garvan, C. W., Wobie, K., & Eyler, F. D. (2006). Predicting caregiver-reported behavior problems in cocaine-exposed children at 3 years. *Journal of Developmental and Behavioral Pediatrics, 27,* 83–92.

Wasserman, G. A., Liu, X., Pine, D. S., & Graziano, J. H. (2001). Contribution of maternal smoking during pregnancy and lead exposure to early child behavior problems. *Neurotoxicology and Teratology, 23,* 13–21.

Wasserman, G. A., Staghezza-Jaramillo, B., Shrout, P., Popovac, D., & Graziano, J. (1998). The effect of lead exposure on behavior problems in preschool children. *American Journal of Public Health, 88,* 481–486.

Weissman, M. M., Warner, V., Wickramaratne, P. J., & Kandel, D. B. (1999). Maternal smoking during pregnancy and psychopathology in offspring followed to adulthood. *Journal of the American Academy of Child and Adolescent Psychiatry, 38,* 892–899.

Whaley, S. E., O'Connor, M. J., & Gunderson, B. (2001). Comparison of the adaptive functioning of children prenatally exposed to alcohol to a nonexposed clinical sample. *Alcoholism: Clinical and Experimental Research, 25,* 1018–1024.

Williams, G. M., O'Callaghan, M., Najman, J. M., Bor, W., Andersen, M. J., & Richards, D. (1998). Maternal cigarette smoking and child psychiatric morbidity: A longitudinal study. *Pediatrics, 102,* e11.

Wright, J. P., Dietrich, K. N., Ris, M. D., Hornung, R. W., Wessel, S. D., Lanphear, B. P., . . . Rae, M. N. (2008). Association of prenatal and childhood blood lead concentrations with criminal arrests in early adulthood. *PLoS Medicine, 5,* e101.

# CHAPTER 10

# Brain Injury as a Risk Factor for Psychopathology

KATHERINE E. SHANNON BOWEN AND LISA M. GATZKE-KOPP

## HISTORICAL CONTEXT

THE 1848 ACCIDENT OF railroad worker Phineas Gage is legendary in psychology and neuroscience, described commonly in introductory textbooks. Gage attained fame after surviving an extraordinary accident in which an explosion propelled a 3-foot-long iron rod through the frontal portion of his skull and brain. Merely surviving such an accident is uncommon, but more remarkable was his apparent recovery of memory, communication, and most other basic mental functions. However, reports from those close to Gage indicate that the injury conferred permanent changes to his personality, resulting in self-destructive and socially inappropriate behaviors stemming from poor judgment (see Macmillan, 2002). Continued fascination with this story over the past 150 years follows from its demonstration that the brain is responsible for fundamental aspects of our individuality. This story illustrates both the importance of brain function for cardinal components of psychological health, and its vulnerability to trauma.

## TERMINOLOGICAL AND CONCEPTUAL ISSUES

Gage's story is an incontrovertible example of open head brain trauma. More recently, scientists have also gained increased understanding of the consequences of traumatic force occurring without skull penetration—referred to as *closed head injury*. Closed head injuries and their sequelae continue to be a prominent focus of medical research. This is especially the case for minor head injuries, commonly known as *concussions*. A concussion is usually defined as neurological impairment caused by biomechanical strain on central nervous system (CNS) tissue. It is important to note, however, that the term *concussion* has no standardized definition and that it is used inconsistently among clinicians and parents to refer to varying severities of brain injury and may even be used to ease parental concern and imply a lack of lasting consequences (Dematteo et al., 2010). Yet despite no formal definition, concussions are usually associated with symptoms in one or more of the following domains: (a) cognitive, including confusion, poor concentration, inability to follow directions or answer questions, amnesia and/or loss of consciousness; (b) medical, including headaches, nausea and/or vomiting; (c) sensory, including dizziness, poor coordination and/or loss of balance, alterations in vision or hearing (seeing stars or hearing ringing); and (d) psychological, including irritability, changes in personality, and/or emotions inappropriate for their context (McCrory et al., 2005).

Concussions were long believed to be transient physical states with complete resolution of symptoms expected within 3 months. Thus, it was believed that no permanent changes in brain structure, function, or behavior characterized concussion victims (Gaetz, Goodman, & Weinberg, 2000). However, recent research indicates that detrimental effects can persist for many individuals for extended periods of time even in cases classified as mild (see Yeates, 2010). Some evidence also suggests that impairments can increase rather than decrease in the weeks following injury (Scherwath et al., 2011).

Importantly, detrimental effects of mild head injuries are extended and exacerbated when experienced repeatedly. Repetitive head injuries are common among athletes at both the amateur and professional levels, from childhood through adulthood. High-contact sports such as football and hockey, where head-to-head contact can occur between athletes, and even soccer, where the head may collide with other athletes, hit the ground, or strike the ball, are associated with high concussion rates (Delaney, Puni, & Rouah, 2006). Consequently, organized sports have become a focus of both research and policy developments with regard to brain injury. In 2009, the Zackery Lystedt law (2009) was passed prohibiting young athletes from returning to play after a suspected concussion without approval from a medical professional. This law follows in part from evidence that concussions result in metabolic changes that temporarily enhance susceptibility of the brain to further damage. Unfortunately, recent neuroimaging research suggests that resolution of these metabolic changes may not coincide with remission of cognitive symptoms or recovery time (Vagnozzi et al., 2008). Considerably more work is needed before precise decisions can be made about when vulnerability subsides.

In addition to traumatic head injury, the brain is susceptible to insults from other sources, most notably teratogenic substances (i.e., substances ingested by the mother that affect the developing brain; see Chapter 9) and insufficient supply of oxygen (hypoxia) or blood flow (ischemia). The brain may be especially vulnerable to these influences prenatally. In particular, hypoxia and ischemia result in extensive cell death (see Ment, Hirtz, & Hüppi, 2009; Vannucci, 2000), although the behavioral and psychological consequences are not specific or well understood. In this chapter, we review basic brain injury mechanisms, discuss specific developmental aspects of brain injury, and consider how injury contributes to the development of psychopathology.

PREVALENCE

Children between the ages of 0 and 4 years, and adolescents between the ages of 15 and 19 years, are most likely to sustain a brain injury (Faul, Xu, Wald, & Coronado, 2010). Each year an estimated half million children are brought to emergency rooms for treatment of traumatic brain injury (TBI), of whom fewer than 1% die. An unknown number of additional individuals sustain injuries that are unreported and receive no medical attention (Faul et al., 2010). Abuse is a common cause of head injuries among infants and toddlers, representing an estimated 22% of all TBIs among those 0 to 3 years old (Leventhal, Martin, & Asnes, 2010). Factors resulting in even mild levels of oxygen desaturation—including medical conditions such as congenital heart disease, sleep-disordered breathing, and severe or poorly treated asthma, as well as accidents such as near drownings or carbon monoxide poisoning—can also result in significant cell death (Bass et al., 2004; Hori, 1985). However, such injuries are difficult to quantify and may go unrecognized in mild cases, making occurrence rates difficult to estimate.

In addition to age, other individual differences are also associated with susceptibility to brain injuries. Rates of occurrence are higher in males and among individuals of lower socioeconomic status (Bruns & Hauser, 2003; Faul et al., 2010). Researchers reviewing medical charts across more than 70 hospitals found that children with high levels of impulsivity, such as those with attention deficit/hyperactivity disorder (ADHD), are more likely to sustain injuries to all areas of the body, with head injuries being no exception. In this study, children with ADHD were also more likely to sustain severe injuries (DiScala, Lescohier, Barthel, & Li, 1998). However, other studies have failed to report these associations (see Davidson, 1987; Olsson, Le Brocque, Kenardy, Anderson, & Spence, 2008), and some authors have suggested that the apparent link is due in large part to poor parental supervision commonly experienced by externalizing children (Schwebel, Hodgens, & Sterling, 2006). Furthermore, although impulsivity is highly heritable (see Chapter 6), child-specific environment factors are a better predictor of injury frequency than genetic or family environment factors, suggesting little support for a heritable "injury/accident proneness" trait among children (Ordoñana, Caspi, & Moffitt, 2008). Given these conflicting findings, debate continues regarding impulsivity as a risk factor for head injuries, including whether head injuries and externalizing behaviors are multifinal consequences of other environmental risks.

## ETIOLOGICAL FORMULATION

Causes of brain injury include accidental trauma (i.e., falls, car or bicycle accidents, sports collisions), non-accidental trauma (i.e., child abuse), and hypoxic-ischemic events (i.e., medical conditions that interfere with oxygen availability, including pregnancy and birth complications, infection, or damage secondary to trauma). Developments in research over the past several decades have highlighted the fact that injury to the brain can occur at any time during development, and multiple causes of injury can result in similar types of brain damage. Animal models, postmortem studies with humans, and advanced neuroimaging techniques have helped to elucidate the mechanisms and pathophysiology underlying brain injury. In the sections that follow, we focus on the most common and basic injurious factors resulting in brain cell death, trauma and hypoxia, and describe neuroimaging methods that are sensitive to detecting various types of injuries and causes of brain cell death.

## Mechanisms of Brain Injury

*Trauma.* Traumatic brain injury is defined as a change in brain function that manifests as confusion, altered level of consciousness, coma, seizure, acute sensory or motor neurological deficit, neuropsychological deficit, or behavioral change, resulting from any blunt or penetrating force to the head (Bruns & Hauser, 2003). TBI occurs when rapid deceleration of the brain against the bony inner surface of the skull produces tissue compression, resulting in neuronal and vascular damage (Finnie & Blumbergs, 2002). The nature of the mechanical force applied to the head produces different types of tissue damage, most commonly classified as focal or diffuse (Gennarelli & Meaney, 1996). Focal tissue damage occurs most often in injuries resulting from a translational force applied along the linear axis of the brain (Yeates, 2000). Under conditions insufficient to penetrate the skull, the force results in a localized deformation of the bone and compression of the underlying tissue (Gennarelli & Meaney, 1996). When the brain compresses against the skull, small hemorrhages develop on the gyral surfaces of the brain, causing a contusion or focal tissue damage (Finnie & Blumbergs, 2002). Such injuries also result in contrecoup contusions, constituting compressive tissue damage at regions remote from the initial contact point. This occurs when the force applied to the head causes the brain to rebound, contacting the skull a second time at a point opposite the initial contact (Gennarelli & Meaney, 1996). These types of injuries can result in significant tissue damage, most commonly without a loss of consciousness (Gennarelli & Meaney, 1996). Given the degree of tissue damage that can occur without a consequent loss of consciousness, the neurological indicator of unconsciousness is a poor surrogate for radiological or neuropsychological assessment (Schutzman & Greenes, 2001).

In contrast to focal damage caused by translational injuries, diffuse damage results from rotational forces, producing angular movement around the brain's center of gravity. This occurs when the head strikes against a broad object, such as the interior of a car, diffusing the force across the surface of the skull (Gennarelli & Meaney, 1996). The rotational force produces a shearing strain on the brain, tearing axonal tissue. By destroying axons, afferent and efferent activity can be interrupted in any brain region. The destruction of axonal communications between and across regions can produce functionally similar impairments as direct focal damage to the disrupted region. For instance, a disruption in the connection between the frontal cortex and subcortical structures can produce frontally mediated impairment without observable damage to the frontal lobe (Schnider & Gutbrod, 1999). In fact, axonal damage is frequently undetectable by standard neuroimaging protocols, requiring advanced imaging techniques such as volumetric analysis and diffusion tensor imaging (Ashwal, Holshouser, & Tong, 2006; Van Boven et al., 2009). Because of disrupted connections between brain areas, these types of injuries often lead to widespread damage and can affect deeper anatomical structures than are vulnerable to focal contusions.

Regardless of the form of injury, TBI severity is most commonly classified into categories of mild, moderate, or severe based on acute neurological impairment using the Glasgow Coma Scale (GCS; Teasdale & Jennett, 1974). Past estimates of hospitalized brain injured patients indicate that as many as 80% suffer injuries classified as mild based on GCS ratings (Kraus & Nourjah, 1988). Mild injuries can include loss of consciousness, concussive symptoms, and the need for short-term hospitalization, but they may also present with sequelae mild enough to be dismissed by the patient (Gabriel & Turner, 1996; Rimel, Giordani, Barth, Boll, & Jane, 1981). Although clinical neuroimaging may appear normal, suggestive of no lasting damage, recent diffusion imaging studies with children and adolescents reveal microscopic damage (see Ashwal, Wycliffe, & Holshouser, 2010; Chu et al., 2010). Acquisition of small lesions resulting from mild injuries may be especially dangerous if they accumulate over time through repeated injury exposure (Collins et al., 2003; Prins, Hales, Reger, Giza, & Hovda, 2010).

In addition to the primary effects of damage in response to the biomechanical strain placed on tissue, secondary injuries frequently evolve from brain trauma. Most commonly edema, or swelling, occurs at the site of focal injuries, increasing intracranial pressure and restricting blood flow, which leads to metabolic failures, resulting in cell death (Bigler, 2001b). This type of cell death (see hypoxia section, below) can lead to apoptosis, or signaling of one cell to induce death in neighboring cells. Secondary brain injury in response to trauma develops over time and can occur among those whose injuries are initially classified as mild and whose clinical evaluations in the immediate aftermath of the injury appear normal (Schutzman & Greenes, 2001). Because of the extent of secondary injuries, tissue damage is often more global than local. Studies of both children and adults indicate that reductions in total gray and white matter follow even mild injuries and appear to increase linearly with injury severity (Bigler, 2001a; Wilde et al., 2005).

*Hypoxia.* Hypoxia refers to a reduction in the supply of oxygen necessary for normal cellular function and can occur through both respiratory and circulatory failures (Nyakas, Buwalda, & Luiten, 1996). Hypoxia leads to brain damage through both acute and protracted pathways. Acute reduction in oxygen inhibits metabolic processes in cells and results in release of neurotransmitters with excitotoxic effects (Golan & Huleihel, 2006). This cytotoxic process then induces a stress response that propagates chemical signaling of the self-destructive process known as apoptosis. The extended activation of programmed cell death can occur up to several weeks beyond the original hypoxic insult. The accumulation of cell loss over these several weeks is often what leads to behavioral deficits (Golan & Huleihel, 2006). Although research has focused on medical interventions that may arrest this process and alleviate damage induced by acute hypoxic events, such procedures vary widely in their use, often with uncertain clinical utility, particularly for pediatric patients (see Morrow & Pearson, 2010).

Hypoxia occurring in conjunction with a variety of medical conditions can cause adverse neurological effects (Bass et al., 2004). However, the majority of hypoxic events occur pre- and perinatally. Consequently, pre- and perinatal effects have dominated the study of hypoxia, with far less attention paid to the effects of acute hypoxic events later in life. Hypoxia is a common complication of compromised pregnancies and can result from a variety of causes including premature birth and placental insufficiency (Vannucci, 2000). Hypoxia is also a complication of restricted blood flow to the umbilical artery, which occurs during episodes of maternal alcohol consumption (Mukherjee & Hodgen, 1982) and smoking (Socol, Manning, Murata, & Druzin, 1982). In cases of prenatal hypoxic exposure, infants are often characterized by low birth weight for their gestational age, an overt indication of maldevelopment (McClure, Peiffer, Rosen, & Fitch, 2005). In addition to prenatal damage, hypoxia can also occur during the birthing process from restricted oxygen flow to the fetus during a prolonged or complicated delivery, resulting in respiratory difficulties requiring resuscitation on delivery. Hypoxic damage ranks among the top 10 causes of death in neonates (Martin, Kochanek, Strobino, Guyer, & MacDorman, 2005) and is a common complication in babies born preterm. The incidence of preterm birth accounted for 12.3% of U.S. births in 2003 (Martin et al., 2005). Fortunately, in recent years, increasing survival rates have been accompanied by decreases in medical complications, negative neurological sequelae, and adverse cognitive effects (Baron & Rey-Casserly, 2010).

The regions of tissue damage and resultant behavioral implications in response to hypoxia are dependent on a wide range of factors, complicating clinical efforts to generate a prognosis (Golan & Huleihel, 2006). Factors such as developmental maturation of the neural tissue, duration and degree of hypoxic exposure, and the degree of neuroprotective factors intrinsic to an individual are difficult to identify and quantify in clinical practice. Thus, sequelae of hypoxia are variable and range from mild impairments in cognition and behavior to deficits in motor coordination and the development of cerebral palsy in extreme cases. If ischemia is also present, more severe atrophy of brain regions including the motor cortex, hippocampus, and striatum may occur (Decker & Rye, 2002). When extreme and overt compromise is evident—resulting in such conditions as motor disabilities, cerebral palsy, and even epilepsy—the extent of damage may be revealed with neuroimaging techniques. Using magnetic resonance imaging, white matter damage is the most commonly identified pathology in infants suffering hypoxia prenatally, with additional reductions in overall cortical gray matter (Robinson, 2005; see Ment et al., 2009).

However, more subtle variations in neurochemical function affecting cellular communication occur in response to hypoxia that is insufficient to produce gross structural damage. For instance, researchers have found decrements in dopamine receptors in the striatum following experimental induction of hypoxia/ischemia, despite normal structural appearance (Zouakia, Guilloteau, Zimmer, Besnard, & Chalon, 1997). Striatal cells are the most vulnerable to cell death resulting from mild hypoxia (Rothstein & Levison, 2005; see Gatzke-Kopp, 2011). Subtle neurochemical disruptions are thought to result in psychological and behavioral disturbances, such as ADHD, which are observed with higher frequency in cases of fetal hypoxia, even in the absence of marked neurological dysfunction (Nyakas et al., 1996). Such findings are consistent with theories identifying striatal mesolimbic dopamine deficiency as a primary etiological contribution to the development of ADHD (Gatzke-Kopp, 2011; Gatzke-Kopp & Beauchaine, 2007; Sagvolden, Johansen, Aase, & Russell, 2005).

## ADVANCES IN NEUROIMAGING AND PEDIATRIC TBI

Traditional clinical imaging techniques include computed tomography (CT) and magnetic resonance imaging (MRI). Because MRI does not require radioactive exposure, it has advantages for pediatric patients when repeated scans are necessary. MRI volumetric analysis identifies both gray and white matter total and regional volume loss, which correlate with injury severity (Levine et al., 2008; Van Boven et al., 2009). However, findings from the past 5 to 10 years, in which the use of advanced imaging techniques has become increasingly common, suggest that volumetric MRI may be insufficiently sensitive to neuronal damage associated with mild head injuries.

Structural measures such as susceptibility-weighed imaging (SWI) and diffusion tensor imaging (DTI) allow for increased sensitivity to hemorrhagic and axonal injury, respectively (Van Boven et al., 2009). SWI capitalizes on the different magnetic susceptibilities of discrete tissue types, and can be calibrated to preferentially enhance sensitivity to the detection of blood (Van Boven et al., 2009). SWI can identify 4 to 6 times as many microhemorrhages in pediatric TBI than standard clinical imaging protocols, and is useful in predicting neurologic and neuropsychiatric outcomes (Ashwal et al., 2010). DTI measures the diffusion of water molecules indirectly, and is most commonly thought to index integrity of white matter tracts. DTI is sensitive to microstructural abnormalities, and is especially useful in mild TBI, where structural abnormalities may not be detected with standard imaging protocols. However, this method is nonspecific and abnormalities may represent a variety of conditions, including axonal sheering, demyelenation, inflammation, and edema (Van Boven et al., 2009). Regardless of etiology, changes in diffusivity identified with DTI predict working memory and executive deficits among children (Wozniak et al., 2007). In fact, in assessing diffuse prefrontal injury, DTI may be more predictive of neurological outcome than traditional MRI techniques (Oni et al., 2010). Other measures, such as magnetic resonance spectroscopy (MRS), may be better suited for detecting metabolic changes in cell function related to brain injury and vulnerability. MRS allows for the assessment of metabolites that mark injury, even in clinical scans that are deemed "normal." In children, altered metabolite ratios (i.e., lower *N*-acetylaspartate (NAA)/creatine (CR), lower NAA/choline (Cho), higher Cho/Cr) are related to poorer neurological and neurobehavioral outcomes (see Ashwal et al., 2010).

Advances in statistical analyses have also provided better understanding of the sequelae of damage, but only recently have these methods been used with children. Functional connectivity analyses have begun to provide information about interrelationships between brain regions rather than simple independent levels of activation within given regions. Functional connectivity can refer to any correlational measure of regional activation, but is most often used to refer to correlations in blood-oxygen-level dependent (BOLD) activation either during task or resting states. It provides an indirect measure of coordination between brain regions without assuming anatomical connectivity (Fox & Raichle, 2007). To date, functional connectivity studies with children are sparse. However, in one study, task related functional connectivity between Wernicke's area and other bilateral language areas during passive listening was stronger for children born preterm than for controls, suggesting a broader and less specialized functional brain network for language processing among preterm children (Gozzo et al., 2009). Research also demonstrates that resting-state patterns in brain functional integration, or "default mode" networks, change across development (Fair et al., 2009). Abnormalities in resting-state connectivity have been identified among children born preterm (Damaraju et al., 2010) and among adults who have sustained TBI (Johnson et al., 2011). Advanced imaging techniques have allowed for greater detection of injury and predictive utility in pediatric populations. These measures are not only more sensitive to changes that result from both primary and secondary injury, but in conjunction with traditional imaging modalities, hold promise for better detection of pediatric brain injury (Ashwal et al., 2006).

## DEVELOPMENTAL CONSIDERATIONS

Researchers have begun to acknowledge that injuries sustained by children confer different vulnerabilities than similar injuries sustained by adults. For example, rodent models demonstrate that the same dopamine depleting lesions that produce severe motor impairment in mature rats can result in motor hyperactivity when induced in juvenile rats (Davids, Zhang, Tarazi, & Baldessarini, 2003). Among humans, children who experience frontal lobe damage exhibit greater loss of psychosocial function than adults who sustain similar injuries (Anderson, Bechara, Damasio, Tranel, & Damasio, 1999).

Developmental factors affect the nature and degree of injury sustained, and the degree of functional recovery likely to follow. Children's relatively large heads and weaker neck muscles increase their vulnerability to rotational movements implicated in diffuse axonal injuries. Furthermore, the greater flexibility of their skulls allows force to be distributed over greater surface area, favoring diffuse over focal injuries (Anderson, Catroppa, Morse, Haritou, & Rosenfeld, 2005).

The developmental state of the tissue is also implicated in the extent of damage these mechanical forces have on the brain. Unlike any other organ in the human body, brain development is substantially incomplete at birth with developmental changes continuing well into the postnatal period through adolescence and early adulthood (Johnson, 1999; Nowakowski & Hayes, 2002; Sowell, Thompson, Holmes, Jernigan, & Toga, 1999). Developmental changes taking place in the brain also differ across tissue types. White matter develops its characteristic appearance only after birth as axons connecting cells across anatomical regions become myelinated (Andersen, 2003). Myelination occurs rapidly in the first few years of life (McKinstry, 2011) but continues to take place throughout childhood and adolescence (Giedd et al., 1999).

The overall lower level of axonal myelination in children increases the susceptibility of these fibers to shearing strain, making them more vulnerable to diffuse injuries (Lea & Faden, 2001). Furthermore, hypoxia can induce failure of myelination (see Ment et al., 2009).

In contrast to white matter development, gray matter development includes processes that refine synaptic relationships between neurons. Immature brains contain excess neurons. Based on an individual's experience, neurons used regularly form connections with other neurons to develop efficient circuits, whereas neurons that are not used are eliminated. Despite this pruning process, the brain continues to grow through early childhood. This growth is due in part to arborization, or branching of neurons to increase the number of neighboring cells with which they communicate. Gray matter develops at different rates across each of the four lobes (Giedd, 2004), with regions of the frontal lobe continuing to develop well into adulthood (Diamond, 2002). Gray matter tissue in children is more susceptible to secondary injuries following trauma, such as edema (Aldrich et al., 1992). This susceptibility is likely to be related to the immaturity of neurochemical receptors in young brains, which increases vulnerability to excitotoxic damage associated with hypoxia and contributes to extensive apoptotic cell death (Lea & Faden, 2001).

Despite these anatomical characteristics that confer increased vulnerability to children following brain trauma, the relative immaturity of the brain at birth is also an asset in human development, because the brain remains plastic. The structure of neural tissue is not determined entirely by genetic or chemical signals taking place during development. Experience-dependent specialization also emerges (Johnson, 1999). Thus, when structure is compromised through injury prior to the specialization of cortical tissue, alternate brain regions may assume functions of lost tissue. For instance, portions of the auditory cortex may respond to visual stimuli when the visual cortex is damaged prior to neuronal specialization (Johnson, 1999). However, despite the remarkable compensatory ability of younger brains, there are clear limits to plasticity, and functional recovery is often far from absolute. Furthermore, early damage often carries a substantial cost over the course of development. Damage to the brain that results in an inability to acquire basic functions may affect wide-ranging higher-order processes that depend on that initial component (Bachevalier & Loveland, 2003; Black, Jones, Nelson, & Greenough, 1998). For example, children who sustain brain injuries prior to age 4 exhibit worse cognitive and social outcomes than children who sustained injuries just 2 years later (Sonnenberg, Dupuis, & Rumney, 2010). Thus, the younger a child is when an injury is sustained, the less severe the injury needs to be to result in lifelong effects on cognitive functioning (Anderson et al., 2005).

Even when recovery occurs for some functions, it may be at the expense of acquiring other abilities (Luciana, 2003). In rodents, early brain tissue damage results in neural organizational compensations that allow for recovery of motor control not seen in animals damaged in adulthood, yet diminished cognitive functioning is observed (Kolb & Gibb, 2001). Brain plasticity in childhood therefore may not predict full recovery. Rather, extensive brain damage may prevent acquisition of new skills necessary to traverse the developmental landscape (see Anderson et al., 2011).

Contradictory predictions offered by increased plasticity versus increased vulnerability are complex and cannot be accounted for fully by severity or age at injury alone. Recently, Anderson, Spencer-Smith, and Wood (2011) proposed a hierarchical model to account for the high degree of variability in outcomes and considerable clinical challenges in prognosis. They suggest that functional and neural recovery from early brain injury is influenced by the independent and interacting effects of developmental, constitutional, and environmental factors. Developmentally, the brain is characterized by sensitive periods. In general sensitive periods refer to any developmental epoch during which plasticity is heightened to facilitate skill acquisition across certain regions of the brain. Damage sustained during peak periods of developmental sensitivity may be most likely to induce long-term deficits (Ewing-Cobbs, Prasad, Landry, Kramer, & DeLeon, 2004). This may occur because damage incurred prior to periods of developmental sensitivity allows time for alternative brain regions to be recruited, whereas damage occurring later allows for the preservation skills that were acquired prior to the injury.

Individual differences in biological susceptibility and resilience to injury are also being identified (see later). Furthermore, individual factors such as cognitive ability and sex appear to moderate outcome. For example, cognitive ability, measured within 3 weeks of injury among children with mild TBI, moderates postconcussive symptoms 3 months later (Fay et al., 2010). Females are at greater risk for postconcussive symptoms after mild TBI, but may be protected from social skills and processing speed deficits post injury (see Stavinoha, Butcher, & Spurgin, 2011). In addition, animal research suggests that the less-lateralized female brain may have a greater potential for plasticity and transfer of function between hemispheres after injury. However, other research indicates that male animals show greater neural and behavioral recovery after injury in response to enriched environments (Anderson et al., 2011; Kolb, Gibb, & Gorny, 2000). Finally, environmental factors including both interpersonal support and medical intervention also affect prognosis (Anderson et al., 2011).

## BRAIN INJURY AND THE FRONTAL LOBE

Regionally, the temporal and frontal lobes are especially vulnerable to damage (Mendelsohn et al., 1992; Wilde et al., 2005). The susceptibility of these regions is a consequence of their proximal location to the jagged inner surface of the skull (Schnider & Gutbrod, 1999). In addition, these regions readily sustain contrecoup contusions regardless of the initial site of impact (Gennarelli & Meaney, 1996). Although many brain regions are developmentally stable at adult levels by adolescence, maturational changes in frontal regions continue through adolescence and into early adulthood, supporting emotional and cognitive development across this age range (Sowell et al., 1999). This protracted maturation indicates that prefrontal structures may be vulnerable longer than other anatomical sites. The functions attributed to the frontal lobe are critical to mental health, and their compromise is of substantial clinical importance. This anatomical region is frequently divided into dorsal and orbital cortical subregions, which have unique yet interactive psychological functions (Duncan & Owen, 2000). The orbital frontal cortex (OFC) is the ventral-most region of the frontal cortex and maintains extensive reciprocal connectivity with the limbic region, whereas the dorsolateral prefrontal cortex (DLPFC) occupies the lateral region above the OFC.

## DORSOLATERAL PREFRONTAL CORTEX

The dorsolateral prefrontal cortex (DLPFC) and middorsal cortices respond to a wide array of cognitive demands requiring problem solving and executive functioning (Duncan & Owen, 2000). The DLPFC operates through a network of interconnected structures including the dorsal caudate, global pallidus, dorsomedial thalamic nucleus, and cerebellum (Heyder, Suchan, & Daum, 2004). The integrity of this network is essential for future planning toward attainment of distal goals (Anderson & Catroppa, 2005; Levin & Hanten, 2005). Thus, this region is implicated in inhibitory control, and the ability to integrate environmental feedback into ongoing behavior to make rapid behavioral changes. This skill is often deficient in children with frontal brain injuries (Ornstein et al., 2009).

Because executive functions are crucial in allowing children to adapt to changing developmental demands, early damage to this region may establish cascading effects of decrements across multiple domains. These skills begin to emerge in preschool and undergo rapid development thereafter (Diamond, 2002). Because frontal regions are not well developed in young children, damage is less likely to reveal immediate behavioral deficits, whereas such damage would be readily detected among adults. Thus, in the immediate aftermath of injury, behavioral deficits may be minimal in children, as the functions associated with this region have not yet developed and therefore cannot be lost. However, the interrupted developmental progression in self-control is likely to reveal itself increasingly over time, as children fail to acquire skills that are developing in their peers (Eslinger, Biddle, & Grattan, 1997).

## ORBITOFRONTAL CORTEX

In contrast to executive function deficits, damage to orbitofrontal regions are associated with social/emotional functioning important in interpersonal relationships, including the ability to read social and emotional cues and to use this information in a self-regulatory manner (Bachevalier & Loveland, 2003). Damage in this region is also associated with an inability to develop and/or use internal cues of potential punishment to guide behavior (Damasio, Tranel, & Damasio, 1990). Interestingly, behavior and personality deficits associated with damage to this region frequently exist in the absence of neuropsychological deficits (Schnider & Gutbrod, 1999). Hemispheric localization of orbitofrontal lesions is influential in the clinical presentation of symptoms. Lesions localized to the left hemisphere are associated with depressive symptoms, apathy, emotional blunting, and poor planning, whereas right hemisphere lesions are associated with hyperactivity, disinhibition, socially inappropriate behavior, irritability, and lack of empathy (Schnider & Gutbrod, 1999). When damage extends across both hemispheres, characteristics of both syndromes coexist (Schnider & Gutbrod, 1999).

Orbitofrontal damage acquired by children often results in more extensive deficits in social behavior than lesions acquired in adulthood (Anderson et al., 1999; Bachevalier & Loveland, 2003). In a case study of two individuals who sustained significant orbitofrontal damage before age 16 months, recovery and function appeared very positive in the immediate aftermath of the lesion, and cognitive and motoric development proceeded normally. However, many years later these individuals were brought to medical attention because of their significant psychopathological behaviors. These individuals were insensitive to punishment, unresponsive to future consequences, and unlike adults with similar damage, they showed extensive impairment in moral and social reasoning (Anderson et al., 1999). Furthermore, recent work with DTI in children has shown that disruption of the uncinate fasciculus, which connects the orbital frontal cortex to temporal regions, predicted poor social/behavioral outcomes (Johnson et al., 2011). The increased deficits in comparison to adult-onset lesions indicate impairment in the acquisition of normal social behavior leading to more global dysfunction.

## GENETICS AND HERITABILITY

In addition to factors including developmental state and injury severity, marked individual differences in functional and structural deficits incurred in response to brain injury may be influenced by genetic factors (Blackman, Worley, & Strittmatter, 2005; see McAllister, 2010, for review). Research addressing genetically mediated differences in susceptibility to postinjury outcome has expanded rapidly in the past 5 years. Allelic variants of genes associated with cognitive function, as well as variants of genes that are known to enhance or impede post-injury cellular recovery, moderate outcomes following neurological insult (Jordan, 2007; McAllister et al., 2008; McAllister, 2010). The latter category has received the majority of attention to date, with a significant emphasis on the apolipoprotein E (ApoE) gene, which has at least 3 well-characterized allelic variants. Extensive research on the function of the ApoE proteins indicates a role in neurologic repair, with variability between alleles implicated in the degree of neural damage suffered from oxidative, circulatory, and traumatic type injuries over the lifespan (Blackman et al., 2005; Laskowitz et al., 2010). In contrast to the $\varepsilon 2$ and possibly the $\varepsilon 3$ allele, the $\varepsilon 4$ allele appears less effective in conferring neuroprotection and leads to increased damage due to post-injury inflammation, edema, and excitotoxicity (Aono et al., 2002; Lee, Aono, Laskowitz, Warner, & Pearlstein, 2004; Lynch et al., 2002). Thus, genes appear to be critical in the degree of pathological response to brain injury, establishing the potential for important Gene $\times$ Environment interactions applicable to psychological function.

Interestingly, research examining ApoE $\varepsilon 4$ in children, although sparse, has been contradictory. Some studies indicate a neuroprotective function of $\varepsilon 4$ as opposed to $\varepsilon 2$, the opposite finding from studies with adults (Blackman et al., 2005; Oria et al., 2005). Other studies have identified a marked discrepancy between the amount of cerebral perfusion pressure post injury and severity of outcome for children with the ε4 allele (Lo et al., 2009). Despite showing the lowest degree of cerebral perfusion, these children evidence paradoxically far worse outcomes, whereas the opposite was true for children with the ε3 allele. Discrepancies in the literature to date are likely to be a function of small sample sizes.

Research also indicates the potential for genotypes to interact with environmental trauma exposure in ways that produce specific psychiatric outcomes (see, e.g., Beauchaine, Neuhaus, Zalewski, Crowell, & Potapova, 2011). For example, a range of perinatal traumatic factors, many of which are thought to contribute to hypoxic damage in neonates, have been associated repeatedly with later development of schizophrenia (Rosso & Cannon, 2003). Cannon and colleagues (2002) found that a history of fetal hypoxia was associated with a distinct pattern of brain abnormalities visible on MRI in patients with schizophrenia and in their nonaffected siblings, but not in a control sample. One component of the genetic risk for schizophrenia might be a heightened sensitivity to hypoxic events, putting those who experience hypoxia during neural development at greater risk for developing the disorder (Cannon et al., 2002).

In fact, as many as 50% of reported schizophrenia-related genes may be regulated in part by hypoxia/ischemia (Schmidt-Kastner, van Os, Steinbusch, & Schmitz, 2006). Furthermore, animal models indicate that these genes are likely expressed during development and may contribute to the pathogenesis of schizophrenia. The authors postulate that vulnerability genes responding to oxidative stress may confer risk by producing defective gene products normally serving neuroprotective functions. Recently, other lines of research have also supported this model. In a large-scale study, the relationship between genetic risk for depression and offspring externalizing behavior appeared to be moderated through pregnancy risk (Pemberton et al., 2010). Thus, one mechanism through which genetic risk confers vulnerability to various forms of psychopathology is through susceptibility to injurious influences on neural development.

Dopamine functioning is also highly sensitive to environmental insults such as hypoxia. Changes in dopamine function following hypoxic insults may be especially detrimental for individuals whose dopaminergic function is genetically compromised (McAllister et al., 2005).

## CLINICAL CONSIDERATIONS

Brain injury can play a causal role in the pathogenesis of specific psychological disorders by compromising neural systems directly. Changes in behavior and personality are common in response to brain injury as a consequence of the high prevalence of orbitofrontal damage. Children with a history of mild TBI prior to age 5 are more likely to evidence clinical impairment in adolescence, with a 4.2-fold increase in ADHD, a 6.2-fold increase in conduct and oppositional defiant disorders, a 3.6-fold increase in the development of substance abuse, and a 3.1-fold increase in prevalence of a mood disorders (McKinlay, Grace, Horwood, Fergusson, & MacFarlane, 2009). Low-grade hypoxia may also contribute directly to the development of psychopathology. In animal experiments, intermittent hypoxia results in attenuation of extracellular dopamine in nigrostriatal regions, which is implicated in behavioral hyperactivity and increased responding to novelty (Decker, Jones, Solomon, Keating, & Rye, 2005). Interestingly, evidence suggests that male and female brains differ in the degree of vulnerability to ischemia/hypoxia induced damage, with females showing less severe pathological outcomes (Hurn, Vannucci, & Hagberg, 2004; see Anderson et al., 2011).

Although psychological symptoms may develop as a direct result of lesions to a damaged area, brain injury also contributes to psychopathology in indirect ways through the exacerbation of preexisting pathology or in the development of post-traumatic stress disorder in reaction to the injurious situation (Middleton, 2001). This observation is especially salient when considering that factors such as low socioeconomic status and poor family functioning increase the risk of sustaining a brain injury (Bruce, 1996), and some research suggests that brain-injured patients show higher levels of premorbid psychological and behavioral disturbances (Catte-lani, Lombardi, Brianti, & Mazzucchi, 1998). Premorbid functioning also contributes significantly to the development of adverse outcomes post injury (Donders & Strom, 2000). Brain injury is also likely to increase stress in family systems, leading to further contextual risk factors for suboptimal recovery and development. Greater family-level distress and caregiver burden are observed among families of children who sustain a brain injury in comparison to other injuries requiring hospitalization (Stancin, Wade, Walz, Yeates, & Taylor, 2010). High-family functioning moderates the relationship between injury and long-term functioning (Gerrard-Morris et al., 2010; Yeates et al., 1997). Young children (3 to 6 years) who sustain mild- to moderate head injuries demonstrate lower social competence post injury than matched controls who sustain orthopedic injuries (Yeates, Taylor, Walz, Stancin, & Wade, 2010). In addition, outcomes for children with mild/moderate TBI are exacerbated for individuals exposed to high levels of authoritarian or permissive parenting. Individuals with severe brain injury evidence the worst outcomes regardless of parenting practices, indicating that parents are an especially important influence in children's coping with, and compensating for, functional impairments resulting from more mild brain injuries (Yeates et al., 2010). These findings highlight the importance of postinjury clinical support with parents and the injured child in order to maximize recovery and prepare parents for behavioral challenges. Brain injury establishes vulnerability, and when such vulnerability is met with environmental risk, the likelihood of developing psychopathology may be increased.

Identifying the effects of brain injury on psychopathological development may also have important implications for treatment. For instance, research suggests that methylphenidate is less effective when ADHD emerges after traumatic brain injury than when ADHD follows a traditional developmental course (Jin & Schachar, 2004). When brain injury is identified, treatment should focus not only on the child's level of functioning, but also on the quality of the familial environment. Because premorbid functioning is frequently compromised, dysfunctional family systems may already be in place, limiting the potential effectiveness of the family to cope with the injury and contribute to successful recovery. These factors are especially important to consider given that head injuries may result from abuse or neglect.

Unfortunately, assessing the role that head injuries play in the development of psychopathology is extremely challenging because brain injury can be difficult to detect in cases where it exists primarily at a microscopic or neurochemical level. Furthermore, a long interval between the acquisition of injury and the onset of psychopathology may obscure the causal relation between the injury and later behavior. As many as 75% of infants surviving acute perinatal asphyxia are classified as *nonimpaired* because they fail to show neurological indicators of encephalopathic damage in the weeks after injury. However, impairments in cognitive, memory, and socioemotional behavior often are not evident until later in life when the child fails to meet increasing developmental demands (de Haan et al., 2006). Even cases of mild insults may produce lasting alterations in development, which may take years to recognize (Gronwall, Wrightson, & McGinn, 1997). In addition, mild damage, such as the low-grade hypoxia associated with snoring, may result in reductions in attention and intelligence, despite the fact that children continue to score within the normal range and are thus overlooked medically (Blunden, Lushington, Kennedy, Martin, & Dawson, 2000). Therefore, careful consideration of potential contributions of brain injury to presenting psychological symptoms should be undertaken so that appropriate comprehensive treatment plans can be developed.

## SYNTHESES AND FUTURE DIRECTIONS

Although children with acute brain injuries present and are treated in medical settings, the effects of their injuries may be lifelong and include psychopathology. Severe injury affects multiple domains of functioning, and presents serious challenges to both the child and his or her caretakers. However, brain injuries can also be subtle, as in mild TBI or hypoxia. Such injuries may be difficult to detect even though they can often potentiate psychopathology. In addition to environmental and genetic factors that are becoming increasingly well characterized in the development of psychopathology, early brain injury should not be overlooked, particularly as an environmental potentiator of genetic susceptibility. Because injuries can be difficult to detect and their sequelae may take years to manifest, the association with injury and psychopathological outcomes may be overlooked in clinical practice. However, brain injury as an etiological factor may be important in informing treatment strategies, and as such, should be assessed adequately.

Research aimed at addressing these challenges involves improving the ability to assess brain damage resulting from concussions. In the past decade, advances in neuroimaging have allowed for increased detection of microscopic injury that have the potential to cause lasting effects, but these methods have not been readily adopted into clinical practice. Standard neuroimaging protocols and acute neuropsychological testing continue to dominate current postinjury assessments and recommendations for return to play for athletes, both of which have limited sensitivity in quantifying the extent of neurological damage (Ellemberg, Henry, Macciocchi, Guskiewicz, & Broglio, 2009.) Further research on the genetics of brain injury may also assist in identifying individuals at high risk but more importantly in characterizing biological processes involved in injury and in developing appropriate pharmaceutical approaches to arresting these processes to reduce the severity of their effects. The next steps in understanding pediatric brain injury should focus on multidisciplinary, translational research, which capitalizes on recent advances in neuroimaging, behavioral research, and clinical practice (Anderson et al., 2011).

## REFERENCES

Aldrich, E. F., Eisenberg, H. M., Saydjari, C., Luerssen, T. G., Foulkes, M. A., Jane, J. A., . . . Young, H. F. (1992). Diffuse brain swelling in severely head-injured children. A report from the NIH traumatic coma data bank. *Journal of Neurosurgery, 76*, 450–454.

Andersen, S. L. (2003). Trajectories of brain development: Point of vulnerability or window of opportunity? *Neuroscience and Biobehavioral Reviews, 27*, 3–18.

Anderson, S. W., Bechara, A., Damasio, H., Tranel, D., & Damasio, A. R. (1999). Impairment of social and moral behavior related to early damage in human prefrontal cortex. *Nature Neuroscience, 2*, 1032–1037.

Anderson, V., & Catroppa, C. (2005). Recovery of executive skills following paediatric traumatic brain injury (TBI): A 2 year follow-up. *Brain Injury, 19*, 459–470.

Anderson, V., Catroppa, C., Morse, S., Haritou, F., & Rosenfeld, J. (2005). Functional plasticity of vulnerability after early brain injury? *Pediatrics, 116*, 1374–1382.

Anderson, V., Spencer-Smith, M., & Wood, A. (2011). Do children really recover better? Neurobehavioural plasticity after early brain insult. *Brain, 134*, 2197–2221.

Aono, M., Lee, Y., Grant, E. R., Zivin, R. A., Pearlstein, R. D., Warner, D. S., . . . Laskowitz, D. T. (2002). Apo-lipoprotein E protects against NMDA excitotoxicity. *Neurobiology of Disease, 11*, 214–220.

Ashwal, S., Holshouser, B. A., & Tong, K. (2006). Use of advanced neuroimaging techniques in the evaluation of pediatric traumatic brain injury. *Developmental Neuroscience, 28*, 309–326.

Ashwal, S., Wycliffe, N. D., & Holshouser, B. A. (2010). Advanced neuroimaging in children with nonaccidental trauma. *Developmental Neuroscience, 32*, 33–342.

Bachevalier, J., & Loveland, K. A. (2003). Early orbitofrontal-limbic dysfunction and autism. In D. Cicchetti & W. Walker (Eds.), *Neurodevelopmental mechanisms in psychopathology* (pp. 215–236). New York, NY: Cambridge University Press.

Baron, I. S., & Rey-Casserly, C. (2010). Extremely preterm birth outcome: A review of four decades of cognitive research. *Neuropsychology Review, 20*, 430–452.

Bass, J. L., Corwin, M., Gozal, D., Moore, C., Nishida, H., Parker, S., . . . Kinane, T. B. (2004). The effect of chronic or intermittent hypoxia on cognition in childhood: A review of the evidence. *Pediatrics, 114*, 805–816.

Beauchaine, T. P., Neuhaus, E., Zalewski, M., Crowell, S. E., & Potapova, N. (2011). The effects of allostatic load on neural systems subserving motivation, mood regulation, and social affiliation. *Development and Psychopathology, 23*, 975–999.

Bigler, E. D. (2001a). The lesion(s) in traumatic brain injury: Implications for clinical neuropsychology. *Archives of Clinical Neuropsychology, 16*, 95–131.

Bigler, E. D. (2001b). Quantitative magnetic resonance imaging in traumatic brain injury. *Journal of Head Trauma Rehabilitation, 16,* 117–134.

Black, J. E., Jones, T. A., Nelson, C. A., & Greenough, W. T. (1998). Neuronal plasticity and the developing brain. In N. Alessi, J. Coyle, S. Harrison, & S. Eth (Eds.), *The handbook of child and adolescent psychiatry* (Vol. 6, pp. 31–53). New York, NY: Wiley.

Blackman, J. A., Worley, G., & Strittmatter, W. J. (2005). Apolipoprotein E and brain injury: Implications for children. *Developmental Medicine & Child Neurology, 47,* 64–70.

Blunden, S., Lushington, K., Kennedy, D., Martin, J., & Dawson, D. (2000). Behavior and neurocognitive performance in children aged 5–10 years who snore compared to controls. *Journal of Clinical and Experimental Neuropsychology, 22,* 554–568.

Bruce, D. A. (1996). Pediatric head injury. In R. Wilkins & S. Rengachary (Eds.), *Neurosurgery* (2nd ed., pp. 2709–2715). New York, NY: McGraw-Hill.

Bruns, J., & Hauser, A. (2003). The epidemiology of traumatic brain injury: A review. *Epilepsia, 44*(Suppl. 10), 2–10.

Cannon, T. D., van Erp, T. G. M., Rosso, I. M., Huttunen, M., Lonnqvist, J., Pirkola, T., . . . Standertskjold-Nordenstam, C. G. (2002). Fetal hypoxia and structural brain abnormalities in schizophrenic patients, their siblings, and controls. *Archives of General Psychiatry, 59,* 35–41.

Cattelani, R., Lombardi, F., Brianti, R., & Mazzucchi, A. (1998). Traumatic brain injury in childhood: Intellectual, behavioral, and social outcome into adulthood. *Brain Injury, 12,* 283–296.

Chu, Z., Wilde, E. A., Hunter, J. V., McCauley, S. R., Bigler, E. D., Troyanskaya, M., . . . Levin, H. S. (2010). Voxel-based analysis of diffusion tensor imaging in mild traumatic brain injury in adolescents. *American Journal of Neuroradiology, 31,* 340–346.

Collins, M. W., Lovell, M. R., Iverson, G. L., Cantu, R. C., Maroon, J. C., & Field, M. (2003). Cumulative effects of concussion in high school athletes. *Neurosurgery, 53,* 247–248.

Damaraju, E., Phillips, J. R., Lowe, J. R., Ohls, R., Calhoun, V. D., & Caprihan, A. (2010). Resting-state functional connectivity differences in premature children. *Frontiers in Systems Neuroscience, 4,* 1–13.

Damasio, A. R., Tranel, D., & Damasio, H. (1990). Individuals with sociopathic behavior caused by frontal damage fail to respond autonomically to social stimuli. *Behavioral Brain Research, 41,* 81–94.

Davids, E., Zhang, K., Tarazi, F. I., & Baldessarini, R. J. (2003). Animal models of attention-deficit/hyperactivity disorder. *Brain Research Reviews, 42,* 1–21.

Davidson, L. L. (1987). Hyperactivity, antisocial behavior and childhood injury: A critical analysis of the literature. *Journal of Developmental and Behavioral Pediatrics, 8,* 335–340.

de Haan, M., Wyatt, J. S., Roth, S., Vargha-Khadem, F., Gadian, D., & Mishkin, M. (2006). Brain and cognitive-behavioural development after asphyxia at term birth. *Developmental Science, 9,* 350–358.

Decker, M. J., Jones, K. A., Solomon, I. G., Keating, G. L., & Rye, D. B. (2005). Reduced extracellular dopamine and increased responsiveness to novelty: Neurochemical and behavioral sequelae of intermittent hypoxia. *Sleep, 28,* 165–167.

Decker, M. J., & Rye, D. B. (2002). Neonatal intermittent hypoxia impairs dopamine signaling and executive functioning. *Sleep and Breathing, 6,* 205–210.

Delaney, J. S., Puni, V., & Rouah, F. (2006). Mechanisms of injury for concussions in university football, ice hockey, and soccer – a pilot study. *Clinical Journal of Sports Medicine, 16,* 162–165.

Dematteo, C. A., Hanna, S. E., Mahoney, W. J., Hollenberg, R. D., Scott, L. A., Law, M. C., . . . Xu, L. (2010). My child doesn't have a brain injury, he only has a concussion. *Pediatrics, 125,* 327–334.

Diamond, A. (2002). Normal development of prefrontal cortex from birth to young adulthood: Cognitive functions, anatomy, and biochemistry. In D. Stuss & R. Knight (Eds.), *Principles of frontal lobe function* (pp. 466–503). New York, NY: Oxford University Press.

DiScala, C., Lescohier, I., Barthel, M., & Li, G. (1998). Injuries to children with attention deficit hyperactivity disorder. *Pediatrics, 102,* 1415–1421.

Donders, J., & Strom, D. (2000). Neurobehavioral recovery after pediatric head trauma: Injury, pre-injury, and post-injury issues. *Journal of Head Trauma Rehabilitation, 15,* 792–803.

Duncan, J., & Owen, A. M. (2000). Common regions of the human frontal lobe recruited by diverse cognitive demands. *Trends in Neuroscience, 23,* 475–483.

Ellemberg, D., Henry, L. C., Macciocchi, S. N., Guskiewicz, K. M., & Broglio, S. P. (2009). Advances in sport concussion assessment: From behavioral to brain imaging measures. *Journal of Neurotrauma, 26,* 2365–2382.

Eslinger, P. J., Biddle, K. R., & Grattan, L. M. (1997). Cognitive and social development in children with prefrontal cortex lesions. In N. Krasnegor, G. Lyon, & P. Goldman-Rakic (Eds.), *Development of the prefrontal cortex: Evolution, neurobiology, and behavior.* (pp. 295–335). Baltimore, MD: Brooks.

Ewing-Cobbs, L., Prasad, M. R., Landry, S. H., Kramer, L., & DeLeon, R. (2004). Executive functions following traumatic brain injury in young children: A preliminary analysis. *Developmental Neuropsychology, 26,* 487–512.

Fair, D. A., Cohen, A. L., Power, J. D., Dosenbach, N. U. F., Church, J. A., Miezin, F. M., . . . Petersen, S. E. (2009). Functional brain networks develop from a "local to distributed" organization. *PLoS Computational Biology, 5,* e1000381.

Faul, M., Xu, L., Wald, M. M., & Coronado, V. G. (2010). *Traumatic brain injury in the United States: Emergency department visits, hospitalizations, and deaths.* Atlanta (GA): Centers for Disease Control and Prevention, National Center for Injury Prevention and Control.

Fay, T. B., Yeates, K. O., Taylor, H. G., Bangert, B., Dietrich, A., Nuss, K. E., . . . Wright, M. (2010). Cognitive reserve as a moderator of postconcussive symptoms in children with complicated and uncomplicated mild traumatic brain injury. *Journal of the International Neuropsychological Society, 16,* 94–105.

Finnie, J. & Blumbergs, P. (2002). Traumatic brain injury. *Veterinary Pathology, 39,* 679–689.

Fox, M. D., & Raichle, M. E. (2007). Spontaneous fluctuations in brain activity observed with functional magnetic resonance imaging. *Nature Reviews Neuroscience, 8*, 700–711.

Gabriel, E., & Turner, D. (1996). Minor head injury management and outcome. In R. Wilkin & S. Rengachary (Eds.), *Neurosurgery* (2nd ed., pp. 2723–2726). New York, NY: McGraw-Hill.

Gaetz, M., Goodman, D., & Weinberg, H. (2000). Electrophysiological evidence for the cumulative effects of concussion. *Brain Injury, 14*, 1077–1088.

Gatzke-Kopp, L. M. (2011). The canary in the coalmine: The sensitivity of mesolimbic dopamine to environmental adversity during development. *Neuroscience and Biobehavioral Reviews, 35*, 794–803.

Gatzke-Kopp, L. M., & Beauchaine, T. P. (2007). Central nervous system substrates of impulsivity: Implications for the development of attention-deficit/hyperactivity disorder and conduct disorder. In D. Coch, G. Dawson, & K. Fischer (Eds.), *Human behavior and the developing brain: Atypical development.* New York, NY: Guilford Press.

Gennarelli, T. A., & Meaney, D. F. (1996). Mechanisms of primary head injury. In R. Wilkin & S. Rengachary (Eds.), *Neurosurgery* (2nd ed., pp. 2611–2621). New York, NY: McGraw-Hill.

Gerrard-Morris, A., Taylor, H. G., Yeates, K. O., Walz, N. C., Stancin, T., Minich, N., & Wade, S. L. (2010). Cognitive development after traumatic brain injury in young children. *Journal of International Neuropsychological Society, 16*, 157–168.

Giedd, J. N. (2004). Structural magnetic resonance imaging of the adolescent brain. *Annals of the New York Academy of Sciences, 1021*, 77–85.

Giedd, J. N., Blumenthal, J., Jeffries, N. O., Castellanos, F. X., Liu, H., Zijdenbos, A., . . . Rapoport, J. L. (1999). Brain development during childhood and adolescence: A longitudinal MRI study. *Nature Neuroscience, 2*, 861–863.

Golan, H., & Huleihel, M. (2006). The effect of prenatal hypoxia on brain development: Short- and long-term consequences demonstrated in rodent models. *Developmental Science, 9*, 338–349.

Gozzo, Y., Vohr, B., Lacadie, C., Hampson, M., Katz, K. H., Maller-Kesselman, J., . . . Ment, L. R. (2009). Alterations in neural connectivity in preterm children at school age. *NeuroImage, 48*, 458–463.

Gronwall, D., Wrightson, P., & McGinn, V. (1997). Effect of mild head injury during the preschool years. *Journal of the International Neuropsychological Society, 3*, 592–597.

Heyder, K., Suchan, B., & Daum, I. (2004). Cortico-subcortical contributions to executive control. *Acta Psychologica, 115*, 271–289.

Hori, T. (1985). Pathophysiology analysis of hypoxaemia during acute severe asthma. *Archives of Diseases in Childhood, 60*, 640–643.

Hurn, P. D., Vannucci, S. J., & Hagberg, H. (2004). Adult or perinatal brain injury: Does sex matter? *Stroke, 36*, 193–195.

Jin, C., & Schachar, R. (2004). Methylphenidate treatment of attention-deficit/hyperactivity disorder secondary to traumatic brain injury: A critical appraisal of treatment studies. *CNS Spectrums, 9*, 217–226.

Johnson, B., Zhang, K., Gay, M., Horovitz, S., Hallett, M., Sebastianelli, W., & Slobounov, S. (2011). Alteration of brain default network in subacute phase of injury in concussed individuals: Resting-state fMRI study. *Neuroimage.* Epub ahead of print.

Johnson, C. P., Juranek, J., Kramer, L. A., Prasad, M. R., Swank, P. R., & Ewing-Cobbs, L. (2011). Predicting behavioral deficits in pediatric traumatic brain injury through uncinate fasciculus integrity. *Journal of the International Neuropsychological Society, 17,* 663–673.

Johnson, M. H. (1999). Cortical plasticity in normal and abnormal cognitive development: Evidence and working hypotheses. *Development and Psychopathology, 11,* 419–437.

Jordan, B. D. (2007). Genetic influences on outcome following traumatic brain injury. *Neurochemical Research, 32,* 905–915.

Kolb, B., & Gibb, R. (2001). Early brain injury, plasticity and behavior. In C. Nelson & M. Luciana (Eds.), *Handbook of developmental cognitive neuroscience* (pp. 175–190). Cambridge, MA: MIT Press.

Kolb, B., Gibb, R., & Gorny, G. (2000). Cortical plasticity and the development of behavior after early frontal cortical injury. *Developmental Neuropsychology, 18,* 423–444.

Kraus, J. F., & Nourjah, P. (1988). The epidemiology of mild, uncomplicated brain injury. *Journal of Trauma, 28,* 1637–1643.

Laskowitz, D. T., Song, P., Wang, H., Mace, B., Sullivan, P. M., Vitek, M. P., & Dawson, H. N. (2010). Traumatic brain injury exacerbates neurodegenerative pathology: Improvement with an apolipoprotein E-based therapeutic. *Journal of Neurotrauma, 27,* 1983–1995.

Lea, P. M., & Faden, A. I. (2001). Traumatic brain injury: Developmental differences in glutamate receptor response and the impact on treatment. *Mental Retardation and Developmental Disabilities Research Reviews, 7,* 235–248.

Lee, Y., Aono, M., Laskowitz, D., Warner, D. S., & Pearlstein, R. D. (2004). Apolipoprotein E protects against oxidative stress in mixed neuronal-glial cell cultures by reducing glutamate toxicity. *Neurochemistry International, 44,* 107–118.

Leventhal, J. M., Martin, K. D., & Asnes, A. G. (2010). Fractures and traumatic brain injuries: Abuse versus accidents in a U.S. database of hospitalized children. *Pediatrics, 126,* e104–e115.

Levin, H. S., & Hanten, G. (2005). Executive functions after traumatic brain injury in children. *Pediatric Neurology, 33,* 79–93.

Levine, B., Kovacevic, N., Nica, E. L., Cheung, G., Gao, F., Schwartz, M. L., & Black, S. E. (2008). The Toronto traumatic brain injury study: Injury severity and quantified MRI. *Neurology, 70,* 771–778.

Lo, T. Y. M., Jones, P. A., Chambers, I. R., Beattie, T. F., Forsyth, R., Mendelow, A. D., & Minns, R. A. (2009). Modulating effects of apolipoprotein E polymorphisms on secondary brain insult and outcome after childhood brain trauma. *Child's Nervous System, 25,* 47–54.

Luciana, M. (2003). Cognitive development in children born preterm: Implications for theories of brain plasticity following early injury. *Development and Psychopathology, 15,* 1017–1047.

Lynch, J. R., Pineda, J. A., Morgan, D., Zhang, L., Warner, D. S., Benveniste, H., & Laskowitz, D. T. (2002). Apolipoprotein E affects the central nervous system response to injury and the development of cerebral edema. *Annals of Neurology, 51,* 113–117.

Macmillan, M. (2002). *An odd kind of fame: Stories of Phineas Gage.* Cambridge, MA: MIT Press.

Martin, J. A., Kochanek, K. D., Strobino, D. M., Guyer, B., & MacDorman, M. F. (2005). Annual summary of vital statistics—2003. *Pediatrics, 115,* 619–634.

McAllister, T. W., (2010). Genetic factors modulating outcome after neurotrama. *Physical Medicine & Rehabilitation, 2,* S241–S252.

McAllister, T. W., Flashman, L. A., Harker Rhodes, C., Tyler, A. L., Moore, J. H., Saykin, A. J., . . . Tsongalis, G. J. (2008). Single nucleotide polymorphisms in ANKK1 and the dopamine D2 receptor gene affect cognitive outcome shortly after traumatic brain injury: A replication and extension study. *Brain Injury, 22,* 705–714.

McAllister, T. W., Rhodes, C. H., Flashman, L. A., McDonald, B. C., Belloni, D., & Saykin, A. J. (2005). Effect of the dopamine D2 receptor T allele on response latency after mild traumatic brain injury. *American Journal of Psychiatry, 162,* 1749–1751.

McClure, M. M., Peiffer, A. M., Rosen, G. D., & Fitch, R. H. (2005). Auditory processing deficits in rats with neonatal hypoxic-ischemic injury. *International Journal of Developmental Neuroscience, 23,* 351–362.

McCrory, P., Johnston, K., Meeuwisse, W., Aubry, M., Cantu, R., Dvorak, J., . . . Schamasch, P. (2005). Summary and agreement statement of the 2nd international conference on concussion in sport, Prague 2004. *British Journal of Sports Medicine, 39,* 196–204.

McKinlay, A., Grace, R. C., Horwood, L. J., Fergusson, D. M., & MacFarlane M. R. (2009). Adolescent psychiatric symptoms following preschool childhood mild traumatic brain injury: Evidence from a birth cohort. *Journal of Head Trauma Rehabilitation, 24,* 221–227.

McKinstry, R. C. (2011). Advances in pediatric diffusion tensor imaging. *Pediatric Radiology, 41,* S137–S138.

Mendelsohn, D., Levin, H. S., Bruce, D., Lilly, M., Harward, H., Culhane, K. A., & Eisenberg, H. M. (1992). Late MRI after head injury in children: Relationship to clinical features and outcome. *Child Nervous System, 8,* 445–452.

Ment, L. R., Hirtz, D., & Hüppi, S. (2009). Imaging biomarkers of outcome in the developing preterm brain. *Lancet Neurology, 8,* 1042–1055.

Middleton, J. A. (2001). Practitioner review: Psychological sequelae of head injury in children and adolescents. *Journal of Child Psychology and Psychiatry, 42,* 165–180.

Morrow, S. E., & Pearson, M. (2010). Management strategies for severe closed head injuries in children. *Seminars in Pediatric Surgery, 19,* 279–285.

Mukherjee, A. B., & Hodgen, G. D. (1982). Maternal ethanol exposure induces transient impairment of umbilical circulation and fetal hypoxia in monkeys. *Science, 218,* 700–702.

Nowakowski, R. S., & Hayes, N. L. (2002). General principles of CNS development. In M. H. Johnson, Y. Munakata, & R. O. Gilmore (Eds.), *Brain development and cognition: A reader* (2nd Ed.) (pp. 57–82). Malden MA: Blackwell Publishing.

Nyakas, C., Buwalda, B., & Luiten, P. G. M. (1996). Hypoxia and brain development. *Progress in Neurobiology, 49,* 1–51.

Olsson, K. A., Le Brocque, R. M., Kenardy, J. A., Anderson, V., & Spence, S. H. (2008). The influence of pre-injury behavior on children's type of accident, type of injury, and severity of injury. *Brain Injury, 22,* 595–602.

Oni, M. B., Wilde, E. A., Bigler, E. D., McCauley, S. R., Wu, T. C. Yallampalli, R., . . . Levin, H. S. (2010). Diffusion tensor imaging analysis of frontal lobes in pediatric traumatic brain injury. *Journal of Child Neurology, 25,* 976–984.

Ordoñana, J. R., Caspi, A., & Moffitt, T. E. (2008). Unintentional injuries in a twin study of preschool children: Environmental, not genetic, risk factors. *Journal of Pediatric Psychology 33,* 185–194.

Oria, R. B., Patrick, P. D., Zhang, H., Lorntz, B., De Castro Costa, C. M., Brito, G. A. C., Guerrant, R. L. (2005). APOE4 protects the cognitive development in children with heavy diarrhea burdens in northeast Brazil. *Pediatric Research, 57,* 310–316.

Ornstein, T. J., Levin, H. S., Chen, S., Hanten, G., Ewing-Cobbs, L., Dennis, M., . . . Schachar, R. (2009). Performance monitoring in children following traumatic brain injury. *Journal of Child Psychology and Psychiatry, 50,* 506–513.

Pemberton, C. K., Neiderhiser, J. M., Leve, L. D., Natsuaki, M. N., Shaw, D. S., Reiss, D., & Ge, X. (2010). Influence of parental depressive symptoms on adopted toddler behaviors: An emerging developmental cascade of genetic and environmental risks. *Development and Psychopathology, 22,* 1–16.

Prins, M. L., Hales, A., Reger, M., Giza, C. C., & Hovda, D. A. (2010). Repeat traumatic brain injury in the juvenile rat is associated with increased axonal injury and cognitive impairments. *Developmental Neuroscience, 32,* 510–518.

Rimel, R. W., Giordani, B., Barth, J. T., Boll, T. J., & Jane, J. A. (1981). Disability caused by minor head injury. *Neurosurgery, 9,* 221–228.

Robinson, S. (2005). Systematic prenatal insults disrupt telencephalon development: Implications for potential interventions. *Epilepsy & Behavior, 7,* 345–363.

Rosso, I. M., & Cannon, T. D. (2003). Obstetric complications and neurodevelopmental mechanisms in schizophrenia. In D. Cicchetti & E. Walker (Eds.), *Neurodevelopmental mechanisms in psychopathology* (pp. 111–137). New York, NY: Cambridge University Press.

Rothstein, R. P., & Levison, S. W. (2005). Gray matter oligodendrocyte progenitors and neurons die caspase-3 mediated deaths subsequent to mild perinatal hypoxic/ischemic insults. *Developmental Neuroscience, 27,* 149–159.

Sagvolden, T., Johansen, E. B., Aase, H., & Russell, V. A. (2005). A dynamic developmental theory of attention-deficit/hyperactivity disorder (ADHD) predominantly hyperactive/impulsive and combined subtypes. *Behavioral and Brain Sciences, 28,* 397–468.

Scherwath, A., Sommerfeldt, D. W., Bindt, C., Nolte, A., Boiger, A., Koch, U., & Petersen-Ewert, C. (2011). Identifying children and adolescents with cognitive dysfunction following mild traumatic brain injury—preliminary findings on abbreviated neuropsychological testing. *Brain Injury, 25*, 401–408.

Schmidt-Kastner, R., van Os, J., Steinbusch, H. W. M., & Schmitz, C. (2006). Gene regulation by hypoxia and the neurodevelopmental origin of schizophrenia. *Schizophrenia Research, 84*, 253–271.

Schnider, A., & Gutbrod, K. (1999). Traumatic brain injury. In D. Cicchetti, & E. Walker (Eds.), *The human frontal lobes: Functions and disorders* (pp. 487–506). New York, NY: Guilford Press.

Schutzman, S. A., & Greenes, D. S. (2001). Pediatric minor head trauma. *Annals of Emergency Medicine, 37*, 64–74.

Schwebel, D. C., Hodgens, J. B., & Sterling, S. (2006). How mothers parent their children with behavior disorders: Implications for unintentional injury risk. *Journal of Safety Research, 37*, 167–173.

Socol, M. L., Manning, F. A., Murata, Y., & Druzin, M. L. (1982). Maternal smoking causes fetal hypoxia: Experimental evidence. *American Journal of Obstetrics and Gynecology, 15*, 214–218.

Sonnenberg, L. K., Dupuis, A., & Rumney, P. G. (2010). Pre-school traumatic brain injury and its impact on social development at 8 years of age. *Brain Injury, 24*, 1003–1007.

Sowell, E. R., Thompson, P. M., Holmes, C. J., Jernigan, T. L., & Toga, A. W. (1999). In vivo evidence for post-adolescent brain maturation in frontal and striatal regions. *Nature Neuroscience, 2*, 859–861.

Stancin, T., Wade, S. L., Walz, N. C., Yeates, K. O., & Taylor, H. G. (2010). Family adaptation 18 months after traumatic brain injury in early childhood. *Journal of Developmental Behavioral Pediatrics, 31*, 317–325.

Stavinoha, P. L., Butcher, B., & Spurgin, A. A. (2011). Premorbid functional considerations in pediatric concussion. In J. N. Apps & K. D. Valter (Eds.), *Pediatric and adolescent concussion: Diagnosis, management, and outcomes* (pp. 133–150). New York, NY: Springer.

Teasdale, G., & Jennett, B. (1974). Assessment of coma and impaired consciousness. A practical scale. *Lancet, 2*, 81–84.

Vagnozzi, R., Signoretti, S., Tavazzi, B., Floris, R., Ludovici, A., Marziali, S., . . . Lazzarino, G. (2008). Temporal window of metabolic brain vulnerability to concussion: A pilot 1H-magnetic resonance spectroscopic study in concussed athletes—Part III. *Neurosurgery, 62*, 1286–1296.

Van Boven, R. W., Harrington, G. S., Hackney, D. B., Ebel, A., Gauger, G., Bremner, J. D., Weiner, M. W. (2009). Advances in neuroimaging of traumatic brain injury and posttraumatic stress disorder. *Journal of Rehabilitation Research & Development, 46*, 717–757.

Vannucci, R. C. (2000). Hypoxic-ischemic encephalopathy. *American Journal of Perinatology, 17*, 113–120.

Wilde, E. A., Hunter, J. V., Newsome, M. R., Scheibel, R. S., Bigler, E. D., Johnson, J. L., . . . Levin, H. S. (2005). Frontal and temporal morphometric findings on MRI in children after moderate to severe traumatic brain injury. *Journal of Neurotrauma*, 22, 333–344.

Wozniak, J. R., Krach, L., Ward, E., Mueller, B. A., Muetzel, R., Schnoebelen, S., . . . Lim, K. O. (2007). Neurocognitive and neuroimaging correlates of pediatric traumatic brain injury: A diffusion tensor imaging (DTI) study. *Archives of Clinical Neuropsychology*, 22, 555–568.

Yeates, K. O. (2000). Closed-head injury. In K. Yeates, M. Ris, & H. Taylor (Eds.), *Pediatric neuropsychology: Research, theory, and practice* (pp. 92–116). New York, NY: Guilford Press.

Yeates, K. O. (2010). Mild traumatic brain injury and postconcussive symptoms in children and adolescents. *Journal of the International Neuropsychological Society*, 16, 953–960.

Yeates, K. O., Taylor, H. G., Drotar, D., Wade, S. L., Klein, S., Stancin, T., & Schatschneider, C. (1997). Preinjury family environment as a determinant of recovery from traumatic brain injuries in school-age children. *Journal of the International Neuropsychological Society*, 3, 617–630.

Yeates, K. O., Taylor, H. G., Walz, N. C., Stancin, T., & Wade, S. L. (2010). The family environment as a moderator of psychosocial outcomes following traumatic brain injury in young children. *Neuropsychology*, 24, 345–356.

Zackery Lystedt Law, Wash. Rev. Code §§ 28A.600.190 (2009).

Zouakia, A., Guilloteau, D., Zimmer, L., Besnard, J. C., & Chalon, S. (1997). Evolution of dopamine receptors in the rat after neonatal hypoxia-ischemia: Autoradiographic studies. *Life Sciences*, 60, 151–162.

# CHAPTER 11

# Emotion Dysregulation as a Risk Factor for Psychopathology

PAMELA M. COLE, SARAH E. HALL, AND NASTASSIA J. HAJAL

T HE IDEA THAT PEOPLE can become dysregulated emotionally is of keen interest in the mental health sciences despite challenges in (a) defining emotion, emotion regulation, and emotion dysregulation, and (b) knowing whether emotion dysregulation is a causal factor, a correlate, or a consequence of psychopathology. As we have grappled with these thorny issues, we have continued to find that emotion dysregulation is a valuable concept in clinical practice and therefore worthy of study. We adopt a developmental psychopathology framework to conceptualize the role of emotion dysregulation in clinically meaningful trajectories of development as well as the view that emotions are fundamentally adaptive processes. Emotions allow people to adjust to diverse circumstances in which they find themselves, and to modulate their emotional reactions and behavior to fit those circumstances. Over the course of development, individual differences can conspire with life circumstances to lead to maladaptive patterns of emotional functioning. In this chapter, we discuss these issues and offer four characteristics that differentiate emotion dysregulation from emotion regulation.

## HISTORICAL CONTEXT

Emotions, their regulation, and their capacity to interfere with adaptive behavior have been a focus of scholarly thought in both the humanities and the sciences for centuries. For example, Aristotle, like Plato before him, noted the importance of emotion in persuasion (*Rhetoric*, 335–322 B.C.E.) and morality (*Nicomachean Ethics*, 350 B.C.E.). He concluded that emotions serve a functional purpose but are also irrational, and that children must learn to manage their emotions through the logic of deliberative cognition. Aristotle defined emotion, which he conceptualized in terms of physiological changes, as "affectations of the soul" that were "enmattered formulable essences" (*De Anima*, ca. 359 B.C.E.).

These views have been echoed through the centuries in scientific treatments of emotion. Darwin (1872) noted phylogenic patterns in emotion expression that led him to argue for evolutionary consistencies across species. But it was James (1884) who posed the classic question "What is an emotion?" Emphasizing its centrality in human functioning, James concluded that physiological changes constituted emotion (see also Lange's view in Ellsworth, 1994) and that the brain was the seat of emotion. In the next 100 years, debate about the nature of emotion was contentious—particularly regarding the roles of physiological changes and emotion expressions. James thought physiological changes comprise emotion, Cannon (1927) that those changes were caused by emotions, and Schacter and Singer (1962) that emotions were the interpretation of physiological change. Emotion research moved to the background as behaviorism and the cognitive revolution ascended in prominence but by 1980 interest in emotion research was revived. Zajonc (1980), on receiving the 1979 Distinguished Scientific Contribution Award of the American Psychological Association, asserted that emotion and cognition were separate processes and that emotion took precedence over cognition.

In addition to philosophical and scientific debate about the nature of emotion, religious scriptures have echoed the theme that emotions must be controlled. Jewish scriptures, for example, discuss the moral imperative of bringing emotions under control of reason as guided by Jewish law (Bokser, 1981). Christian scriptures conceptualize emotions as desires of the flesh (Galatians 5:16–24), and that rule over emotion was empowering (Proverbs 16:32). Buddhist texts regard emotions as illusory attachments to temporary realities and encourage the mental fortitude to be emotionally detached (Goleman, 2003). Yet no one more than Freud (1901) brought the public to see emotions as subterranean influences that interfere with human functioning. Most contemporary views now acknowledge that emotions have been conserved over time because of their adaptive value in survival and maintenance of well-being, that they often operate out of conscious awareness, and that emotional reactions that are poorly managed compromise behavioral functioning. Advances in our understanding of behavior, cognition, and neurophysiology have not resolved the complicated issues about the nature of emotion, yet they have enlightened the discussion.

## TERMINOLOGICAL AND CONCEPTUAL ISSUES

In the following sections we discuss the concepts of emotion, emotion regulation, and emotion dysregulation. There have been many debates about the nature of these constructs and their scientific utility—debates we do not resolve. Because of their critical importance to understanding the development of psychopathology, we describe the ways we have used the literature and the debates to guide our thinking.

### EMOTION

Before discussing emotion dysregulation, we state our understanding of the nature of emotion. Emotions comprise two integrated processes, appraisal and action preparation, which constitute a kind of psychological radar and response readiness system (e.g., Arnold, 1960; Frijda, 1986; Lazarus, 1991). Appraising is the radar by which we evaluate the significance of circumstances vis-à-vis our goals for well-being. Action preparation is readiness to respond in a particular way that enables us to regain or maintain well-being. Emotions therefore do not deter reasonable action; rather they organize responses to perceived circumstances (Frijda, 1986; Lazarus, 1991). Furthermore, they are adaptive because they permit rapid detection of threats to well-being and ability to act on our own behalf without delay. At the same time, most human beings are well equipped to regulate reactions such that the readiness to act does not dictate action. Emotions entail ongoing processes of relating to changing environments (both actual and perceived) in terms of their significance for well-being (e.g., Barrett & Campos, 1987).

An implication of this model is that emotion itself is inherently regulatory and regulated. Changes in emotion organize how we relate to the environment (Frijda, 1986); they focus attention, facilitate or limit memory processes, and facilitate specific motor activities (e.g., Hajcak, Molnar, George, Bolger, Koola, & Najas, 2007; Hamann, 2001; Isen, Shalker, Clark, & Karp, 1978; Ochsner & Schacter, 2000). Advances in affective neuroscience also indicate that emotional functioning involves dynamic, ongoing organismic adjustments to situational changes (Davidson, 2000) that usually operate out of conscious awareness (e.g., LeDoux, 1986). Neural transmission occurs in feed-forward and feedback networks involving limbic structures and prefrontal and orbitofrontal regions, which support regulatory processes such as deliberate reallocation of attention and inhibiting action. Studies using methods such as functional magnetic resonance imaging (fMRI), eye blink startle, positron emission tomography (PET), and electrophysiology (EEG and ERP) to study these neural processes suggest that individuals with psychopathology regulate their emotions differently than nonpsychiatric controls. However, these techniques are limited in their ability to inform our knowledge of psychopathology and its development. EEG and ERP, for example, measure the summation of electrical activity at the scalp, and are not well suited for precise localization of activation, particularly in subcortical regions. Although fMRI can assess spatial distributions of neural activity, including subcortical connections, it requires constrained experimental conditions that are many steps removed from ecologies in which emotion dysregulation occurs. Nevertheless, fMRI research is helping us understand brain function, which will ultimately allow specific hypotheses for testing the respective roles of different neural networks in emotion regulation and dysregulation (Ochsner & Gross, 2007). In short, affective neuroscience underscores the systemic, inherently regulatory nature of the central nervous system and holds promise for our ability to better understand how emotions are regulated, and the brain's role in the development of emotion dysregulation.

The autonomic nervous system (ANS), which plays an important role in action readiness, is also a self-regulatory system. When emotions change (e.g., a person feels angry), neural information directs the heart to increase output, pumping blood to other muscles and bringing increased oxygen to them, thereby fortifying their readiness to contract. This increased cardiac output, facilitated by reduced parasympathetic and increased sympathetic ANS activation, readies a person for action. The vagus nerve of the parasympathetic nervous system regulates much of the cardiovascular response. As we breathe, heart rate fluctuates in response to cyclic activation and deactivation of parasympathetic input, under the control of the vagus nerve. Parasympathetic efference to the heart, often referred to as vagal tone, is indexed by measures of heart rate variability (e.g., respiratory sinus arrhythmia). Individuals with greater heart rate variability are better regulated emotionally (Porges, 2001), perhaps due to greater autonomic control over responding. For instance, children with higher heart rate variability are less negative in response to lab-based frustrations (Calkins & Dedmon, 2000; Calkins & Keane, 2004) and appear to be buffered from the negative sequelae of family adversity (El-Sheikh, Harger, & Whitson, 2001; Katz & Gottman, 1995; Katz & Hunter, 2007; Shannon, Beauchaine, Brenner, Neuhaus, & Gatzke-Kopp, 2007). In sum, being emotional entails continual processes of evaluating the meaning of, and readying responses to, ever-changing circumstances, a set of processes that both regulate other psychological systems and are inherently self-regulatory.

## EMOTION REGULATION

This definition of emotion creates a challenge for defining emotion regulation (Cole, Martin, & Dennis, 2004). How—if at all—does emotion regulation differ from emotion (Cicchetti, Ackerman, & Izard, 1995; Thompson, 2011)? This is a particular challenge for the study of psychopathology, which often involves judgments about the adaptiveness of behavior. At the behavioral level, the mental operations that underlie emotion cannot be observed. Behavior is a product of both a response to changing circumstances and the inherent regulation of the response at levels that are beyond the individual's awareness and ordinary observation.

Despite these limitations, there is clinical utility in using behavioral methods to gauge emotion regulation. To this end, we conceptualize emotion regulation as *changes* in an initial, measurable emotional response (Cole et al., 2004). If an emotion is an appraisal and readiness to act to the changing environment, then emotion regulation refers to the modulation of that appraisal/action readiness response. As an emotional response unfolds, psychological processes can be recruited to modulate it—we can shift attention, recall memories that intensify or reduce the emotion, reappraise the situation, or take instrumental action. These in turn can alter the valence or temporal dynamics of the emotion (Davidson, 2000; Thompson, 1994). Given the adaptive nature of emotion is derived from its permitting quick, intense, and sustained emotion, it is the ability to *regulate* emotional responses that allows us to vary and modulate a response to a situation. Appropriate inferences about emotion regulation can be gleaned from meticulous observations of behavior, including examination of emotion-behavior-emotion sequences, convergence of data from multiple levels of measurement (behavioral, self-report, and physiological), and strategic manipulations of situational context (Cole et al., 2004). Ultimately, evidence from studies of neurophysiological processes, along with field and lab research of children's emotion-related behavior in situational context, can provide a fuller picture of emotional development and of trajectories that lead to emotional competence and disorder. This is particularly important for studies of very young children, during age periods when patterns of emotion regulation are being established (e.g., Tarullo & Gunnar, 2006).

In sum, despite the complex nature of emotion, emotion regulation can be conceptualized as changes in initial appraisal/action readiness responses to circumstances that can be modulated by other processes (attentional, cognitive, social, and behavioral; Cole et al., 2004). Mental health and emotional competence require both emotional responsiveness and regulation of responses such that behavior accords to social standards (Saarni, 1999).

## Emotion Dysregulation

Given that emotions are adaptive, it might seem paradoxical that emotion dysregulation figures prominently in conceptualizations of psychopathology. Emotions are neither irrational nor disruptive; they are organizing, regulated processes. Fear, anger, sadness, joy, interest, guilt, and other emotions are all advantageous for dealing with the complexity of a social world that is constantly changing and often challenging. The elegance of emotional processes is that there are multiple points at which emotions can be modified, even without awareness (Frijda, 1986; Gross & Thompson, 2007). Nonetheless, individuals can develop patterns of emotion regulation that appear emotionally dysregulated.

We all have times when our emotions get the better of us. Within a developmental psychopathology framework, such instances of feeling emotionally "out of control" contrast with atypical functioning. The contrast is important; these common instances do not disrupt and compromise lives in persistent ways. Emotion dysregulation occurs when patterns of emotion regulation compromise longer term functioning *even as they serve the goal of achieving an immediate sense of well-being.* For instance, a person with borderline personality disorder may fend off feeling rejected by being hostile to others. In this and other clinical examples, emotions are not unregulated but they are dysregulated (Cole, 1994). They are regulated in that they diminish psychological discomfort but they do so at a cost: they jeopardize relationships, productivity, and future achievements. These patterns of emotion dysregulation develop when biology and circumstances conspire to compromise the development of, or override, patterns of emotion regulation that achieve well-being and promote the longer-term goals of becoming a competent, healthy person. Emotion dysregulation then refers to dysfunctional patterns of emotion regulation. But how do we distinguish these from emotion regulation?

## Emotion Dysregulation From a Clinical Perspective

We regard emotion dysregulation as a general feature of psychopathology (Cicchetti, Ackerman, & Izard, 1995; Cole, Michel, & Teti, 1994; Gross & Muñoz, 1995). It is treated as central to many different disorders (e.g., Barkley, 1997; Beauchaine, Gatzke-Kopp, & Mead, 2007; Gotlib, Joormann, Minor, & Cooney, 2006; Kovacs et al., 2006; Leibenluft, Charney, & Pine, 2003; Linehan, 1993; Mennin, Heimberg, Turk, & Fresco, 2002; Suveg, Morelen, Brewer, & Thomassin, 2010), and featured in descriptions of several disorders in the *Diagnostic and Statistical Manual of Mental Disorders* (*DSM-IV-TR*; American Psychiatric Association, 2000).

The centrality of emotion dysregulation in psychopathology has led to studies of the developmental links between early emotional functioning and later symptoms (e.g., Calkins, Dedmon, Gill, Lomax, & Johnson, 2002; Cole, Zahn-Waxler, Fox, Usher, & Welsh, 1996; Gilliom, Shaw, Beck, Schonberg, & Lukon, 2002). In general, higher levels of negative emotion earlier in life are associated with both concurrent and later symptoms and disorders, suggesting emotion dysregulation is a risk factor rather than a consequence of mental health problems (McLaughlin, Hatzenbuehler, Mennin, & Nolen-Hoeksema, 2011). This leads to an urgent need to understand emotional competence and the ways it develops and is derailed.

Emotional competence is defined by being able to experience a full range of emotions, to be responsive to others' emotional states, to value one's own and others' emotions, to appreciate the need to regulate emotion and the ability to do so in ways that fit situational constraints, and to achieve a sense of emotional self-efficacy (Halberstadt, Denham, & Dunsmore, 2001; Saarni, 1999). Emotion dysregulation can be distinguished from emotionally competent patterns of regulation in the following ways:

- Emotions endure and regulatory attempts are ineffective.
- Emotions interfere with appropriate behavior.
- Emotions are context inappropriate.
- Emotions change too abruptly or too slowly.

These qualities are not mutually exclusive. As a group, they share qualities of being unpredictable, inappropriate, and maladaptive. Thus, dysregulation stems not from strong anger or shame or other emotion, but from deviations in how emotion is regulated (see Cole, Dennis, Martin, & Hall, 2008, for a clinical example) and from the failure of regulatory efforts to meet goals appropriately (Thompson, 2011).

## Emotions Are Enduring and Regulatory Attempts Are Ineffective

Intense or persisting emotions are not necessarily dysfunctional if they are regulated well. One partner in a couple may be very angry for days due to something the other partner did; he may even actively work to maintain anger in order to emphasize the perceived seriousness of the problem. If the couple has a good relationship, the other partner will come to see how great the concern is; then through both mutual and self-regulatory behavior the anger is resolved.

In other instances, sustained emotion such as prolonged irritability and generalized anxiety interfere with rather than foster effective problem solving and healthy relationship maintenance (Carthy, Horesh, Apter, & Gross, 2010; Sheeber et al., 2009; Suveg, Hoffman, Zeman, & Thomassin, 2009). In the case of dysregulation, sustained and/or intense emotion loses any initial value and begins to interfere with functioning, both intra- and inter-personal. Dysfunctional sustained emotion is often unresponsive to regulatory efforts because the person has an insufficient repertoire of regulatory strategies, lacks skill at executing strategies, is undermined by faulty biological systems that ordinarily support emotion and coping, or receives secondary or partial gains for sustaining the emotion. Sustained but dysfunctional emotion occurs if strategies to modify the emotion are either ineffective (e.g., ruminating about a failure) or are used ineffectively (e.g., distraction is used when action is needed).

A variety of regulatory strategies are known to modify the temporal and intensive dynamics of emotional responses—delaying a reaction, reducing intensity, shortening duration, or shifting from one emotion to another (Davidson, 2000; Thompson, 1994). Active problem-solving, cognitive reappraisal, exercise, information-seeking, and support-seeking are generally adaptive strategies; avoidance, denial, emotion suppression, rumination, substance use, aggression, and venting are less optimal (e.g., Aldao, Nolen-Hoeksema, & Schweizer, 2010; Grolnick, Bridges, & Connell, 1996; Hayes, Wilson, Gifford, Follette, & Strosahl, 1996). Mentally healthy, emotionally competent children have a repertoire of strategies from which to choose, are able to select and deploy them effectively and flexibly to fit personal needs and situational constraints, and respond to the regulatory efforts of others (Halberstadt et al., 2001; Saarni, 1999).

*Individual differences.* In early and middle childhood, children with externalizing problems do not regulate frustration as well as asymptomatic children (e.g., Bar-Haim, Bar-Av, & Sadeh, 2011; Calkins & Dedmon, 2000; Cole, Zahn-Waxler, & Smith, 1994; Eisenberg et al., 2001; Gilliom et al., 2002), suggesting they have less adaptive or less effective strategies. They are less likely to use effective strategies (e.g., Calkins & Dedmon, 2000; Calkins et al., 2002; Eisenberg et al., 2001; Melnick & Hinshaw, 2000). Internalizing symptoms in children and adolescents are also linked with use of ineffective strategies (Hughes, Gullone, & Watson, 2011). This work, however, did not evaluate whether children attempted effective strategies without success.

Particularly compelling evidence for the clinical importance of effective strategies in the face of high levels of negative emotion comes from a study in which three-year-old boys with oppositional defiant symptoms who used effective strategies to immediately reduce anger were better adjusted at later ages than those who could not do this (Gilliom et al., 2002); that is, attention shifting at age 3 predicted more cooperativeness and fewer externalizing symptoms at age 6, and information seeking predicted later assertiveness. In a different study, 4- to 7-year-old daughters of depressed mothers, a group of children who are at risk for later psychopathology, engaged in strategies but less actively than children whose mothers were asymptomatic (Silk, Shaw, Skuban, Oland, & Kovacs, 2006). Finally, highly anxious, sad, and angry children and adolescents use less effective strategies and are less confident in their strategy use (Burwell & Shirk, 2007; Carthy et al., 2010; Suveg & Zeman, 2004).

We do not know the degree to which children with specific symptoms or disorders deploy different strategies, have fewer strategies available, use less-mature or appropriate strategies, or use strategies less effectively or flexibly. Nevertheless, evidence suggests that (a) attention-shifting, problem-focused information seeking, and appropriate, instrumental actions regulate children's emotions, at least in the short term; (b) greater reliance on these strategies is associated with better adjustment from infancy to adolescence; and (c) children with symptoms of anxiety, depression, and oppositionality are less likely to use these strategies and lack confidence that they can use them effectively. With a repertoire of effective strategies that are deployed flexibly to match situational demands, a person should experience enduring or intense emotion only as needed and without being disabled by it.

## Emotions Interfere With Appropriate Behavior

Emotions are defined in part by readiness to act in a particular way—to approach a blocked goal with force (anger), approach a goal with eagerness and openness (joy), withdraw from perceived threat (fear), and relinquish a lost goal (sadness), to name a few. This is a crucial part of the adaptive nature of emotions—they quickly (without requiring awareness) ready us to act on the environment to maintain and regain well-being. Indeed, young children can stay focused on a task despite being frustrated. For example, if typically developing 3- and 4-year-olds' anger is modulated, it is followed by *appropriate* action, such as persistently and flexibly solving a problem (Dennis, Cole, Wiggins, Cohen, & Zalewski, 2009). The world, however, is complex, and many situations involve multiple and sometimes conflicting goals and social constraints. Although emotion makes certain actions more likely, those actions can be appropriate or inappropriate. Emotionally competent, mentally healthy children who feel strong emotions have learned to behave in ways that take into account these constraints. Actions that are understandable and effective in the short run (a child hits another child to get a toy) compromise functioning if they become a stable pattern that interferes with friendship formation or self-control. A poignant illustration is that of incest victims who may dissociate from their overwhelming emotions. At first, this strategy is not linked to symptoms but if it becomes a generalized coping strategy it has detrimental effects on long-term mental health (e.g., Marx & Sloan, 2002). In sum, emotion dysregulation occurs when emotions lead to behaviors that violate social standards or compromise developmental goals.

*Individual differences.* The discussion implies that emotion-behavior sequences differentiate typically developing children from those at risk for psychopathology. Research, however, that examines correlations between emotions and behaviors rather than behavior sequences cannot address whether emotions organize or disorganize behavior (Dagne & Snyder, 2011). Anger followed by inappropriate acts is seen in school-aged children with behavior problems, whereas this sequence is not observed in asymptomatic children (Casey, 1996); after exposure to background anger, 86.7% of children with oppositional defiant disorder either stopped playing (i.e., shut down) or became disruptive, but 60% of asymptomatic children continued to behave appropriately. Adolescent females with difficulty regulating emotion engage in more self-injury (Adrian, Zeman, Erdley, Lisa, & Sim, 2011), which may be a maladaptive strategy borne from inability to tolerate negative emotion (Klonsky, 2007).

*Emotions about emotions.* One way that emotion can lead to inappropriate action is when a person has an emotional reaction to an initial emotional response. Clinicians, for example, note that clients may feel guilty about getting angry, but emotions about emotions are rarely studied. Children may have feelings about their emotional reactions.

Consider youth who engage in serious misconduct. Some of them will have grown up in highly stressed families, experiencing acute vulnerability as young children and without the adult support they need to help them cope with their emotions (see Cole, Hall, & Radzioch, 2009). Their parents may have had poorly regulated emotions, modeling inadequate emotion regulation as well as their emotions distressing their children. Clinically, we form the view that these children regulated their feelings of vulnerability as best they could but could not resolve them. Yet when the clinician tries to help them experience, understand and resolve those feelings, they encounter the youth's avoidance of feeling vulnerable, and anger, even hostility, when feelings of sadness, rejection, and/or anxiety are stirred.

We know little about "emotions about emotions" in either typically developing or at-risk children. However, it is known that parents who have negative attitudes and emotions about feelings have children who are symptomatic (Hunter et al., 2011; Katz & Hunter, 2007). Saarni (1998) points out that the emotionally competent person is aware of all emotions (i.e., does not selectively attend to certain emotions), appreciates that mixed emotions often occur, and realizes one can be unaware of emotions (see also Halberstadt et al., 2001). A body of developmental work on understanding mixed emotions provides a point of departure for a deeper understanding of the development of emotional dysregulation.

By about age 8 to 9 years, typically developing children have a fairly differenti-ated understanding of multiple emotions, including mixed and conflicting emotions (Harter & Buddin, 1987; Harter & Whitesell, 1989; Pons, Harris, & de Rosnay, 2004; Wintre & Vallance, 1994). Appreciation that one emotion influences another emotion, however, appears to be more sophisticated, not appearing until the preadolescent period (Donaldson & Westerman, 1986). Adolescents who disavow having mixed emotions endorse repressive coping styles (Sincoff, 1992). Moreover, youth with externalizing problems, compared to internalizing and asymptomatic youth, have less complex, differentiated understanding of their emotional responses, but inter-nalizing youth are less differentiated in understanding their reactions to perceived threat, and are more confused about their emotions (O'Kearney & Dadds, 2005).

In sum, the study of temporal emotion-behavior sequences and emotion-emotion sequences helps us understand an important aspect of emotion dysregulation. In considering how the unfolding of an emotional response influences behavior, we need both basic and applied developmental work on emotions about emotions.

## EMOTIONS THAT ARE CONTEXT INAPPROPRIATE

A third feature of emotion dysregulation involves the goodness of fit between an emotional response and the situation in which it occurs. In contrast to inappropriate action that results from an emotional response, an emotional response, experienced or expressed, may deviate from how individuals usually feel in a given context.

In considering context appropriateness, there are 3 points to keep in mind. First, positive as well as negative emotions can be contextually inappropriate, as when a person enjoys something that would distress most people. Second, situations alone do not dictate emotional responses. The functional perspective contends that emotions reflect the personal meaning ascribed to a situation; emotional responses to the same situation can and do vary among individuals. Nonetheless, many contexts generally elicit emotions from a particular emotion family (Ekman, 1994), which allows a means of studying atypical emotional responses. Third, a major source of individual differences in appraising situations is a child's developmental level. A child's ability to understand a situation and appreciate its complexity will influence if the child finds a specific situation frightening, funny, frustrating, or inconsequential.

*Socially inappropriate emotion expression.* An expressed emotion is inappropriate when it violates social or cultural norms for the situation, such as laughing when someone is hurt. Although it may be understandable to feel like laughing, doing so is inconsiderate or disrespectful. The expression of socially inappropriate emotion is linked to a variety of psychological risk factors and problems (Casey, 1996; Cole, Zahn-Waxler, & Smith, 1994; Shields & Cicchetti, 1998; Suveg & Zeman, 2004; Weisbrot, Gadow, DeVincent, & Pomeroy, 2005). In contrast, the ability to modulate emotion expression according to social standards is linked to social competence. As early as age 3, typically developing children spontaneously attempt to modulate disappointment (anger and sadness) according to social standards (Cole, 1986). Preschoolers (Garner & Power, 1996; Liew, Eisenberg, & Reiser, 2004) and school-aged children (McDowell, O'Neill, & Parke, 2000) who try to smile although disappointed have better emotion knowledge and are more socially competent.

A consistent pattern of socially inappropriate emotion expression interferes with relationships (e.g., Halberstadt et al., 2001). Might inappropriately expressed fear predict a different developmental outcome than inappropriately expressed anger? Are certain ways of modulating emotion preferable? Cole et al. (1994) found that oppositional preschool-aged girls, in contrast to asymptomatic girls, suppressed disappointment even without the social pressure to mask disappointment. Research on children's expressive control has not explored these potentially important aspects of emotion regulation and the mechanisms that cause them to develop. Inappropriate emotion expression may involve poor social awareness, disregard for social display rules, or inability to regulate expression even when the individual wishes to do so.

*Atypical emotional responses to specific contexts.* A second form of context-inappropriate emotion involves atypical emotional responses, such as feeling sad or afraid in situations that most children enjoy. Excessive distrust, pleasure at another's distress, and emotional reactions for no apparent reason embody the idea of emotion-context mismatch. An example is hostile attribution bias, in which malevolent intent attributed to an ambiguous interpersonal situation leads to context-inappropriate anger (Crick & Dodge, 1994).

Few studies address the role of context-inappropriate emotion in child psychopathology but a link is suggested. Aggressive children, who typically have difficulty regulating anger, may respond with positive emotions to situations in which most children feel angry, anxious, or subdued. Oppositional preschoolers laughed at their mothers' anger more than asymptomatic children did (Cole, Teti, & Zahn-Waxler, 2003). They did not seem anxious about the harm to the relationship or of negative consequences; they may have derived a sense of mastery or power from their misconduct (Cole et al., 2009). Indeed, aggressive children identify more positive and fewer negative consequences of aggression (Boldizar, Perry, & Perry, 1989; Slaby & Guerra, 1988). They are also less accurate in reading peers' negative emotions, particularly sadness and fear (Blair & Coles, 2000; Bowen & Dixon, 2010; Casey, 1996). Unknown is the timing and conditions under which such atypical emotional reactions develop and how they relate to the lack of remorse and empathy. Notably, externalizing males may appear sad or empathic in regard to another's distress but may not show the autonomic responses that typically developing children do (Marsh, Beauchaine, & Williams, 2008). Dyssynchrony between expressive and physiological aspects of emotional responding may reveal information about emotion regulation and mark risk for psychopathology.

Context-inappropriate emotion has also been linked with anxiety symptoms. Toddlers who react fearfully to situations that other children enjoy may be exhibiting dysregulated fear (Buss, Kiel, Williams, & Leuty, 2005), which may forecast risk for the development of anxiety symptoms (see also Chapter 7). Similarly, emotion-context mismatch has been reported in depressed adults; they report high levels of sadness while watching films that evoke happiness in control participants (Rottenberg, Gross, & Gotlib, 2005). Lastly, infants who react to a blocked goal with sadness rather than anger have higher cortisol responses (Lewis & Ramsay, 2005).

*Emotional unresponsiveness.* A third form of context-inappropriate emotion is emotional unresponsiveness to situations that usually evoke emotion. Flat affect is seen in schizophrenia, depression, and posttraumatic stress disorder. Inexpressivity in children is also linked to both externalizing and internalizing symptoms (Cole et al., 1996; Frick, Lilienfeld, Ellis, Loney, & Silverthorn, 1999; Hayden, Klein, & Durbin, 2005).

Emotional unresponsiveness in situations that anger or frustrate most children has been observed in children with disruptive behavior or general difficulties with emotion regulation. These include the absence of sympathy, empathy, or guilt when another is distressed (Cole et al., 1996; Eisenberg, Fabes, Murphy, Karbon, Smith, & Maszk, 1996; Frick et al., 1999; Liew, Eisenberg, Losoya, Fabes, Guthrie, & Murphy, 2003). Such unresponsiveness may have a biological basis, as these children often lack the physiological responsiveness to emotional stimuli that typical children have (Fung et al., 2005; Marsh et al., 2008) and have morphological differences in their brains that are linked with emotional deficits (Raine et al., 2003). Emotional unresponsiveness to situations that elicit positive emotions in most children is linked with internalizing problems. Preschoolers who express low levels of positive emotion during usually enjoyable tasks appear depressed or disruptive as preschoolers and later develop helplessness and negative self-views (Hayden, Klein, Durbin, & Olino, 2006; Luby et al., 2006).

Emotional inexpressivity also predicts self-harm among female college students (Gratz, 2006), consistent with the idea that nonsuicidal self-injury evokes feeling in individuals whose ability to experience emotion is impaired (Crowell, Beauchaine, &

Linehan, 2009; Chapter 18). Distressed individuals may also actively limit the experience of negative emotion (Hayes et al., 1996). Although healthy individuals occasionally avoid negative emotions (e.g., avoid discussing a sad event), generalized avoidance of negative interferes with relationships and paradoxically increases stress (Hayes et al., 1996; Marx & Sloan, 2002). Experiential avoidance is linked to a variety of disorders, including depression, anxiety, obsessive-compulsive disorder, and borderline personality disorder (Hayes et al., 1996, 2004).

In sum, context-inappropriate emotion is a form of emotion dysregulation that includes socially inappropriate emotional expressions, mismatches between emotional reactions and situational context, and unresponsiveness to particular or a range of situations. Research on context-inappropriate emotion and the development of psychopathology is quite limited.

## Emotions Change Too Abruptly or Too Slowly

Finally, emotional reactions may deviate in how they ebb and flow. If you have coded emotion second by second, you have seen considerable variation across individuals and situations. These expressions can appear and fade in a matter of seconds, but even then they usually begin at a low level of intensity, reach a peak, and then steadily fade. Moreover, between codable emotion expressions there are longer periods of neutral (nonemotional) expressions. This pattern contrasts with emotions that linger (do not recover quickly) or that change abruptly or frequently. Slow emotional recovery (e.g., unremitting dysphoria or anxiety) and lability (i.e., affective instability) are symptomatic of psychopathology.

*Individual differences.* Rapid changes in emotion are common in infancy (Camras, 1994), but in children are linked to ADHD (Anastopoulos et al., 2011; Sobanski et al., 2010), externalizing symptoms (Martin, Boekamp, McConville, & Wheeler, 2010) and bullying (Garner & Hinton, 2010). Emotional lability is especially common among youth with comorbid internalizing and externalizing disorders and hospitalized adolescents (Gerson et al., 1996; Stringaris & Goodman, 2009). Self-reported lability is associated with adolescent depression, aggression, and anxiety and with adult borderline personality disorder (Koenigsburg et al., 2002; Larsen, Raffaelli, Richards, & Ham, 1990; Neumann, van Lier, Frijns, Meeus, & Koot, 2011; Silk, Steinberg, & Morris, 2003). Childhood lability in some cases may lead to adult bipolar disorder and borderline personality disorder (Fergus et al., 2003; Kochman et al., 2005).

*Emotional responses that resist change.* Emotional lability is usually not contrasted with emotions that resist change. We place them together to underscore that the temporal dynamics of emotions are at least as important as their valence. Emotional responses normally develop and resolve in short periods of time and the ability to recover from negative emotion is one hallmark of emotional health (Davidson, 2000).

*Individual differences.* Aggressive kindergartners have difficulty shifting to positive emotion states after a difficult task (Wilson, 2003). Yet little is known about the development of the ability to recover emotionally and the significance of individual differences in latency to regain a calm or content state after being upset or to enjoy activities after being distressed. Regulating negative emotion may deplete psychological resources (Baumeister, Bratslavsky, Murven, & Tice, 1998) but in adults the experience of positive emotion after being frustrated seems to restore the ability to self-regulate (Tice, Baumeister, & Zhang, 2004).

Resistance to emotional change is a feature of mood and anxiety disorders. Prolonged sadness or irritability is the central symptom of adult and childhood depression. Furthermore, inability to resolve anger and sadness is a main concern of parents who try, unsuccessfully, to soothe distress of depressed children or encourage them to feel better (Cole, Luby, & Sullivan, 2008). Enduring negative emotion and anhedonia may be related. Prolonged anxiety, even when immediate threats to well-being have subsided, is a central symptom of anxiety disorders. Oppositional children endure in being angry even when asymptomatic children's anger is resolved (Cole et al., 1994). Thus, emotions that resist change may signal dysregulation.

## ETIOLOGICAL FORMULATIONS

### NORMAL DEVELOPMENT

Initially, negative infant emotional expressions appear undifferentiated (Bridges, 1931; Lewis & Haviland-Jones, 2000) but by the end of the first year anger, sadness, and fear are discernible (Bennett, Bendersky, & Lewis, 2002; Camras, Oster, Campos, & Bakeman, 2003; Izard, 2002). At first, infant emotions switch quickly (Camras, 1994)—a crying infant can quickly smile at a parent's intervention—yet by 6 months facial expressions change less rapidly or frequently (Malatesta & Haviland, 1982). Emotional lability appears to follow a normative decline across development (Gerson et al., 1996).

Caregivers help infants maintain and regain calm and pleasant states, which fosters the development of more autonomous emotion regulation (Diener & Mangelsdorf, 1999; Kopp, 1989; Thompson, 1994). Infants can spontaneously engage in behaviors that immediately reduce negative emotions, but with limited effectiveness. Infant self-comforting and attention redirection reduce distress (Crockenberg & Leerkes, 2004; Stifter & Braungart, 1995), but very young children resume being distressed if the situation is unchanged (Buss & Goldsmith, 1998). With age and experience, the variety and effectiveness of regulatory strategies increase (Grolnick et al., 1996; Mangelsdorf, Shapiro, & Marzolf, 1995; Stansbury & Sigman, 2000). By age three, low level anger appears to motivate task persistence and flexible problem solving (Dennis et al., 2009), and children can delay and modulate frustration and disappointment (Cole, 1986; Cole et al., 2011).

By the time children enter school, most deal with ordinary, familiar frustrations and disappointments without becoming dysregulated. They use distraction and cognitive reappraisal effectively (Reijntjes et al., 2006; Silk et al., 2003). Being fear- or anger-prone or experiencing family adversity appears to compromise the development of emotion regulation (Morris, Silk, Steinberg, Meyers, & Robinson, 2007).

## Temperament

Temperament, defined as predispositions involving reactivity and regulation (Derryberry & Rothbart, 1988; Rothbart & Bates, 2006), predicts difficulties with emotion regulation even from early childhood (Calkins & Fox, 2002). Six-month-olds disposed to both high activity and low attention control are more readily frustrated and use less effective strategies than other infants (Calkins et al., 2002). In preschoolers, high-negative affectivity is linked to the use of fewer constructive and more maladaptive regulation strategies (Blair, Denham, Kochanoff, & Whipple, 2004; Santucci, Silk, Shaw, Gentzler, Fox, & Kovacs, 2008). Links have also been found between inhibitory control and emotion regulation in preschoolers (Carlson & Wang, 2007), and emotional dysregulation is associated with low temperamental reactivity and low persistence (Yagmurlu & Altan, 2010). Temperamental characteristics also predict school age children's regulatory strategies (Jaffe, Gullone, & Hughes, 2010). Overall, biologically based dispositions seem to influence the development of emotion regulation and dysregulation (Rothbart & Sheese, 2007). In addition, children are influenced by their interactions with their caregivers. Temperament may render a child more susceptible to caregiving quality (Ellis, Boyce, Belsky, Bakermans-Kranenburg, & Van Ijzendoorn, 2011).

## Parenting and Parent–Child Relationships

Attachment quality has been linked with emotion dysregulation. Children who are classified as securely attached are better able to rely on their mothers and also on objects as regulatory aids when they are stressed in situations that do not activate the attachment system whereas insecurely attached children exhibit poorer emotion regulation (e.g., Brody & Flor, 1998; Contreras, Kerns, Weimer, Gentzler, & Tomich, 2000; Crugnola et al., 2011; Kidwell et al., 2010). Secure attachment is linked to parent–child discussion and validation of children's emotions when they are upset (Waters et al., 2010).

In addition, warm, supportive parental responses, and firm discipline when needed, appear to support the development of healthy emotion regulation (Bocknek, Brophy-Herb, & Banerjee, 2009; Chang, Schwartz, Dodge, & McBride-Chang, 2003). Still, little is known about the *specific* practices that foster self-regulation of emotion; parental emotion expressions, reactions to children's emotions, and teaching opportunities may all play a role (Eisenberg et al., 1998; Morris et al., 2007). For example, mothers who express both positive and negative emotions have children with better self-regulation (Eisenberg et al., 2003), and maternal emotional reactions to child emotion predict the quality of child emotion regulation strategies (Garner, 2006) and exacerbate or remediate child anger control problems (Cole et al., 2003). Toddlers whose mothers minimize or reject their children's emotions display more context-inappropriate emotion (Tonyan, 2005), whereas parents who use distraction and cognitive reframing strategies have children who self-regulate effectively (Morris et al., 2011). Most of this work, however, has not examined the effects of parenting qualities and practices as a function of child disposition. Certain children may benefit from active and early intervention, while for others such parenting may be distressing and interfere with the development of self-reliance in emotion regulation (Grolnick, Kurowski, McMenamy, Rivkin, & Bridges, 1998; Mirabile, Scaramella, Sohr-Preston, & Robison, 2009).

## PARENTAL PSYCHOPATHOLOGY

Parents' ability to foster healthy emotion regulation in a child depends on their ability to regulate their own emotions (Teti & Cole, 2011). This may explain links between parental mental health problems and child emotion dysregulation. Evidence comes from work on maternal depression (Goodman & Gotlib, 2002). Maternal depression is not always associated with poorer child emotion regulation (Silk, Shaw, Forbes, Lane, & Kovacs, 2006), but emotional dysregulation is more common among children of depressed mothers, even as early as infancy (Dagne & Snyder, 2011; Feldman et al., 2009; Hoffman, Crnic, & Baker, 2006). Child characteristics, such as temperamental proclivity for negative reactivity, may heighten effects (Blandon, Calkins, Keane, & O'Brien, 2008; Tronick & Weinberg, 2000).

The timing of parental depression relative to the child's developmental status must be considered (Feng et al., 2008; Maughan, Cicchetti, Toth, & Rogosch, 2007; Silk et al., 2006). In infancy, maternal depression influences how mothers and infants respond to one another (Gianino & Tronick, 1988; Tronick & Cohn, 1989). Depressed mothers misread infant emotions, increasing the chance of emotional mismatches and insensitive responses by the mother, which may cause infant emotional dysregulation, such as disengaging from the mother or being hard to soothe (Tronick & Reck, 2009). In older children, parent–child interaction may also be affected by the history of the child's exposure to the parent's depression. Maternal depression–historic or current–affects parenting behaviors (Feng, Shaw, Skuban, & Lane, 2007) but a history of maternal childhood-onset depression affects her parenting above and beyond effects of her current depression status (Shaw et al., 2006).

Changes in maternal behavior, in turn, change the way children engage emotionally with a depressed parent. Toddlers whose mothers have depressive symptoms sometimes display more negative affect in their interactions with their mothers but they may also show diminished negative affect (Cole, Barrett, & Zahn-Waxler, 1992; Dagne & Snyder, 2011; NICHD Early Child Care Network, 2004). At least some children may even try to care for the withdrawn or irritable parent (Radke-Yarrow, Zahn-Waxler, Richardson, Susman, & Martinez, 1994), which could restrict their own emotions and learning to regulate them in a healthy manner.

## MALTREATMENT AND VIOLENCE EXPOSURE

Maltreatment is associated with child emotion dysregulation as early as the first three years of life and into young adulthood (Burns, Jackson, & Harding, 2010; Kim & Cicchetti, 2010; Maughan & Cicchetti, 2002; Robinson et al., 2009; Shields & Cicchetti, 1997, 1998; Shipman, Zeman, Penza, & Champion, 2000). Maltreatment may interfere with the development of healthy emotion regulation in several ways. First, the trauma of maltreatment affects children neurologically (Wilson, Hansen, & Li, 2011). Neural regions involved in processing emotion are altered by neurochemical responses to prolonged stress. Second, maltreating parents are less sensitive to their children's needs and may lack the skills to both teach and model effective emotion regulation (Shipman et al., 2007). Third, maltreatment affects child emotion processing. Children who are maltreated are quicker to detect anger in others (Pollak, Messner, Kistler, & Cohn, 2009). Their negative internal representations of their parents may interfere with how well they regulate emotion in any interpersonal situation (Shields, Ryan, & Cicchetti, 2001). Finally, the way a child copes with maltreatment may require emotion dysregulation (Cole et al., 1994; Maughan & Cicchetti, 2002). Overregulating one's negative affect may avoid parental anger, which promotes safety in the short term but can lead to a style of emotional functioning that is dysregulated in other relationships.

Exposure to unresolved marital conflict, particularly domestic violence, affects child emotion regulation (Koss et al., 2011). Exposure to adult anger distresses children, and they respond in varying ways. Exposure may threaten a child's sense of security (Cummings & Davies, 2010), which interferes with the ability to emotionally engage fully and appropriately with activities and relationships (El-Sheikh, Cummings, Kouros, Elmore-Staton, & Buckhalt, 2008). Maltreatment and interadult violence often co-occur, and evidence suggests that the effect of marital conflict on child emotion regulation could be accounted for by maltreatment (Maughan & Cicchetti, 2002).

## GENETICS AND HERITABILITY OF EMOTION DYSREGULATION

Behavioral (e.g., adoption, twin, and sibling studies) and molecular genetics studies suggest there are genetic effects on the etiology of emotion dysregulation. Genes influence the psychological processes that support or hinder adaptive emotion regulation, both directly (are heritable) and indirectly (e.g., via gene-environment correlation; Scarr & McCartney, 1983). Genes directly influence physiology, which enables emotional responsiveness and regulation. Furthermore, genetic influences interact with environmental influences at multiple levels (e.g., gene-environment correlations).

Specific gene polymorphisms are associated with neural measures of recovery from unpleasant stimuli (Larson, Taubitz, & Robinson, 2010), hormonal responses to stress (e.g., cortisol; Armbruster et al., 2009), and indicators of physiological regulation, such as respiratory sinus arrhythmia (Kupper et al., 2005; Propper et al., 2008). One way that child development researchers have approached genetic influences on emotion regulation and dysregulation is through the construct of temperament. Although infant temperament is influenced by the prenatal environment (Di-Pietro, Ghera, & Costigan, 2008), individual differences in temperament are also attributable to genetic heritability.

Individual differences in temperament vary in their heritability, ranging from 20 to 60% (Auerbach et al., 1999; Goldsmith, Buss, & Lemery, 1997; Goldsmith,

Lemery, Buss, & Campos, 1999; Lakatos et al., 2003; see Saudino, 2005, for a review). Some basic cognitive processes that are (1) implicated in temperamental differences and (2) support emotion regulation are also genetically influenced, such as: (a) attention control (Holmboe et al., 2010; Sheese, Voelker, Posner, & Rothbart, 2009), with implications for regulating attention when distressed (e.g., averting gaze from aversive stimuli; Soussignan et al., 2009); (b) verbal and non-verbal communication (Hardy-Brown & Plomin, 1985), which contribute to young children's ability to reflect on their circumstances, to communicate needs, and to guide their own behavior (Cole, Armstrong, & Pemberton, 2010); and (c) the capacity to control pre-potent responses (inhibitory control) and to activate sub-dominant responses (effortful control; Gagne & Saudino, 2010; Goldsmith et al., 1997). In regard to the development of emotion dysregulation, temperament may create risk for developing healthy emotion regulation if it predisposes a child to strong, intense emotional reactions that are difficult to modulate and may overwhelm inchoate regulatory strategy development or limits a child's development of attention control, communicative skills, or the ability to inhibit or activate behavior.

Genetic influences on the etiology of emotion dysregulation may also operate *indirectly* through relational processes that are central to the development of emotion regulation. These associations may arise because (1) caregiver genetic characteristics influence their interactions with their children, (2) children's genetic characteristics elicit specific types of responses from adults (i.e., evocative gene-environment correlation, or, *r*GE), and (3) certain types of child–parent interactions influence the expression of genetic risk (e.g., gene-environment interaction).

For example, we know that depression is heritable (Kendler, Gatz, Gardner, & Pedersen, 2006; Kendler & Prescott, 1999; Philibert et al., 2003) and is related to parenting behaviors that undermine children's emotional development (Goodman, 2007; Lovejoy, Graczyk, O'Hare, & Neuman, 2000). Thus, one indirect way that genes operate in the etiology of emotion dysregulation is through the influence of *parents'* genes on how they behave with their children. In addition, children's genes may influence parents' behaviors via *r*GE. Genetically informed studies show that specific parenting behaviors (e.g., harsh parenting) are associated with children's genetic characteristics (Ge et al., 1996; Hajal et al., 2011; Mills-Koonce et al., 2007; Narusyte et al., 2008; Neiderhiser, Reiss, Lichtenstein, Spotts, & Ganiban, 2007; O'Connor, Deater-Deckard, Fulker, Rutter, & Plomin, 1998). Finally, parent–child relational processes influence the development of emotion regulation through gene-environment interaction. For instance, the short allele of the serotonin transporter gene interacts with attachment security to predict infant and adolescent self-regulation (Kochanska, Philibert, & Barry, 2009; Zimmerman, Mohr, & Spangler, 2009). In terms of emotion dysregulation, child temperament and parental depression, both of which are influenced by genetic characteristics, interact to compromise normal growth in child emotion regulation (Blandon et al., 2008). Thus, in addition to the direct effects of genes on the etiology of emotion dysregulation, parents' and children's genes may also operate *indirectly* on the development of emotion dysregulation through parent–child interactions.

## SUMMARY AND CONCLUSIONS

Emotion dysregulation is a general feature of psychopathology. Dysregulation is not simply a matter of a person being emotionally negative. Four characteristics of emotional functioning that occur in the presence of psychopathology define dysregulation: (1) emotions that endure due to ineffective strategies, (2) emotions that lead to inappropriate behavior, (3) emotions that are contextually inappropriate, and (4) aberrations in how emotions change. These are not exclusive categories, yet each is associated with specific types of symptoms. The empirical evidence is limited, especially from a developmental viewpoint, and does not address when emotion dysregulation as defined is a precursor, a correlate, or an outcome of psychopathology. It is critical to have a clinically informed, developmental approach to conceptualizing and studying emotion regulation and dysregulation. Therefore, there is an acute need for studies that examine how skillful emotion regulation develops typically, how children with and without specific clinical problems differ in this development, how emotion regulation and dysregulation patterns relate to symptoms, and which conditions lead to skillful emotion regulation and emotion dysregulation outcomes. Such research has promise not only for understanding childhood disorders but may be crucial for understanding the emergence of adult disorders that are thought to have their origins in early childhood, such as personality disorders (Linehan, 1993; Rogosch & Cicchetti, 2005). In addition, this approach to research will inform early identification of risk and both early and crisis intervention (Tolan & Dodge, 2005).

## REFERENCES

Adrian, M., Zeman, J., Erdley, C., Lisa, L., & Sim, C. (2011). Emotional dysregulation and interpersonal difficulties as risk factors for nonsuicidal self-injury in adolescent girls. *Journal of Abnormal Child Psychology*, *39*, 389–400.

Aldao, A., Nolen-Hoeksema, S., & Schweizer, S. (2010). Emotion-regulation strategies across psychopathology: A meta-analytic review. *Clinical Psychology Review*, *30*, 217–237.

American Psychiatric Association. (2000). *Diagnostic and statistical manual of mental disorders* (4th ed., text revision). Washington, DC: American Psychiatric Association.

Anastopoulos, A. D., Smith, T. F., Garrett, M. E., Morrissey-Kane, E., Schatz, N. K., Sommer, J. L., & Ashley-Koch, A. (2011). Self-regulation of emotion, functional impairment, and comorbidity among children with AD/HD. *Journal of Attention Disorders*, *15*, 583–592.

Armbruster, D., Mueller, A., Moser, D. A., Lesch, K. P., Brocke, B., & Kirschbaum, C. (2009). Interaction effect of D4 dopamine receptor gene and serotonin transporter promoter polymorphism on the cortisol stress response. *Behavioral Neuroscience*, *123*, 1288–1295.

Arnold, M. B. (1960). *Emotion and personality*. New York, NY: Columbia University Press.

Auerbach, J., Geller, V., Lezer, S., Shinwell, E., Belmaker, R. H., Levine, J., & Ebstein, R. P. (1999). Dopamine D4 receptor (D4DR) and serotonin transporter promoter (5-HTTLPR) polymorphisms in the determination of temperament in 2-month-old infants. *Molecular Psychiatry, 4*, 369–373.

Bar-Haim, Y., Bar-Av, G., & Sadeh, A. (2011). Measuring children's regulation of emotion-expressive behavior. *Emotion, 11*, 215–223.

Barkley, R. A. (1997). *ADHD and the nature of self-control.* New York, NY: Guilford Press.

Barrett, K. C., & Campos, J. J. (1987). Perspectives on emotional development II: A functionalist approach to emotions. In J. D. Osofsky (Ed.), *Handbook of infant development* (2nd ed. pp. 555–578). Oxford, United Kingdom: Wiley.

Baumeister, R. F., Bratslavsky, E., Muraven, M., & Tice, D. M. (1998). Ego depletion: Is the active self a limited resource? *Journal of Personality and Social Psychology, 74*, 1252–1265.

Beauchaine, T. P., Gatze-Kopp, L., & Mead, H. K. (2007). Polyvagal theory and developmental psychopathology: Emotion dysregulation and conduct problems from preschool to adolescence. *Biological Psychology, 74*, 174–184.

Bennett, D. S., Bendersky, M., & Lewis, M. (2002). Facial expressivity at 4 months: A context by expression analysis. *Infancy, 3*, 97–113.

Blair, R., & Coles, M. (2000). Expression recognition and behavioural problems in early adolescence. *Cognitive Development, 15*, 421–434.

Blair, K. A., Denham, S. A., Kochanoff, A., & Whipple, B. (2004). Playing it cool: Temperament, emotion regulation, and social behavior in preschoolers. *Journal of School Psychology, 42*, 419–443.

Blandon, A. Y., Calkins, S. D., Keane, S. P., & O'Brien, M. (2008). Individual differences in trajectories of emotion regulation processes: The effects of maternal depressive symptomatology and children's physiological regulation. *Developmental Psychology, 44*, 1110–1123.

Bocknek, E., Brophy-Herb, H. E., & Banerjee, M. (2009). Effects of parental supportiveness on toddlers' emotion regulation over the first three years of life in a low-income African American sample. *Infant Mental Health Journal, 30*, 452–476.

Bokser, B. (1981). *The Jewish mystical tradition.* New York, NY: Pilgrim Press

Boldizar, J. P., Perry, D. G., & Perry, L. C. (1989). Outcome values and aggression. *Child Development, 60*, 571–579.

Bowen, E., & Dixon, L. (2010). Concurrent and prospective associations between facial affect recognition accuracy and childhood antisocial behavior. *Aggressive Behavior, 36*, 305–314.

Bridges, K. M. B. (1931). *The social and emotional development of the pre-school child.* Oxford, United Kingdom: Kegan Paul.

Brody, G. H., & Flor, D. L. (1998). Maternal resources, parenting practices, and child competence in rural, single-parent African American families. *Child Development, 69*, 803–816.

Burns, E. E., Jackson, J. L., & Harding, H. G. (2010). Child maltreatment, emotion regulation, and posttraumatic stress: The impact of emotional abuse. *Journal of Aggression, Maltreatment & Trauma, 19*, 801–819.

Burwell, R. A., & Shirk, S. R. (2007). Subtypes of rumination in adolescence: Associations between brooding, reflection, depressive symptoms, and coping. *Journal of Clinical Child and Adolescent Psychology, 36*, 56–65.

Buss, K. A., & Goldsmith, H. H. (1998). Fear and anger regulation in infancy: Effects on the temporal dynamics of affective expression. *Child Development, 69*, 359–374.

Buss, K. A., Kiel, E. J., Williams, N. A., & Leuty, M. (2005). *Using context to identify toddlers with dysregulated fear responses.* Paper presented at the Society for Research in Child Development Conference, Atlanta, GA.

Calkins, S. D., & Dedmon, S. E. (2000). Physiological and behavioral regulation in two-year-old children with aggressive/destructive behavior problems. *Journal of Abnormal Child Psychology, 28*, 103–118.

Calkins, S. D., Dedmon, S. E., Gill, K. L., Lomax, L. E., & Johnson, L. M. (2002). Frustration in infancy: Implications for emotion regulation, physiological processes, and temperament. *Infancy, 3*, 175–197.

Calkins, S. D., & Fox, N. A. (2002). Self-regulatory processes in early personality development: A multilevel approach to the study of childhood social withdrawal and aggression. *Development and Psychopathology, 14*, 477–498.

Calkins, S. D., & Keane, S. P. (2004). Cardiac vagal regulation across the preschool period: Stability, continuity, and implications for childhood adjustment. *Developmental Psychobiology, 45*, 101–112.

Camras, L. A. (1994). Two aspects of emotional development: Expression and elicitation. In P. Ekman & R. J. Davidson (Eds.), *The nature of emotions: Fundamental questions* (pp. 347–351). New York, NY: Oxford University Press.

Camras, L. A., Oster, H., Campos, J. J., & Bakeman, R. (2003). Emotional facial expressions in European-American, Japanese, and Chinese infants. In P. Ekman, J. J. Campos, R. J. Davidson, & F. B. M. de Waal (Eds.), *Emotions inside out: 130 years after Darwin's the expression of the emotions in man and animals. Annals of the New York of Sciences: Vol. 1000* (pp. 135–151). New York, NY: New York University Press.

Cannon, W. B. (1927). The James-Lange theory of emotion: A critical examination and an alternative theory. *American Journal of Psychology, 36*, 106–124.

Carlson, S. M., & Wang, T. S. (2007). Inhibitory control and emotion regulation in preschool children. *Cognitive Development, 22*, 489–510.

Carthy, T., Horesh, N., Apter, A., & Gross, J. J. (2010). Patterns of emotional reactivity and regulation in children with anxiety disorders. *Journal of Psychopathology and Behavioral Assessment, 32*, 23–26.

Casey, R. J. (1996) Emotional competence in children with externalizing and internalizing disorders. In M. Lewis (Ed.), *Emotional development in atypical children* (pp. 161–183). Mahwah, NJ: Erlbaum.

Chang, L., Schwartz, D., Dodge, K. A., & McBride-Chang, C. (2003). Harsh parenting in relation to child emotion regulation and aggression. *Journal of Family Psychology, 17*, 598–606.

Cicchetti, D., Ackerman, B. P., & Izard, C. E. (1995). Emotions and emotion regulation in developmental psychopathology. *Development and Psychopathology, 7*, 1–10.

Cole, P. M. (1986). Children's spontaneous control of facial expression. *Child Development, 57,* 1309–1321.

Cole, P. M., Armstrong, L. M., & Pemberton, C. K. (2010). The role of language in the development of emotion regulation. In S. D. Calkins & M. A. Bell (Eds.), *Development at the intersection of emotion and cognition* (pp. 59–77). Washington, DC: American Psychological Association.

Cole, P. M., Barrett, K. C., & Zahn-Waxler, C. (1992). Emotion displays in two-year-olds during mishaps. *Child Development, 63,* 314–324.

Cole, P. M., Dennis, T. A., Martin, S. E., & Hall, S. E. (2008). Emotion regulation and the early development of psychopathology. In M. Vandekerckhove, C. von Scheve, S. Ismer, S. Jung, & S. Kronast (Eds.), *Regulating emotions: Culture, social necessity, and biological inheritance* (pp. 171–188). Malden, MA: Blackwell Publishing.

Cole, P. M., Hall, S. E, & Radzioch, A. M. (2009). Emotional dysregulation and the development of serious misconduct. In S. L. Olson & A. J. Sameroff (Eds.), *Biopsychosocial regulatory processes in the development of childhood behavioral problems* (pp. 186–211). New York, NY: Cambridge University Press.

Cole, P. M., Luby, J., & Sullivan, M. W. (2008). Emotions and the development of childhood depression: Bridging the gap. *Child Development Perspectives, 2,* 141–148.

Cole, P. M., Martin, S. E., & Dennis, T. A. (2004). Emotion regulation as a scientific construct: Methodological challenges and directions for child development research. *Child Development, 75,* 317–333.

Cole, P. M., Michel, M. K., & Teti, L. O. (1994). The development of emotion regulation and dysregulation: A clinical perspective. In N. A. Fox (Ed.), The development of emotion regulation: Biological and behavioral considerations. *Monographs of the Society for Research in Child Development, 59* (2–3, Serial No. 240), 73–100.

Cole, P. M., Tan, P. Z., Hall, S. E., Zhang, Y., Crnic, K. A., Blair, C. B., & Li, R. (2011). Developmental changes in anger expression and attention focus: Learning to wait. *Developmental Psychology, 47,* 1078–1089.

Cole, P. M., Teti, L. O., & Zahn-Waxler, C. (2003). Mutual emotion regulation and the stability of conduct problems between preschool and early school age. *Development and Psychopathology, 15,* 1–18.

Cole, P. M., Zahn-Waxler, C., Fox, N. A., Usher, B. A., & Welsh, J. D. (1996). Individual differences in emotion regulation and behavior problems in preschool children. *Journal of Abnormal Psychology, 105,* 518–529.

Cole, P. M., Zahn-Waxler, C., & Smith, K. D. (1994). Expressive control during a disappointment: Variations related to preschoolers' behavior problems. *Developmental Psychology, 30,* 835–846.

Contreras, J. M., Kerns, K. A., Weimer, B. L., Gentzler, A. L., & Tomich, P. L. (2000). Emotion regulation as a mediator of associations between mother–child attachment and peer relationships in middle childhood. *Journal of Family Psychology, 14,* 111–124.

Crick, N. R., & Dodge, D. K. (1994). A review and reformulation of social information-processing mechanisms in children's social adjustment. *Psychological Bulletin, 115,* 74–101.

Crockenberg, S. C., & Leerkes, E. M. (2004). Infant and maternal behaviors regulate infant reactivity to novelty at 6 months. *Developmental Psychology, 40,* 1123–1132.

Crowell, S. E., Beauchaine, T. P., & Linehan, M. M. (2009). A biosocial developmental model of borderline personality: Elaborating and extending Linehan's theory. *Psychological Bulletin, 135,* 495–510.

Crugnola, C., Tambelli, R., Spinelli, E. M., Gazzotti, S., Caprin, C., & Albizzati, A. (2011). Attachment patterns and emotion regulation strategies in the second year. *Infant Behavior and Development, 34,* 136–151.

Cummings, M., & Davies, P. T. (2010). *Marital conflict and children: An emotional security perspective.* New York, NY: Guilford Press.

Dagne, G. A., & Snyder, J. (2011). Relationship of maternal negative moods to child emotion regulation during family interaction. *Development and Psychopathology, 23,* 211–223.

Darwin, C. (1872). *The expression of the emotions in man and animals.* New York, NY: Oxford.

Davidson, R. J. (2000). Affective style, psychopathology, and resilience: Brain mechanisms and plasticity. *American Psychologist, 55,* 1196–1214.

Dennis, T. A., Cole, P. M., Wiggins, C. N., Cohen, L. H., & Zalewski, M. (2009). The functional organization of preschool age children's emotion expressions and actions in challenging situations. *Emotion, 9,* 520–530.

Derryberry, D., & Rothbart, M. K. (1988). Arousal, affect, and attention as components of temperament. *Journal of Personality and Social Psychology, 55,* 958–966.

Diener, M. L., & Mangelsdorf, S. C. (1999). Behavioral strategies for emotion regulation in toddlers: Associations with maternal involvement and emotional expressions. *Infant Behavior and Development, 22,* 569–583.

DiPietro, J. A., Ghera, M. M., & Costigan, K. A. (2008). Prenatal origins of temperamental reactivity in early infancy. *Early Human Development, 84,* 569–575.

Donaldson, S. K., & Westerman, M. A. (1986). Development of children's understanding of ambivalence and causal theories of emotions. *Developmental Psychology, 22,* 655–662.

Eisenberg, N., Cumberland, A., Spinrad, T. L., Fabes, R. A., Shepard, S. A., Reiser, M . . . Guthrie, I. K. (2001). The relations of regulation and emotionality to children's externalizing and internalizing problem behavior. *Child Development, 72,* 1112–1134.

Eisenberg, N., Fabes, R. A., Murphy, B., Karbon, M., Smith, M., & Maszk, P. (1996). The relations of children's dispositional empathy-related responding to their emotionality, regulation, and social functioning. *Developmental Psychology, 32,* 195–209.

Eisenberg, N., Cumberland, A., & Spinrad, T. L. (1998). Parental socialization of emotion. *Psychological Inquiry, 9,* 241–273.

Eisenberg, N., Valiente, C., Morris, A., Fabes, R. A., Cumberland, A., Reiser, M., & . . . Losoya, S. (2003). Longitudinal relations among parental emotional expressivity, children's regulation, and quality of socioemotional functioning. *Developmental Psychology, 39,* 3–19.

Ekman, P. (1994). Strong evidence for universals in facial expressions: A reply to Russell's mistaken critique. *Psychological Bulletin, 115*, 268–287.

Ellis, B. J., Boyce, W., Belsky, J., Bakermans-Kranenburg, M. J., & Van Ijzendoorn, M. H. (2011). Differential susceptibility to the environment: An evolutionary–neurodevelopmental theory. *Development and Psychopathology, 23*, 7–28.

Ellsworth, P. C. (1994). William James and emotion: Is a century of fame worthy a century of misunderstanding? *Psychological Review, 101*, 222–229.

El-Sheikh, M., Cummings, E., Kouros, C. D., Elmore-Staton, L., & Buckhalt, J. (2008). Marital psychological and physical aggression and children's mental and physical health: Direct, mediated, and moderated effects. *Journal of Consulting and Clinical Psychology, 76*, 138–148.

El-Sheikh, M., Harger, J., & Whitson, S. M. (2001). Exposure to interparental conflict and children's adjustment and physical health: The moderating role of vagal tone. *Child Development, 72*, 1617–1636.

Feldman, R., Granat, A., Pariente, C., Kanety, H., Kuint, J., & Gilboa-Schechtman, E. (2009). Maternal depression and anxiety across the postpartum year and infant social engagement, fear regulation, and stress reactivity. *Journal of the American Academy of Child and Adolescent Psychiatry, 48*, 919–927.

Feng, X., Shaw, D. S., Kovacs, M., Lane, T., O'Rourke, F. E., & Alarcon, J. H. (2008). Emotion regulation in preschoolers: The roles of behavioral inhibition, maternal affective behavior, and maternal depression. *Journal of Child Psychology and Psychiatry, 49*, 132–141.

Feng, X., Shaw, D. S., Skuban, E. M., & Lane, T. (2007). Emotional exchange in mother-child dyads: Stability, mutual influence, and associations with maternal depression and child problem behavior. *Journal of Family Psychology, 21*, 714–725.

Fergus, E. L., Miller, R. B., Luckenbaugh, D. A., Leverich, G. S., Findling, R. L., Speer, A. M., & Post, R. M. (2003). Is there progression from irritability/dyscontrol to major depressive and manic symptoms? A retrospective community survey of parents of bipolar children. *Journal of Affective Disorders, 77*, 71–78.

Folkman, S., & Lazarus, R. S. (1980). Coping and emotion. In N. L. Stein, B. Leventhal, & T. Trabasso (Eds.), *Psychological and biological approaches to emotion* (pp. 313–332). Hillsdale, NJ: Erlbaum.

Freud, S. (1901/1965). *The psychopathology of everyday life*. New York, NY: Norton.

Frick, P. J., Lilienfeld, S. O., Ellis, M., Loney, B., & Silverthorn, P. (1999). The association between anxiety and psychopathy dimensions in children. *Journal of Abnormal Child Psychology, 27*, 383–392.

Frijda, N. H. (1986). *The emotions: Studies in emotion and social interaction*. New York, NY: Cambridge University Press.

Fung, M. T., Raine, A., Loeber, R., Lynam, D. R., Steinhauer, S. R., Venables, P. H., & Stouthamer-Loeber, M. (2005). Reduced electrodermal activity in psychopathy-prone adolescents. *Journal of Abnormal Psychology, 114*, 187–196.

Gagne, J. R., & Saudino, K. J. (2010). Wait for it! A twin study of inhibitory control in early childhood. *Behavior Genetics, 40*, 327–337.

Garner, P. W. (2006). Prediction of prosocial and emotional competence from maternal behavior in African American preschoolers. *Cultural Diversity and Ethnic Minority Psychology, 12,* 179–198.

Garner, P. W., & Hinton, T. (2010). Emotional display rules and emotion self-regulation: Associations with bullying and victimization in community-based after school programs. *Journal of Community and Applied Social Psychology, 20,* 480–496.

Garner, P. W., & Power, T. G. (1996). Preschoolers' emotional control in the disappointment paradigm and its relation to temperament, emotional knowledge, and family expressiveness. *Child Development, 67,* 1406–1419.

Ge, X., Conger, R. D., Cadoret, R. J., Neiderhiser, J. M., Yates, W., Troughton, E., & Stewart, M. A. (1996). The developmental interface between nature and nurture: A mutual influence model of child antisocial behavior and parent behaviors. *Developmental Psychology, 32,* 574–589.

Gerson, A. C., Gerring, J. P., Freund, L., Joshi, P., Capozzoli, J., Brady, K., & Denckla, M. B. (1996). The Children's Affective Lability Scale: A psychometric evaluation of reliability. *Psychiatry Research, 65,* 189–197.

Gianino, A., & Tronick, E. Z. (1988). The mutual regulation model: The infant's self and interactive regulation and coping and defensive capacities. In T. M. Field, P. M. McCabe, & N. Schneiderman (Eds.), *Stress and coping across development* (pp. 47–68). Hillsdale, NJ: Erlbaum.

Gilliom, M., Shaw, D. S., Beck, J. E., Schonberg, M. A., & Lukon, J. L. (2002). Anger regulation in disadvantaged preschool boys: Strategies, antecedents, and the development of self-control. *Developmental Psychology, 34,* 222–235.

Goldsmith, H. H., Buss, K. A., & Lemery, K. S. (1997). Toddler and childhood temperament: Expanded context, stronger genetic evidence, new evidence for the importance of the environment. *Developmental Psychology, 33,* 891–905.

Goldsmith, H. H., Lemery, K. S., Buss, K. A., & Campos, J. J. (1999). Genetic analyses of focal aspects of infant temperament. *Developmental Psychology, 35,* 972–985.

Goleman, D. (2003). *Destructive emotions: A scientific dialogue with the Dalai Lama.* New York, NY: Bantam Books.

Goodman, S. H. (2007). Depression in mothers. *Annual Review of Clinical Psychology, 3,* 107–135.

Goodman, S., & Gotlib, I. (Eds.). (2002). *Children of depressed parents: Mechanisms of risk and implications for treatment.* Washington, DC: American Psychological Association.

Gotlib, I. H., Joormann, J., Minor, K. L., & Cooney, R. E. (2006). Cognitive and biological functioning in children at risk for depression. In T. Canli (Ed.), *Biology of personality and individual differences* (pp. 353–382). New York, NY: Guilford Press.

Gratz, K. L. (2006). Risk factors for deliberate self-harm among female college students: The role and interaction of childhood maltreatment, emotional inexpressivity, and affect intensity/reactivity. *American Journal of Orthopsychiatry, 76,* 238–250.

Grolnick, W. S., Bridges, L. J., & Connell, J. P. (1996). Emotion regulation in two-year-olds: Strategies and emotional expression in four contexts. *Child Development, 67*, 928–941.

Grolnick, W. S., Kurowski, C. O., McMenamy, J. M., Rivkin, I., & Bridges, L. J. (1998). Mothers' strategies for regulating their toddlers' distress. *Infant Behavior and Development, 21*, 437–450.

Gross, J. J., & Muñoz, R. F. (1995). Emotion regulation and mental health. *Clinical Psychology: Science and Practice, 2*, 151–164.

Gross, J. J., & Thompson, R. A. (2007). Emotion regulation: Conceptual foundations. In J. J. Gross (Ed.), *Handbook of emotion regulation* (pp. 3–24). New York, NY: Guilford Press.

Hajal, N. J., Neiderhiser, J. M., Shaw, D., Moore, G. A., Leve, L. D., & Reiss, D. (2011, April). Evocative effects on parenting over time: *Similarities and differences between adoptive mothers and fathers.* Paper presented at the Biennial Meeting of the Society for Research in Child Development, Montreal Quebec.

Hajcak, G., Molnar, C., George, M. S., Bolger, K., Koola, J., & Nahas, Z. (2007). Emotion facilitates action: A transcranial magnetic stimulation study of motor cortex excitability during picture viewing. *Psychophysiology, 44*, 91–97.

Halberstadt, A. G., Denham, S. A., & Dunsmore, J. C. (2001). Affective social competence. *Social Development, 10*, 79–119.

Hamann, S. (2001). Cognitive and neural mechanisms of emotional memory. *Trends in Cognitive Sciences, 5*, 394–400.

Hardy-Brown, K., & Plomin, R. (1985). Infant communicative development: Evidence from adoptive and biological families for genetic and environmental influences on rate differences. *Developmental Psychology, 21*, 378–385.

Harter, S., & Buddin, B. J. (1987). Children's understanding of the simultaneity of two emotions: A five-stage developmental acquisition sequence. *Developmental Psychology, 23*, 388–399.

Harter, N. R., & Whitesell, S. (1989). Children's reports of conflict between simultaneous opposite-valence emotions. *Child Development, 60*, 673–682.

Hayden, E. P., Klein, D. N., & Durbin, C. E. (2005). Parent reports and laboratory assessments of child temperament: A comparison of their associations with risk for depression and externalizing disorders. *Journal of Psychopathology and Behavioral Assessment, 27*, 89–100.

Hayden, E. P., Klein, D. N., Durbin, C. E., & Olino, T. M. (2006). Positive emotionality at age 3 predicts cognitive styles in 7-year-old children. *Development and Psychopathology, 18*, 409–423.

Hayes, S. C., Strosahl, K., Wilson, K. G., Bissett, R. T., Pistorello, J., Toarmino, D., . . . McCurry, S. M. (2004). Measuring experiential avoidance: A preliminary test of a working model. *Psychological Record, 54*, 553–578.

Hayes, S. C., Wilson, K. G., Gifford, E. V., Follette, V. M., & Strosahl, K. D. (1996). Experiential avoidance and behavioral disorders: A functional dimensional approach to diagnosis and treatment. *Journal of Consulting and Clinical Psychology, 64*, 1152–1168.

Hoffman, C., Crnic, K. A., & Baker, J. K. (2006). Maternal depression and parenting: Implications for children's emergent emotion regulation and behavioral functioning. *Parenting: Science and Practice, 6*, 271–295.

Holmboe, K., Nemoda, Z., Fearon, R. M. P., Csibra, G., Sasvari-Szekely, M., & Johnson, M. H. (2010). Polymorphisms in dopamine system genes are associated with individual differences in attention in infancy. *Developmental Psychology, 46*, 404–416.

Hughes, E. K., Gullone, E., & Watson, S. D. (2011). Emotional functioning in children and adolescents with elevated depressive symptoms. *Journal of Psychopathology and Behavioral Assessment, 33*, 335–345.

Hunter, E. C., Katz, L., Shortt, J., Davis, B., Leve, C., Allen, N. B., & Sheeber, L. B. (2011). How do I feel about feelings? Emotion socialization in families of depressed and healthy adolescents. *Journal of Youth and Adolescence, 40*, 428–441.

Isen, A. M., Shalker, T. E., Clark, M., & Karp, L. (1978). Affect, accessibility of material in memory, and behavior: A cognitive loop? *Journal of Personality and Social Psychology, 36*, 1–12.

Izard, C. E. (2002). Translating emotion theory and research into preventive interventions. *Psychological Bulletin, 128*, 796–824.

Jaffe, M., Gullone, E., & Hughes, E. K. (2010). The roles of temperamental dispositions and perceived parenting behaviours in the use of two emotion regulation strategies in late childhood. *Journal of Applied Developmental Psychology, 31*, 47–59.

James, W. (1884). What is an emotion? *Mind, 9*, 188–205.

Katz, L. F., & Gottman, J. M. (1995). Vagal tone protects children from marital conflict. *Development and Psychopathology, 7*, 83–92.

Katz, L., & Hunter, E. C. (2007). Maternal meta-emotion philosophy and adolescent depressive symptomatology. *Social Development, 16*, 343–360.

Kendler, K. S., Gatz, M., Gardner, C. O., & Pedersen, N. L. (2006). A Swedish national twin study of lifetime major depression. *American Journal of Psychiatry, 163*, 109–114.

Kendler, K. S., & Prescott, C. A. (1999). A population-based twin study of lifetime major depression in men and women. *Archives of General Psychiatry, 56*, 39–44.

Kidwell, S. L., Young, M. E., Hinkle, L. D., Ratliff, A. D., Marcum, M. E., & Martin, C. N. (2010). Emotional competence and behavior problems: Differences across preschool assessment of attachment classifications. *Clinical Child Psychology and Psychiatry, 15*, 391–406.

Kim, J., & Cicchetti, D. (2010). Longitudinal pathways linking child maltreatment, emotion regulation, peer relations, and psychopathology. *Journal of Child Psychology and Psychiatry, 51*, 706–716.

Klonsky, E. D. (2007). The functions of deliberate self-injury: A review of the evidence. *Clinical Psychology Review, 27*, 226–239.

Kochanska, G., Philibert, R. A., & Barry, R. A. (2009). Interplay of genes and early mother-child relationship in the development of self-regulation from toddler to preschool age. *Journal of Child Psychology and Psychiatry, 50*, 1331–1338.

Kochman, F. J., Hantouche, E. G., Ferrari, P., Lencrenon, S., Bayart, D., & Akiskal, H. S. (2005). Cyclothymic temperament as a prospective predictor of bipolarity and suicidality in children and adolescents with major depressive disorder. *Journal of Affective Disorders, 85,* 181–189.

Koenigsburg, H. W., Harvey, P. D., Mitropoulou, V., Schmeidler, J., New, A. S., Goodman, M. et al. (2002). Characterizing affective instability in borderline personality disorder. *American Journal of Psychiatry, 159,* 784–788.

Kopp, C. B. (1989). Regulation of distress and negative emotions: A developmental view. *Developmental Psychology, 25,* 343–354.

Koss, K. J., George, M. W., Bergman, K. N., Cummings, E. M., Davies, P. T., & Cicchetti, D. (2011). Understanding children's emotional processes and behavioral strategies in the context of marital conflict. *Journal of Experimental Child Psychology, 109,* 336–352.

Kovacs, M., Sherrill, J., George, C. J., Pollock, M., Tumuluru, R. V., & Ho, V. (2006). Contextual emotion-regulation therapy for childhood depression: Description and pilot testing of a new intervention. *Journal of the American Academy of Child & Adolescent Psychiatry, 45,* 892–903.

Kupper, N., Willemsen, G., Posthuma, D., DeBoer, D., Boomsma, D. I., & DeGeus, E. J. C. (2005). A genetic analysis of ambulatory cardiorespiratory coupling. *Psychophysiology, 42,* 202–212.

Lakatos, K., Nemoda, Z., Birkas, E., Ronai, Z., Kovacs, E., Ney, K., . . . Gervai, J. (2003). Associations of D4 dopamine receptor gene and serotonin transporter promoter polymorphisms with infants' response to novelty. *Molecular Psychiatry, 8,* 90–97.

Lange, C. (1922). The emotions. Cited by Ellsworth, P.C. (1994). William James and emotion: Is a century of fame worth a century of misunderstanding? *Psychological Review, 101,* 222–229.

Larsen, R. W., Raffaelli, M., Richards, M. H., & Ham, M. (1990). Ecology of depression in late childhood and early adolescence: A profile of daily states and activities. *Journal of Abnormal Psychology, 99,* 92–102.

Larson, C. L., Taubitz, L. E., & Robinson, J. S. (2010). MAOA T941G polymorphism and the time course of emotional recovery following unpleasant pictures. *Psychophysiology, 47,* 857–862.

Lazarus, R. S. (1991). *Emotion and adaptation.* New York, NY: Oxford University Press.

LeDoux, J. E. (1986). Sensory systems and emotion: A model of affective processing. *Integrative Psychiatry, 4,* 237–243.

Leibenluft, E., Charney, D. S., & Pine, D. S. (2003). Researching the pathophysiology of pediatric bipolar disorder. *Biological Psychiatry, 53,* 1009–1020.

Lewis, M., & Haviland-Jones, J. M. (2000). *Handbook of emotions* (2nd ed.). New York, NY: Guilford Press.

Lewis, M., & Ramsay, D. (2005). Infant emotional and cortisol responses to goal blockage. *Child Development, 76,* 518–530.

Liew, J., Eisenberg, N., Losoya, S. H., Fabes, R. A., Guthrie, I. K., & Murphy, B. C. (2003). Children's physiological indices of empathy and their socioemotional adjustment: Does caregivers' expressivity matter? *Journal of Family Psychology, 17,* 584–597.

Liew, J., Eisenberg, N., & Reiser, M. (2004). Preschoolers' effortful control and negative emotionality, immediate reactions to disappointment, and quality of social functioning. *Journal of Experimental Child Psychology, 89*, 298–313.

Linehan, M. M. (1993). *Cognitive-behavioral treatment of borderline personality disorder.* New York, NY: Guilford Press.

Lovejoy, M. C., Graczyk, P. A., O'Hare, E., & Neuman, G. (2000). Maternal depression and parenting behavior: A meta-analytic review. *Clinical Psychology Review, 20*, 561–592.

Luby, J. L., Sullivan, J., Belden, A., Stalets, M., Blankenship, S., & Spitznagel, E. (2006). An observational analysis of behavior in depressed preschoolers: Further validation of early-onset depression. *Journal of the American Academy of Child & Adolescent Psychiatry, 45*, 203–212.

Malatesta, C. Z., & Haviland, J. M. (1982). Learning display rules: The socialization of emotion expression in infancy. *Child Development, 53*, 991–1003.

Mangelsdorf, S. C., Shapiro, J. R., & Marzolf, D. (1995). Developmental and temperamental differences in emotion regulation in infancy. *Child Development, 66*, 1817–1828.

Marsh, P., Beauchaine, T. P., & Williams, B. (2008). Dissociation of sad facial expressions and autonomic nervous system responding in boys with disruptive behavior disorders. *Psychophysiology, 45*, 100–110.

Martin, S. E., Boekamp, J. R., McConville, D. W., & Wheeler, E. E. (2010). Anger and sadness perception in clinically referred preschoolers: Emotion processes and externalizing behavior symptoms. *Child Psychiatry and Human Development, 41*, 30–46.

Marx, B. P., & Sloan, D. M. (2002). The role of emotion in the psychological functioning of adult survivors of childhood sexual abuse. *Behavior Therapy, 33*, 563–577.

Maughan, A., & Cicchetti, D. (2002). Impact of child maltreatment and interadult violence on children's emotion regulation abilities and socioemotional adjustment. *Child Development, 73*, 1525–1542.

Maughan, A., Cicchetti, D., Toth, S. L., & Rogosch, F. A. (2007). Early-occurring maternal depression and maternal negativity in predicting young children's emotion regulation and socioemotional difficulties. *Journal of Abnormal Child Psychology, 35*, 685–703.

McDowell, D. J., O'Neill, R., & Parke, R. D. (2000). Display rule application in a disappointing situation and children's emotional reactivity: Relations with social competence. *Merrill-Palmer Quarterly, 46*, 306–324.

McLaughlin, K. A., Hatzenbuehler, M. L., Mennin, D. S., & Nolen-Hoeksema, S. (2011). Emotion dysregulation and adolescent psychopathology: A prospective study. *Behaviour Research and Therapy, 49*, 544–554.

Melnick, S. M., & Hinshaw, S. P. (2000) Emotion regulation and parenting in AD/HD and comparison boys: Linkages with social behaviors and peer preference. *Journal of Abnormal Child Psychology, 28*, 73–86.

Mennin, D. S., Heimberg, R. G., Turk, C. L., & Fresco, D. M. (2002). Applying an emotion regulation framework to integrative approaches to generalized anxiety disorder. *Clinical Psychology: Science and Practice, 9*, 85–90.

Mills-Koonce, W. R., Propper, C. B., Gariepy, J., Blair, C., Garrett-Peters, P., & Cox, M. J. (2007). Bidirectional genetic and environmental influences on mother and child behavior: The family system as the unit of analysis. *Development and Psychopathology, 19,* 1073–1087.

Mirabile, S. P., Scaramella, L. V., Sohr-Preston, S. L., & Robison, S. D. (2009). Mothers' socialization of emotion regulation: The moderating role of children's negative emotional reactivity. *Child and Youth Care Forum, 38,* 19–37.

Morris, A., Silk, J. S., Morris, M. S., Steinberg, L., Aucoin, K. J., & Keyes, A. W. (2011). The influence of mother–child emotion regulation strategies on children's expression of anger and sadness. *Developmental Psychology, 47,* 213–225.

Morris, A., Silk, J. S., Steinberg, L., Myers, S. S., & Robinson, L. (2007). The role of the family context in the development of emotion regulation. *Social Development, 16,* 361–388.

Narusyte, J., Neiderhiser, J. M., D'Onofrio, B., Reiss, D., Spotts, E. L., Ganiban, J., & Lichtenstein, P. (2008). Testing different types of genotype-environment correlation: An extended children-of-twins model. *Developmental Psychology, 44,* 1591–1603.

Neiderhiser, J. M., Reiss, D., Lichtenstein, P., Spotts, E. L., & Ganiban, J. (2007). Father-adolescent relationships and the role of genotype-environment correlation. *Journal of Family Psychology, 21,* 560–571.

Neumann, A., van Lier, P. C., Frijns, T., Meeus, W., & Koot, H. M. (2011). Emotional dynamics in the development of early adolescent psychopathology: A one-year longitudinal study. *Journal of Abnormal Child Psychology, 39,* 657–669.

NICHD Early Child Care Network. (2004). Affect dysregulation in the mother-child relationship in the toddler years: Antecedents and consequences. *Development and Psychopathology, 16,* 43–68.

Ochsner, K. N., & Gross, J. J. (2007). The neural architecture of emotion regulation. In J. J. Gross (Ed.), *Handbook of emotion regulation* (pp. 87–109). New York, NY: Guilford Press.

Ochsner, K. N., & Schacter, D. L. (2000). A social cognitive neuroscience approach to emotion and memory. In J. C. Borod (Ed.), *The neuropsychology of emotion* (pp. 163–193). New York, NY: Oxford University Press.

O'Connor, T. G., Deater-Deckard, K., Fulker, D., Rutter, M., & Plomin, R. (1998). Genotype-environment correlations in late childhood and early adolescence: Antisocial behavioral problems and coercive parenting. *Developmental Psychology, 34,* 970–981.

O'Kearney, R., & Dadds, M. R. (2005). Language for emotions in adolescents with externalizing and internalizing disorders. *Development and Psychopathology, 17,* 529–548.

Philibert, R., Caspers, K., Langbehn, D., Troughton, E. P., Yucuis, R., Sandhu, H. K., & Cadoret, R. J. (2003). The association of the D2S2944 124 bp allele with recurrent early onset major depressive disorder in women. *American Journal of Medical Genetics, 121B,* 39–43.

Pollak, S. D., Messner, M., Kistler, D. J., & Cohn, J. F. (2009). Development of perceptual expertise in emotion recognition. *Cognition, 110,* 242–247.

Pons, F., Harris, P. L., & de Rosnay, M. (2004). Emotion comprehension between 3 and 11 years: Developmental periods and hierarchical organization. *European Journal of Developmental Psychology, 1*, 127–152.

Porges, S. W. (2001). The polyvagal theory: Phylogenetic substrates of a social nervous system. *International Journal of Psychophysiology, 42*, 123–146.

Propper, C., Moore, G. A., Mills-Koonce, W. R., Halpern, C. T., Hill-Soderlund, A. L., Calkins, S. D.,...Cox, M. (2008). Gene-environment contributions to the development of infant vagal reactivity: The interaction of dopamine and maternal sensitivity. *Child Development, 79*, 1377–1394.

Radke-Yarrow, M., Zahn-Waxler, C., Richardson, D. T., & Susman, A. (1994). Caring behavior in children of clinically depressed and well mothers. *Child Development, 65*, 1405–1414.

Raine, A., Lencz, T., Taylor, K., Hellige, J. B., Bihrle, S., Lacasse, L.,...Colletti, P. (2003). Corpus callosum abnormalities in psychopathic antisocial individuals. *Archives of General Psychiatry, 60*, 1134–1142.

Reijntjes, A., Stegge, H., Meerum Terwogt, M., Kamphuis, J. H., & Telch, M. J. (2006). Emotion regulation and its effects on mood improvement in response to an in vivo peer rejection challenge. *Emotion, 6*, 543–552.

Robinson, L. R., Morris, A., Heller, S., Scheeringa, M. S., Boris, N. W., & Smyke, A. T. (2009). Relations between emotion regulation, parenting, and psychopathology in young maltreated children in out of home care. *Journal of Child and Family Studies, 18*, 421–434.

Rogosch, F. A., & Cicchetti, D. (2005). Child maltreatment, attention networks, and potential precursors to borderline personality disorder. *Development and Psychopathology, 17*, 1071–1089.

Rothbart, M. K., & Bates, J. E. (2006). Temperament. In N. Eisenberg, W. Damon, R. M. Lerner (Eds.), *Handbook of child psychology: Vol. 3, Social, emotional, and personality development* (6th ed., pp. 99–166). Hoboken, NJ: Wiley.

Rothbart, M. K., & Sheese, B. E. (2007). Temperament and emotion regulation. In J. J. Gross (Ed.), *Handbook of emotion regulation* (pp. 331–350). New York, NY: Guilford.

Rottenberg, J., Gross, J. J., & Gotlib, I. H. (2005). Emotion context insensitivity in major depressive disorder. *Journal of Abnormal Psychology, 114*, 627–639.

Saarni, C. (1999). *The development of emotional competence.* New York, NY: Guilford Press.

Santucci, A. K., Silk, J. S., Shaw, D. S., Gentzler, A., Fox, N. A., & Kovacs, M. (2008). Vagal tone and temperament as predictors of emotion regulation strategies in young children. *Developmental Psychobiology, 50*, 205–216.

Saudino, K. J. (2005). Behavioral genetics and child temperament. *Journal of Developmental and Behavioral Pediatrics, 26*, 214–224.

Scarr, S., & McCartney, K. (1983). How people make their own environments: A theory of genotype → environment effects. *Child Development, 54*, 424–435.

Schacter, S., & Singer, J. E. (1962). Cognitive, social, and physiological determinants of emotional state. *Psychological Review, 69*, 379–399.

Shannon, K. E., Beauchaine, T. P., Brenner, S. L., Neuhaus, E., & Gatzke-Kopp, L. (2007). Familial and temperamental predictors of resilience in children at risk for conduct disorder and depression. *Development and Psychopathology, 19,* 701–727.

Shaw, D. S., Schonberg, M., Sherrill, J., Huffman, D., Lukon, J., Obrosky, D., & Kovacs, M. (2006). Responsivity to offspring's expression of emotion among childhood-onset depressed mothers. *Journal of Clinical Child and Adolescent Psychology, 35,* 490–503.

Sheeber, L. B., Allen, N. B., Leve, C., Davis, B., Shortt, J. W., & Katz, L. F. (2009). Dynamics of affective experience and behavior in depressed adolescents. *Journal of Child Psychology and Psychiatry, 50,* 1419–1427.

Sheese, B. E., Voelker, P., Posner, M. I., & Rothbart, M. K. (2009). Genetic variation influences on the early development of reactive emotions and their regulation by attention. *Cognitive Neuropsychiatry, 14,* 332–355.

Shields, A., & Cicchetti, D. (1997). Emotion regulation among school-age children: The development and validation of a new criterion Q-sort scale. *Developmental Psychology, 33,* 906–916.

Shields, A., & Cicchetti, D. (1998). Reactive aggression among maltreated children: The contributions of attention and emotion dysregulation. *Journal of Clinical Child Psychology, 27,* 381–395.

Shields, A., Ryan, R. M., & Cicchetti, D. (2001). Narrative representations of caregivers and emotion dysregulation as predictors of maltreated children's rejection by peers. *Developmental Psychology, 37,* 321–337.

Shipman, K. L., Schneider, R., Fitzgerald, M. M., Sims, C., Swisher, L., & Edwards, A. (2007). Maternal emotion socialization in maltreating and non-maltreating families: Implications for children's emotion regulation. *Social Development, 16,* 268–285.

Shipman, K., Zeman, J., Penza, S., & Champion, K. (2000). Emotion management skills in sexually maltreated and nonmaltreated girls: A developmental psychopathology perspective. *Development and Psychopathology, 12,* 47–62.

Silk, J. S., Shaw, D. S., Forbes, E. E., Lane, T. L., & Kovacs, M. (2006). Maternal depression and child internalizing: The moderating role of child emotion regulation. *Journal of Clinical Child and Adolescent Psychology, 35,* 116–126.

Silk, J. S., Shaw, D. S., Skuban, E. M., Oland, A. A., & Kovacs, M. (2006). Emotion regulation strategies in offspring of childhood-onset depressed mothers. *Journal of Child Psychology and Psychiatry, 47,* 69–78.

Silk, J. S., Steinberg, L., & Morris, A. S. (2003). Adolescents' emotion regulation in daily life: Links to depressive symptoms and problem behavior. *Child Development, 74,* 1869–1880.

Sincoff, J. B. (1992). Ambivalence and defense: Effects of a repressive style on normal adolescents' and young adults' mixed feelings. *Journal of Abnormal Psychology, 101,* 251–256.

Slaby, R. G., & Guerra, N. G. (1988). Cognitive mediators of aggression in adolescent offenders: I. *Assessment. Developmental Psychology, 24,* 580–588.

Sobanski, E., Banaschewski, T., Asherson, P., Buitelaar, J., Chen, W., Franke, B., . . . Faraone, S. V. (2010). Emotional lability in children and adolescents with attention deficit hyperactivity disorder (ADHD): Clinical correlates and familial prevalence. *Journal of Child Psychology and Psychiatry, 51,* 915–923.

Soussignan, R., Boivin, M., Girard, A., Pérusse, D., Liu, X., & Tremblay, R. E. (2009). Genetic and environment etiology of emotional and social behaviors in 5-month-old infant twins: Influence of the social context. *Infant Behavior and Development*, *32*, 1–9.

Stansbury, K., & Sigman, M. (2000). Responses of preschoolers in two frustrating episodes: Emergence of complex strategies for emotion regulation. *Journal of Genetic Psychology*, *161*, 182–202.

Stifter, C. A., & Braungart, J. M. (1995). The regulation of negative reactivity in infancy: Function and development. *Developmental Psychology*, *31*, 448–455.

Stringaris, A. A., & Goodman, R. R. (2009). Mood lability and psychopathology in youth. *Psychological Medicine: A Journal of Research in Psychiatry and the Allied Sciences*, *39*, 1237–1245.

Suveg, C., Hoffman, B., Zeman, J. L., & Thomassin, K. (2009). Common and specific emotion-related predictors of anxious and depressive symptoms in youth. *Child Psychiatry and Human Development*, *40*, 223–239.

Suveg, C., Morelen, D., Brewer, G. A., & Thomassin, K. (2010). The emotion dysregulation model of anxiety: A preliminary path analytic examination. *Journal of Anxiety Disorders*, *24*, 924–930.

Suveg, C., & Zeman, J. (2004). Emotion regulation in children with anxiety disorders. *Journal of Clinical Child and Adolescent Psychology*, *33*, 750–759.

Tarullo, A. R., & Gunnar, M. R. (2006). Child maltreatment and the developing HPA axis. *Hormones and Behavior*, *50*, 632–639.

Teti, D. M., & Cole, P. M. (2011). Parenting at risk: New perspectives, new approaches. *Journal of Family Psychology*, *25*, 625–634.

Thompson, R. A. (1994). Emotion regulation: A theme in search of definition. In N. A. Fox (Ed.), The development of emotion regulation: Biological and behavioral considerations. *Monographs of the Society for Research in Child Development*, *59*, 25–52.

Thompson, R. A. (2011). Methods and measures in developmental emotions research: Some assembly required. *Journal of Experimental Child Psychology*, *110*, 275–285.

Tice, D. M., Baumeister, R. F., & Zhang, L. (2004). The role of emotion in self-regulation: Differing role of positive and negative emotions. In P. Philippot & R. S. Feldman (Eds.), *The regulation of emotion* (pp. 213–226). Mahwah, NJ: Erlbaum.

Tolan, P. H., & Dodge, K. A. (2005). Children's mental health as a primary care and concern: A system for comprehensive support and service. *American Psychologist*, *60*, 601–614.

Tonyan, H. A. (2005). Coregulating distress: Mother-child interactions around children's distress from 14 to 24 months. *International Journal of Behavioral Development*, *29*, 433–444.

Tronick, E. Z., & Cohn, J. F. (1989). Infant-mother face-to-face interaction: Age and gender differences in coordination and the occurrence of miscoordination. *Child Development*, *60*, 85–92.

Tronick, E., & Reck, C. (2009). Infants of depressed mothers. *Harvard Review of Psychiatry*, *17*, 147–156.

Tronick, E. Z., & Weinberg, M. (2000). Gender differences and their relation to maternal depression. In S. L. Johnson, A. M. Hayes, T. M. Field, N. Schneiderman, & P. M. McCabe (Eds.), *Stress, coping, and depression* (pp. 23–34). Mahwah, NJ: Erlbaum.

Waters, S. F., Virmani, E. A., Thompson, R. A., Meyer, S., Raikes, H., & Jochem, R. (2010). Emotion regulation and attachment: Unpacking two constructs and their association. *Journal of Psychopathology and Behavioral Assessment, 32,* 37–47.

Weisbrot, D. M., Gadow, K. D., DeVincent, C. J., & Pomeroy, J. (2005). The presentation of anxiety in children with pervasive developmental disorders. *Journal of Child and Adolescent Psychopharmacology, 15,* 477–496.

Wilson, B. J. (2003). The role of attentional processes in children's prosocial behavior with peers: Attention shifting and emotion. *Development and Psychopathology, 15,* 313–329.

Wilson, K. R., Hansen, D. J., & Li, M. (2011). The traumatic stress response in child maltreatment and resultant neuropsychological effects. *Aggression and Violent Behavior, 16,* 87–97.

Wintre, M. G., & Vallance, D. D. (1994). A developmental sequence in the comprehension of emotions: Intensity, multiple emotions, and valence. *Developmental Psychology, 30,* 509–514.

Yagmurlu, B., & Altan, O. (2010). Maternal socialization and child temperament as predictors of emotion regulation in Turkish preschoolers. *Infant and Child Development, 19,* 275–296.

Zajonc, R. B. (1980). Feeling and thinking: Preferences need no inferences. *American Psychologist, 35,* 151–175.

Zimmerman, P., Mohr, C., & Spangler, G. (2009). Genetic and attachment influences on adolescents' regulation of autonomy and aggressiveness. *Journal of Child Psychology and Psychiatry, 50,* 1339–1347.

# PART III

# EXTERNALIZING BEHAVIOR DISORDERS

# CHAPTER 12

# Attention-Deficit/Hyperactivity Disorder

JOEL NIGG

## HISTORICAL CONTEXT

EW CHILD DIFFICULTIES GENERATE as much controversy and concern in our society as problems with attention and impulse control, especially the syndrome of attention-deficit/hyperactivity disorder (ADHD; APA, 1994, 2013). Such concern is fueled in part by rates of medication treatments for children in the United States, which rose dramatically in the 1990s (Robison, Sclar, Skaer, & Galin, 1999) and have continued to climb (Setlik, Bond, & Ho, 2009). This concern is often combined with inadequate mental health and educational services for children with special needs in this country, raising worries that medication is the lowest cost but not the best treatment. The debate is important: ADHD is a highly impairing syndrome affecting a large number of children for much of their lives. Although probably no definitive conclusion is possible about whether there is a true secular trend of rising incidence or prevalence of ADHD in the United States, diagnostic prevalence is clearly rising (Boyle et al., 2011; Morbidity and Mortality Weekly Report, 2010).

The disorder, by different names, was mentioned in the medical literature as early as 1800 (Rush, 1812 [1962]) (as cited in Taylor, 2011), but only occasionally noted for the next 100 years (for a detailed historical review see Taylor, 2011). By the early 20th century, the medical literature referenced children with "minimal brain damage," followed by references to "hyperkinetic reaction of childhood," "hyperkinesis," "minimal brain dysfunction" (not to be confused with minimal brain damage), "attention deficit disorder" (ADD), and "attention-deficit/hyperactivity disorder" (ADHD). Each of these refers to largely the same group of children.

In the 1930s, it was discovered that Benzedrine (an amphetamine-like stimulant) seemed to "calm" hyperkinetic children (Bradley, 1937), and by the 1950s, stimulants were coming into regular use to treat hyperactivity (FDA approval was granted

*Author Note.* Work on this chapter was supported by NIMH grant 2R01-MH59105.

for Ritalin in the early 1960s). By the 1970s, treating inattentive and hyperactive children with stimulants began to spark controversy, a theme that continues in Western societies to the present time. Treatment rates rose markedly again from 1990 to the present, attributable in part to changes in educational policy that facilitated identification of children with ADHD in the United States. This rise has also been influenced by a widening definition of the ADHD phenotype.

In the nomenclature of the U.S. American Psychiatric Association in the *DSM-III* (APA, 1980), the condition was labeled attention deficit disorder (ADD with two types: with and without hyperactivity). These subtypes were eliminated and the condition was renamed as ADHD in the *DSM-III-R* (APA, 1987). In the *DSM-IV* (APA, 1994), ADHD was retained, but subtypes were reintroduced in modified form: a predominantly inattentive type (ADHD-PI, similar to *DSM-III* ADD without hyperactivity), a predominantly hyperactive-impulsive type (ADHD-PH, unprecedented in previous nomenclatures), and a combined type (ADHD-C). Subsequent work suggested that these types were not stable, leading the forthcoming *DSM-5* workgroup to downgrade them to indicators of current course rather than distinct subtypes. *DSM-5* also proposes a fourth presentation to capture children who are markedly inattentive with essentially no symptoms of hyperactivity.

As this abbreviated history suggests, appropriate breadth and delineation of the ADHD phenotype has been a persistent concern. For instance, historically, motor control problems were a part of the overinclusive term "minimal brain dysfunction" used in the mid-century. They were removed from *DSM-III-R* and *DSM-IV*, to the diagnostic category *developmental coordination disorder*. However, data continue to appear on motor control problems, clumsiness, and motor output in ADHD (Piek, Pitcher, & Hay, 1999).

Traditionally considered a disorder of childhood, by the end of the 20th century it became clear that ADHD often persists into adolescence and adulthood (Mannuzza & Klein, 2000). Accordingly, data on adults with ADHD have accumulated in the past 20 years. Following from these data, considerable debate was undertaken in formation of *DSM-5* regarding the appropriateness of changing the criteria set for adults.

In this chapter, I emphasize mechanistic theories about within-child psychological and/or cognitive dysfunction in ADHD, and a multilevel perspective on etiology. I conclude by emphasizing that ADHD is not a unitary syndrome but reflects important heterogeneity among affected children. For more detailed discussions of ADHD see Barkley (2006), Nigg (2006b), and Nigg, Hinshaw, and Huang-Pollock (2006).

## TERMINOLOGICAL AND CONCEPTUAL ISSUES

Despite periodic public controversy, there is substantial evidence for validity of the ADHD syndrome with regard to factor structure, impairment, and family patterns (Faraone et al., 2005; Willcutt et al., in press). It is important to note that symptom domains are divided into distinct dimensions in the *DSM-IV*, including (a) inattentive-disorganized, and (b) hyperactive-impulsive. Despite some debate as to whether impulsivity and hyperactivity should count as one dimension or as separate subdimensions among adults, at least in children the two-factor solution has received strong support in terms of divergent external validity. Inattentive behaviors are most strongly associated with academic problems and a range of other impairments, whereas hyperactive/impulsive behaviors aggregate with peer rejection and disruptive tendencies in school and at home (Willcutt et al., in press). Distinct molecular genetic influences also accrue for inattention/disorganization versus hyperactivity/impulsivity (Nikolas & Burt, 2010). Thus, ADHD is best understood not as unitary, but as a two-dimensional syndrome.

Less clear is whether, from a conceptual standpoint, it is more accurate to view ADHD as a discrete syndrome, or as reflecting extreme standing on a normal-varying trait. Although this is a difficult question to answer in terms of underlying causal factors, evidence to date indicates fairly clearly that the syndrome usually reflects extreme standing on a continuously varying trait in the population (Willcutt, Pennington, & DeFries, 2000). Clinicians still need to make diagnostic decisions, however, and the cut points in the *DSM* have empirical support as efficiently identifying impaired children in need of services. However, when we consider models of etiology, a dimensional model is likely to be most useful.

As noted earlier, the subtypes proposed in *DSM-IV* have not attained strong empirical support. In part this is due to a shortage of research on children who present as primarily inattentive, particularly if they have no evidence of symptoms of hyperactivity. Recent data raise the tantalizing possibility that if a child has two or fewer symptoms of hyperactivity-impulsivity, but otherwise meets *DSM* criteria for ADHD, this could be a meaningful type. This group emerges in latent class analyses (Volk, Todorov, Hay, & Todd, 2009) and has worse problems with some types of attention than more symptomatic children with both inattentive and hyperactive impulsive symptoms (Carr, Henderson, & Nigg, 2010; Goth-Owens, Martinez-Torteya, Martel, & Nigg, 2010). This literature is still in its infancy and it may turn out that this group of children lack a stable "type" presentation over time. This will be an interesting area for future study.

Note that studies of ADHD sometimes use the *DSM-IV* criteria, sometimes the *International Classification of Disease-10th Edition* (*ICD-10*) criteria (WHO, 1993) for hyperkinetic disorder, and sometimes merely extreme rating scale scores. Herein, I use the term "ADHD" throughout to avoid tedious cataloguing of differences in phenotype definition across studies.

## DIAGNOSTIC ISSUES AND *DSM* CRITERIA

As of this writing, *DSM-5* and *ICD-11* criteria for ADHD (all easily located on the World Wide Web along with the *DSM-IV* and *ICD-10* criteria) are still being finalized. Students should find it interesting to compare these criteria sets. *DSM-5* is due out in 2013 and *ICD-11* in 2014. Despite much interest in reconciling these two systems, they are likely to remain somewhat divergent for ADHD. Although the symptom lists are similar, several distinctions can be seen between *DSM-IV* ADHD and *ICD-10* hyperkinetic disorder, reflecting ongoing differences in how this syndrome is defined in the United States versus Europe. The most important difference is that the two systems have different rules about comorbid disorders as rule-outs, with *ICD-10* being more restrictive and *DSM-IV* being more inclusive. Additional criteria include onset by age 7 years (likely to be dropped or modified in *DSM-5*), cross-situational display, and impairment (a general requirement for most mental disorders in the *DSM* system).

Whereas guidelines about age of onset lack consistent empirical support (Kieling et al., 2010), guidelines requiring cross-situational problems and impairment have strong empirical support. Failure to assess impairment, in particular, is quite likely to inflate prevalence estimates (Gordan et al., 2005) and inclusion of parent and teacher standardized ratings greatly enhances assessment validity (Pelham, Fabiano, & Massetti, 2005).

Thus, appropriate assessment requires a careful history, data from multiple adult informants with well-normed rating instruments, distinguishing ADHD from either normal developmental variation or any of several medical and psychiatric conditions that feature inattention and impulse control problems (e.g., anxiety and mood disorders, sleep and other health-related disorders, and some types of learning disorders), and, when possible, direct observation. Careful consideration of functional adjustment in multiple domains can further assist with treatment tailoring (Pelham et al., 2005). Assessing these issues becomes difficult in preschool children due to the high base rate of impulsive or hyperactive behavior. However, ADHD can be identified reliably and validly in research settings as early as age 3 to 4 years, prompting many clinicians to attempt to do the same. Medical guidelines now exist for assessment and treatment in 4- to 5-year-old children (American Academy of Pediatrics, 2011 [epub ahead of print]). Assessment is more difficult in adults, because retrospective history is difficult to obtain reliably and because some of the extant *DSM-IV* symptoms are rarely endorsed by adults.

## PREVALENCE

In the past decade, systematic population-based national surveys were conducted for the first time. Because of different methods, these did not yield identical results but they still give a consistent picture of ADHD as a common condition. In one national survey a 1-year prevalence rate for children and adolescents of 8.5% was reported (Merikangas et al., 2010). Among U.S. adults, the prevalence of ADHD is 4.4% (Kessler et al., 2006). Practitioner surveys by the Centers for Disease Control indicate a rising prevalence of ADHD in the United States from the late 1990s to the late 2000s (Boyle et al., 2011), but it is unclear whether this increase is due to true secular trends or to various identification changes. Worldwide, or when data from different countries are pooled, meta-analytic reviews suggest a 1-year prevalence rate of ADHD in children and adolescents of around 5.3% (Polanczyk, de Lima, Horta, Biederman, & Rohde, 2007) and 2.5% in adults (Simon, Czobor, Balint, Meszaros, & Bitter, 2009). Although these figures seem somewhat lower than the latest U.S. figures outlined above, differences in study methodologies make it impossible to determine, to date, whether there are true variations in ADHD prevalence rates across societies or nations. Most developed nations have been studied, but no attempt has been made to study a syndrome like ADHD among original aboriginal peoples (i.e., untouched by modern technology or disease) to address the common lay speculation that ADHD is a contemporary ailment. However, ADHD-like problems are certainly seen among Native American and Innuit peoples, though confounded with other health conditions.

Although convergent, all of these figures may be high estimates. Few studies used *full DSM-IV* criteria, obtained multiple informants, carefully assessed impairment, or ruled out comorbid conditions. Prevalence rates were much lower for *ICD-10* criteria, typically around 1%, due largely to its exclusion of children with comorbid mood or behavioral conditions. It is unknown what the prevalence will be for the revised definition in *ICD-11*.

## RISK FACTORS AND ETIOLOGICAL FORMULATIONS

I now turn to etiological approaches, emphasizing both (a) within-child correlates that may elucidate etiology and help explain the behavioral problems observed, and (b) risk factors that may contribute to the disorder, perhaps via these internal mechanisms. I bypass a range of psychological mechanisms such as self-esteem and locus of control and instead focus primarily on neurally mediated models.

### GENETIC INFLUENCES ON LIABILITY TO ADHD

Family studies established long ago that ADHD "breeds true," with a two- to fourfold increased risk among first-degree relatives. How much of this familial similarity is due to genes versus common family experiences? More than a dozen behavioral genetic (twin and/or adoption) studies of ADHD have established that in parent ratings, substantial portions of liability are carried by genetic variation, with a heritability coefficient, averaged across many studies, exceeding .8 (Burt, 2009; Willcutt, in press). Heritability estimates are somewhat lower, however, when teacher ratings are examined, although the heritability of a latent variable for shared parent and teacher agreement was .78 in a large Dutch sample (Derks, Hudziak, Van Beijsterveldt, Dolan, & Boomsma, 2006). Relatively few studies have examined twin concordance of ADHD diagnoses derived from full clinical evaluation or the combining of parent and teacher input on symptoms and impairment.

The variation in results for teacher versus parent ratings raises questions of rater bias (known as contrast effects) as an influence on heritability estimates. Contrast bias (parents emphasizing differences more in DZ than MZ twins) is known to inflate heritability estimates of activity level in preschoolers (Saudino, 2003). Such effects in ADHD ratings appear to depend on what rating scale is used. Reitveld et al. (2004) reported on a longitudinal study of a large sample of twins in Europe, with maternal CBCL ratings at four age points (3, 7, 10, and 12 years). Even with rater contrast effects controlled, heritability was above .7 at each age. Simonoff et al. (1998) confirmed maternal contrast effects but also noted biases in teacher ratings due to twin confusion (known as correlated errors), especially for MZ twins. In other words, many twins have the same teacher, and teachers have more difficulty keeping MZ twins straight in their minds. When these effects are accounted for, heritability is between .6 and .7.

In sum, the heritability of ADHD is likely to be around .7. Nonshared environmental effects account for the remainder of variance in ADHD liability. In response to these findings, researchers aggressively pursued molecular genetic studies during the period from 2000 to 2010.

The most common approach to studying molecular correlates in ADHD initially was to look at candidate genes—that is, selected markers on genes believed for theoretical reasons to be of interest, such as dopamine receptor genes (see Chapters 3, 6). A meta-analysis of that literature indicated that six genes have common markers that have been reliably associated with ADHD to date: dopamine transporter (DAT1), dopamine D4 and D5 receptors (DRD4, DRD5), serotonin transporter (5HTTPLR), HTR1B, and SNAP25 (Gizer et al., 2008). However, these in combination account for only 1% of phenotypic variance in ADHD—a common problem in psychiatric genetics (see Chapter 3).

A second approach is to conduct genome-wide scans (GWAS). With this approach searches are conducted across hundreds of thousands of common markers (called *single nucleotide repeats* or *SNPs*). Somewhat to the surprise and disappointment of many scientists, genome-wide scans have failed to identify important new genes in ADHD (Franke et al., 2011). In part, such failures occur because a large number of statistical tests are required (hundreds of thousands), resulting in low statistical power. Yet, pending studies appear likely to identify genome-wide significant markers in psychiatric illness. Further, the GWA studies identified additional candidates that warrant follow up, including one that is under a genome-wide significant linkage peak in a meta-analysis, CDH13 (Lasky-Su et al., 2008). This gene is expressed in nicotinic receptors and neurite outgrowth (Poelmans, Pauls, Buitelaar, & Franke, 2011).

A third approach is to organize common gene variants into their chemical and physiological groupings, called *pathways*. This approach tests for significant association with an over- or underexpressed pathway and thus has more power than searches for individual markers. To date, only two studies have attempted this approach with ADHD and both used a limited approach of examining only already-known pathways (the existing catalog of biological gene pathways is notably incomplete). Still, results were intriguing. Poelmans et al. (2011) identified a coherent network related to nicotinic receptors (already one of the biochemical theories of ADHD) and related to neural growth (relevant to newer theories of neurodevelopmental delay). Stergiakouli et al. (2012) also identified relevant biological pathways, most interestingly in those metabolic systems related to CNS development and choleresterol metabolism (essential for neural development). Once again, the findings, although only a first look at this type of approach and likely to be updated in coming years, provoke new ideas about pathophysiology. It is likely that more gene-pathway-based approaches will be fruitful in the future.

A fourth approach, which has been somewhat successful in schizophrenia and autism spectrum disorder, is to examine rare structural variants, many of which are copy number variants (meaning the only difference in the gene is that a given nucleotide sequence is repeated too many times). This can be accomplished by reanalyzing GWAS data. For example, a recent study using this method found evidence of a rare copy number variation at locus related to ADHD on chromosome 15 at q13.3 occurring in a little under 1% of the population that doubles the risk of ADHD (Williams et al., 2012). New variants can be discovered by sequencing exomal regions of the genome (nonsynonymous variants) or by sequencing the entire genome. These types of studies are now underway in ADHD on a large scale and are likely to yield new discoveries in the coming decade. As of this writing, an international consortium has assembled 15,000 samples of ADHD and control children for an analysis of nonsynonymous (functional) variants, most of which are relatively rare in the population. Sequencing is just getting underway but is expected to identify some causal variants, similar to the picture already going on in autism research (see Chapter 20).

In short, the molecular genetics of ADHD remains a vibrant, exciting area of research despite some surprising and disappointingly small results to date. Our inability to explain most of the variance in the ADHD phenotype has several possible explanations. Perhaps the most interesting include the possibilities of Gene × Environment (G × E) interaction and/or epigenetic effects (see Chapter 3).

## GENE × ENVIRONMENT EFFECTS

In the past decade, studies of G × E effects have become the norm in psychiatric research. Most of these studies examine one or two selected genetic markers (candidates) in relation to selected measures of the environment. The hazards in such studies are many. In particular, (a) the environmental measure may itself be influenced by variation in unmeasured genes, and (b) if variables are not properly scaled, artifactual or "false positive" effects are easily found. Nonetheless, initial efforts in this area have been interesting. A recent meta-analysis (Nigg, Nikolas, & Burt, 2010) indicated interactions of psychosocial distress measures and genotype, particularly for dopamine transporter (DAT1) and serotonin transporter, are reliable in predicting ADHD. However, these effects remain reliant on a few small studies and could still be overturned. Yet, more work on Gene × Environment interaction in ADHD is likely to be of considerable interest in coming years.

Further, the past decade has seen exciting developments in epigenetics, that is, the recognition that experience can alter the genome—and thus the phenotype—sometimes dramatically. This occurs through methylation (modification of chromatin, the material in which DNA is "housed"), to alter gene expression. That is, the expression of much of human variation may not depend only on DNA structure but on the regulatory markings that control whether and how a gene is expressed.

These two insights (the importance of G × E and the importance of epigenetic effects) have sparked a renaissance in studies of environmental contributions to ADHD (as well as several other psychiatric conditions) that is changing the face of research in the second decade of the 21st century and may potentially also change the face of clinical practice in the decades that follow.

## Environmental Risks and Triggers

When G × E and epigenetic mechanisms are recognized, many possible environmental contributors to the etiology of ADHD emerge as potentially important. A fruitful way to think about the etiology of ADHD is to consider structural DNA (the part that, as far as we know, cannot be changed except by mutations) as conveying liability or susceptibility to ADHD. Experiences then activate the condition, either by causing direct changes in the brain or physiology or via epigenetic markings that change gene expression. This model suggests that a given environmental risk will not affect all children: Some are "immune" to the effect but other children will be susceptible and develop ADHD in the presence of this risk.

G × E empirical studies tend to support such possibilities. For example, it is known that (1) neurotoxic pesticide clearance rates from the body depend on genotype (Engel et al., 2011); (2) blood lead levels are modulated by iron uptake, in turn controlled by genotype (Hopkins et al., 2008); and (3) responses to dietary additives may be modulated by genotype (Stevenson et al., 2010). It also appears from neuroimaging studies of discordant identical twins in which one has ADHD and one does not, that major changes in the brain associated with ADHD are not accounted for genetically (Castellanos et al., 2002). Thus it appears likely that a susceptibility-plasticity model will ultimately fit best for ADHD (and probably for other kinds of psychopathology and complex disease generally), rather than a genetic main-effect model.

As for specific environments, several are notable. First, commentators have suggested that inadequate schooling, rapid societal tempo, and family stress are contributing to an alleged increase in ADHD incidence. Many of these sociological ideas are interesting but untested (or untestable) and some (like schooling) occur too late in development to account for ADHD onset.

Regarding other potential environmental potentiators of genetic liability, biological context, both pre- and postnatally, may be especially important. For example, low birth weight (<2500 grams) is a specific risk factor for inattention/hyperactivity and certain learning and motor problems but not other behavioral or emotional problems at age 6 (Breslau & Chilcoat, 2000). However, low birth weight is itself multiply determined by factors such as maternal health and nutrition, maternal smoking, maternal weight, low SES, stress, and other factors, making identification of specific biological mechanisms difficult. On the other hand, an extensive literature indicates that some prenatal teratogens increase risk of ADHD (see Chapter 9). For example, alcohol exposure, at least for women in the United States at moderate levels of drinking (S. W. Jacobson, Jacobson, Sokol, Chiodo, & Corobana, 2004; Mick, Biederman, Faraone, Sayer, & Kleinman, 2002), increases risk of offspring ADHD. However, these children may have a somewhat distinct neuropsychological profile from typical ADHD, with particular problems in visual attention and mathematics. Prospective population studies implicate household and outdoor pesticide exposures during critical periods in pregnancy as predictive of ADHD (Marks et al., 2010; Sagiv et al., 2010). A crucial challenge is to determine if such correlates, even though they emerge in prospective population-based studies, are causal. Although G × E as well as gene-environment correlation can mask environmental effects, they can also mask genetic effects. Teratogens and toxins could be proxies for genetic risk because of gene-environment correlation (see Chapter 9).

Although experimental proof among humans is difficult to obtain, it is not impossible. A recent meta-analysis of randomized experimental data concluded that dietary factors provide a clinically meaningful causal influence on ADHD (Nigg, Lewis, Edinger, & Falk, 2012). In contrast, two clever family designs, one using surrogate mothers who were related and unrelated to their offspring and one using siblings who differed in whether their mother smoked during pregnancy, both concluded that causal effects of prenatal smoking on ADHD were likely smaller than previously believed (D'Onofrio et al., 2008; Thapar et al., 2009). It is also possible that prenatal nicotine exposure is linked more specifically with conduct problems rather than ADHD (e.g., Gatzke-Kopp & Beauchaine, 2007).

It is unclear into which category neurotoxicants will fall. However, because they are fairly universally distributed in the population, exposure to them, unlike maternal smoking, is unlikely to be a proxy for genetic risk. In addition to early household pesticide exposure, particularly well studied are effects of lead exposure. It has been known for centuries that lead is neurotoxic and for decades that at sufficiently high exposure can cause hyperactivity and other health problems. However, more unexpected in the past decade has been the discovery that even at background level exposure—which is near-universal in the U.S. population (about 1 ug/dL of blood)—blood lead level is correlated with ADHD symptoms (Braun et al., 2006; Chiodo, Jacobson, & Jacobson, 2004; Nigg et al., 2008; Nigg, Nikolas, Knottnerus, Cavanagh, & Friderici, 2010). It will be extremely difficult to prove causal effects, but from a precautionary point of view these findings are of significant public health concern, because the levels of lead being studied remain common in the United States and are epidemic in many nations around the world.

Many other experiential factors have been hypothesized to influence ADHD, from general sociological claims such as "faster pace of life" to more testable effects of early electronic media on brain development. Although no conclusive evidence has been reported for those various ideas, it remains possible that important discoveries will emerge regarding experiential triggers.

## MECHANISMS I: NEUROIMAGING FINDINGS

Whether we discuss genetic contributors to liability or environmental triggers, these effects are presumably expressed in the brain. Thus, isolation of causal mechanisms suggests that we consider brain circuitry and associated abilities. I therefore review neuroimaging findings before turning to psychological functioning in ADHD.

The most striking findings in the brain-imaging literature to date comes from a large nationally representative sample of several hundred children, some of them scanned several times, undertaken by the intramural branch at NIMH from the 1990s to the present. First, that cohort revealed that smaller volume of key brain structures was apparent at the earliest ages studied (4 to 5 years old) and remained stable in relation to comparison children throughout development (Castellanos et al., 2002). Second, it revealed that ADHD was associated with altered timing of posterior-to-anterior cortical thinning, which normally happens with development due to the pruning and shaping of brain circuits (Shaw et al., 2006). Although the effects remain too small to be helpful in diagnosing individual cases, they confirm that at a group level, ADHD is a neurodevelopmental condition that is associated with reliable, persistent, and widespread alterations in brain maturation throughout development.

These findings complement a host of smaller studies of brain structure and function. Structural findings demonstrate that on average, children with ADHD evidence a 5% reduction in overall brain volume and a 12% reduction in volume of key frontal and subcortical structures, particularly the prefrontal cortex (PFC), which is crucial to complex, planned behavior, keeping goals in mind, and over-riding inappropriate responses; the basal ganglia/striatum, a group of subcortical structures important in response control; the cerebellum, which is important in temporal information processing and motor control; and the corpus callosum, which is involved in integrating information for efficient responding. The most compelling evidence points to a neural circuit that links the prefrontal cortex and a subcortical region known as the striatum, a circuit thought to be important in response output control. Additionally, notably smaller structural sizes are observed in the cerebellum (especially the cerebellar vermis), a region important for temporal information processing and executive functioning, which is connected via long fiber projections with the prefrontal cortex.

Task-based functional imaging studies seem to support this view. A meta-analysis of 16 functional imaging studies of ADHD revealed consistent brain-activation deficits in virtually all regions of the prefrontal cortex, as well as other brain regions (Dickstein, Bannon, Castellanos, & Milham, 2006). These findings support abnormal functioning in fronto-striatal as well as frontal-parietal neural circuitry in ADHD (see also Durston et al., 2003).

It must be noted, however, that in the past decade, newer imaging methods have begun to sweep the field and to change the face of psychiatric neuroimaging. Most notable in relation to ADHD and other child disorders is the emergence of more robust methods for evaluating neural circuits directly (rather than via inference). The first of these methods is diffusion tensor imaging (DTI). Conducted with MRI, this method traces the directional flow of water molecules in the brain. These molecules generally "diffuse" in line with the tissue in which they are located. This principle makes it possible to trace the integrity of axonal connections (white matter tracts). The DTI signal is altered when white matter microstructure is altered (e.g., due to reduced development of glial cells, reduced axonal size, or other physiological changes). More than a dozen studies have been conducted in ADHD using DTI. All show multiple areas of altered white matter microstructure in ADHD. One of the most comprehensive analyses, conducted with the youngest group of children studied with this method to date, showed that by age 7 to 8 years, widespread (brain-wide) microstructural alterations are observable in ADHD (Nagel et al., 2011). Many questions remain about the reproducibility, clinical utility, and reliability of these white matter findings, so they require scrutiny, longitudinal follow-up, and explanation in any theory of ADHD. In particular, the widespread nature of the findings calls into question theories of ADHD that focus on single brain circuits or neurotransmitters and boosts theories that address brain-wide mechanisms such as synaptic signaling, myelin formation, and the like.

Second, a promising new technique is known as resting state functional connectivity MRI. In this method, functional MRI is used and the key measure is the BOLD signal (a measure of blood flow, which is assumed to reflect neuronal activity; so long as that assumption can be supported, the inferences are of interest). Traditionally, fMRI studies have examined changes in the BOLD signal during different task conditions. However, that method suffers at times in reproducibility and clinical application because results are heavily dependent on specific task characteristics. The hope is that resting-state functional connectivity MRI (rs_fcMRI) can transcend this limitation and produce more cross-site reproducible results. The intriguing idea behind the rs_fcMRI signal is that instead of subtracting the massive background "noise" of neural activity that goes on outside of task-specific activation, such main neural action in the brain is now the focus of study. Spontaneous neural firing occurs throughout the brain when people are not engaged in any particular task (as well as when they are). However, that firing is not random—it is synchronized across different brain regions. When those synchronized signals are mapped, they create functional maps of both known and novel brain circuits. It is as if the Hebbian signal has been mapped—as if neurons are firing together to maintain their connection in case it is needed. Questions remain about the potential for artifact in this method; some circuits may appear connected to participant head motion, for example, and these effects are still being understood. Even so, studies using this method also show particular patterns of altered functional connectivity in ADHD and can potentially provide new tools to map subcortical circuits (Castellanos et al., 2008; Fair et al., 2010; Uddin et al., 2008). Although it is too early to draw firm conclusions about results from this method, the insights it generates are likely to inform ADHD theory in coming years.

## Mechanism II: Performance Studies of Neuropsychological and Cognitive Abilities

In understanding the psychological mechanisms that are involved, which might correspond to what is known about neural findings, four key functional systems in the brain are implicated in ADHD: (1) nonexecutive attention and arousal, (2) executive functioning and cognitive control, (3) motivation and reinforcement, and (4) temporal information processing.

*Attention* can be defined as the facilitated processing of one piece or source of information over others—in other words, the ability to focus or filter information. Usually considered a cognitive process, attention can be influenced by emotion as

**Table 12.1**

Summary of Brain Imaging Findings in ADHD

| Structure | Key Findings |
|---|---|
| Prefrontal cortex | Reduced right > left asymmetry, with relatively smaller right side; reduced dorsolateral prefrontal cortex volume; underactivation of right medial prefrontal cortex and ventrolateral prefrontal cortex to challenge |
| Dorsal anterior cingulated cortex | Few structural studies of this region; functional studies indicate possible hypoactivation during challenge tasks, need replication |
| Basal ganglia | Reduced volume of the caudate, but not putamen; decreased volume of the pallidum, reduced size of globus pallidus in preliminary studies; hypoactivation of left caudate during executive task performance; reduced blood flow to the putamen in reflexometric MRI study |
| Cerebellum | Reduced size of vermis, especially posterior-inferior lobules; overall decreased right cerebellar volumes |
| Corpus callossum | Smaller rostrum (anterior and inferior region); abnormalities of the posterior regions linked to temporal and parietal cortices in the splenium |
| Exploratory findings | Decreased volume of the parietal lobe, reduced occipital gray and white matter, significantly larger posterior lateral ventricles bilaterally |
| Caveats | Insufficient data on subregions of key structures; insufficient control of confounds; lack of data on key subcortical regions |

Data from Castellanos et al., 2002; Giedd, Blumenthal, Molloy, & Castellanos, 2001; Seidman, Valera, & Makris, 2005.

well (as when anxiety narrows attentional focus). Attentional selection (whether by location, movement, timing, or other features) is influenced both by bottom-up stimulus-driven processes that are relatively automatic and early developing, and by top-down goal-driven processes that are strategic, relatively deliberate, related to the concept of executive control, and later developing. In contrast, a posterior network involved in reflexive orienting and perceptual filtering is apparently not involved in ADHD (Huang-Pollock & Nigg, 2003; Huang-Pollock, Nigg, & Carr, 2005; Sergeant & van der Meere, 1998).

On the other hand, aspects of a system responsible for attentional alerting (immediate focus of attention on something important, related to the older concept of arousal) and vigilance (maintaining the alert state over time, also called *sustained attention*) are salient for ADHD. This system involves a right-lateralized network of neural structures that include the noradrenergic system originating in the locus coeruleus, the cholinergic system of the basal forebrain, the intralaminar thalamic nuclei, the right prefrontal cortex (Posner & Petersen, 1990), and possibly the ascending reticular activating system (related to wakefulness). Sustained attention (vigilance) appears to be affected only under certain task conditions (such as different event rates), potentially implicating a process known as activation or response readiness (Sergeant et al., 1999). In contrast, abnormalities in the alerting function in ADHD are apparent in the form of (a) poor signal detection on continuous performance tasks (Losier, McGrath, & Klein, 1996); (b) a tendency to respond too slowly on "fast as you can" reaction time tasks (apparently due to an excess of extremely slow responses, suggesting failures of alertness); and (c) excess slow-wave activity in brain EEG observations (Barry, Clarke, & Johnstone, 2003).

*Cognitive control* (related to the older but widely used term, *executive function*) refers to strategic or deliberate allocation of both attention and response. When in the service of a later goal held in mind we suppress an unwanted thought (I am anxious but I focus on the exam question), or behavior (I am eager to interrupt but I want to keep my New Year's resolution not to), we engage in cognitive control. Children must use this ability to study first and play later, to pay attention in class even when other children are talking, to keep track of their materials when returning home from school, and to wait their turn. Such behaviors depend in large part on dopaminergic and noradrenergic circuits in dorsolateral, orbital-prefrontal, and anterior cingulate cortices and their projections to and from the basal ganglia and parietal cortex. These circuits track whether what has occurred is consistent with expectations—and adjust behavior accordingly. Yet also relevant are prefrontal-cerebellar circuits, which may be important for determining if the timing of events is consistent with what was expected and then modulating behavior (Nigg & Casey, 2005). We parse this broad domain into (a) working memory, which depends on maintaining attentional control; (b) response suppression (executive inhibition); and (c) shifting (involving parietal activity).

*Working memory* refers to a limited capacity system for keeping something in mind while doing something else, such as remembering a phone number while completing a conversation. It is supported by simple passive storage or "short-term" memory (holding something in mind for a moment). It includes separate neural loops for handling verbal information (the left-lateralized phonological loop) and spatial information (right lateralized). Most of the 20 or so studies on working memory and ADHD have taken place in the last decade and were evaluated in two recent meta-analyses (Martinussen, Hayden, Hogg-Johnson, & Tannock, 2005; Willcutt, Doyle, Nigg, Faraone, & Pennington, 2005). Both reviews estimated effect sizes for verbal working memory and storage in the small to medium range, at $d = .43$ (Martinussen et al., 2005) to $d = .54$ (Willcutt et al., 2005). In contrast to these modest effects, spatial working memory weaknesses were medium to large, in the range of $d = .72$ (Willcutt et al., 2005) to $d = 1.06$ (Martinussen et al., 2005). Effects were nearly as large for short-term memory ($d = .85$, in Martinussen et al., 2005). The small number of studies included (6 to 8) must be kept in mind, but results indicate a meaningful ADHD effect for spatial tasks.

*Response suppression* (executive inhibition) refers to the ability to interrupt a response during dynamic moment-to-moment behavior. Although often associated conceptually with impulsivity, this ability may be equally or more related to inattention-disorganization, in that maintaining focused behavior requires continually suppressing alternative behaviors that may be activated by context. Imagine a "check-swing" in baseball as an index of being able to keep behavior immediately responsive to a rapidly changing context (Logan, 1994). Several experimental computer-based paradigms, brain imaging results, and brain-injury studies converge on links between this ability and a right-lateralized neural circuit involving the inferior frontal gyrus and, subcortically, the caudate, a structure in the basal ganglia, and possibly parts of the thalamus. Key measurement paradigms include the go/no-go task, the anti-saccade task (an eye-movement experiment), and the Logan (1994) stopping task. All converge on some ADHD-related weakness in this ability. More than 30 studies have been conducted on the stopping task alone, making it perhaps the most heavily studied paradigm in ADHD. Willcutt et al. (2005) reviewed 27 of these studies and noted a composite effect size for ADHD versus control of $d = .61$ (a medium-effect size).

*Set shifting* refers to shifting one's mental focus within a task such as sorting by color versus sorting by number; whereas task switching refers to alternating tasks, such as counting objects versus naming objects. These abilities involve attentional networks in the parietal cortex (particularly for set shifting) and are likely to involve executive control and perhaps cerebellar control for task switching. Most neuropsychological studies of ADHD appear to involve set shifting, using tasks such as the Wisconsin Card Sort, and these yield only small to medium ADHD effects that do not replicate well ($d = .46$ across 24 studies; Willcutt et al., 2005). On the other hand, task-switching paradigms have only recently begun to be examined in ADHD.

Overall, difficulties in cognitive control are relevant to ADHD. They appear to be right-lateralized, involving in particular spatial working memory (and the dorsolateral prefrontal cortex) and response suppression (and inferior right prefrontal cortex and projection zones). In contrast, other executive abilities, such as verbal working memory and set shifting, exhibit smaller weaknesses, suggesting that they are less likely to be core mechanisms.

## Motivation, Approach, and Reinforcement Response

The central motivational processes involved in ADHD have been approached from a temperament perspective (for reviews see Nigg, 2006a; Rothbart & Bates, 1998), as well as from an experimental perspective examining response to reinforcement. I begin with temperament, synthesizing several models to focus on two key traits.

Withdrawal or reactive control is anchored in limbic structures including the amygdala, the hippocampus, and their interconnections. This form of control implements reactions of anxiety and fear that trigger spontaneous inhibition of some or all behaviors in response to novelty or threat. A rich literature suggests that such reactive control of behavior is related to anxiety and anxiety disorders (Kagan & Snidman, 2004). Low responses of this system (failure of fear response) appear to be related to psychopathy (Blair, Peschardt, Budhani, Mitchell, & Pine,

**Table 12.2**
Summary of Neuropsychological Findings in ADHD

| Domain | Status | Meta-Analytic Effect Size |
|---|---|---|
| **Attention** | | |
| Perceptual selection | 4 | na |
| Reflexive orienting | 4 | $d = .20$ |
| Alerting/Vigilance system | 1 | $d = .75$ |
| **Cognitive Control/Executive Functioning** | | |
| Interference control | 4 | $d = .20$ |
| Working memory verbal | 2 | $d = .45$ |
| Working memory spatial | 1 | $d = 1.0$ |
| Planning | 2 | $d = .55$ |
| Response inhibition | 1 | $d = .60$ |
| Set shifting | 2 | $d = .50$ |
| Activation | 3 | na |
| **Motivational Response** | | |
| Reactive (anxious) inhibition | 4 | na |
| Reward response (approach) | 2 | na |
| Motor and temporal response | | |
| Motor control | 2 | na |
| Temporal processing | 2 | na |

Ratings of status: 1 = replicated deficit, substantial in size (reliably larger than .50 based on number of studies, confidence interval around pooled effect size); 2 = deficit probably exists, but aggregate effects are modest in size (not reliably larger than .50) or consistent results rely on a small number of studies (so pooled effect size has wide confidence interval); 3 = possible deficit but findings are mixed across different indicators, and positive findings rest on small number of studies; 4 = spared or effect is too trivial in size to be clinically meaningful). Na = not available or not applicable. Effect sizes are rounded off estimates. Reprinted from Nigg (2006b), where detailed review is also available.

2006) and perhaps conduct disorder but not ADHD. As reviewed in detail by Nigg (2001), experimental paradigms designed to elicit caution in response to potential punishment cues do not yield a reliable set of responses in relation to ADHD.

Approach, or willingness to approach possible incentive or reward/reinforcement, is associated with speed of reinforcement learning. It is conceptualized as related to the appetitive, dopaminergic systems, including the nucleus accumbens and ascending limbic-frontal dopaminergic networks. At the level of the autonomic nervous system, it is linked with sympathetic activation during the performance of rewarded behaviors. One crucial index is heart rate acceleration in response to the application of effort or the appearance of incentive (Beauchaine, 2001). Goldsmith, Lemery, and Essex (2004) followed children from birth through first grade, with multisource temperament measures and parent and teacher ratings of ADHD symptoms. Observational data linked hyperactivity/impulsivity primarily to high approach, though magnitudes of associations were modest ($r$s in the .2 to .3 range). Other studies of personality and temperament have yielded mixed results for this trait (Nigg, Blaskey, Huang-Pollock, & Rappley, 2002), although cross sectional ratings of children suggest it is related to hyperactivity/impulsivity but not inattention (Martel & Nigg, 2006).

Another line of work has considered ADHD from the viewpoint of reinforcement response—mechanistic activation levels in the appetitive and reinforcement learning systems of the midbrain ascending DA network. These neurons appear to signal unexpected responses to the PFC and to be heavily involved in reinforcement learning, as well as in triggering cognitive control in a bottom-up process. Relying heavily on a series of elegant animal studies, Sagvolden, Johansen, Aase, and Russell (2005) suggested that ADHD may be linked to a weakened reinforcement-delay gradient—that is, as the time to wait for an outcome increases, children with ADHD lose interest in earning the reward more precipitously than do other children. The result is difficulty in learning and in unlearning behaviors that are linked to reinforcers. Human studies to evaluate this theory are needed.

A large literature on reward response in ADHD has yielded complex findings that are difficult to link to any one theory. A comprehensive review by Luman, Oosterlaan, and Sergeant (2005) concluded that ADHD is associated with (a) increased weighting of near-term over long-term (but larger) reward, (b) possible positive response to high-intensity reinforcement, (c) lack of physiological response (e.g., heart rate acceleration) to potential rewards. However, comorbid conditions, notably conduct disorder, have not been adequately considered in this literature.

## Temporal Information Processing and Motor Control

The field of ADHD research has focused also on temporal information processing. This idea emanates both from (a) recent theories of executive functioning, which emphasize the importance of temporal integration for both behavioral control (Barkley, 1997) and learning and modulation of behavior (Nigg & Casey, 2005), and (b) imaging findings of cerebellar alterations, as noted earlier. The cerebellum is now thought to be involved not only in learning of complex motor behaviors but also in timing of behavior and temporal-dependent learning. In short, the mind's internal "clock" may depend on the cerebellum. Implications of faulty time perception for behavioral control are extensive (Barkley, 1997). Toplak et al. (2005) reviewed some 20 extant studies and concluded that ADHD is associated with poor time estimation and poor time reproduction. Although more work in this area is needed, implications for a complete understanding of neurobiology in ADHD are substantial. Problems in cerebellar functioning and temporal information processing could contribute to poor reinforcement learning, poor executive functioning, and even poor motor coordination.

## DEVELOPMENTAL PROGRESSION

Despite questions about the appropriate age of onset criterion (if any) for diagnosing ADHD, the early school years are the modal age of case identification. It may be possible to reliably identify ADHD in children as young as age 3 (Lahey et al., 1998; see also Campbell, 2002), although this is controversial. Even earlier in development, it is likely that consolidation of regulatory capacities in the toddler years and the influence of temperament in the first year of life may interact with the social environment to shape vulnerability to ADHD (Nigg, 2006b; see also Chapter 6). However, diagnostic prediction from these early temperamental precursors remains uncertain, and many at-risk toddlers do not develop ADHD in later childhood.

Some of the variation in subtype status is related to normal developmental trajectories. That is, motoric hyperactivity is more pronounced in preschool, and tends to decline with time, whereas problems with inattention can become more pronounced with age as peers undergo rapid maturation of prefrontal cortical structures and accompanying cognitive abilities at the same time that school demands intensify. Many children with ADHD-HI during the preschool years develop ADHD-C (or remit) as they enter the school years. Correspondingly, the inattentive type becomes more common later in childhood and through adolescence (Hart, Lahey, Loeber, Applegate, & Frick, 1995). Moreover, heterotypic continuity is not well addressed in the diagnostic system. That is, most behavioral symptoms are designed to describe school-age children; corresponding criteria for adolescence or adulthood are lacking, although this issue is beginning to be addressed by empirical work by Achenbach (1991), Conners et al. (1997), and others. Adult findings are emerging, suggesting a syndrome with clinical validity in terms of impairment and cognitive deficits (Barkley, Murphy, & Fischer, 2008; Murphy, Barkley, & Bush, 2001; Nigg et al., 2005).

## COMORBIDITY

ADHD is highly likely to exist in concert with one or more disruptive behavior disorders (oppositional defiant disorder, conduct disorder) as well as other conditions. In children, this rate is about 50% for ODD and about 22% for CD (Willcutt et al., in press). *DSM-5* is likely to introduce a new disorder known as *disruptive mood dysregulation disorder*. It is intended to describe children who have extreme irritability (e.g., temper tantrums and anger). Such children have been too frequently labeled as bipolar in the past two decades (see Chapter 19). Most of these children will also meet criteria for ADHD, although the prevalence of this disorder in ADHD samples is unclear. Anxiety co-occurs with ADHD, but any one anxiety disorder is seen only in a minority of cases (e.g., 10% to 15% of children with ADHD will have a generalized anxiety disorder; Willcutt et al., in press), and only 8% of adults (Kessler et al., 2006). However, by adulthood, when all anxiety disorders are combined, nearly half of adults with ADHD have experienced at least one type of anxiety disorder or phobia in the past year (Kessler et al., 2006). In addition, about one quarter of children with ADHD meet criteria for a learning disorder (Willcutt et al., in press), underscoring the value of cognitive evaluation in these samples. Some studies also indicate above chance association with obsessive compulsive disorder, tic disorders, and autism spectrum disorder.

Comorbid profiles may provide clues to etiology. For example, consistent with the nosology in *ICD-10*, when ADHD co-occurs with clinically significant

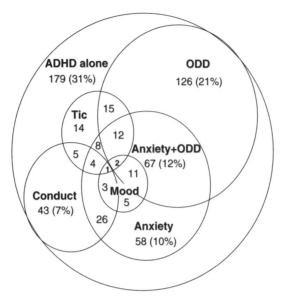

Data from *Archives of General Psychiatry,*1999 (n= 579)
courtesy of JimSwanson

**Figure 12.1**  Patterns of comorbidity in the MTA study.

Data from the MTA Cooperative Group, 1999. "A 14-month randomized clinical trial of treatment strategies for attention-deficit/hyperactivity disorder." The MTA Cooperative Group, Multimodal Treatment
Study of Children with ADHD.

aggression or with major internalizing (anxious, depressed) features, it may constitute a substantially different condition than when it exists alone (e.g., Jensen
et al., 2001). Alternatively, G × E interactions (see earlier) may facilitate progression
from ADHD to more severe externalizing conduct for some vulnerable children
(Beauchaine, Hinshaw, & Pang, 2010).

Figure 12.1 illustrates patterns of comorbidity for boys with ADHD-C in the large,
multisite, multimodal treatment study of ADHD (hereafter referred to as the MTA).
As can be seen, even after accounting for oppositional defiant disorder (the most co-
occurring condition), more than two thirds of the children had at least one additional
*DSM-IV* syndrome. Thus, clinical assessment must include comorbid disorders in
case formulation. Similarly, a complete nosological account of heterogeneity must
take into account patterns of comorbid problems. It is important to recognize that
many studies of etiology have not adequately considered comorbid conditions.
Thus, degree of specificity of many of these effects to ADHD versus other disorders
remains under dispute.

## SEX DIFFERENCES

As with most psychiatric/developmental disorders of childhood onset, ADHD
shows a male preponderance, on the order of 2:1 or higher (Polanczyk et al., 2007),
which drops somewhat, to only 1.6:1, by adulthood (Kessler et al., 2006), perhaps due

in part to underidentification of girls in childhood. Boys are referred for treatment at much higher rates than girls. In addition, the larger sex difference in childhood may be an artifact of criteria that were developed based on predominately male samples. Girls may be more likely to display inattentive behaviors, yet whether they show a greater number of comorbid internalizing problems is controversial. Studies of clinically referred girls and boys with ADHD indicate that they show comparable levels of impairment in academic and social functioning, but girls with the disorder may have greater intellectual deficits (Gaub & Carlson, 1997). In community samples, however, girls are less likely to have comorbid externalizing problems than boys, and they do not show greater intellectual impairment (Gaub & Carlson, 1997). With regard to cognitive and biological correlates, girls with ADHD show similar patterns of impairments in executive functioning and cognitive control as their male counterparts (Hinshaw, Carte, Sami, Treuting, & Zupan, 2002; Rucklidge & Tannock, 2001). In a major series of clinical cases, girls and boys with ADHD showed similar patterns of impairment on measures of set-shifting and interference control, and both groups performed significantly worse than sex-matched controls (Seidman et al., 2005). In the same sample at Massachusetts General Hospital, Doyle et al. (2005) reported patterns of neuropsychological impairment in family members of girls with ADHD similar to those in the relatives of boys with the disorder. These types of data suggest important similarities between manifestation of ADHD in boys and girls and suggest that the same construct is being captured.

However, key issues remain. It is unclear whether sex-specific cutoffs should be considered when diagnosing ADHD in girls (see Hinshaw & Blachman, 2005). Girls are less active and disruptive than boys overall, yet symptom counts used to diagnose ADHD are the same for both sexes. Hence, it is possible that some impaired girls are missed by current criteria. Second, girls may have greater resistance to the etiological factors that cause ADHD. In a twin study, Rhee, Waldman, Hay, and Levy (1999) found evidence consistent with this differential threshold model, suggesting that girls with ADHD need more risk genes before manifesting ADHD. Further studies that incorporate studies of hormonal and other sex-specific effects in early development will be important to a complete understanding of ADHD. Despite recent advances, ADHD in girls remains less well understood than in boys, and the apparent equalizing of prevalence in adolescence and adulthood is not well explained.

## CULTURAL CONSIDERATIONS

A pooled meta-regression analysis by Polanczyk et al. (2007) included data from more than 170,000 participants in 102 studies on all populated continents (although the majority of studies have been conducted in North America and Europe), with a pooled worldwide prevalence rate of 5.3%, as noted earlier. Cross-nationally, significant variation exists: Prevalence was highest in South America (11.8%) and Africa (8.5%) and lowest in the Middle East (2.4%), though these differences were nonsignificant after adjustment for methodology differences (i.e., differences in how ADHD was assessed). Few studies were available in these regions, so confidence intervals encompassed too wide of a range to enable differentiation across these regions. Continents with enough data for narrow confidence intervals all had similar prevalences (North America, 6.3%, Europe, 4.7%, Oceania, 4.6%, Asia, 3.7%). Within-country data were not analyzed due to the reduced $N$ of available studies. Thus, additional local prevalence data will be important to etiological theories. For example, if lead exposure, anemia, or malnutrition contribute to ADHD, then prevalence should be somewhat higher in nations with higher exposures (e.g., South Africa), unless these effects are countered by alternative etiologies in developed nations (e.g., higher rates of surviving children with low birth weight). Even so, rates of stimulant treatment are higher in the United States than in many nations due to differences in historical approach, laws, and professional practice (Scheffler, Hinshaw, Modrek, & Levine, 2007), although other wealthy nations are on a similar use trajectory (Lang, Scheffler, & Hu, 2010). Nevertheless, several complexities are worthy of comment.

First, ADHD-related behaviors may not have the same meaning in the eyes of teachers and parents across cultural groups. For example, Mann et al. (1992) and Mueller et al. (1995) found that clinicians of different cultures rated the same child actors at significantly different symptom levels even when faced with identical behaviors (independent of race of the child). On the other hand, Epstein et al. (2005) found that teacher's ratings of excess ADHD symptoms in African American children were consistent with behavioral observations of the same classrooms. This main effect of race was partially due to the fact that African American children were more often in classrooms where the average child had more misbehavior. The paucity of research on these issues represents a gaping hole in our knowledge base.

Second, it is unclear to what extent the ADHD syndrome has similar internal validity across ethnic or cultural groups, or under what conditions this might change. Data suggest that the ADHD symptom factor structure is essentially the same across nations (Toplak et al., 2012). Yet Reid et al. (1998) examined the factor loadings of ADHD symptoms in African American and Euro-American children in the United States. Although the general two-factor symptom structure was preserved across groups, the item loadings differed, suggesting that the syndrome might have a different meaning in the two groups. It is not difficult to imagine how the same behavior could have different meanings across racial groups in the United States (for instance, one might speculate that an African American child more often may be socialized to call out in groups, whereas a European American child may be socialized to remain quiet or wait his or her turn in large groups). Different meanings across nations are also plausible.

Still, countering such suppositions, the major review by Rohde et al. (2005) concluded that studies in nondeveloped nations yield similar factor structures, treatment responses, prevalences, and biological correlates as studies in developed nations, supporting the cross-cultural validity of ADHD. Likewise, Yang, Schaller, and Parker (2000) found similar factor loadings in Taiwan and the United States. Such evidence raises the question of when, if at all, racially or culturally specific norms should be included in the assessment of ADHD. Again, a paucity of research signifies ripe opportunities for future investigators in this area to clarify local variation or boundary conditions, if any, on the cross-cultural validity of ADHD and thus to provide a more differentiated map of construct validity.

Third, treatment rates vary radically across nations (Hinshaw et al., 2011), and approaches to treatment may be different across cultural groups even within the United States (Visser, Bitsko, Danielson, & Perou, 2010). Data are lacking as to the important issue of whether this discrepancy leads to excess poor outcomes among minority children. These differences in services may reflect reduced access to care, or they may reflect distinct attitudes toward the diagnostic and treatment infrastructure. Further empirical work is needed on such issues as costs, access to care, attitudes and beliefs, and differential outcomes.

## PROTECTIVE FACTORS

Aside from obvious and global protections such as strong prenatal care and avoidance of early risk factors (e.g., severe trauma, low birth weight), little is known about protective factors against ADHD. However, some clues have come from recent studies of Risk × Experience interactions. For example, when children are exposed to environmental contaminants early in life (typically prenatally), effects on intellectual and ADHD outcomes are moderated by family context (those who breast fed, a proxy for more well-prepared parents, do not show associations of exposure to later problem outcome; (J. Jacobson & S. Jacobson, 2003). Similarly, Tully et al. (2004) found that parental warmth moderated the effect of low birth weight on ADHD outcomes. This result is consistent with Breslau and Chilcoat's (2000) finding that the effect of low birth weight on ADHD was smaller in suburban than urban communities, suggesting that additional family resources or better health care may have prevented these risk factors from having their full effect.

Second, recent findings regarding biological, genetic, and cognitive protective factors suggest that children exposed to multiple indicators of adversity (low SES, parental Axis I disorders, marital conflict, family stress)—but who are below clinical cutoffs for ADHD symptoms (classified as the resilient group)—are more effective in neuropsychological response inhibition and have fewer "risk" catecholamine genotypes (defined by a count of risk markers across three catecholamine genes expressed in the brain (Nigg, Nikolas, Friderici, Park, & Zucker, 2007). Notably, higher IQ did not serve as such a protective factor.

Third, what about secondary protection? That is, once a child has ADHD, what are protective factors that prevent the worst outcomes? Here, we are on firmer empirical footing, although protective factors often appear to be simply the converse of risk factors. These include (a) stronger reading ability, (b) absence of aggressive behavior, and (c) positive peer relations (for a review, see Barkley, 2006). Additionally, effective parenting may have some effect in reducing persistence of ADHD from preschool into childhood (Campbell, 2002).

## THEORETICAL SYNTHESIS

ADHD is a syndrome that reflects multiple developmental pathways and causal processes. A range of early risks during development apparently affects a minority of these children via neural injury (e.g., prenatal substance exposure)—effects that could be preventable (if society so desired) through adequate prenatal care and reduction in exposure to environmental toxins. A percentage may represent extreme temperaments interacting with a society demanding tight conformity to indoor, desk-type work in childhood. However, findings of neuropsychological weaknesses in many of these children argue against this subgroup's constituting the modal group. Another unknown percentage is likely to reflect the confluence or interaction of vulnerable constitution (genetic liability) and environmental risks (e.g., contaminants or teratogens). Identifying such interactions is a major objective.

The primary internal mechanism driving ADHD appears to involve various types of breakdown in the striatal-prefrontal neural circuitry that supports cognitive control. However, whether the primary element here is a problem in top-down control, or in bottom-up signaling of the need for control, remains in debate. One possible resolution lies in the idea that each is involved in a distinct aspect of the disorder. Sonuga-Barke (2005) suggested a dual pathway approach. Within the framework advanced here, it may be that the inattentive-disorganized symptom domain reflects breakdowns in top-down control mechanisms (anchored in a frontal-striatal neural circuit), whereas hyperactivity-impulsivity reflects breakdowns in bottom-up signaling, perhaps involving reactive control or motivational response processes (anchored in frontal-limbic circuitry). Additional pathways have been suggested (Nigg, 2006a, 2006b). Thus, more than one mechanism may lead to ADHD, exemplifying equifinality, and multiple influences may converge to create the full syndrome. For example, it was noted earlier that distinct external correlates accompany ADHD with and without aggression.

What remains to be clarified is the extent to which distinct etiological influences (e.g., lead exposure, teratogens) operate independently of or interactively with genetic susceptibility. One promising model is that genes confer susceptibility to ADHD and that a range of biological and perhaps experiential stressors in the pre- and postnatal environment set the vulnerable child on a course toward ADHD. In other instances, ADHD may reflect an extreme temperament (e.g., high approach, activity level, or extraversion) that plays out in recursive loops in a particular socialization context to lead to the requisite set of symptoms. Defining and mapping of these distinct routes and pathways is an exciting challenge for researchers in the coming generation.

In summary, ADHD is a complex syndrome, with substantial genetic influence that involves early departures from normal maturation of prefrontal-subcortical and cerebellar brain circuitry. In many instances, this pathway may reflect activating effects of early pre- or perinatal insult; in other instances, it may reflect an extreme genotype. These child characteristics serve as a liability or vulnerability to ADHD. Effects are then likely to be mediated through socialization (genotype-experience correlations), to culminate in breakdowns or failure in the learning of self-regulation and cognitive control, which manifest as persistent problems with adaptation and regulation of cognition and motor control—that is, symptoms of ADHD.

## FUTURE DIRECTIONS

Key issues for future directions can be summed under three broad domains. First, how will the phenotype best be defined, and how will heterogeneity and specificity issues be resolved? This clarification will require a shift from variable-centered to person-centered approaches, and greater attention to mechanistic variability within ADHD samples. Nearly all biological and genetic findings are nonspecific—that is, similar genes, neural regions, and cognitive problems are seen in other disorders. This nonspecificity suggests that either very subtle differences in neural effects are extremely important or, more likely, that these neural or temperamental susceptibilities are shaped by particulars of the learning environment that are yet to be fully specified. The critical roles of integration of functions and of socialization in the development of regulatory control supports this supposition.

Second, what are the specific etiologies of the expected subgroups currently defined as having ADHD? Most research has focused on specifying within-child mechanisms, but these are not adequately linked with causes (be they specific genotypes, specific perinatal or toxic events, or specific epigenetic processes in socialization). Thus, whereas genetic work on ADHD is in its infancy, its ultimate integration with likely experiential etiologies will be essential. These include both direct gene-experience interactions (such as effects of low-level lead or low birth weight on genetically vulnerable children) and epigenetic effects in which the nature of the socialization environment or the nature of biological insult may alter or instantiate expression of genetic liability.

Third, what are key moderators of the meaning and outcome of these behaviors? Here, we can point particularly to the need to understand cultural variation in the meaning of the behaviors and their external correlates, as we map validity with greater precision. Relatedly, it is clear that this syndrome, like many child psychopathologies, will not be fully understood without an adequate explanation of sex differences in incidence and risk. More generally, interactions with widespread societal risk factors also remain unknown. Distinct neuropsychological and temperamental pathways are emerging, and a key goal for the next generation of research is to map those to specific etiologies.

Following from this emphasis on etiology, in addition to identifying prevention opportunities, there remains a need to identify long-term treatments that can alter the developmental course for these children, so that self-regulation is more easily at their command. Current treatments ameliorate symptoms but it is not clear that they reverse the developmental course of regulatory problems. A better understanding of the early developmental origins and dynamics of etiology and mechanism may be helpful in this regard.

In conclusion, ADHD is an important and fascinating syndrome, with multiple routes to its final endpoint. Despite controversies about misdiagnosis, which may emanate from inadequate mental health services, the multiple impairments and strong psychobiological underpinnings seen in these children argue against the idea that ADHD is merely a cultural construct. Furthermore, the complexity of the syndrome's mechanisms and causes is becoming tractable. Still, these effects are likely interacting with poorly understood biological activators and, perhaps, cultural moderators. Their understanding will require describing experiential and genetic effects in integrative studies. The study and treatment of ADHD are characterized by energy and optimism on the part of researchers and practitioners, as their efforts begin to show promise of bearing further fruit.

# REFERENCES

Achenbach, T. (1991). *Manual for the young adult self report and young adult behavior checklist*. Burlington, VT: University of VT Psychiatry.

American Academy of Pediatrics. (2011). ADHD: Clinical practice guideline for the diagnosis, evaluation, and treatment of attention-deficit/hyperactivity disorder in children and adolescents. *Pediatrics, 128*, 1–16.

American Psychiatric Association. (1980). *Diagnostic and statistical manual of mental disorders* (3rd ed.). Washington, DC: Author.

American Psychiatric Association. (1987). *Diagnostic and statistical manual of mental disorders* (3rd ed., rev.).Washington, DC: Author.

American Psychiatric Association. (1994). *Diagnostic and statistical manual of mental disorders* (4th ed.). Washington, DC: Author.

Barkely, R. A. (2006). *Attention-deficit hyperactivity disorder: A handbook for diagnosis and treatment* (3rd ed). New York, NY: Guilford Press.

Barkley, R. A. (1997). Behavioral inhibition, sustained attention, and executive functions: Constructing a unifying theory of ADHD. *Psychological Bulletin, 121*, 65–94.

Barkley, R. A., Murphy, K. R., & Fischer, M. (2008). *ADHD in adults: What the science says*. New York, NY: Guilford Press.

Barry, R. J., Clarke, A. R., & Johnstone, S. J. (2003). A review of electrophysiology in attention-deficit/hyperactivity disorder: I. Qualitative and quantitative electroencephalography. *Clinical Neurophysiology, 114*, 171–183.

Beauchaine, T. (2001). Vagal tone, development, and Gray's motivational theory: Toward an integrated model of autonomic nervous system functioning in psychopathology. *Development and Psychopathology, 13*, 183–214.

Blair, R. J., Peschardt, K. S., Budhani, S., Mitchell, D. G., & Pine, D. S. (2006). The development of psychopathy. *Journal of Child Psychology and Psychiatry, 47*, 262–276.

Boyle, C. A., Boulet, S., Schieve, L. A., Cohen, R. A., Blumberg, S. J., Yeargin-Allsopp, M.,... Kogan, M. D. (2011). Trends in the prevalence of developmental disabilities in US children, 1997–2008. *Pediatrics, 127*, 1034–1042.

Bradley, C. (1937). The behaviour of children receiving Benzedrine. *American Journal of Psychiatry, 94*, 577–585.

Braun, M. U., Rauwolf, T., Bock, M., Kappert, U., Boscheri, A., Schnabel, A., & Strasser, R. H. (2006). Percutaneous lead implantation connected to an external device in stimulation-dependent patients with systemic infection—A prospective and controlled study. *Pacing Clinical Electrophysiology, 29,* 875–879.

Breslau, N., & Chilcoat, H. D. (2000). Psychiatric sequelae of low birth weight at 11 years of age. *Biological Psychiatry, 47,* 1005–1011.

Burt, S. A. (2009). Rethinking environmental contributions to child and adolescent psychopathology: A meta-analysis of shared environmental influences. *Psychological Bulletin, 135,* 608–637.

Campbell, S. B. (2002). *Behavior problems in preschool children* (2nd ed.). New York, NY: Guilford Press.

Carr, L., Henderson, J., & Nigg, J. T. (2010). Cognitive control and attentional selection in adolescents with ADHD versus ADD. *Journal of Clinical Child and Adolescent Psychology, 39,* 726–740.

Castellanos, F. X., Lee, P. P., Sharp, W., Jeffries, N. O., Greenstein, D. K., Clasen, L. S., . . . Rapoport, J. L. (2002). Developmental trajectories of brain volume abnormalities in children and adolescents with attention-deficit/hyperactivity disorder. *Journal of the American Medical Association, 288,* 1740–1748.

Castellanos, F. X., Margulies, D. S., Kelly, C., Uddin, L. Q., Ghaffari, M., Kirsch, A., . . . Milham, M. P. (2008). Cingulate-precuneus interactions: A new locus of dysfunction in adult attention-deficit/hyperactivity disorder. *Biological Psychiatry, 63,* 332–337.

Chiodo, L. M., Jacobson, S. W., & Jacobson, J. L. (2004). Neurodevelopmental effects of postnatal lead exposure at very low levels. *Neurotoxicology and Teratology, 26,* 359–371.

Conners, C. K., Wells, K. C., Parker, J. D., Sitarenios, G., Diamond, J. M., & Powell, J. W. (1997). A new self-report scale for assessment of adolescent psychopathology: Factor structure, reliability, validity, and diagnostic sensitivity. *Journal of Abnormal Child Psychology, 25,* 487–497.

Derks, E. M., Hudziak, J. J., Van Beijsterveldt, C. E., Dolan, C. V., & Boomsma, D. I. (2006). Genetic analyses of maternal and teacher ratings on attention problems in 7-year-old Dutch twins. *Behavioral Genetics, 36,* 833–844.

Dickstein, S. G., Bannon, K., Castellanos, F. X., & Milham, M. P. (2006). The neural correlates of attention deficit hyperactivity disorder: An ALE meta-analysis. *Journal of Child Psychology and Psychiatry, 47,* 1051–1062.

D'Onofrio, B. M., Van Hulle, C. A., Waldman, I. D., Rodgers, J. L., Harden, K. P., Rathouz, P. J., & Lahey, B. B. (2008). Smoking during pregnancy and offspring externalizing problems: An exploration of genetic and environmental confounds. *Development and Psychopathology, 20,* 139–164.

Doyle, A. E., Wilens, T. E., Kwon, A., Seidman, L. J., Faraone, S. V., Fried, R., . . . Biederman, J. (2005). Neuropsychological functioning in youth with bipolar disorder. *Biological Psychiatry, 58,* 540–548.

Durston, S., Tottenham, N. T., Thomas, K. M., Davidson, M. C., Eigsti, I. M., Yang, Y., . . . Casey, B. J. (2003). Differential patterns of striatal activation in young children with and without ADHD. *Biological Psychiatry, 53*, 871–878.

Engel, S. M., Wetmur, J., Chen, J., Zhu, C., Barr, D. B., Canfield, R. L., & Wolff, M. S. (2011). Prenatal exposure to organophosphates, paraoxonase 1, and cognitive development in childhood. *Environmental Health Perspectives, 119*, 1182–1188.

Epstein, J. N., Willoughby, M., Valencia, E. Y., Tonev, S. T., Abikoff, H. B., Arnold, L. E., & Hinshaw, S. P. (2005). The role of children's ethnicity in the relationship between teacher ratings of attention-deficit/hyperactivity disorder and observed classroom behavior. *Journal of Consulting and Clinical Psychology, 73*, 424–434.

Fair, D. A., Posner, J., Nagel, B. J., Bathula, D., Dias, T. G., Mills, K. L., . . . Nigg, J. T. (2010). Atypical default network connectivity in youth with attention-deficit/hyperactivity disorder. *Biological Psychiatry, 68*, 1084–1091.

Faraone, S. V., Perlis, R. H., Doyle, A. E., Smoller, J. W., Goralnick, J. J., Holmgren, M. A., & Sklar, P. (2005). Molecular genetics of attention-deficit/hyperactivity disorder. *Biological Psychiatry, 57*, 1313–1323.

Franke, B., Faraone, S. V., Asherson, P., Buitelaar, J., Bau, C. H., Ramos-Quiroga, J. A., . . . Reif, A. (2011). The genetics of attention deficit/hyperactivity disorder in adults, a review. *Molecular Psychiatry, 18*, 1–28.

Gatzke-Kopp L. M., & Beauchaine T. P. (2007). Direct and passive prenatal nicotine exposure and the development of externalizing psychopathology. *Child Psychiatry Hum Dev, 38*, 255–269.

Gaub, M., & Carlson, C. L. (1997). Gender differences in ADHD: A meta-analysis and critical review. *Journal of the American Academy of Child and Adolescent Psychiatry, 36*, 1036–1045.

Giedd, J. N., Blumenthal, J., Molloy, E., & Castellanos, F. X. (2001). Brain imaging of attention deficit/hyperactivity disorder. *Annals of the New York Academy of Sciences, 931*, 33–49.

Gizer, I. R., Waldman, I. D., Abramowitz, A., Barr, C. L., Feng, Y., Wigg, K. G., . . . Rowe, D. C. (2008). Relations between multi-informant assessments of ADHD symptoms, DAT1, and DRD4. *Journal of Abnormal Psychology, 117*, 869–880.

Goldsmith, H. H., Lemery, K. S., & Essex, M. J. (Eds.). (2004). *Temperament as a liability factor for childhood behavior disorders: The concept of liability.* Washington, DC: APA Press.

Gordan, M., Shtshel, K., Faraone, S. V., Barkely, R., Lewandowski, L., & Hudziak, J. (2005). Symptoms versus impairment: The case for respecting DSM-IV's criterion D. *ADHD Report, 13*, 1–9.

Goth-Owens, T. L., Martinez-Torteya, C., Martel, M. M., & Nigg, J. T. (2010). Processing speed weakness in children and adolescents with non-hyperactive but inattentive ADHD (ADD). *Child Neuropsychology, 16*, 577–591.

Hart, E. L., Lahey, B. B., Loeber, R., Applegate, B., & Frick, P. J. (1995). Developmental change in attention-deficit hyperactivity disorder in boys: A four-year longitudinal study. *Journal of Abnormal Child Psychology, 23*, 729–749.

Hinshaw, S. P., & Blachman, D. R. (Eds.). (2005). *Attention-deficit/hyperactivity disorder.* New York, NY: Kluwer Academic/Plenum.

Hinshaw, S. P., Carte, E. T., Sami, N., Treuting, J. J., & Zupan, B. A. (2002). Preadolescent girls with attention-deficit/hyperactivity disorder: II. Neuropsychological performance in relation to subtypes and individual classification. *Journal of Consulting and Clinical Psychology, 70,* 1099–1111.

Hinshaw, S. P., Scheffler, R. M., Fulton, B. D., Aase, H., Banaschewski, T., Cheng, W., . . . Weiss, M. D. (2011). International variation in treatment procedures for ADHD: Social context and recent trends. *Psychiatric Services, 62,* 459–464.

Hopkins, M. R., Ettinger, A. S., Hernandez-Avila, M., Schwartz, J., Tellez-Rojo, M. M., Lamadrid-Figueroa, H., . . . Wright, R. O. (2008). Variants in iron metabolism genes predict higher blood lead levels in young children. *Environmental Health Perspectives, 116,* 1261–1266.

Huang-Pollock, C. L., & Nigg, J. T. (2003). Searching for the attention deficit in attention deficit hyperactivity disorder: The case of visuospatial orienting. [Meta-Analysis Research Support, U.S. Gov't, P.H.S.]. *Clinical Psychology Review, 23,* 801–830.

Huang-Pollock, C. L., Nigg, J. T., & Carr, T. H. (2005). Deficient attention is hard to find: Applying the perceptual load model of selective attention to attention deficit hyperactivity disorder subtypes. [Research Support, N.I.H., Extramural]. *Journal of Child Psychology and Psychiatry and Allied Disciplines, 46,* 1211–1218.

Jacobson, J. L., & Jacobson, S. W. (2003). Prenatal exposure to polychlorinated biphenyls and attention at school age. *Journal of Pediatrics, 143,* 780–788.

Jacobson, S. W., Jacobson, J. L., Sokol, R. J., Chiodo, L. M., & Corobana, R. (2004). Maternal age, alcohol abuse history, and quality of parenting as moderators of the effects of prenatal alcohol exposure on 7.5-year intellectual function. *Alcohol Clinical and Experimental Research, 28,* 1732–1745.

Jensen, P. S., Hinshaw, S. P., Kraemer, H. C., Lenora, N., Newcorn, J. H., Abikoff, H. B., . . . Vitiello, B. (2001). ADHD comorbidity findings from the MTA study: Comparing comorbid subgroups. *Journal of the American Academy of Child and Adolescent Psychiatry, 40,* 147–158.

Kagan, J., & Snidman, N. (2004). *The long shadow of temperament.* Cambridge, MA: Harvard University Press.

Kessler, R. C., Adler, L., Barkley, R., Biederman, J., Conners, C. K., Demler, O., . . . Zaslavsky, A. M. (2006). The prevalence and correlates of adult ADHD in the United States: Results from the national comorbidity survey replication. *American Journal of Psychiatry, 163,* 716–723.

Kieling, C., Kieling, R. R., Rohde, L. A., Frick, P. J., Moffitt, T., Nigg, J. T., . . . Castellanos, F. X. (2010). The age at onset of attention deficit hyperactivity disorder. *American Journal of Psychiatry, 167,* 14–16.

Lahey, B. B., Pelham, W. E., Stein, M. A., Loney, J., Trapani, C., Nugent, K., . . . Baumann, B. (1998). Validity of DSM-IV attention-deficit/hyperactivity disorder for younger children. *Journal of the American Academy of Child and Adolescent Psychiatry, 37,* 695–702.

Lang, H. C., Scheffler, R. M., & Hu, T. W. (2010). The discrepancy in attention deficit hyperactivity disorder (ADHD) medications diffusion: 1994–2003—A global pharmaceutical data analysis. *Health Policy, 97,* 71–78.

Lasky-Su, J., Anney, R. J., Neale, B. M., Franke, B., Zhou, K., Maller, J. B., . . . Faraone, S. V. (2008). Genome-wide association scan of the time to onset of attention deficit hyperactivity disorder. *American Journal of Medical Genetics Part B, Neuropsychiatric Genetics, 147B,* 1355–1358.

Logan, G. D. (Ed.). (1994). *A user's guide to the stop signal paradigm.* San Diego, CA: Academic Press.

Losier, B. J., McGrath, P. J., & Klein, R. M. (1996). Error patterns on the continuous performance test in non-medicated and medicated samples of children with and without ADHD: A meta-analytic review. *Journal of Child Psychology and Psychiatry, 37,* 971–987.

Luman, M., Oosterlaan, J., & Sergeant, J. A. (2005). The impact of reinforcement contingencies on AD/HD: A review and theoretical appraisal. *Clinical Psychology Review, 25,* 183–213.

Mann, E. M., Ikeda, Y., Mueller, C. W., Takahashi, A., Tao, K. T., Humris, E., . . . Chin, D. (1992). Cross-cultural differences in rating hyperactive-disruptive behaviors in children. *American Journal of Psychiatry, 149,* 1539–1542.

Mannuzza, S., & Klein, R. G. (2000). Long-term prognosis in attention-deficit/ hyperactivity disorder. *Child and Adolescent Psychiatric Clinics of North America, 9,* 711–726.

Marks, A. R., Harley, K., Bradman, A., Kogut, K., Barr, D. B., Johnson, C., . . . Eskenazi, B. (2010). Organophosphate pesticide exposure and attention in young Mexican-American children: The CHAMACOS study. *Environmental Health Perspectives, 118,* 1768–1774.

Martel, M. M., & Nigg, J. T. (2006). Child ADHD and personality/temperament traits of reactive and effortful control, resiliency, and emotionality. *Journal of Child Psychololgy and Psychiatry, 47,* 1175–1183.

Martinussen, R., Hayden, J., Hogg-Johnson, S., & Tannock, R. (2005). A meta-analysis of working memory impairments in children with attention-deficit/hyperactivity disorder. *Journal of the American Academy of Child and Adolescent Psychiatry, 44,* 377–384.

Merikangas, K. R., He, J. P., Brody, D., Fisher, P. W., Bourdon, K., & Koretz, D. S. (2010). Prevalence and treatment of mental disorders among US children in the 2001–2004 NHANES. *Pediatrics, 125,* 75–81.

Mick, E., Biederman, J., Faraone, S. V., Sayer, J., & Kleinman, S. (2002). Case–control study of attention-deficit hyperactivity disorder and maternal smoking, alcohol use, and drug use during pregnancy. *Journal of the American Academy of Child and Adolescent Psychiatry, 41,* 378–385.

Morbidity and Mortality Weekly Report. (2010). Increasing prevalence of parent-reported attention-deficit/hyperactivity disorder among children: United States, 2003 and 2007. *Morbidity and Mortality Weekly Report, 59,* 1439–1443.

MTA Cooperative Group. (1999). A 14-month randomized clinical trial of treatment strategies for attention-deficit/hyperactivity disorder. *Archives of General Psychiatry, 56,* 1073–1086.

Mueller, C. W., Mann, E. M., Thanapum, S., Humris, E., Ikeda, Y., & Takahashi, A. (1995). Teachers ratings of disruptive behavior in five countries. *Journal of Clinical Child Psychology, 24,* 434–442.

Murphy, K. R., Barkley, R. A., & Bush, T. (2001). Executive functioning and olfactory identification in young adults with attention deficit-hyperactivity disorder. *Neuropsychology, 15,* 211–220.

Nagel, B. J., Bathula, D., Herting, M., Schmitt, C., Kroenke, C. D., Fair, D., & Nigg, J. T. (2011). Altered white matter microstructure in children with attention-deficit/hyperactivity disorder. *Journal of the American Academy of Child and Adolescent Psychiatry, 50,* 283–292.

Nigg, J. T. (2001). Is ADHD a disinhibitory disorder? *Psychological Bulletin, 127,* 571–598.

Nigg, J. T. (2006a). Temperament and developmental psychopathology. *Journal of Child Psychology and Psychiatry, 47,* 395–422.

Nigg, J. T. (2006b). *What causes ADHD?: Understanding what goes wrong and why.* New York, NY: Guilford Press.

Nigg, J. T., Blaskey, L. G., Huang-Pollock, C. L., & Rappley, M. D. (2002). Neuropsychological executive functions and DSM-IV ADHD subtypes. [Research Support, U.S. Gov't, P.H.S.]. *Journal of the American Academy of Child and Adolescent Psychiatry, 41,* 59–66.

Nigg, J. T., & Casey, B. J. (2005). An integrative theory of attention-deficit/hyperactivity disorder based on the cognitive and affective neurosciences. *Development and Psychopathology, 17,* 785–806.

Nigg, J. T., Hinshaw, S. P., & Huang-Pollack, C. (Eds.). (2006). *Disorders of attention and impulse regulation.* New York, NY: Wiley.

Nigg, J. T., Knottnerus, G. M., Martel, M. M., Nikolas, M., Cavanagh, K., Karmaus, W., & Rappley, M. D. (2008). Low blood lead levels associated with clinically diagnosed attention-deficit/hyperactivity disorder and mediated by weak cognitive control. [Research Support, N.I.H., Extramural Research Support, Non-U.S. Gov't]. *Biological Psychiatry, 63,* 325–331.

Nigg, J. T., Lewis, K., Edinger, T., & Falk, M. (2012). Meta-analysis of attention-deficit/hyperactivity disorder or attention-deficit/hyperactivity disorder symptoms, restriction diet, and synthetic food color additives. *Journal of the American Academy of Child and Adolescent Psychiatry, 51,* 86–97.

Nigg, J. T., Nikolas, M., & Burt, S. A. (2010a). Measured gene-by-environment interaction in relation to attention-deficit/hyperactivity disorder. *Journal of the American Academy of Child and Adolescent Psychiatry, 49,* 863–873.

Nigg, J. T., Nikolas, M., Friderici, K., Park, L., & Zucker, R. A. (2007). Genotype and neuropsychological response inhibition as resilience promoters for ADHD, ODD, and CD under conditions of psychosocial adversity. *Development and Psychopathology, 19,* 767–786.

Nigg, J. T., Nikolas, M., Knottnerus, G., Cavanagh, K., & Friderici, K. (2010b). Confirmation and extension of association of blood lead with attention-deficit/hyperactivity disorder (ADHD) and ADHD symptom domains at population-typical exposure levels. *Journal of Child Psychology and Psychiatry, 51*, 58–65.

Nigg, J. T., Stavro, G., Ettenhofer, M., Hambrick, D. Z., Miller, T., & Henderson, J. M. (2005). Executive functions and ADHD in adults: Evidence for selective effects on ADHD symptom domains. *Journal of Abnormal Psychology, 114*, 706–717.

Nikolas, M. A., & Burt, S. A. (2010). Genetic and environmental influences on ADHD symptom dimensions of inattention and hyperactivity: A meta-analysis. *Journal of Abnormal Psychology, 119*, 1–17.

Pelham, W. E. Jr., Fabiano, G. A., & Massetti, G. M. (2005). Evidence-based assessment of attention deficit hyperactivity disorder in children and adolescents. *Journal of Clinical Child and Adolescent Psychology, 34*, 449–476.

Piek, J. P., Pitcher, T. M., & Hay, D. A. (1999). Motor coordination and kinaesthesis in boys with attention deficit-hyperactivity disorder. *Developments in Medical Child Neurology, 41*, 159–165.

Poelmans, G., Pauls, D. L., Buitelaar, J. K., & Franke, B. (2011). Integrated genome-wide association study findings: Identification of a neurodevelopmental network for attention deficit hyperactivity disorder. *American Journal of Psychiatry, 168*, 365–377.

Polanczyk, G., de Lima, M. S., Horta, B. L., Biederman, J., & Rohde, L. A. (2007). The worldwide prevalence of ADHD: A systematic review and metaregression analysis. *American Journal of Psychiatry, 164*, 942–948.

Posner, M. I., & Petersen, S. E. (1990). The attention system of the human brain. *Annual Review of Neuroscience, 13*, 25–42.

Reid, R., DuPaul, G. J., Power, T. J., Anastopoulos, A. D., Rogers-Adkinson, D., Noll, M. B., & Riccio, C. (1998). Assessing culturally different students for attention deficit hyperactivity disorder using behavior rating scales. *Journal of Abnormal Child Psychology, 26*, 187–198.

Rhee, S. H., Waldman, I. D., Hay, D. A., & Levy, F. (1999). Sex differences in genetic and environmental influences on DSM-III-R attention-deficit/hyperactivity disorder. *Journal of Abnormal Psychology, 108*, 24–41.

Rietveld, M. J., Hudziak, J. J., Bartels, M., van Beijsterveldt, C. E., & Boomsma, D. I. (2004). Heritability of attention problems in children: Longitudinal results from a study of twins, age 3 to 12. *Journal of Child Psychology and Psychiatry, 45*, 577–588.

Robison, L. M., Sclar, D. A., Skaer, T. L., & Galin, R. S. (1999). National trends in the prevalence of attention-deficit/hyperactivity disorder and the prescribing of methylphenidate among school-age children: 1990–1995. *Clinical Pediatrics, 38*, 209–217.

Rohde, L. A., Szobot, C., Polanczyk, G., Schmitz, M., Martins, S., & Tramontina, S. (2005). Attention-deficit/hyperactivity disorder in a diverse culture: Do research and clinical findings support the notion of a cultural construct for the disorder? *Biological Psychiatry, 57*, 1436–1441.

Rothbart, M. K., & Bates, J. E. (Eds.). (1998). *Temperament*. New York, NY: Wiley.

Rucklidge, J. J., & Tannock, R. (2001). Psychiatric, psychosocial, and cognitive functioning of female adolescents with ADHD. *Journal of the American Academy of Child and Adolescent Psychiatry, 40,* 530–540.

Rush, B. (1812/1962). *Medical inquiries and observations upon the diseases of the mind.* New York, NY: Macmillan-Hafner Press.

Sagiv, S. K., Thurston, S. W., Bellinger, D. C., Tolbert, P. E., Altshul, L. M., & Korrick, S. A. (2010). Prenatal organochlorine exposure and behaviors associated with attention deficit hyperactivity disorder in school-aged children. *American Journal of Epidemiology, 171,* 593–601.

Sagvolden, T., Johansen, E. B., Aase, H., & Russell, V. A. (2005). A dynamic developmental theory of attention-deficit/hyperactivity disorder (ADHD) predominantly hyperactive/impulsive and combined subtypes. *Behavioral and Brain Sciences, 28,* 397–419; discussion 419–368.

Saudino, K. J. (2003). Parent ratings of infant temperament: Lessons from twin studies. *Infant Behavior and Development, 26,* 118–120.

Scheffler, R. M., Hinshaw, S. P., Modrek, S., & Levine, P. (2007). The global market for ADHD medications. *Health Affairs, 26,* 450–457.

Seidman, L. J., Biederman, J., Monuteaux, M. C., Valera, E., Doyle, A. E., & Faraone, S. V. (2005). Impact of gender and age on executive functioning: Do girls and boys with and without attention deficit hyperactivity disorder differ neuropsychologically in preteen and teenage years? *Developmental Neuropsychology, 27,* 79–105.

Seidman, L. J., Valera, E. M., & Makris, N. (2005). Structural brain imaging of attention-deficit/hyperactivity disorder. *Biological Psychiatry, 57,* 1263–1272.

Sergeant J. A., Oosterlaan J., & van der Meere J. (1999). Information processing and energetic factors in attention-deficit/hyperactivity disorder. In H. C. Quay & A. E. Hogan (Eds.), *Handbook of disruptive behavior disorders* (pp. 75–104). NY: Kluwer Academic/Plenum.

Sergeant, J. A., & van der Meere, J. J. (1998). What happens after a hyperactive child commits an error? *Psychological Research, 24,* 157–164.

Setlik, J., Bond, G. R., & Ho, M. (2009). Adolescent prescription ADHD medication abuse is rising along with prescriptions for these medications. *Pediatrics, 124,* 875–880.

Shaw, P., Greenstein, D., Lerch, J., Clasen, L., Lenroot, R., Gogtay, N., . . . Giedd, J. (2006). Intellectual ability and cortical development in children and adolescents. *Nature, 440,* 676–679.

Simon, V., Czobor, P., Balint, S., Meszaros, A., & Bitter, I. (2009). Prevalence and correlates of adult attention-deficit hyperactivity disorder: Meta-analysis. *British Journal of Psychiatry, 194,* 204–211.

Simonoff, E., Pickles, A., Hervas, A., Silberg, J. L., Rutter, M., & Eaves, L. (1998). Genetic influences on childhood hyperactivity: Contrast effects imply parental rating bias, not sibling interaction. *Psychological Medicine, 28,* 825–837.

Sonuga-Barke, E. J. (2005). Causal models of attention-deficit/hyperactivity disorder: From common simple deficits to multiple developmental pathways. *Biological Psychiatry, 57,* 1231–1238.

Stergiakouli, E., Hamshere, M., Holmans, P., Langley, K., Zaharieva, I., Hawi, Z., . . . Thapar, A. (2012). Investigating the contribution of common genetic variants to the risk and pathogenesis of ADHD. *American Journal of Psychiatry, 169*, 186–194.

Stevenson, J., Sonuga-Barke, E., McCann, D., Grimshaw, K., Parker, K. M., Rose-Zerilli, M. J., . . . Warner, J. O. (2010). The role of histamine degradation gene polymorphisms in moderating the effects of food additives on children's ADHD symptoms. *American Journal of Psychiatry, 167*, 1108–1115.

Taylor, E. (2011). Antecedents of ADHD: A historical account of diagnostic concepts. *Attention Deficit Hyperactivity Disorder, 3*, 69–75.

Thapar, A., Rice, F., Hay, D., Boivin, J., Langley, K., van den Bree, M., . . . Harold, G. (2009). Prenatal smoking might not cause attention-deficit/hyperactivity disorder: Evidence from a novel design. *Biological Psychiatry, 66*, 722–727.

Toplak M. E., Dockstader C., & Tannock R. (2006). Temporal information processing in ADHD: Findings to date and new methods. *J. Neurosci. Methods, 151*, 15–29.

Toplak, M. E., Sorge, G. B., Flora, D. B., Chen, W., Banaschewski, T., Buitelaar, J., . . . Faraone, S. V. (2012). The hierarchical factor model of ADHD: Invariant across age and national groupings? *Journal of Child Psychology and Psychiatry, 53*, 292–303.

Toplak, M. E., & Tannock, R. (2005). Time perception: Modality and duration effects in attention-deficit/hyperactivity disorder (ADHD). *Journal of Abnormal Child Psychology, 33*, 639–654.

Tully, L. A., Arseneault, L., Caspi, A., Moffitt, T. E., & Morgan, J. (2004). Does maternal warmth moderate the effects of birth weight on twins' attention-deficit/hyperactivity disorder (ADHD) symptoms and low IQ? *Journal of Consulting Clinical Psychology, 72*, 218–226.

Uddin, L. Q., Kelly, A. M., Biswal, B. B., Margulies, D. S., Shehzad, Z., Shaw, D., . . . Milham, M. P. (2008). Network homogeneity reveals decreased integrity of default-mode network in ADHD. *Journal of Neuroscientific Methods, 169*, 249–254.

Visser, S. N., Bitsko, R. H., Danielson, M. I., & Perou, R. (2010). Increasing prevalence of parent-reports attention-deficit/hyperactivity disorder among children—United States, 2003 and 2007. *Morbidity and Mortality Weekly Report, 59*, 1439–1443.

Volk, H. E., Todorov, A. A., Hay, D. A., & Todd, R. D. (2009). Simple identification of complex ADHD subtypes using current symptom counts. *Journal of the American Academy of Child and Adolescent Psychiatry, 48*, 441–450.

Willcutt, E. G. (in press). Genetics of ADHD. In D. M. Barch (Ed.), *Cognitive and affective neuroscience of psychopathology*. New York, NY: Oxford University Press.

Willcutt, E. G., Doyle, A. E., Nigg, J. T., Faraone, S. V., & Pennington, B. F. (2005). Validity of the executive function theory of attention-deficit/hyperactivity disorder: A meta-analytic review. [Meta-Analysis Research Support, N.I.H., Extramural Research Support, U.S. Gov't, P.H.S. Review]. *Biological Psychiatry, 57*, 1336–1346.

Willcutt, E. G., Nigg, J. T., Pennington, B. F., Solanto, M. V., Rohde, L. A., Tannock, R., . . . Lahey, B. B. (in press). Validity of DSM-IV attention deficit/hyperactivity disorder symptom dimensions and subtypes. *Journal of Abnormal Psychology*.

Willcutt, E. G., Pennington, B. F., & DeFries, J. C. (2000). Etiology of inattention and hyperactivity/impulsivity in a community sample of twins with learning difficulties. *Journal of Abnormal Child Psychology, 28,* 149–159.

Williams, N. M., Franke, B., Mick, E., Anney, R. J., Freitag, C. M., Gill, M., . . . Faraone, S. V. (2012). Genome-wide analysis of copy number variants in attention deficit hyperactivity disorder: The role of rare variants and duplications at 15q13.3. *American Journal of Psychiatry, 169,* 195–204.

World Health Organization. (1993). *International classification of disease* (10th ed.). Geneva, Switzerland.

Yang, K. N., Schaller, J. L., & Parker, R. (2000). Factor structures of Taiwanese teachers' ratings of ADHD: A comparison with U.S. studies. *Journal of Learning Disabilities, 33,* 72–82.

# CHAPTER 13

# Oppositional Defiant Disorder, Conduct Disorder, and Juvenile Delinquency

IRWIN D. WALDMAN AND BENJAMIN B. LAHEY

## INTRODUCTION

NTISOCIAL BEHAVIORS ARE AMONG the most common behavior problems and significant symptoms of psychiatric disorders in childhood and adolescence, and among the most refractory to treatment. Children and adolescents who persistently violate laws and important social rules are seriously impaired in their social relationships and at risk for a range of adverse sequelae, including incarceration and violent death (Loeber & Stouthamer-Loeber, 1998; Moffitt, Caspi, Rutter, & Silva, 2001), marital problems and divorce (Robins, 1966), under- and unemployment (Robins, 1966), and various forms of substance abuse (Robins, 1966). Antisocial behavior also harms others in a variety of ways, from the loss of property to death by homicide (Loeber et al., 2005).

## TERMINOLOGICAL AND CONCEPTUAL ISSUES

A number of constructs have been developed to conceptualize and label antisocial behavior in youth. The term *juvenile delinquency* is used in the criminal justice system to refer to children and adolescents who have broken a law. This is a broad term that refers to anything from sneaking into a movie without a ticket to homicide. In the *Diagnostic and Statistical Manual of Mental Disorders–Fourth Edition (DSM-IV;* American Psychiatric Association, 1994), two diagnoses are directly relevant to antisocial behavior in youth: conduct disorder (CD) and oppositional defiant disorder (ODD).

Preparation of this chapter was supported in part by grants R01 MH070025 and R01 MH53554 from the National Institute of Mental Health.

Conduct disorder refers to engaging in at least 3 from a list of 15 antisocial behaviors within a 12 month period. CD only partially overlaps with delinquency for three reasons. First, not all juvenile crimes are symptoms of CD (e.g., selling drugs, receiving stolen property). Second, some symptoms of CD do not necessarily violate laws (e.g., bullying, staying out late without permission). Third, CD describes youth who frequently engage in a variety (i.e., at least three) of antisocial behaviors in a relatively short time frame, whereas a youth could be considered to be delinquent on the basis of a single criminal act.

Oppositional defiant disorder is also related to antisocial behavior in youth. ODD is defined as frequently engaging in at least 4 disruptive interpersonal behaviors, including arguing with adults, actively defying adult requests, and spiteful or vindictive behavior, for at least 6 months. ODD often severely impairs social relationships of children and adolescents (Lahey et al., 1994) and is intimately linked to CD, often representing a precursor condition.

It is important to note that many researchers believe that the *DSM-IV* diagnoses of both ODD and CD reflect arbitrary dichotomizations of what are probably continua (Boyle et al., 1996; Lahey et al., 1994). That is, youth do not suddenly shift from *normality* to *abnormality* when they engage in their fourth ODD symptom or their third CD symptom. Rather, the more symptoms of ODD or CD that a youth exhibits, the more serious the consequences for the youth and others. Another reason for caution regarding *DSM-IV* diagnostic definitions is that Rowe, Maughan, Costello, and Angold (2005) noted a large "hole" in the diagnosis of ODD. In the 10th edition of the International Classification of Diseases (ICD-10; World Health Organization [WHO], 1993), ODD is defined by the same symptoms as in *DSM-IV*, but in a different way. In ICD-10, if a youth does not meet diagnostic criteria for either ODD or CD, the total number of ODD plus CD symptoms is counted. If there are four such ODD + CD symptoms, the youth meets criteria for ODD. Rowe et al. (2005) found that this large group of youth was as impaired in its social functioning as youth who met *DSM-IV* criteria for ODD. It is not surprising that youth who exhibit three symptoms of ODD and one or two symptoms of CD (i.e., who fall short of the diagnostic criteria for either disorder) would be impaired. Similar findings were obtained in a recent study (Burke, Waldman, & Lahey, 2010) in which treating CD symptoms as ODD symptoms when diagnostic criteria for CD were not met identified more functionally impaired children than the more restrictive *DSM-IV* definition of ODD, thus showing the validity and virtue of plugging this diagnostic "hole."

Although there are important differences among the constructs of juvenile delinquency, ODD, and CD, it is necessary to refer collectively to all three constructs in this chapter for the sake of brevity and clarity. For this purpose, the terms *conduct problems* and *antisocial behavior* refer collectively to juvenile delinquency, ODD, and CD. Similarly, the term *youth* refers collectively to both children and adolescents in this chapter.

## COMORBIDITY

One cannot view any form of psychopathology as if it were separate from all others. Youth who meet diagnostic criteria for any mental disorder are considerably more likely than chance to meet criteria for other mental disorders (Angold, Costello, & Erkanli, 1999; Lahey et al., 2004; Nottelmann & Jensen, 1995). That is, co-occurrence of symptoms and diagnoses (or comorbidity) is the rule, not the exception. ODD and CD often co-occur, and both disorders often co-occur with attention-deficit/hyperactivity disorder (ADHD; Angold et al., 1999; Lahey, Miller, Gordon, & Riley, 1999). In addition, ODD and CD often co-occur with depression (Angold et al., 1999; Lahey et al., 2002; Rowe, Maughan, & Eley, 2006).

Some investigators view comorbidity as a problem for taxonomies of mental disorders (Rutter, 1997), whereas others view comorbidity as the inevitable result of the nearly ubiquitous correlations among symptoms of different disorders (Lahey et al., 2008; Lahey, Applegate et al., 2004). In the latter view, comorbidity is informative rather than problematic. For example, CD is impairing and requires intervention regardless of whether it occurs alone or in the presence of symptoms of other disorders. On the other hand, a youth who meets criteria for CD and another disorder such as major depression may well need treatment for each disorder. In addition, viewing comorbidity as informative facilitates the study of both the common and distinct causal influences on different forms of psychopathology. This perspective recently has gained momentum at the National Institute of Mental Health, which is investing in novel research strategies that will examine basic biological and psychological mechanisms that cut across traditional diagnostic boundaries (Insel & Wang, 2010). Such studies should shed new light on the phenomenon and causes of comorbidity.

## THE NEED TO CONSIDER DEVELOPMENTAL AND SEX DIFFERENCES

It is important in discussing any mental disorder to take a *developmental perspective* (see Chapter 1). In this chapter, conduct problems are considered from four different developmental perspectives: (1) developmental trajectories of conduct problems; (2) age differences in the prevalence of conduct problems; (3) childhood characteristics that predict later conduct problems; and (4) the adolescent and adult outcomes of childhood conduct problems.

Similarly, it also is important to consider potential differences between females and males when considering the development of conduct problems. Although conduct problems are prevalent and problematic in both sexes, they are considerably more common in males (Lahey et al., 2006; Moffitt et al., 2001). Because the sex difference in the prevalence of childhood conduct problems is large, especially for aggression, it will be necessary for the field to understand the causes of sex differences to fully understand the causes of conduct problems themselves. For the same reason, a theory of the origins of conduct problems that does not explain the origins of sex differences would be incomplete, if not inaccurate, for one or both sexes.

## PREVALENCE AND AGE OF ONSET

### DEVELOPMENTAL TRAJECTORIES OF CONDUCT PROBLEMS

Many have suggested that one can only understand youth conduct problems by distinguishing between different *developmental trajectories* of behavior (e.g., Farrington,

1991; Hinshaw, Lahey, & Hart, 1993; Loeber, 1988; Moffitt, 1993; Patterson, Reid, & Dishion, 1992; Quay, 1987). In this context, a *trajectory* is a more or less distinct temporal pattern of conduct problems that each youth engages in from early childhood through adolescence. For example, two 17-year-olds arrested for shoplifting might have very different developmental trajectories. One may have exhibited no symptoms of CD as a child and had never broken a law until skipping school and shoplifting for the first time at age 17. The other might have continuously met criteria for CD since early childhood, shoplifted dozens of times before, and committed many other crimes since middle childhood. Such differences in developmental trajectories may reveal a great deal about differences in the causes of those conduct problems.

Moffitt (1993, 2003) proposed that youth who follow two different trajectories engage in delinquency for qualitatively different reasons. According to Moffitt, a relatively small number of youth follow a *childhood-onset* (or *life-course persistent*) trajectory in which they exhibit symptoms of ADHD, ODD, and CD in childhood and engage in persistent conduct problems through adolescence and into adulthood. A larger group of youth follow an *adolescent-onset* (or *adolescence-limited*) trajectory in which they engage in relatively few conduct problems during childhood, first break laws during adolescence, and often desist from offending in early adulthood. Adolescent delinquency is common, but the exact numbers depend on how juvenile delinquency is defined. Approximately 10% to 21% engage in what Moffitt (1993) refers to as adolescent-onset delinquency, whereas 5% to 14% of youth exhibit childhood-onset delinquency (Lahey et al., 2006; Moffitt et al., 2001).

Moffitt (1993, 2003) hypothesized that childhood-onset conduct problems are caused by neurodevelopmental deficits, inadequate parenting, and adverse social influences, whereas adolescent-onset conduct problems are caused by peer influences during the transition to adulthood. For this reason, Moffitt has argued that studies of the causes of delinquency that do not distinguish these trajectories may produce disinformation that does not apply to either trajectory. In considering developmental trajectories, it also is important to note that many children who engage in high levels of childhood conduct problems do not do so in adolescence (Coté, Vaillancourt, Le Blanc, Nagin, & Tremblay, 2006; Moffitt, 2007; Moffitt, Caspi, Dickson, Silva, & Stanton, 1996; Raine et al., 2005) and that many adolescence-limited youth do not completely desist by adulthood (Chapter 14; Moffitt, 2007).

## ARE THERE SEX DIFFERENCES IN DEVELOPMENTAL TRAJECTORIES?

Essentially equal numbers of females and males exhibit adolescent-onset delinquency, but males outnumber females at least 3:1 in the childhood-onset trajectory (Lahey et al., 2006; Moffitt et al., 2001). Silverthorn and Frick (1999) suggested that females rarely follow the childhood-onset trajectory, but rather follow a trajectory unique to girls. Although this hypothesis stimulated research that clarified the nature of sex differences in delinquency, it has not been supported (Coté, Zoccolillo, Tremblay, Nagin, & Vitaro, 2001; Lahey et al., 2006; Moffitt et al., 2001). Instead it appears that girls follow both delinquency trajectories as Moffitt (1993, 2003) defines them, but there are fewer girls on a childhood-onset trajectory.

## ALTERNATIVE TO QUALITATIVE DEVELOPMENTAL TRAJECTORY MODELS

Lahey and Waldman (2003, 2005) suggest a different view of developmental trajectories. They agree with Moffitt (1993, 2003) that adolescent delinquents with high or low levels of childhood conduct problems tend to be antisocial for different reasons, but hypothesize a *continuum* of such differences rather than two qualitatively distinct trajectories. According to our view, there is a continuum ranging from those who were well behaved as children to those who were poorly behaved from the toddler years onward, with every gradation in levels and consistency of childhood behavior problems in between. It appears that there are two distinct groups of adolescent delinquents only when researchers arbitrarily divide them into two such groups. Nonetheless, because the notion of two distinct developmental trajectories is a useful heuristic, Moffitt's dichotomous terms are often used in this chapter for simplicity.

## RELATIONS AMONG ODD, CD, AND DEVELOPMENTAL TRAJECTORIES OF DELINQUENCY

Nearly all studies of developmental trajectories have examined delinquent behavior rather than ODD or CD. Thus, there currently is not enough information to know how many youth in Moffitt's two developmental trajectories of delinquency would meet diagnostic criteria for ODD or CD. Because most definitions of delinquency require only the commission of a single delinquent act, and because CD requires a variety of antisocial behaviors during the past 12 months, many delinquent youth do not meet criteria for CD. One study of CD suggested that most clinic-referred adolescents who meet criteria for CD reported that their CD behaviors began in childhood, with only a small percent reporting adolescent onset of CD (Lahey et al., 1998). In a stronger longitudinal study of a representative sample of girls, Coté et al. (2001) found that nearly all adolescent females who met criteria for CD had childhood-onset CD. These studies may suggest that the majority of youth who meet criteria for CD follow what Moffitt (1993, 2003) would define as a childhood-onset trajectory. On the other hand, there may be a group of youth who meet criteria for CD who have later ages of onset and who share risk factors and outcomes with adolescent-onset delinquency. Indeed, *DSM-IV* distinguishes between childhood- and adolescent-onset CD based on this premise. Unfortunately, the validity of these subtypes has not been studied extensively in large longitudinal studies (Lahey et al., 1998). There also is evidence that most youth on a childhood-onset trajectory of delinquency met criteria for ODD during childhood (Lahey et al., 2006), but more remains to be learned. This issue is also complicated by the overlap of the early- versus late-onset distinction with other possible criteria for subtyping, such as aggressive versus nonaggressive, and showing high versus low levels of callous unemotional traits, issues to which we return later in this chapter.

## AGE, SEX, AND PREVALENCE OF CONDUCT PROBLEMS

There are marked age differences in the numbers of youth who meet diagnostic criteria for ODD and CD from early childhood through adolescence. Although it is difficult to estimate the exact prevalence of ODD and CD in the general population, there is good evidence that ODD is more prevalent than CD during early childhood, but by adolescence the numbers of youth who meet criteria for ODD and CD are close to equal (Lahey, Miller et al., 1999; Loeber, Burke, Lahey, Winters, & Zera, 2000; Maughan, Rowe, Messer, Goodman, & Meltzer, 2004). This is because the prevalence of ODD either stays constant or declines somewhat from early childhood through adolescence (Lahey et al., 2000; Maughan et al., 2004), whereas the prevalence of CD increases from early childhood through adolescence. The age-related increase in the prevalence of CD is much greater in boys than girls, which means that the sex difference in CD is greatest during late adolescence (Lahey et al., 2000; Maughan et al., 2004; Moffitt et al., 2001), whereas boys appear to be somewhat more likely to meet criteria for ODD at all ages (Lahey et al., 2000; Maughan et al., 2004).

Rates of delinquency increase steeply with age until they peak at 16 or 17 years of age and then decline with increasing age almost as steeply, a developmental pattern known as the *age-crime curve* (Hirschi & Gottfredson, 1983). Given the age-crime curve, more than half of all crime is juvenile crime. This curve is consistent with Moffitt's (1993, 2003) view that youth on a childhood-onset trajectory are joined by the larger number of youth on an adolescent-onset trajectory, swelling the total number of adolescents who engage in delinquency. Males are more likely to engage in delinquency than females at all ages, but like the diagnosis of CD, the sex difference in delinquency is greatest when males are at the peak of their age-crime curve at 16 or 17 years of age (Farrington & Painter, 2004; Lahey et al., 2006; Moffitt et al., 2001). Current evidence is sketchy, but the age-crime curve might be flatter for females, with an earlier peak (Farrington & Painter, 2004; Lahey et al., 2006; Moffitt et al., 2001).

# CHILDHOOD CHARACTERISTICS THAT PREDICT CD AND DELINQUENCY

Many emotional and behavioral characteristics predict later CD and delinquency in children. In some cases, these behavioral characteristics may be viewed as *developmental precursors* that appear to be "juvenile forms" of later conduct problems. Other childhood characteristics do not resemble later conduct problems but are still useful predictors of future serious conduct problems. Knowledge of these predictors makes it possible to study children who are likely to develop a disorder *before* it emerges, facilitating both studies of the early causes of conduct problems and efforts to prevent them.

## CHILDHOOD PREDICTORS

The following early childhood characteristics predict serious conduct problems during later childhood and adolescence. It should be kept in mind, however, that none predicts adolescent antisocial behavior with a high degree of certainty.

*Temperament.* Several aspects of young children's temperamental dispositions predict later conduct problems (see Chapter 6). These include a tendency for young children to resist control by adults (Keily, Bates, Dodge, & Pettit, 2001), a tendency to respond to threat and frustrations with excessive negative emotions (Gilliom & Shaw, 2004; Waldman et al., 2011), a tendency to engage in daring and sensation seeking behaviors (Gilliom & Shaw, 2004; Raine, Reynolds, Venables, Mednick, & Farrington, 1998; Waldman et al., 2011), low levels of prosocial behavior (Coté et al., 2002; Waldman et al., 2011), and impulsivity/lack of persistence (Beauchaine, Hinshaw, & Pang, 2010; Henry, Caspi, Moffitt, & Silva, 1996).

*ODD and ADHD.* Although ODD is an important disorder in its own right, it also may be a developmental precursor to CD. ODD symptoms typically emerge earlier in childhood than most but not all CD symptoms, and the presence of ODD in early childhood predicts meeting criteria for CD in the future (Lahey, McBurnett, & Loeber, 2000; Rowe, Maughan, Pickles, Costello, & Angold, 2002). The percentage of children with ODD who go on to meet criteria for CD is not known precisely, but it appears to be $\geq 25\%$ (Lahey, Loeber, Quay, Frick, & Grimm, 1992). Conversely, it is likely that many children with ODD never meet criteria for CD (Lahey et al., 2000; Rowe et al., 2002). Some studies suggest that ADHD in early childhood also is an independent developmental precursor to later conduct problems (Beauchaine et al., 2010; Mannuzza et al., 1991; Mannuzza, Klein, Abikoff, & Moulton, 2004; Mannuzza, Klein, Bessler, Malloy, & LaPadula, 1993), whereas other longitudinal studies indicate that childhood ADHD does not predict future antisocial behavior when childhood CD is controlled (Lahey et al., 2000; Lilienfeld & Waldman, 1990). The hypothesis that childhood ADHD predicts later antisocial personality disorder (ASPD) is plausible, as ASPD is defined partly by impulsivity and irresponsibility—which are similar to key symptoms of ADHD—but the support for this hypothesis is quite inconsistent (see Chapter 12). One possible explanation for these confusing findings is that it may well be that the *combination* of childhood ADHD and CD is the key developmental precursor to adult ASPD (Beauchaine et al., 2010; Hinshaw et al., 1993; Lynam, 1998). More evidence is needed to resolve this, however.

*Early shyness and anxiety.* There is evidence that in the absence of early conduct problems, shyness and fearfulness in early childhood *decrease* risk for later conduct problems (Graham & Rutter, 1973; Kohlberg, Ricks, & Snarey, 1984; Mitchell & Rosa, 1981; Moffitt, Caspi, Harrington, & Milne, 2002; Sanson, Pedlow, Cann, Prior, & Oberklaid, 1996; see Chapter 7). In addition, delinquents with higher levels of anxiety are less likely to commit future crimes (Quay & Love, 1977). These findings are puzzling, as other studies show that anxiety disorders co-occur with conduct problems at greater than chance rates (Loeber & Keenan, 1994; Zoccolillo, 1992). It is possible that anxiety is heterogeneous and some aspects of anxiety (e.g., social inhibition) foster conduct problems whereas other aspects (e.g., high constraint) inhibit conduct problems (Lahey & Waldman, 2003). In addition, children with conduct problems and aggression who are socially withdrawn are at increased risk for persistent and serious conduct problems (Blumstein, Farrington, & Moitra, 1985; Kerr, Tremblay, Pagani-Kurtz, & Vitaro, 1997), as well as other forms of serious psychopathology and maladjustment as adolescents or adults (Serbin et al., 1998).

It seems likely, however, that "socially withdrawn" in these studies refers to a lack of interaction with other children, perhaps due to lack of interest in or rejection by others, and not to shyness that is secondary to social anxiety and fear (Rutter & Giller, 1983).

*Childhood cognitive skills and language.* Considerable research indicates that children with lower cognitive abilities are more likely to develop conduct problems (Elkins, Iacono, Doyle, & McGue, 1997; Fergusson, Horwood, & Ridder, 2005; Ge, Donnellan, & Wenk, 2001; Kratzer & Hodgins, 1999; Lynam, Moffitt, & Stouthamer-Loeber, 1993; Moffitt & Silva, 1988). This does not appear to be an artifact of low socioeconomic status (SES), the likelihood that more-intelligent youth avoid detection of their antisocial behavior, or low test motivation (Lynam et al., 1993; Moffitt & Silva, 1988). At this time it is not clear if deficits in specific cognitive abilities, such as executive functions (e.g., Morgan & Lilienfeld, 2000), versus lower general intelligence, are associated with conduct problems. There is some evidence, however, that a specific cluster of executive functions, memory, and language abilities may be associated with early onset conduct problems and aggression, even controlling for general intelligence (Giancola, Martin, Tarter, Pelham, & Moss, 1996; Raine et al., 2005; Seguin, Boulerice, Harden, Tremblay, & Pihl, 1999; Waldman, 1996).

Lower verbal intelligence is correlated with slower language development in early childhood (Sparks, Ganschow, & Thomas, 1996), and the latter is associated with the development of conduct problems (Baker & Cantwell, 1987; Beitchman et al., 2001; Cohen et al., 1998; Stattin & Klackenberg-Larsson, 1993). Keenan and Shaw (1997) suggested that slowly developing language makes the process of parental socialization of their toddler more difficult and more frustrating for both parent and child. Toddlers with better language skills can communicate their needs more clearly and are more likely to understand the rules and requests of adults, both of which facilitate socialization. Language development is slower on average in boys, which may be one reason why boys exhibit more conduct problems from age 4 on (Keenan & Shaw, 1997).

## Developmental Trajectories and Child Characteristics That Predict Serious Conduct Problems

It is revealing to examine childhood characteristics that predict future conduct problems while viewing developmental trajectories as continua (Lahey & Waldman, 2003) rather than as the two distinct groups defined by Moffitt (1993). A large longitudinal study of the offspring of a nationally representative sample of mothers found that adolescents who engaged in high levels of delinquency varied considerably in their levels of the childhood characteristics that predict later delinquency (Lahey et al., 2006). Youth who were highly delinquent during adolescence and who exhibited increasingly higher levels of childhood conduct problems had increasingly lower scores on cognitive ability tests, were progressively less sociable with interviewers and less compliant with adult instructions, and exhibited increasingly higher levels of ADHD and ODD symptoms. Thus, two qualitatively distinct trajectory groups did not emerge; rather, at each progressively higher number of childhood conduct problems, delinquent adolescents exhibited more maladaptive levels of the child characteristics that predict later delinquency.

A provocative finding is that preadolescent children who exhibit high levels of conduct problems during childhood exhibit similar levels of childhood precursors, including ADHD, ODD, maladaptive temperament, and cognitive ability scores (Lahey et al., 2006; Raine et al., 2005), *regardless of whether they improve* (i.e., are not delinquent during adolescence) *or go on to exhibit childhood-onset delinquency.* Thus, much remains to be learned about the factors that differentiate children with childhood conduct problems who improve from those who progress to engage in adolescent delinquency.

## ADOLESCENT AND ADULT OUTCOMES OF CHILDHOOD ODD AND CD

Another way to understand conduct problems in a developmental perspective is to examine the later mental health outcomes of children and adolescents with conduct problems. Although ODD and CD are important because they cause serious impairment during childhood, they also are important because they increase the likelihood of other serious mental disorders in adolescence and adulthood. It is crucial to remember that not all children with high levels of childhood conduct problems continue to manifest them or develop other problems (i.e., follow a life-course persistent trajectory); many children with childhood conduct problems outgrow them and do not develop serious mental disorders (Moffitt et al., 1996).

CD in childhood increases risk for criminal behavior in adolescence and adulthood (Fergusson et al., 2005; Kjelsberg, 2002) and for adult ASPD (Lahey, Loeber, Burke, & Applegate, 2005; Maughan & Rutter, 2001). ASPD is a pernicious syndrome characterized by irresponsible behavior, persistent crime, and aggression and violence. Children with CD who are from low-income families and exhibit more *nonaggressive* symptoms are particularly at risk for adult ASPD (Lahey et al., 2005). Nonetheless, the majority of children and adolescents with CD (perhaps 60% to 70%) do not progress to ASPD (Lahey et al., 2005; Maughan & Rutter, 2001; see Chapter 14).

It is also clear that adolescents who engage in high levels of delinquent behavior are at increased risk for criminal behavior during early adulthood (Piquero, Brame, & Moffitt, 2005), even though many such adolescents desist. Crime is not the only adverse outcome associated with CD and serious adolescent delinquency, however, as antisocial adolescents are also at increased risk for reduced education, substance dependence, early parenthood, poor work records, dependence on welfare, unsuccessful family relationships, incarceration and criminal records, dangerous driving, and accidental injuries and early death (Loeber et al., 2005; Loeber, Farrington, Stouthamer-Loeber, & Van Kammen, 1998; Moffitt et al., 2001). Moffitt et al. (1996) hypothesized that many of these outcomes "ensnare" youth in an antisocial and nonproductive future. Unfortunately, this provocative hypothesis has not yet been extensively tested.

Childhood ODD is associated with increased risk for later depressive disorders, whereas CD appears to indirectly increase risk for depression by causing stressful life events—such as expulsion from school, peer rejection, and incarceration—that precipitate depression (Burke, Loeber, Lahey, & Rathouz, 2005; Little & Garber, 2005; Patterson & Stoolmiller, 1991). Nonetheless, there is mounting evidence that CD and depression might also share a common neural vulnerability via orbitofrontal-limbic dysfunction (e.g., Rubia, 2011). Children who meet criteria for CD also are at increased risk for adolescent drug and alcohol abuse (Marshal & Molina, 2006). This is important because the risk of suicide is greatest among adolescents with comorbid CD, depression, and substance abuse (Brent et al., 2002; Fombonne, Wostear, Cooper, Harrington, & Rutter, 2001).

Adolescent and adult outcomes of serious conduct problems are quite poor for both males and females (Bardone, Moffitt, Caspi, & Dickson, 1996; Bardone et al., 1998; Moffitt et al., 2001). Nonetheless, there are sex differences in the extent to which females and males are impaired in each specific area of adult functioning (Moffitt et al., 2001). Males are particularly likely to exhibit criminal behavior, work problems, and substance abuse, whereas females are more likely to experience depression and suicidal behavior and have poor physical health.

## RISK FACTORS AND CAUSES OF CONDUCT PROBLEMS

An important goal for developmental psychopathologists in the 21st century is to move from cataloging lists of risk factors for conduct problems to understanding their underlying causal mechanisms (Lahey, Moffitt, & Caspi, 2003). There are many ways of doing this, but behavior genetics provides a particularly helpful framework (Rutter, 2006; see Chapter 3). It is possible to use genetically informative designs—various types of twin and adoption studies—to distinguish heritable from environmental influences on behavior (Rutter, 2006). For example, contrasting the similarity for a trait between pairs of identical (monozygotic) twins, who share all of their segregating genes, and fraternal (dizygotic) twins, who share on average 50% of their segregating genes, allows one to estimate the magnitude of genetic and environmental influences on a trait or disorder. When certain assumptions are met, finding greater resemblance among monozygotic than dizygotic twin pairs suggests genetic influences on the trait (Rutter, 2006).

Rhee and Waldman (2002) conducted a meta-analytic review of 51 twin and adoption studies of conduct problems. They found that genetic influences account for 41% of the variation in broadly defined antisocial behavior among individuals in the population. For the diagnosis of CD in particular, the magnitude of genetic influences was slightly higher (i.e., 50%). A small proportion (11%) of the variance in CD is attributable to aspects of the environment that siblings share in common and make them more similar (e.g., the family's financial resources), with the remainder (39%) attributable to aspects of the environment that siblings experience uniquely and make them different (e.g., only one sibling's being abused; different peer groups for different siblings) and to measurement error. There is evidence that the early childhood characteristics that predict later serious conduct problems, including difficult temperament and ADHD and ODD, are substantially influenced by genes (Saudino, 2005; Simonoff, 2001; Waldman, Rhee, Levy, & Hay, 2001).

Interestingly, findings from a recent study (Meier, Slutske, Heath, & Martin, 2011) suggest that although the *magnitude* of genetic and shared and nonshared environmental influences on childhood CD are highly similar for boys and girls, the *specific* genetic or shared environmental risk factors that predispose to CD may differ somewhat for boys and girls.

Thus, there is strong evidence that genetic influences account for a substantial proportion of the causal influences on conduct problems. It is unlikely, however, that genes influence complex human traits such as conduct problems in simple and direct ways alone (see Chapter 3). Rather, genes are likely to influence human behavior through complex interactions with the environment (Rutter, 2006). By understanding something of the interplay between genes and environments, we are in a better position to evaluate what is known about possible genetic and environmental influences later in the chapter.

## GENE–ENVIRONMENT CORRELATIONS

Genetic and environmental influences on conduct problems or other traits may be correlated in three ways (Plomin, DeFries, & Loehlin, 1977; Rutter, 2006; Scarr & McCartney, 1983). *Passive gene–environment correlation* ($r_{GE}$) describes situations in which genetic and environmental influences that are transmitted from parents to children are correlated. This is likely to occur for childhood conduct problems because children with high levels of such problems often have antisocial parents who transmit genes that predispose to antisocial behavior as well as provide aspects of the environment (e.g., young parental age at childbirth, lower parental supervision, increased use of harsh discipline) that represent risk factors for the development of childhood conduct problems (Lahey et al., 1988; Lahey, Russo, Walker, & Piacentini, 1989; Nagin, Pogarsky, & Farrington, 1997). Passive $r_{GE}$ is important because children who are genetically at risk for conduct problems are raised by antisocial parents who are unlikely to provide the skilled child rearing that attenuates the development of conduct problems.

*Evocative or reactive* $r_{GE}$ describes a situation in which the child's genetically influenced characteristics change the environment in ways that make it more likely (positive reactive $r_{GE}$) or less likely (negative reactive $r_{GE}$) that he or she will manifest a particular trait or disorder. Several inappropriate methods of parenting are associated with conduct problems in children (Patterson et al., 1992) and likely represent examples of reactive $r_{GE}$. Unfortunately, young children with ODD and early conduct problems—conditions that are at least moderately genetically influenced—tend to *evoke* exactly the kinds of coercive, harsh, rejecting, and inconsistent parenting behaviors that appear to contribute to the development of their later conduct problems (Anderson, Lytton, & Romney, 1986; Ge et al., 1996; Sanson & Prior, 1999). In this way, genes that influence childhood temperament and ODD become evocatively correlated with adverse parenting environmental risk factors.

*Active* $r_{GE}$ describes a situation in which the child's genetically influenced characteristics lead them to seek out environments that are related to a particular trait or disorder. For example, some children selectively form friendships with delinquent peers who foster their delinquent behavior. There is evidence that a child's association with delinquent peers is itself genetically influenced (Rowe & Osgood, 1984), suggesting this as an instance of active $r_{GE}$ (see Chapter 14).

## Gene × Environment Interaction

There also are three kinds of evidence that conduct problems are influenced by *gene–environment interactions* (G × E). First, genetic influences on childhood conduct problems can be mitigated by favorable social learning environments. Evidence for this kind of G × E comes from adoption studies, which show that the adopted-away offspring of antisocial biological parents have fewer conduct problems when they are raised by well-adjusted adoptive parents than by antisocial adoptive parents (Bohman, 1996; Cadoret, Yates, Troughton, Woodward, & Stewart, 1995). Second, in the aforementioned meta-analysis (Rhee & Waldman, 2002), the magnitude of genetic and environmental influences on antisocial behavior differed by a host of moderators, including operationalization, assessment method, zygosity determination method, and age, suggesting that the causal influences on antisocial behavior are highly malleable as a function of personal, situational, or methodological characteristics. Third, there is growing evidence that different individuals respond in different ways to the same experiences partly because of differences in their genes. Findings on this kind of G × E will be summarized in the section below on molecular genetics.

## Potential Environmental Causes of Conduct Problems

In this section, findings on aspects of the child's environment that are potential causes of conduct problems are reviewed. In reading this section one should keep in mind that correlation does not imply causation; thus, conduct problems may be correlated with a variable that is not itself causal, but that is correlated due to the effects of some common causal influence.

*Birth weight and birth complications.* A number of pregnancy and birth factors are correlated with the development of serious conduct problems (Brennan, Grekin, & Mednick, 2003), including birth complications (e.g., lack of oxygen to the fetus during labor) and low birth weight (Brennan et al., 2003; see Chapter 10), particularly in disorganized families with few resources (Arseneault, Tremblay, Boulerice, & Saucier, 2002). This finding might indicate that better-functioning families provide environments that lessen the negative effects of birth complications, but it is not usually possible to determine whether birth complications have a causal effect, or are related to various outcomes because of the many genetically and environmentally influenced variables that are correlated with them. Nonetheless, studies of genetically informative samples have provided evidence that at least some perinatal factors appear to have a causal effect on risk for conduct problems (Raz, Shah, & Sander, 1996). For example, because monozygotic twins share all of their segregating genes and share all aspects of the environment that are common to twins who grow up in the same home, finding differences between monozygotic twins in their conduct problems that are related to differentially experiencing a particular birth complication would provide strong evidence that it plays a causal role. For example, van Os et al. (2001) found that the monozygotic twin with the lower birth weight was more likely to develop conduct problems. The suggestion is that low birth weight itself (or some prenatal complication that gives rise to low birth weight) may play a causal role, perhaps because low birth weight is associated with alterations in brain systems involved in risk for conduct problems (Brennan et al., 2003). Yet the magnitude of this relation throughout the full range of birth weight is likely to be quite small (Ficks, Lahey, & Waldman, manuscript submitted for publication), although there may be a stronger relation at the extremes. Other studies suggest that birth complications interact with genetic risk for conduct problems (Wichers et al., 2002). There is also inconsistent evidence that the correlation between birth complications and conduct problems may be stronger among males (Brennan et al., 2003).

*Maternal cigarette smoking and substance use during pregnancy.* Women who smoke, drink alcohol, or use drugs such as cocaine during pregnancy are considerably more likely to have children who develop conduct problems, even when other maternal characteristics known to be associated with conduct problems in their children are controlled (Brennan et al., 2003; Wakschlag, Pickett, Cook, Benowitz, & Leventhal, 2002; see Chapter 9). This suggests that toxic substances such as carbon monoxide in tobacco, which crosses the placental barrier to the fetus, may affect fetal brain development in ways that increase risk for conduct problems. The difficulty with this research is that embryos are not randomly assigned to develop in women who smoke during pregnancy versus women who don't, and women who smoke during pregnancy differ from women who do not smoke in many ways, including characteristics that have not been controlled in previous studies. A large study that controlled extraneous background genetic and environmental risk factors has raised questions about whether the apparent effects of prenatal exposure to smoking are truly causal. D'Onofrio et al. (2008) found that on average, women who smoked more during their pregnancies gave birth to children with more conduct problems. On the other hand, when mothers who smoked during one pregnancy smoked less (or not at all) during their other pregnancies, the level of conduct problems in their offspring did not vary with their level of smoking during each pregnancy. Thus, these findings suggest that mother's smoking during pregnancy is correlated with child conduct problems because of some other characteristic of the mothers that has yet to be identified, which is itself causal of both the maternal smoking and the childhood conduct problems. Yet regardless of what maternal characteristic accounts for the apparent effect of maternal smoking, it is robustly related to conduct problems. Further findings by D'Onofrio et al. (2008) suggest that it is an environmental factor, but more research is needed.

There is much stronger evidence that maternal alcohol use during pregnancy plays a causal role in the development of children's conduct problems (see Chapter 9). In the same sample used to study maternal cigarette smoking, D'Onofrio et al. (2007) found a linear dose–response effect: the greater the amount of alcohol consumed, including even moderate levels of drinking, the greater the risk of conduct problems was in the offspring. Because this relation with alcohol use was clear even when mothers drank at different levels during the multiple pregnancies of their children, these results strongly suggest an adverse causal effect of drinking alcohol during pregnancy. If a causal effect of maternal alcohol consumption is confirmed, this would offer a preventable environmental cause of childhood conduct problems.

*Socioeconomic status (SES).* Children and adolescents from families with lower incomes and less parental education are more likely to exhibit serious conduct problems (Coté et al., 2006; Lahey, Miller et al., 1999; Lahey & Waldman, 2003). Poverty may create circumstances that foster conduct problems; alternatively, antisocial parents who live in poverty because they did not succeed educationally and occupationally might transmit conduct problems to their offspring through common genetic and environmental mechanisms that are related to both poverty in the parents and conduct problems in the children. Extant studies suggest that both explanations may be correct (Dohrenwend et al., 1992; Miech, Caspi, Moffitt, Wright, & Silva, 1999). Low SES is more strongly associated with childhood-onset delinquency than adolescent-onset delinquency (Lahey et al., 2006; Moffitt et al., 2001). It is not clear if there are sex differences in the magnitude of the association between SES and conduct problems, however (Lahey et al., 2006; Moffitt et al., 2001).

*Parental characteristics, family characteristics, and parenting.* Many studies indicate that a set of correlated characteristics of parents is related to conduct problems in their offspring. Risk for conduct problems is highest among children of mothers and fathers with histories of antisocial behavior and substance abuse, mothers with low intelligence, and mothers who first gave birth at younger ages (Lahey et al., 2003, 2006; Lahey, Miller et al., 1999; Moffitt et al., 2001). In addition, women who have multiple partners and/or discordant partner relationships are more likely to have children with conduct problems (Keenan, Loeber, & Green, 1999; Lahey, Miller et al., 1999). According to social learning theory (Patterson et al., 1992), these and other parent and family characteristics cause child conduct problems by disrupting aspects of parenting behavior per se, and there is considerable support for this view (Jaffee, Belsky, Harrington, Caspi, Moffitt, 2006; Patterson, DeGarmo, & Knutson, 2000). Furthermore, there is robust evidence that inadequate supervision and inconsistent, coercive, and punitive discipline—including physical and sexual abuse and neglect—are correlated with offspring conduct problems (Lahey, Miller et al., 1999; Patterson & Stouthamer-Loeber, 1984). It is also clear that interventions that change these aspects of parenting behavior reduce child conduct problems (Beauchaine, Webster-Stratton, & Reid, 2005; Nock, 2003).

*Deviant peer influence and gang membership.* Two robust findings suggest the importance of peers in the origins of juvenile delinquency. First, almost all crime committed by adolescents is committed in the company of other youth (Conger & Simons, 1997). Second, association with delinquent peers is perhaps the strongest correlate of adolescent delinquency (Conger & Simons, 1997). Some evidence from longitudinal studies indicates that developing friendships with delinquent peers leads to increases in delinquency in youth who had not previously been delinquent (Keenan, Loeber, & Zhang, 1995), which suggests a causal influence (see Chapter 14). More can be learned from studies of membership in antisocial gangs, which is a special case of delinquent peer influence. Although it is clear that engaging in conduct problems during childhood increases the likelihood that a male child will join an antisocial gang (Lahey, Gordon, Loeber, Stouthamer-Loeber, & Farrington, 1999), drug selling, violent behavior, and vandalism all increase sharply after a youth joins a gang, compared to before gang entry and after leaving the gang (Gordon et al., 2004). This temporal pattern suggests but does not prove a causal effect of peer influence. In Moffitt's (1993, 2003) model, peer influence is particularly important for delinquent adolescents who did not engage in high levels of conduct problems as children, but much remains to be learned about peer influences. Furthermore, a child's association with delinquent peers is itself partly genetically influenced (Rowe & Osgood, 1984). In addition, little is currently known about sex differences in peer influences on delinquency.

*Neighborhoods and urbanicity.* Juvenile delinquency is far more common among youth who live in neighborhoods that are characterized by poverty and social disorganization (Loeber et al., 1998). Sampson, Raudenbush, and Earls (1997) suggested that the most important aspects of high-crime neighborhoods are a lack of social connectedness among neighbors and the absence of working together to supervise youth and reduce crime. Meier, Slutske, Arndt, and Cadoret (2008) found that the relation of delinquency with impulsivity and callous-unemotional traits was greater in neighborhoods low in collective efficacy compared to neighborhoods high in collective efficacy. Tuvblad, Grann, and Lichtenstein (2006) found that the proportion of variance in adolescent conduct problems attributable to genetic influences was lower, and the proportion attributable to environmental influences shared by siblings was greater, in such high-risk neighborhoods. If replicated, this interaction provides support for the hypothesis that neighborhood factors play some causal role in the origins of conduct problems.

In addition, juvenile crime is highly concentrated in high-density cities (Laub, 1983). European studies indicate that youth living in big cities report rates of delinquent behavior that are twice those of rural youth (Rutter et al., 1975; Wichström, Skogen, & Oia, 1996), but evidence from North America is inconsistent (Costello et al., 1996; Offord et al., 1987). More research on neighborhood and urban–rural differences in conduct problems is needed.

## STUDIES OF NEURAL MECHANISMS

It is important to relate individual differences in antisocial behavior to variations in the anatomy and physiology of neural systems because such links can illuminate our understanding of conduct problems via what we know about those neural systems. The first physiological studies examined correlations between conduct problems and peripheral markers of neural activity, with the most consistent and robust finding being that lower resting heart rate predicts adolescent conduct problems (Ortiz & Raine, 2004). Low-resting heart rate is interesting partly because it also is related to the temperamental trait of fearless stimulation-seeking (Raine, 2002). In addition, there is evidence that higher autonomic arousal is inversely related to conduct problems and positively related to desistance from childhood conduct problems (Lahey, Hart, Pliszka, & Applegate, 1993; Popma et al., 2006; Quay, 1993; Raine,

Venables, & Williams, 1995). Similarly, individual differences in hypothalamic-pituitary-adrenal (HPA) activity may be related to conduct problems (McBurnett et al., 2005; McBurnett, Lahey, Rathouz, & Loeber, 2000; Popma et al., 2006).

Recent advances in brain imaging have led to studies relating brain anatomy function to conduct problems. These studies suggest that structural and functional deficits of the anterior cingulate and prefrontal cortices are related to conduct problems (Beauchaine, Sauder, Gatzke-Kopp, Shannon, & Aylward, in press; Gatzke-Kopp et al., 2009; Ishikawa & Raine, 2003; Raine, 2002). The prefrontal cortex, which continues to develop through adolescence and beyond, plays a major role in the origin of conduct problems (Ishikawa & Raine, 2003; Morgan & Lilienfeld, 2000; Raine, 2002). In addition, functional connectivity between neural structures involved in impulse control (e.g., caudate) and those involved in behavioral regulation (e.g., medial frontal cortex) appears to be altered among youth with conduct problems, suggesting deficits in top-down control over impulsive behavior (Shannon, Sauder, Beauchaine, & Gatzke-Kopp, 2009).

There are some intriguing links among these research domains, which could lead to a more integrated theory of the neural mechanisms underlying conduct problems. Low-resting heart rate may be correlated with conduct problems because the prefrontal cortex, particularly the insular cortex, plays a role in regulating autonomic arousal (Raine, 2002). It is also interesting that maternal alcohol consumption during pregnancy results in smaller frontal cortices in children (Brennan et al., 2003).

## PROGRESS IN MOLECULAR GENETICS

The past 10 years have witnessed the first steps in the search for genetic variants that increase risk for conduct problems. Some of the first replicated findings will undoubtedly be refined or refuted in the future, but enough has been learned to represent early progress in the molecular genetics of conduct problems. These findings are exciting both in supporting hypotheses regarding the role of specific neurotransmitter systems in the etiology of conduct problems and in fleshing out hypotheses regarding gene–environment interplay (Rutter, 2006).

One of the best examples of gene–environment interplay is a study by Caspi et al. (2002) in which they reported an interaction between childhood maltreatment and a variant in the promoter of the gene that encodes the enzyme monoamine oxidase-A (*MAOA*). *MAOA* is of interest because it regulates the availability of all monoamine neurotransmitters, including serotonin, dopamine, and norepinephrine, all of which have been implicated in animal studies of aggression (Rutter, Moffitt, & Caspi, 2006). Caspi et al. (2002) found that early childhood maltreatment predicted the development of serious conduct problems regardless of *MAOA* genotype, but maltreated children with the low-activity *MAOA* genotype exhibited significantly higher levels of conduct problems than maltreated children with the high-activity genotype. This genetic moderation of the apparent effect of maltreatment has been replicated in several studies (Foley et al., 2004; Kim-Cohen et al., 2006; Nilsson et al., 2006), given that another study closely replicated the *pattern* of differences but the interaction did not reach statistical significance (Haberstick et al., 2005), whereas a study of a clinic-referred sample did not replicate the finding (Young et al., 2006). Nonetheless, a meta-analysis of extant studies confirmed the interaction of *MAOA* with childhood maltreatment in predicting serious antisocial behavior (Kim-Cohen et al., 2006).

It should be noted that the Caspi et al. (2002) findings could reflect gene–gene interaction instead of G × E. That is, a different gene (or set of genes) transmitted from parent to child (manifested in the parent as risk for harsh discipline and in the child as risk for aggressive conduct problems) could interact with *MAOA* to result in the increased risk for serious conduct problems in maltreated children, even if childhood maltreatment had no causal environmental effect. On the other hand, evidence from two other types of studies, which are not subject to the same alternative explanation, support Caspi et al.'s (2002) hypothesis of G × E. First, Newman et al. (2005) found that rhesus monkeys randomly assigned to be raised in isolation as opposed to with their mothers were more aggressive if they had the homologous low-activity *MAOA* genotype. Second, imaging studies in humans show that when presented with emotion-provoking stimuli, persons with the low-activity *MAOA* genotype exhibit a pattern of greater arousal in the amygdala and less arousal in the prefrontal cortex that is associated with aggression (Meyer-Lindberg et al., 2006; Meyer-Lindberg & Weinberger, 2006).

*MAOA* is not the only gene that underlies the neural systems related to aggression. Catechol-O-methyl transferase (*COMT*), a gene that codes for an enzyme involved in the breakdown of synaptic dopamine, epinephrine, and norepinephrine, has been linked with variations in frontal cortex functioning. Thapar et al. (2005) found evidence for a G × E interaction, as *COMT* was associated with increased risk for childhood conduct problems and the association between low birth weight and conduct problems was stronger among children with the high-risk (i.e., val/val) *COMT* genotype. There also are several findings relating conduct problems to variants in the gene encoding the dopamine transporter (*DAT1*), which is involved in the reuptake of dopamine from the synapse (Lee et al., 2007; Young et al., 2002), and of an interaction between *DAT1* and positive and negative parenting (Lahey et al., 2011), as well as an interaction between maternal insensitivity and variants of the D4 receptor gene (Bakermans-Kranenburg & van Ijzendoorn, 2006), in predicting childhood conduct problems. There also is a report linking a commonly studied polymorphism in the serotonin transporter gene (the *5HTTLPR*) to oppositional and aggressive behavior (Haberstick, Smolen, & Hewitt, 2006). A recent meta-analysis (Ficks & Waldman, in preparation) found a significant association between antisocial behavior and the *5HTTLPR* short allele but not the aforementioned promoter variant in *MAOA*, although there was substantial heterogeneity in the effect sizes across studies. A vast amount undoubtedly remains to be learned about genetic influences and gene-environment interplay, but molecular genetic studies of conduct problems are already producing intriguing findings.

Despite the promise of molecular genetic research, it is important to note that to date, the proportion of variance in behavior accounted for by specific genetic markers remains quite low (on the order of a few percent), compared with research from behavioral genetic studies, which consistently suggest that genetic influences account for large proportions of the variance in various behaviors and traits, including conduct problems (see above). For extended discussion, see Chapter 3.

## TOWARD A THEORETICAL SYNTHESIS

Lahey and Waldman (2003, 2005) proposed a theoretical model that integrates current findings on the development of conduct problems. Other theoretical models of youth antisocial behavior are presented in Lahey et al. (2003). In the Lahey and Waldman model, children are born with individual differences in dispositions to respond socially and emotionally to the environment. Variation in these dispositions among children are influenced by genes and prenatal influences and are shaped by the postnatal environment from birth onward. Although the definitions and labels of the dispositions vary somewhat across studies, three dispositions have been identified across many studies as being reliably related to childhood conduct problems:

*Prosociality versus callousness.* Children who care about the feelings of other children and want to please adults are less likely to develop serious conduct problems than children who callously disregard the wishes and feelings of others (e.g., Frick, 2006; Messer, Goodman, Rowe, Meltzer, & Maughan, 2006). In the Lahey and Waldman (2003, 2005) model, this is because the natural consequences of common early childhood misbehaviors such as hitting and taking things from others (e.g., seeing the other child cry) are *punishing* to children who care about the feelings of the other child, but are either neutral or *reinforcing* to more callous children. These individual differences lead to differential reinforcement histories that either increase or decrease the likelihood of future antisocial behavior. Callous children are particularly likely to acquire a pattern of planful, goal-directed aggression (Frick, 2006; Kempes, Matthys, Maassen, van Goozen, & van Engeland, 2006).

*Daring/sensation-seeking versus fearful inhibition.* Children who find novelty and danger attractive and exciting are more likely to develop conduct problems than children who react fearfully to novel, loud, and risky situations (Biederman et al., 2001; Raine et al., 1998; Quay, 1965). Lahey and Waldman (2003, 2005) hypothesized that getting into fights and engaging in transgressions that could lead to apprehension and punishment is reinforcing to daring children, but punishing to less daring children.

*Emotional lability versus emotional stability (negative emotionality).* Children who react with intense negative emotions to even minor frustrations and threats are hypothesized to be at increased risk for conduct problems (Lahey & Waldman, 2003, 2005). When adults attempt to control or discipline highly emotional children, their children are likely to respond with intensely oppositional, defiant, and coercive responses, often prompting the adults to back down from their requests. The net result of such parent–child interactions is negative reinforcement that increases the likelihood of future oppositional-defiant behavior by the child (Patterson et al., 1992). In addition, negative emotional responses to minor frustrations and provocations from other children (e.g., someone is playing with a toy that the child wants to play with) increase the likelihood of reacting in an antisocial manner (e.g., grabbing the toy), leading to negative reinforcement of the antisocial behavior through the removal of the frustration or threat (i.e., the aggressive child gets the toy).

Thus, in a multitude of ways, individual differences in these three early socio-emotional dispositions are hypothesized to increase or decrease the likelihood that a child will develop childhood-onset conduct problems and persist in them as he or she interacts with the social environment over time. In addition, slowly developing cognitive skills and language are hypothesized to interfere with socialization and thereby increase risk for conduct problems (Keenan & Shaw, 1997; Lahey & Waldman, 2003, 2005). Lahey and Waldman (2003, 2005) posit that the three socio-emotional dispositions and cognitive ability play less of a role in the development of adolescent-onset conduct problems. On the other hand, the inverse of these pre-dispositions (prosociality, fearfulness, calm response to frustration and threat, and higher intelligence) may protect adolescents from the development of delinquent behavior in the absence of a history of childhood conduct problems.

At a different level of analysis, individual differences in these predispositions and abilities can be understood as the manifestations of individual differences in brain structure and function that are caused by the same genetic and environmental influences. Genes are hypothesized to influence conduct problems partly because they influence the neural systems related to the dispositions and abilities that affect the likelihood that conduct problems will develop. Genes also influence environments that foster or reduce the likelihood of conduct problems and to interact with those environments. Thus, this theoretical model and others like it can and should incorporate variables at biological, environmental, and behavioral levels of analysis.

The Lahey and Waldman (2003, 2005) model was advanced not only to integrate the vast accumulation of empirical findings on the etiology and origins of youth antisocial behavior, but also to stimulate empirical research that might refute its hypotheses. Many tests will be required, but an early prospective test confirmed the prediction that children high in both negative emotionality and daring are at increased risk for childhood conduct problems (Gilliom & Shaw, 2004). Prosociality was not measured in that study, however. More recently, Waldman et al. (2011) confirmed several key predictions of the model regarding the phenotypic and etiological relations of the three socioemotional dispositions with youth conduct problems. First, conduct disorder symptoms were uniquely related to prosociality, negative emotionality, and daring, which explained 21%, 8%, and 2% of the variance respectively in conduct problems, and which jointly explained a total of 46% of the variance, Second, each of the socioemotional dispositions shared genetic influences in common with childhood conduct problems, and as a set explained 39% of the overall variance in conduct problems. The genetic influences shared with prosociality accounted for 20% of the variance in conduct problems, those shared with negative emotionality accounted for 16% of the variance, and those shared with daring accounted for 3%. Viewed another way, common genetic influences accounted for 73%, 86%, and 100% of the covariance of conduct problems with prosociality, negative emotionality, and daring, respectively (Waldman et al., 2011). These results are consistent with the hypothesis that a substantial proportion of the genetic influences on youth conduct problems are mediated by the three socioemotional dispositions, and suggest that future research on the genetic basis of youth conduct problems should also focus on these socioemotional dispositions as target phenotypes. The ultimate goal of such models is advanced understanding of the causes of youth conduct problems which will facilitate early prevention efforts.

## UNRESOLVED QUESTIONS AND FUTURE DIRECTIONS FOR CLASSIFICATION AND DIAGNOSIS

### MAPPING THE FINE STRUCTURE OF YOUTH ANTISOCIAL BEHAVIOR: ODD AND CD

*Is ODD distinguishable from CD?* As noted earlier, for many years there have been two different views in the literature of the relation between ODD and CD. The first view, perhaps embodied best in the ICD-10 approach to diagnostic classification, is that ODD is part of a CD diagnostic spectrum, characterizes a less severe form of CD, and is often a developmental precursor to CD (WHO, 1993). The second perspective, which is represented in *DSM-IV*, is that although ODD frequently overlaps with CD and their symptoms are highly correlated (Angold et al., 1999; Angold & Costello, 2009; Lahey, Rathouz et al., 2008), ODD and CD are relatively distinct dimensions of psychopathology with some distinct correlates and sequelae (Boden, Fergusson, & Horwood, 2010; Burke et al., 2010; Petty et al., 2009; Rowe, Costello, Angold, Copeland, & Maughan, 2010).

A number of published studies are relevant to evaluating these two alternative hypotheses regarding ODD and CD. The *DSM-IV* field trials for the disruptive behavior disorders identified two nonoverlapping sets of symptoms with greater diagnostic utility for ODD or CD, respectively (Frick et al., 1994). Many studies have subsequently supported the distinction between the *DSM-IV* symptoms lists for ODD and CD using factor analysis, although some ODD symptoms (intentionally bothers others and spiteful and vindictive) may poorly discriminate ODD and CD (Lahey, Applegate et al., 2004; Lahey, Rathouz et al., 2008). In addition, several recent studies suggest partitioning ODD symptoms into those that reflect affect dysregulation (e.g., "loses temper," "is touchy or easily annoyed," "is angry and resentful," and "is spiteful or vindictive") versus those that reflect more "acting-out" behavior (e.g., "argues with adults," "actively defies," "deliberately annoys people," and "blames others for his or her mistakes or behaviors") (Burke, Hipwell & Loeber, 2010; Stringaris & Goodman, 2009). A meta-analysis was conducted of 60 exploratory factor analyses of a range of childhood conduct problem behaviors from 44 separate studies using multidimensional scaling (Frick et al., 1993). This meta-analysis found that two orthogonal bipolar dimensions, overt versus covert and destructive versus nondestructive, best described the factor loadings of these items. The conjunction of these two orthogonal dimensions gives rise to the four symptom dimensions of oppositionality, aggression, property violations, and status offenses. The authors used data from a separate clinically referred sample to both cross-validate these meta-analytic findings regarding the dimensional structure of childhood conduct problems using factor analyses, and to extend them by demonstrating that the four dimensions could be arrayed developmentally based on their retrospectively reported ages-of-onset, with oppositionality having the earliest onset (median age = 6.0 years), followed by aggression (median age = 6.75 years), property violations (median age = 7.25 years), and status offenses (median age = 9.0 years) (Frick et al., 1993). Thus, although they are highly correlated and therefore likely share causal influences and neurobiological mechanisms, ODD and CD are different enough to distinguish as dimensions.

A related issue is whether ODD symptoms are best thought of as reflecting the same dimension as some CD symptoms. A direct comparison has been made between the *DSM-IV* model, in which ODD and CD are separate dimensions, and a model inspired by the structure of the Child Behavioral Checklist (CBCL) (Achenbach, 1978), in which aggressive CD symptoms are on the same dimension as ODD symptoms and nonaggressive CD symptoms are on a separate factor (Lahey, Rathouz et al., 2008). When *DSM-IV* symptoms were used in the comparison of these, a model of ODD and CD based on *DSM-IV* achieved a closer fit than a model inspired by the CBCL (Lahey, Rathouz et al., 2008). In the same study, the *DSM-IV* model achieved a significantly better fit than a model based on ICD-10, in which the ODD and CD symptoms loaded together on a single dimension (Lahey, Rathouz et al., 2008). Taken together, these findings suggest that ODD and CD might best be considered as distinguishable yet highly correlated dimensions of psychopathology, but further studies are needed to see if this distinction holds in both additional large population-based samples as well as in clinically referred samples. Also, few factor analytic studies, and no behavior genetic studies, have investigated the validity of partitioning ODD symptoms into the "affect dysregulation" and "acting-out" dimensions, implying that further such analyses are needed.

*Is the distinction between aggressive and nonaggressive CD symptoms useful?* It is possible that the dimension of CD symptoms also should be further partitioned. In particular, aggressive (e.g., fighting, bullying, and threat with confrontation of the victim) and nonaggressive CD behaviors (e.g., lying to con, truancy, and theft without confrontation of the victim) are highly correlated, but there may be value in distinguishing between them. There is a small but informative literature in which confirmatory factor analyses (CFAs) and behavior genetic analyses have been used to test whether aggressive and nonaggressive CD symptoms are meaningfully distinguishable. As described earlier, a meta-analysis of factor analytic studies and examination of differences in median ages-of-onset supported the distinction of aggression from oppositionality on the one hand, and from property violations and status offenses (i.e., nonaggressive CD symptoms) on the other (Frick et al., 1993). More recently, CFAs of CD symptoms revealed greater statistical support for a model in which aggressive and nonaggressive CD symptoms loaded on two separate, but highly correlated dimensions ($r = .73$) than on a single CD symptom dimension (Tackett, Krueger, Iacono, & McGue, 2005). Researchers also have demonstrated differences between aggressive and nonaggressive conduct problems in personality dimensions. In two nonreferred samples of undergraduate students, Burt and Donnellan (2008) found that several measures of aggression were uniquely correlated with higher levels on the stress reaction scale of the multidimensional personality questionnaire (Patrick, Curtin, & Tellegen, 2002), whereas nonaggressive conduct problems were uniquely correlated with lower levels on the control scale. Taken together, these results suggest that the distinction between aggressive and nonaggressive CD symptoms may be useful for some purposes. A potentially important issue for future research, however, is whether nonaggressive CD behaviors are homogeneous in nature or there are important differences between nonaggressive property violations (e.g., theft without confrontation and vandalism) and nonaggressive status offenses (e.g., truancy and staying out late without parental permission) (Frick et al., 1993; Lahey et al., 2000).

Several multivariate behavior genetic studies have examined common and unique genetic and environmental influences on aggressive and nonaggressive conduct problems, using a variety of measures including the CBCL and both questionnaire and interview assessments of *DSM* symptoms. Early biometric studies of aggressive and nonaggressive conduct problems (e.g., Edelbrock et al., 1995; Eley et al., 1999, 2003) yielded three important findings. First, there were substantial genetic influences on both aggressive and nonaggressive conduct problems (as defined by the CBCL), although these were of greater magnitude for aggressive conduct problems. Second, shared environmental influences were either only present for nonaggressive conduct problems or were of much greater magnitude for nonaggressive conduct problems than for aggression (although the magnitude of shared environmental influences on aggression appears to increase during adolescence; Eley et al., 2003). Third, although there were substantial common genetic influences on aggressive and nonaggressive conduct problems, each dimension of conduct problems showed additional unique genetic influences.

The results of more recent biometric studies of aggressive and nonaggressive conduct problems, using both the CBCL and *DSM-IV* CD symptoms, have largely supported these early findings. Tackett and colleagues found that genetic and nonshared environmental influences underlie both aggressive CD symptoms and the overlap between aggressive and nonaggressive CD symptoms, whereas substantial shared environmental influences (which were of the same magnitude as the genetic influences) also underlie nonaggressive CD symptoms (Tackett et al., 2005). A similar biometric study found that both additive genetic and nonshared environmental influences contribute to the overlap of aggressive and nonaggressive CD symptoms, each of which also show unique genetic and nonshared environmental influences, with the former greater in magnitude for aggressive CD symptoms (Gelhorn et al., 2006). A recent meta-analysis of biometric studies (Burt, 2009) found that genetic influences are more substantial on aggressive conduct problems than on nonaggressive conduct problems (heritabilities = 65% and 48%, respectively), and that only the latter showed substantial shared environmental influences (accounting for 18% of the variance). Furthermore, there is evidence from one study that the level of genetic influence on aggressive CD behaviors is stable from childhood through adolescence, but the genetic influences on nonaggressive CD behaviors increases with increasing age (Burt & Klump, 2009). These findings suggest that it may be useful to distinguish between aggressive and nonaggressive CD behaviors (and perhaps between property and status offenses) in future versions of the *DSM*, but further research is needed to see if these distinctions hold in additional large population-based samples as well as in clinically referred samples.

*Is there sufficient breadth of coverage of antisocial behavior in the symptoms of ODD and CD?* Another important but unresolved taxonomic issue is whether the extant ODD and CD criteria are broad enough to cover the full range of impairing antisocial behaviors. In particular, recent factor analytic and behavior genetic studies of reactive, proactive, and relational aggression have raised the possibility that these facets of antisocial behavior may not be sufficiently represented in the current taxonomy.

*Proactive and reactive aggression.* Several factor analytic studies of reactive and proactive aggression have been conducted (Dodge & Coie, 1987; Raine et al., 2006) and have suggested that these represent two distinct yet correlated dimensions. Although this distinction has been challenged (Bushman & Anderson, 2001), several studies have demonstrated distinct correlates of proactive and reactive aggression. For example, proactive aggression has been uniquely associated with delinquency, poor school motivation, poor peer relationships, single-parent status, psychosocial adversity, substance-abusing parents, and hyperactivity during childhood and with psychopathic personality, blunted affect, delinquency, and serious violent offending in adolescence (Kempes, Matthys, de Vries, & van Engeland, 2005; Raine et al., 2006). In contrast, reactive aggression has been associated with impulsivity, hostility, social anxiety, problems encoding and interpreting social cues, lower peer status, and lack of close friends in adolescence (Kempes et al., 2005; Raine et al., 2006).

Several biometric studies of reactive and proactive aggression have been conducted and have examined common and unique genetic and environmental influences on proactive and reactive aggression, with differing results. A study of 172 6-year-old twin pairs (Brendgen, Vitaro, Boivin, Dionne, & Perusse, 2006) found a similar magnitude of genetic influences on proactive and reactive aggression, with a high correlation between the genetic influences on each dimension of aggression ($r = .87$). A study of 1,219 9- to 10-year-old twins (Baker, Raine, Liu, & Jacobson, 2008) found significant sex differences in the magnitude of genetic and environmental influences on aggression, in which moderate genetic influences were found for boys but not for girls, whereas moderate shared environmental influences were found for girls but not boys. In contrast, no sex differences were found for mother or teacher reports of reactive and proactive aggression. Common genetic and environmental influences were both responsible for the correlation between proactive and reactive aggression, with the former being moderate-to-high and the latter being small-to-moderate in magnitude.

Although these CFA and behavior genetic findings are promising, there are two strong *a priori* arguments against including separate dimensions of proactive and/or reactive aggression to the *DSM-5*. First, because many of the items defining reactive aggression are similar to ODD items, any distinction between reactive and proactive aggression may overlap substantially with the distinction between ODD and CD. Second, when items defining proactive and reactive aggression were included with symptoms of psychopathology in the assessment of a large representative sample, exploratory factor analyses supported *DSM-IV*-like symptom dimensions of ODD and CD. Some reactive and proactive aggression items did not load on any psychopathology factor, and the ones that did loaded on either the ODD or the CD factors (Lahey, Applegate et al., 2004). Thus, although it is reasonable to consider some reactive and proactive aggression items as possible new symptoms of ODD or CD, currently there is not sufficient evidence that independent dimensions of proactive or reactive aggression should be included in the *DSM-5*. Nonetheless, given that so few extant studies have examined these issues, further studies are necessary to address whether reactive and proactive aggression can meaningfully increase the breadth of childhood disruptive disorders in the *DSM* over and above ODD and CD.

*Relational aggression.* Unfortunately, even less research is available on relational aggression. The term relational aggression refers to behaviors that are intended to hurt others by damaging their social relationships, reputation, or self-esteem, but that do not involve physical harm (Archer & Coyne, 2005; Crick & Zahn-Waxler, 2003). Researchers have begun to entertain the possibility that relational aggression should be included in the *DSM-5*, either as part of the definition of CD or as a new form of psychopathology (Keenan, Coyne, & Lahey, 2008; Keenan, Wroblewski, Hipwell, Loeber, & Stouthamer-Loeber, 2011; Moffitt et al., 2008). Recent biometric studies have examined the structure of causal influences on relational aggression and its relations with physical aggression. In a sample of 1,981 6- to 18-year-old twin pairs (Tackett, Waldman, & Lahey, 2009), substantial additive genetic influences and moderate shared environmental influences were found on a latent relational aggression factor that comprised both mother and child ratings, and which more strongly reflected mother than child ratings (i.e., accounting for 66% versus 9% of the variance). A study of 172 6-year-old twin pairs (Brendgen et al., 2005) examined the association between physical and relational aggression and found that genetic influences were greater in magnitude for physical than for relational aggression. It is noteworthy that there were shared environmental influences on relational but not physical aggression, and that these were equal in magnitude to the genetic influences underlying relational aggression. Phenotypic overlap between the two forms of aggression was mainly due to common genetic influences. In a sample of 7,449 7-year-old twin pairs (Ligthart, Bartels, Hoekstra, Hudziak, & Boomsma, 2005), genetic, shared environmental, and nonshared environmental influences were found on both relational and direct aggression. The phenotypic correlation between relational and direct aggression was due mainly to common genetic influences and to a lesser extent to shared and nonshared environmental influences (55% to 58% genetic, 30% to 33% shared environmental, and 12% nonshared environmental influences).

As with proactive and reactive aggression, the ultimate question is whether there is an incremental contribution of relational aggression in identifying children with impairing antisocial behavior. Two analyses of data from a large representative sample of children and adolescents are relevant to this question. First, measuring symptoms of relational aggression appeared to add little to the identification of children and adolescents with impairing antisocial behavior over and above symptoms of ODD and CD (Keenan et al., 2008; Keenan et al., 2011). Second, when items defining relational aggression were included with *DSM-IV* symptoms in factor analyses, a relational aggression factor distinct from ODD and CD did not emerge (Lahey, Applegate et al., 2004). Nonetheless, some relationally aggressive behaviors loaded strongly on CD, suggesting that they should be considered for inclusion as symptoms that broaden our description of CD in the *DSM-5*. It should be noted that the extant literature bearing on these important questions is small, comprising only a few studies, so further research in additional large population-based samples as well as in clinically referred samples is needed to see whether reactive, proactive, and relational aggression can add meaningfully to the classification of childhood disruptive disorders.

*Is there sufficient evidence to distinguish subtypes of CD?* There is widespread agreement that CD is a highly heterogeneous diagnostic category, both phenotypically and etiologically (Rhee & Waldman, 2002), but there is no consensus on the best way to reduce that heterogeneity through subtyping the diagnosis. Thus, an important issue is whether subtypes of CD should be distinguished in the *DSM-5* and, if so, which subtypes are most valid and useful. Previous subtyping schemes in the *DSM* distinguished between socialized and undersocialized CD and between aggressive and nonaggressive CD. These were abandoned and replaced in *DSM-IV* because no clear operationalization of the socialized/undersocialized distinction had been proposed and studied and because inspection of data from a longitudinal study of prepubertal children with CD (Lahey et al., 1995b) found that all children who met diagnostic criteria for CD displayed aggression in at least one wave of the study (Lahey, Loeber et al., 1998). In *DSM-IV*, a distinction was instead made between childhood and adolescent age-of-onset subtypes based on the presence of at least one CD symptom prior to age 10. It is crucial to determine whether this or any other subtyping scheme is sufficiently valid to be incorporated into the nosology of CD.

*Validity of subtypes based on age of onset.* Considerable research has documented important differences between childhood-onset, life-course persistent, and adolescence-limited forms of antisocial behavior (Moffitt, 1993, 2003, 2006). Although the prevalence of these forms of antisocial behavior, which range from mild to serious, is far higher than the diagnosis of CD, this research could be relevant to the taxonomy of CD. Childhood-onset (or life-course persistent) antisocial behavior is associated with parental antisocial behavior, serious family dysfunction, perinatal complications, lower IQ and neuropsychological deficits, higher levels of concurrent and earlier ADHD and ODD symptoms, and possibly with greater aggression, and difficulties in school performance and peer relations, whereas adolescence-limited antisocial behavior is associated with greater affiliation with deviant peers and less severe maladjustment and negative outcomes in adulthood (Hinshaw et al., 1993; Lahey et al., 2006; Moffitt, 1993, 2003, 2006; Odgers et al., 2008). The correlates of childhood-onset and adolescent-onset antisocial behavior also are quite different (Lahey et al., 2006; Lahey & Waldman, 2003; Odgers et al., 2008) and, therefore, their causes and mechanisms could differ.

Thus, there is strong evidence that trajectories of broadly defined antisocial behavior differ considerably as a function of age of onset and persistence. A rather different question is whether subtypes of CD based on age of onset should be distinguished as in *DSM-IV*. Challenges have been raised regarding its validity and utility, but evidence for and against the *DSM-IV* subtypes of CD based on age of onset are thin (Moffitt et al., 2008). The primary difficulty is that in the years since the publication of *DSM-IV* no longitudinal study has been published that *prospectively* distinguished between children who met *DSM-IV* criteria for CD and exhibited childhood- versus adolescent-onset CD types. This would require large population-based samples that began in childhood and compared children who met criteria for childhood-onset CD to children who met criteria for adolescent-onset CD in later years of the study. Instead, the only data we have on the distinction are from studies that used *retrospective* ages of onset of symptoms (Lahey, Loeber et al., 1998; McCabe, Hough, Wood, & Yeh, 2001). Although these studies support the *DSM-IV* subtypes, they constitute weak evidence. Given the lack of stronger evidence, it is impossible to evaluate the *DSM-IV* subtypes of CD at this time, and more evidence is necessary.

*Validity of subtypes based on callous-unemotional traits.* Among the alternatives for subtyping CD, that which has received perhaps the most consideration is the use of callous-unemotional traits (CU), a central dimension of psychopathic traits in youth (Dong, Wu, & Waldman, manuscript under review; Frick, 2009; Frick & White, 2008). Children who meet diagnostic criteria for CD would be subtyped based on their levels of CU traits. Although different models for the underlying structure of psychopathic traits in children and adolescents have been proposed (Dong et al., manuscript submitted for publication; Forsman, Lichtenstein, Andershed, & Larsson, 2008; Frick & White, 2008), each has included CU traits as an integral component of psychopathic traits in youth. Biometric studies have suggested that CU traits are moderately heritable (Dong, Ficks, & Waldman, 2011; Forsman et al., 2008; Viding, Blair, Moffitt, & Plomin, 2005; Viding, Jones, Frick, Moffitt, & Plomin, 2008), that they substantially share common genetic influences with CD (Viding, Frick, & Plomin, 2007), and that CD is more heritable when accompanied by high levels of CU (Forsman et al., 2008; Viding et al., 2005; Viding et al., 2008).

There is now consistent evidence that among heterogeneous groups of children and adolescents with conduct problems (i.e., with diagnoses of either ODD or CD), those who are most elevated on CU traits tend to show more persistent CD symptoms, higher levels of proactive aggression (Frick & Viding, 2009; Frick & White, 2008), more serious antisocial outcomes (McMahon, Witkiewitz, & Kotler, 2010), higher psychopathy levels in adulthood (Lynam et al., 2007), and appear to have greater deficits in processing facial emotional expressions of fear and distress (Dadds, El Masry, Wimalaweera, & Guastella, 2008; De Brito et al., 2009; Marsh et al., 2008). These findings strongly imply that CU traits represent an important component of antisocial behavior and therefore could be useful in subtyping CD. Nonetheless, more studies are needed to examine the incremental value of CU traits for subtyping CD, especially for determining whether they represent a more valid and useful basis for subtyping CD than the *DSM-IV* age-of-onset subtypes.

*Overlap of subtype schemas for CD.* In evaluating the validity and utility of alternative ways of subtyping CD, it is important to bear in mind that the various subtyping schemes are highly overlapping and may simply be different ways of identifying the same youth. Specifically, distinctions between aggressive and nonaggressive, undersocialized and socialized, high versus low CU subtypes, and childhood- and adolescent-onset CD may largely identify the same subgroups of individuals with CD. It is possible that children who first meet criteria for CD early in childhood and continue to do so into adolescence exhibit more undersocialized, aggressive, and CU behavior than adolescents whose CD onsets in the absence of a history of childhood conduct problems (Lahey et al., 2006; Moffitt et al., 1996; Odgers et al., 2008). Thus, more research contrasting these subtyping approaches is needed before revising the subtyping of CD in *DSM-5*.

## REFERENCES

Achenbach, T. M. (1978). The child behavior profile: I. Boys aged 6–11. *Journal of Consulting and Clinical Psychology, 46,* 478–488.

American Psychiatric Association. (1994). *Diagnostic and statistical manual of mental disorders* (4th ed.). Washington, DC: American Psychiatric Association.

Anderson, K. E., Lytton, H., & Romney, D. M. (1986). Mothers' interactions with normal and conduct-disordered boys: Who affects whom? *Developmental Psychology, 22,* 604–609.

Angold, A., & Costello, E. J. (2009). Nosology and measurement in child and adolescent psychiatry. *Journal of Child Psychology and Psychiatry, 50,* 9–15.

Angold, A., Costello, E. J., & Erkanli, A. (1999). Comorbidity. *Journal of Child Psychology and Psychiatry, 40,* 57–87.

Archer, J., & Coyne, S. M. (2005). An integrated review of indirect, relational, and social aggression. *Personality and Social Psychology Review, 9,* 212–230.

Arseneault, L., Tremblay, R., Boulerice, B., & Saucier, J. (2002). Obstetrical complications and violent delinquency: Testing two developmental pathways. *Child Development, 73,* 496–508.

Baker, L., & Cantwell, D. P. (1987). A prospective psychiatric follow-up of children with speech/language disorders. *Journal of the American Academy of Child and Adolescent Psychiatry, 26,* 546–553.

Baker, L. A., Raine, A., Liu, J. H., & Jacobson, K. C. (2008). Differential genetic and environmental influences on reactive and proactive aggression in children. *Journal of Abnormal Child Psychology, 36,* 1265–1278.

Bakermans-Kranenburg, M. J., & van Ijzendoorn, M. H. (2006). Gene-environment interaction of the dopamine D4 receptor (DRD4) and observed maternal insensitivity predicting externalizing behavior in preschoolers. *Developmental Psychobiology, 48,* 406–409.

Bardone, A. M., Moffitt, T., Caspi, A., & Dickson, N. (1996). Adult mental health and social outcomes of adolescent girls with depression and conduct disorder. *Development and Psychopathology, 8,* 811–829.

Bardone, A. M., Moffitt, T. E., Caspi, A., Dickson, N., Stanton, W. R., & Silva, P. A. (1998). Adult physical health outcomes of adolescent girls with conduct disorder, depression, and anxiety. *Journal of the American Academy of Child and Adolescent Psychiatry, 37,* 594–601.

Beauchaine, T. P., Hinshaw, S. P., & Pang, K. L. (2010). Comorbidity of attention-deficit/hyperactivity disorder and early-onset conduct disorder: Biological, environmental, and developmental mechanisms. *Clinical Psychology: Science and Practice*, *17*, 327–336.

Beauchaine, T. P., Sauder, C., Gatzke-Kopp, L. M., Shannon, K. E., & Aylward, E. (in press). Neuroanatomical correlates of heterotypic comorbidity in externalizing youth. *Journal of Clinical Child and Adolescent Psychology*.

Beauchaine, T. P., Webster-Stratton, C., & Reid, M. J. (2005). Mediators, moderators, and predictors of one-year outcomes among children treated for early-onset conduct problems: A latent growth curve analysis. *Journal of Consulting and Clinical Psychology*, *73*, 371–388.

Beitchman, J. H., Wilson, B., Johnson, C. J., Atkinson, L., Young, A., Adlaf, E., . . . Douglas, L. (2001). Fourteen-year follow-up of speech/language-impaired and control children: Psychiatric outcome. *Journal of the American Academy of Child and Adolescent Psychiatry*, *40*, 75–82.

Biederman, J., Hirshfeld-Becker, D. R., Rosenbaum, J. F., Herot, C., Friedman, D., Snidman, N., Faraone, S. V. (2001). Further evidence of association between behavioral inhibition and social anxiety in children. *American Journal of Psychiatry*, *158*, 1673–1679.

Blumstein, A., Farrington, D. P., & Moitra, S. (1985), Delinquency careers: Innocents, desisters, and persisters. In M. Tonry & N. Morris (Eds.), *Crime and justice*. Chicago, IL: University of Chicago Press.

Boden, J. M., Fergusson, D. M., & Horwood, L. J. (2010). Risk factors for conduct disorder and oppositional/defiant disorder: Evidence from a New Zealand birth cohort. *Journal of the American Academy of Child and Adolescent Psychiatry*, *49*, 1125–1133.

Bohman, M. (1996). Predispositions to criminality: Swedish adoption studies in retrospect. In G. R. Bock & J. A. Goode (Eds.), *Genetics of criminal and antisocial behavior*. Chichester, United Kingdom: Wiley.

Boyle, M. H., Offord, D. R., Racine, Y., Szatmari, P., Fleming, J. E., & Sanford, M. (1996). Identifying thresholds for classifying childhood psychiatric disorder: Issues and prospects. *Journal of the American Academy of Child and Adolescent Psychiatry*, *35*, 1440–1448.

Brendgen, M., Dionne, G., Girard, A., Boivin, M., Vitaro, F., & Perusse, D. (2005). Examining genetic and environmental effects on social aggression: A study of 6-year-old twins. *Child Development*, *76*, 930–946.

Brendgen, M., Vitaro, F., Boivin, M., Dionne, G., & Perusse, D. (2006). Examining genetic and environmental effects on reactive versus proactive aggression. *Developmental Psychology*, *42*, 1299–1312.

Brennan, P. A., Grekin, E. R., & Mednick, S. (2003). Prenatal and perinatal influences on conduct disorder and serious delinquency. In B. B. Lahey, T. E. Moffitt, & A. Caspi (Eds.), *Causes of conduct disorder and serious delinquency* (pp. 319–344). New York, NY: Guilford Press.

Brent, D. A., Oquendo, M., Birmaher, B., Greenhill, L., Kolko, D., Stanley, B., . . . Mann, J. J. (2002). Familial pathways to early-onset suicide attempt: Risk for suicidal behavior in offspring of mood-disordered suicide attempters. *Archives of General Psychiatry, 59*, 801–807.

Burke, J. D., Hipwell, A. E., & Loeber, R. (2010a). Dimensions of oppositional defiant disorder as predictors of depression and conduct disorder in preadolescent girls. *Journal of the American Academy of Child & Adolescent Psychiatry, 49*, 484–492.

Burke, J. D., Loeber, R., Lahey, B. B., & Rathouz, P. J. (2005). Developmental transitions among affective and behavioral disorders in adolescent boys. *Journal of Child Psychology and Psychiatry, 46*, 1200–1210.

Burke, J. D., Waldman, I. D., & Lahey, B. B. (2010). Predictive validity of childhood oppositional defiant disorder and conduct disorder: Implications for the DSM-V. *Journal of Abnormal Psychology, 119*, 739–751.

Burt, S. A. (2009). Are there meaningful etiological differences within antisocial behavior? Results of a meta-analysis. *Clinical Psychology Review, 29*, 163–178.

Burt, S. A., & Donnellan, M. B. (2008). Personality correlates of aggressive and non-aggressive antisocial behavior. *Personality and Individual Differences, 44*, 53–63.

Burt, S. A., & Klump, K. L. (2009). The etiological moderation of aggressive and nonaggressive antisocial behavior by age. *Twin Research and Human Genetics, 12*, 343–350.

Bushman, B. J., & Anderson, C. A. (2001). Is it time to pull the plug on the hostile versus instrumental aggression dichotomy? *Psychological Review, 108*, 273–279.

Cadoret, R. J., Yates, W. R., Troughton, E., Woodward, G., & Stewart, M. A. (1995). Genetic-environmental interaction in the genesis of aggressivity and conduct disorders. *Archives of General Psychiatry, 52*, 916–924.

Caspi, A., McClay, J., Moffitt, T., Mill, J., Martin, J., Craig, I. W., . . . Poulton, R. (2002). Role of genotype in the cycle of violence in maltreated children. *Science, 297*, 851–854.

Cohen, N. J., Menna, R., Vallance, D. D., Barwick, M. A., Im, N., & Horodezky, N. B. (1998). Language, social cognitive processing, and behavioral characteristics of psychiatrically disturbed children with previously identified and unsuspected language impairments. *Journal of Child Psychology and Psychiatry, 39*, 853–864.

Conger, R. D., & Simons, R. L. (1997). Life-course contingencies in the development of adolescent antisocial behavior: A matching law approach. In T. Thornberry (Ed.), *Developmental theories of crime and delinquency* (pp. 55–100). New Brunswick, NJ: Transaction.

Costello, E. J., Angold, A., Burns, B. J., Stangl, D. K., Tweed, D. L., Erkanli, A., & Worthman C. M. (1996). The Great Smoky Mountains study of youth: Goals, design, methods, and the prevalence of *DSM-III-R* disorders. *Archives of General Psychiatry, 53*, 1129–1136.

Coté, S., Tremblay, R. E., Nagin, D. S., Zoccolillo, M., & Vitaro, F. (2002). Childhood behavioral profiles leading to adolescent conduct disorder: Risk trajectories for boys and girls. *Journal of the American Academy of Child and Adolescent Psychiatry, 41*, 1086–1094.

Coté, S. M., Vaillancourt, T., Le Blanc, J. C., Nagin, D. S., & Tremblay, R. E. (2006). The development of physical aggression from toddlerhood to pre-adolescence:

A nationwide longitudinal study of Canadian children. *Journal of Abnormal Child Psychology, 34*, 71–85.

Coté, S., Zoccolillo, M., Tremblay, R. E., Nagin, D., & Vitaro, F. (2001). Predicting girls' conduct disorder in adolescence from childhood trajectories of disruptive behaviors. *Journal of the American Academy of Child and Adolescent Psychiatry, 40*, 678–684.

Crick, N. R., & Zahn-Waxler, C. (2003). The development of psychopathology in females and males: Current progress and future challenges. *Development and Psychopathology, 15*, 719–742.

Dadds, M. R., El Masry, Y., Wimalaweera, S., & Guastella, A. J. (2008). Reduced eye gaze explains "fear blindness" in childhood psychopathic traits. *Journal of the American Academy of Child and Adolescent Psychiatry, 47*, 455–463.

De Brito, S. A., Hodgins, S., McCrory, E. J. P., Mechelli, A., Wilke, M., Jones, A. P., & Viding, E. (2009). Structural neuroimaging and the antisocial brain: Main finding and methodological challenges. *Criminal Justice and Behavior, 36*, 1173–1186.

Dodge, K. A., & Coie, J. D. (1987). Social-information-processing factors in reactive and proactive aggression in children's peer groups. *Journal of Personality and Social Psychology, 53*, 1146–1158.

Dohrenwend, B. P., Levav, I., Shrout, P. E., Schwartz, S., Naveh, G., Link, B. G.,...Stueve, A. (1992). Socioeconomic status and psychiatric disorders: The causation-selection issue. *Science, 255*, 946–952.

Dong, L., Wu, H., & Waldman, I. D. (submitted). Measurement and structural invariance testing of the antisocial process screening device. *Psychological Assessment*.

Dong, L., Ficks, C. A. & Waldman, I. D. (in preparation). *Behavior genetic analyses of psychopathic trait dimensions in children*.

D'Onofrio, B. M., Van Hulle, C. A., Waldman, I. D., Rodgers, J. L., Harden, K. P., Rathouz, P. J., & Lahey, B. B. (2008). Smoking during pregnancy and offspring externalizing problems: An exploration of genetic and environmental confounds. *Development and Psychopathology, 20*, 139–164.

D'Onofrio, B. M., Van Hulle, C. A., Waldman, I. D., Rodgers, J. L., Rathouz, P. J., & Lahey, B. B. (2007). Causal inferences regarding exposure to prenatal alcohol and childhood conduct problems. *Archives of General Psychiatry, 64*, 1296–1304.

Edelbrock, C., Rende, R., Plomin, R., & Thompson, L. A. (1995). A twin study of competence and problem behavior in childhood and early adolescence. *Journal of Child Psychology and Psychiatry, 36*, 775–785.

Eley, T. C., Lichtenstein, P., & Moffitt, T. E. (2003). A longitudinal behavioral genetic analysis of the etiology of aggressive and nonaggressive antisocial behavior. *Development and Psychopathology, 15*, 383–402.

Eley, T. C., Lichtenstein, P., & Stevenson, J. (1999). Sex differences in the etiology of aggressive and nonaggressive antisocial behavior: Results from two twin studies. *Child Development, 70*, 155–168.

Elkins, I., Iacono, W., Doyle, A., & McGue, M. (1997). Characteristics associated with the persistence of antisocial behavior: Results from recent longitudinal research. *Aggression and Violent Behavior, 2*, 101–124.

Farrington, D. P. (1991). Antisocial personality from childhood to adulthood. *Psychologist, 4*, 389–394.

Farrington, D. P., & Painter, K. A. (2004). *Gender differences in offending: Implications for risk-focused prevention.* London, United Kingdom: Home Office.

Fergusson, D. M., Horwood, L. J., & Ridder, E. M. (2005). Show me the child at seven: The consequences of conduct problems in childhood for psychosocial functioning in adulthood. *Journal of Child Psychology and Psychiatry, 46*, 837–849.

Ficks, C. A., Lahey, B. B., & Waldman, I. D. (submitted). *Does low birth weight share common genetic or environmental risk with childhood disruptive disorders?*

Ficks, C. A., & Waldman, I. D. (in preparation). *Candidate genes for aggression and antisocial behavior: A meta-analysis of the 5-HTTLPR and MAOA-uVNTR.*

Foley, D. L., Eaves, L. J., Wormley, B., Silberg, J. L., Maes, H. H., Kuhn, J., . . . Riley, B., (2004). Childhood adversity, monoamine oxidase A genotype, and risk for conduct disorder. *Archives of General Psychiatry, 61*, 1–7.

Fombonne, E., Wostear, G., Cooper, V., Harrington, R., & Rutter, M. (2001). The Maudsley long-term follow-up of child and adolescent depression: 2. Suicidality, criminality and social dysfunction in adulthood. *British Journal of Psychiatry, 179*, 218–223.

Forsman, M., Lichtenstein, P., Andershed, H., & Larsson, H. (2008). Genetic effects explain the stability of psychopathic personality from mid- to late adolescence. *Journal of Abnormal Psychology, 117*, 606–617.

Frick, P. J. (2006). Developmental pathways to conduct disorder. *Child and Adolescent Psychiatric Clinics of North America, 15*, 311–331.

Frick, P. J. (2009). Extending the construct of psychopathy to youth: Implications for understanding, diagnosing, and treating antisocial children and adolescents. *Canadian Journal of Psychiatry-Revue Canadienne De Psychiatrie, 54*, 803–812.

Frick, P. J., & Viding, E. (2009). Antisocial behavior from a developmental psychopathology perspective. *Development and Psychopathology, 21*, 1111–1131.

Frick, P. J., & White, S. F. (2008). Research Review: The importance of callous-unemotional traits for developmental models of aggressive and antisocial behavior. *Journal of Child Psychology and Psychiatry, 49*, 359–375.

Frick, P. J., Lahey, B. B., Applegate, B., Kerdyck, L., Ollendick, T., Hynd, G. W., & Waldman, I. (1994). DSM-IV field trials for the disruptive behavior disorders: Symptom utility estimates. *Journal of the American Academy of Child and Adolescent Psychiatry, 33*, 529–539.

Frick, P. J., Lahey, B. B., Loeber, R., Tannenbaum, L., Vanhorn, Y., Christ, M. A.G., & Hanson, K. (1993). Oppositional defiant disorder and conduct disorder: A meta-analytic review of factor analyses and cross-validation in a clinic sample. *Clinical Psychology Review, 13*, 319–340.

Gatzke-Kopp, L. M., Beauchaine, T. P., Shannon, K. E., Chipman-Chacon, J., Fleming, A. P., Crowell, S. E., . . . Aylward, E. (2009). Neurological correlates of reward responding in adolescents with and without externalizing behavior disorders. *Journal of Abnormal Psychology, 118*, 203–213.

Ge, X., Conger, R. D., Cadoret, R. J., Neiderhiser, J. M., Yates, W., Troughton, E., . . . Stewart, M. A. (1996). The developmental interface between nature and nurture: A mutual influence model of child antisocial behavior and parent behaviors. *Developmental Psychology, 32,* 574–589.

Ge, X., Donnellan, M. B., & Wenk, E. (2001). The development of persistent criminal offending in males. *Criminal Justice and Behavior, 26,* 731–755.

Gelhorn, H., Stallings, M., Young, S., Corley, R., Rhee, S. H., Hopfer, C., & Hewitt, J. (2006). Common and specific genetic influences on aggressive and nonaggressive conduct disorder domains. *Journal of the American Academy of Child and Adolescent Psychiatry, 45,* 570–577.

Giancola, P. R., Martin, C. S., Tarter, R. E., Pelham, W. E., & Moss, H. B. (1996). Executive cognitive functioning and aggressive behavior in preadolescent boys at high risk for substance abuse/dependence. *Journal of Studies on Alcohol, 57,* 352–359.

Gilliom, M., & Shaw, D. S. (2004). Codevelopment of externalizing and internalizing problems in early childhood. *Development and Psychopathology, 16,* 313–333.

Gordon, R. A., Lahey, B. B., Kawai, E., Loeber, R., Stouthamer-Loeber, M., & Farrington, D. P. (2004). Antisocial behavior and youth gang membership: Selection and socialization. *Criminology, 42,* 55–87.

Graham P., & Rutter, M. (1973). Psychiatric disorders in the young adolescent: A follow-up study. *Proceedings of the Royal Society of Medicine, 66,* 1226–1229.

Haberstick, B., Lessem, J., Hopfer, C., Smolen, A., Ehringer, M., Timberlake, D., & Hewitt, J. K. (2005). Monoamine oxidase A (MAO-A) and antisocial behaviors in the presence of childhood and adolescent maltreatment. *American Journal of Medical Genetics: Neuropsychiatric Genetics, 135,* 59–64.

Haberstick, B. C., Smolen, A., & Hewitt, J. K. (2006). Family-based association test of the 5HTTLPR and aggressive behavior in a general population sample of children. *Biological Psychiatry, 59,* 836–843.

Henry, B., Caspi, A., Moffitt, T. E., & Silva, P. A. (1996). Temperamental and familial predictors of violent and nonviolent criminal convictions: Age 3 to age 18. *Developmental Psychology, 32,* 614–623.

Hinshaw, S. P., Lahey, B. B., & Hart, E. L. (1993). Issues of taxonomy and comorbidity in the development of conduct disorder. *Development and Psychopathology, 5,* 31–50.

Hirschi, T., & Gottfredson, M. (1983). Age and the explanation of crime. *American Journal of Sociology, 89,* 552–584.

Insel, T. R., & Wang, P. S. (2010). Rethinking mental ilness. *JAMA, 303,* 1970–1971.

Ishikawa, S. S., & Raine, A. (2003). Prefrontal deficits and antisocial behavior: A causal model. In B. B. Lahey, T. E. Moffitt, & A. Caspi (Eds.), *Causes of conduct disorder and juvenile delinquency* (pp. 277–304). New York, NY: Guilford Press.

Jaffee, S. R., Belsky, J., Harrington, H., Caspi, A., & Moffitt, T. E. (2006). When parents have a history of conduct disorder: How is the caregiving environment affected? *Journal of Abnormal Psychology, 115,* 309–319.

Keenan, K., Coyne, C., & Lahey, B. B. (2008). Should relational aggression be included in DSM-V? *Journal of the American Academy of Child and Adolescent Psychiatry, 47,* 86–93.

Keenan, K., Loeber, R., & Green, S. (1999). Conduct disorder in girls: A review of the literature. *Clinical Child and Family Psychology Review, 2,* 3–19.

Keenan, K., Loeber, R., & Zhang, Q. (1995). The influence of deviant peers on the development of boys' disruptive and delinquent behavior: A temporal analysis. *Development and Psychopathology, 7*, 715–726.

Keenan, K., & Shaw, D. (1997). Developmental and social influences on young girls' early problem behavior. *Psychological Bulletin, 121*, 95–113.

Keenan, K., Wroblewski, K., Hipwell, A., Loeber, R., & Stouthamer-Loeber, M. (2011). Age of onset, symptom threshold, and expansion of the nosology of conduct disorder for girls. *Journal of Abnormal Psychology, 119*, 689–698.

Keily, M., Bates, J., Dodge, K., & Pettit, G. (2001). Effects of temperament on the development of externalizing and internalizing behaviors over 9 years. In F. Columbus (Ed.), *Advances in psychology research* (Vol. 6, pp. 255–288). Hauppauge, NY: Nova.

Kempes, M., Matthys, W., de Vries, H., & van Engeland, H. (2005). Reactive and proactive aggression in children—A review of theory, findings and the relevance for child and adolescent psychiatry. *European Child and Adolescent Psychiatry, 14*, 11–19.

Kempes, M., Matthys, W., Maassen, G., van Goozen, S., & van Engeland, H. (2006). A parent questionnaire for distinguishing between reactive and proactive aggression in children. *European Child and Adolescent Psychiatry, 15*, 38–45.

Kerr, M., Tremblay, R. E., Pagani-Kurtz, L., & Vitaro, F. (1997). Boy's behavioral inhibition and the risk of later delinquency. *Archives of General Psychiatry, 54*, 809–816.

Kim-Cohen, J., Caspi, A., Taylor, A., Williams, B., Newcombe, R., Craig, I. W., & Moffitt, T. E. (2006). MAOA, maltreatment, and gene-environment interaction predicting children's mental health: New evidence and a meta-analysis. *Molecular Psychiatry, 11*, 903–913.

Kjelsberg, E. (2002). DSM-IV conduct disorder symptoms in adolescents as markers of registered criminality. *European Child and Adolescent Psychiatry, 11*, 2–9.

Kohlberg, L., Ricks, D., & Snarey, J. (1984). Childhood development as a predictor of adaptation in adulthood. *Genetic Psychology Monographs, 110*, 91–172.

Kratzer, L., & Hodgins, S. (1999). A typology of offenders: A test of Moffitt's theory among males and females from childhood to age 30. *Criminal Behaviour and Mental Health, 9*, 57–73.

Lahey, B. B., Applegate, B., Barkley, R. A., Garfinkel, B., McBurnett, K., Kerdyk, L., . . . Shaffer, D. (1994). DSM-IV field trials for oppositional defiant disorder and conduct disorder in children and adolescents. *American Journal of Psychiatry, 151*, 1163–1171.

Lahey, B. B., Applegate, B., Waldman, I. D., Loft, J. D., Hankin, B. L., & Rick, J. (2004). The structure of child and adolescent psychopathology: Generating new hypotheses. *Journal of Abnormal Psychology, 113*, 358–385.

Lahey, B. B., Gordon, R. A., Loeber, R., Stouthamer-Loeber, M., & Farrington, D. P. (1999). *Journal of Abnormal Child Psychology, 27*, 261–276.

Lahey, B. B., Hart, E. L., Pliszka, S., & Applegate, B. (1993). Neurophysiological correlates of conduct disorder: A rationale and a review of research. *Journal of Clinical Child Psychology, 22*, 141–153.

Lahey, B. B., Loeber, R., Burke, J. D., & Applegate, B. (2005). Predicting future antisocial personality disorder in males from a clinical assessment in childhood. *Journal of Consulting and Clinical Psychology, 73*, 389–399.

Lahey, B. B., Loeber, R., Burke, J., Rathouz, P. J., & McBurnett, K. (2002). Waxing and waning in concert: Dynamic comorbidity of conduct disorder with other disruptive and emotional problems over 17 years among clinic-referred boys. *Journal of Abnormal Psychology, 111*, 556–567.

Lahey, B. B., Loeber, R., Hart, E. L., Frick, P. J., Applegate, B., Zhang, Q. W., & Russo, M. F. (1995). 4-Year longitudinal study of conduct disorder in boys: Patterns and predictors of persistence. *Journal of Abnormal Psychology, 104*, 83–93.

Lahey, B. B., Loeber, R., Quay, H. C., Applegate, B., Shaffer, D., & Waldman, I. (1998). Validity of DSM-IV subtypes of conduct disorder based on age of onset. *Journal of the American Academy of Child & Adolescent Psychiatry, 37*, 435–442.

Lahey, B. B., Loeber, R., Quay, H., Frick, P., & Grimm, J. (1992). Oppositional defiant and conduct disorders: Issues to be resolved for the DSM-IV. *Journal of the American Academy of Child and Adolescent Psychiatry, 31*, 539–546.

Lahey, B. B., McBurnett, K., & Loeber, R. (2000). Are attention-deficit hyperactivity disorder and oppositional defiant disorder developmental precursors to conduct disorder? In A. Sameroff, M. Lewis, & S. Miller (Eds.), *Handbook of developmental psychopathology* (2nd ed., pp. 431–446). New York, NY: Plenum.

Lahey, B. B., Miller, T. L., Gordon, R. A., & Riley, A. (1999). Developmental epidemiology of the disruptive behavior disorders. In H. Quay & A. Hogan (Eds.), *Handbook of the disruptive behavior disorders* (pp. 23–48). New York, NY: Plenum.

Lahey, B. B., Moffitt, T. E., & Caspi, A. (Eds.). (2003) *Causes of conduct disorder and serious delinquency*. New York, NY: Guilford Press.

Lahey, B. B., Piacentini, J. C., McBurnett, K., Stone, P. A., Hartdagen, S., & Hynd, G. W. (1988). Psychopathology in the parents of children with conduct disorder and hyperactivity. *Journal of the American Academy of Child and Adolescent Psychiatry, 27*, 163–170.

Lahey, B. B., Rathouz, P. J., Applegate, B., Van Hulle, C. A., Garriock, H. A., Urbano, R. C., & Waldman, I. D. (2008). Testing structural models of DSM-IV symptoms of common forms of child and adolescent psychopathology. *Journal of Abnormal Child Psychology, 36*, 187–206.

Lahey, B. B., Rathouz, P. J., Lee, S. S., Chronis-Tuscano, A., Pelham, W. E., Waldman, I. D., & Cook, E. H. (2011). Interactions between early parenting and a polymorphism of the child's dopamine transporter gene in predicting future child conduct disorder symptoms. *Journal of Abnormal Psychology, 120*, 33–45.

Lahey, B. B., Russo, M. F., Walker, J. L., & Piacentini, J. C. (1989). Personality characteristics of the mothers of children with disruptive behavior disorders. *Journal of Consulting and Clinical Psychology, 57*, 512–515.

Lahey, B. B., Schwab-Stone, M., Goodman, S. H., Waldman, I. D., Canino, G., Rathouz, P. J., Jensen, P. S. (2000). Age and gender differences in oppositional behavior and conduct problems: A cross-sectional household study of middle childhood and adolescence. *Journal of Abnormal Psychology, 109*, 488–503.

Lahey, B. B., Van Hulle, C. A., Waldman, I. D., Rodgers, J. L., D'Onofrio, B. M., Pedlow, S., . . . Keenan, K. (2006). Testing descriptive hypotheses regarding sex differences in the development of conduct problems and delinquency. *Journal of Abnormal Child Psychology, 34,* 737–755.

Lahey, B. B., & Waldman, I. D. (2003). A developmental propensity model of the origins of conduct problems during childhood and adolescence. In B. B. Lahey, T. E. Moffitt, & A. Caspi (Eds.), *Causes of conduct disorder and serious delinquency* (pp. 76–117). New York, NY: Guilford Press.

Lahey, B. B., & Waldman, I. D. (2005). A developmental model of the propensity to offend during childhood and adolescence. In D. P. Farrington (Ed.), *Advances in criminological theory* (Vol. 13, pp. 15–50). Piscataway, NJ: Transaction.

Laub, J. (1983). Urbanism, race, and crime. *Journal of Research in Crime and Delinquency, 20,* 183–198.

Lee, S. S., Lahey, B. B., Waldman, I., Van Hulle, C. A., Rathouz, P., Pelham, W. E., . . . Cook, E. H. (2007). Association of dopamine transporter genotype with disruptive behavior disorders in an eight-year longitudinal study of children and adolescents. *American Journal of Medical Genetics Part B: Neuropsychiatric Genetics, 144,* 310–317.

Ligthart, L., Bartels, M., Hoekstra, R. A., Hudziak, J. J., & Boomsma, D. I. (2005). Genetic contributions to subtypes of aggression. *Twin Research and Human Genetics, 8,* 483–491.

Lilienfeld, S. O., & Waldman, I. D. (1990). The relation between childhood Attention-Deficit Hyperactivity Disorder and adult antisocial behavior reexamined: The problem of heterogeneity. *Clinical Psychology Review, 10,* 699–725.

Little, S. A., & Garber, J. (2005). The role of social stressors and interpersonal orientation in explaining the longitudinal relation between externalizing and depressive symptoms. *Journal of Abnormal Psychology, 114,* 432–443.

Loeber, R. (1988). Natural histories of conduct problems, delinquency, and associated substance abuse: Evidence for developmental progressions. In B. B. Lahey & A. E. Kazdin (Eds.), *Advances in clinical child psychology* (Vol. 11). New York, NY: Plenum.

Loeber, R., Burke, J. D., Lahey, B. B., Winters, A., & Zera, M. (2000). Oppositional defiant and conduct disorder: A review of the past 10 years, Part I. *Journal of the American Academy of Child and Adolescent Psychiatry, 39,* 1468–1484.

Loeber, R., Farrington, D. P., Stouthamer-Loeber, M., & Van Kammen, W. (1998). *Antisocial behavior and mental health problems.* Mahwah, NJ: Erlbaum.

Loeber, R., & Keenan, K. (1994). Interaction between conduct disorder and its comorbid conditions: Effects of age and gender. *Clinical Psychology Review, 14,* 497–523.

Loeber, R., Pardini, D., Homish, D. L., Wei, E. H., Crawford, A. M., Farrington, D. P., . . . Rosenfeld, R. (2005). The prediction of violence and homicide in young men. *Journal of Consulting and Clinical Psychology, 73,* 1074–1088.

Loeber, R., & Stouthamer-Loeber, M. (1998). Development of juvenile aggression and violence: Some common misconceptions and controversies. *American Psychologist, 53,* 242–259.

Lynam, D. R. (1998). Early identification of the fledgling psychopath: Locating the psychopathic child in the current nomenclature. *Journal of Abnormal Psychology, 107*, 566–575.

Lynam, D., Moffitt, T., & Stouthamer-Loeber, M. (1993). Explaining the relation between IQ and delinquency: Class, race, test motivation, school failure or self-control? *Journal of Abnormal Psychology, 102*, 187–196.

Lynam, D. R., Caspi, A., Moffitt, T. E., Loeber, R., & Stouthamer-Loeber, M. (2007). Longitudinal evidence that psychopathy scores in early adolescence predict adult psychopathy. *Journal of Abnormal Psychology, 116*, 155–165.

Mannuzza, S., Klein, R. G., Abikoff, H., & Moulton, J. L. (2004). Significance of childhood conduct problems to later development of conduct disorder among children with ADHD: A prospective follow-up study. *Journal of Abnormal Child Psychology, 32*, 565–573.

Mannuzza, S., Klein, R. G., Bessler, A., Malloy, P., & LaPadula, M. (1993). Adult outcome of hyperactive boys: Educational achievement, occupational rank, and psychiatric status. *Archives of General Psychiatry, 50*, 565–576.

Mannuzza, S., Klein, R. G., Bonagura, N., Malloy, P., Giampino, T. L., & Addalli, K. A. (1991). Hyperactive boys almost grown up: Replication of psychiatric status. *Archives of General Psychiatry, 48*, 77–83.

Marsh, A. A., Finger, E. C., Mitchell, D. G. V., Reid, M. E., Sims, C., Kosson, D. S., & Blair, R. J. R. (2008). Reduced amygdala response to fearful expressions in children and adolescents with callous-unemotional traits and disruptive behavior disorders. *American Journal of Psychiatry, 165*, 712–720.

Marshal, M. P., & Molina, B. S. G. (2006). Antisocial behaviors moderate the deviant peer pathway to substance use in children with ADHD. *Journal of Clinical Child and Adolescent Psychology, 35*, 216–226.

Maughan, B., Rowe, R., Messer, J., Goodman, R., & Meltzer, H. (2004). Conduct disorder and oppositional defiant disorder in a national sample: Developmental epidemiology. *Journal of Child Psychology and Psychiatry, 45*, 609–621.

Maughan, B., & Rutter, M. (2001). Antisocial children grown up. In J. Hill & B. Maughan (Eds.), *Conduct disorders in childhood and adolescence* (pp. 507–552). New York, NY: Cambridge University Press.

McBurnett, K., Lahey, B. B., Rathouz, P. J., & Loeber, R. (2000). Low salivary cortisol and persistent aggression in boys referred for disruptive behavior. *Archives of General Psychiatry, 57*, 38–43.

McBurnett, K., Raine, A., Stouthamer-Loeber, M., Loeber, R., Kumar, A. M., Kumar, M., . . . Lahey, B. B. (2005). Mood and hormone responses to psychological challenge in adolescent males with conduct problems. *Biological Psychiatry, 57*, 1109–1116.

McCabe, K. M., Hough, R., Wood, P. A., & Yeh, M. (2001). Childhood and adolescent onset conduct disorder: A test of the developmental taxonomy. *Journal of Abnormal Child Psychology, 29*, 305–316.

McMahon, R. J., Witkiewitz, K., & Kotler, J. S. (2010). Predictive validity of callous-unemotional traits measured in early adolescence with respect to multiple antisocial outcomes. *Journal of Abnormal Psychology, 119*, 752–763.

Meier, M. H., Slutske, W. S., Arndt, S., & Cadoret, R. J. (2008). Impulsive and callous traits are more strongly associated with delinquent behavior in higher risk neighborhoods among boys and girls. *Journal of Abnormal Psychology, 117,* 377–385.

Meier, M. H., Slutske, W. S., Heath, A. C., & Martin, N. G. (2011). Sex differences in the genetic and environmental influences on childhood conduct disorder and adult antisocial behavior. *Journal of Abnormal Psychology, 120,* 377–388.

Messer, J., Goodman, R., Rowe, R., Meltzer, H., & Maughan, B. (2006). Preadolescent conduct problems in girls and boys. *Journal of the American Academy of Child and Adolescent Psychiatry, 45,* 184–191.

Meyer-Lindenberg, A., Buckholtz, J. W., Kolachana, B., Hariri, A. R., Pezawas, L., Blasi, G., . . . Weinberger, D. R. (2006). Neural mechanisms of genetic risk for impulsivity and violence in humans. *Proceedings of the National Academy of Sciences, 103,* 6269–6274.

Meyer-Lindenberg, A., & Weinberger, D. R. (2006). Intermediate phenotypes and genetic mechanisms of psychiatric disorders. *Nature Reviews Neuroscience, 7,* 818–27.

Miech, R. A., Caspi, A., Moffitt, T. E., Wright, B. R. E., & Silva, P. A. (1999). Low socioeconomic status and mental disorders: A longitudinal study of selection and causation during young adulthood. *American Journal of Sociology, 104,* 1096–1131.

Mitchell, S., & Rosa, P. (1981). Boyhood behavior problems as precursors of criminality: A fifteen year study. *Journal of Child Psychology and Psychiatry, 22,* 19–33.

Moffitt, T. E. (1993). Adolescence-limited and life-course-persistent antisocial behavior: A developmental taxonomy. *Psychological Review, 100,* 674–701.

Moffitt, T. E. (2003). Life-course persistent and adolescence-limited antisocial behavior: A research review and a research agenda. In B. B. Lahey, T. E. Moffitt, & A. Caspi (Eds.), *Causes of conduct disorder and juvenile delinquency* (pp. 49–75). New York, NY: Guilford Press.

Moffitt, T. E. (2007). A review of research on the taxonomy of life-course persistent versus adolescence-limited antisocial behavior. Chapter 3 in D. J. Flannery, A. T. Vazsonyi, & I. D. Waldman. (2007). (Eds.), *The Cambridge handbook of violent behavior.* New York: Cambridge University Press.

Moffitt, T. E., Arseneault, L., Jaffee, S. R., Kim-Cohen, J., Koenen, K. C., Odgers, C. L., & Viding, E. (2008). Research Review: DSM-V conduct disorder: Research needs for an evidence base. *Journal of Child Psychology and Psychiatry, 49,* 3–33.

Moffitt, T. E., Caspi, A., Dickson, N., Silva, P., & Stanton, W. (1996). Childhood-onset versus adolescent-onset antisocial conduct problems in males: Natural history from ages 3 to 18 years. *Development and Psychopathology, 8,* 399–424.

Moffitt, T. E., Caspi, A., Harrington, H., & Milne, B. J. (2002). Males on the life-course-persistent and adolescence-limited antisocial pathways: Follow-up at age 26 years. *Development and Psychopathology, 14,* 179–207.

Moffitt, T. E., Caspi, A., Rutter, M., & Silva, P. (2001). *Sex differences in antisocial behavior.* Cambridge, United Kingdom: Cambridge University Press.

Moffitt, T. E., & Silva, P. A. (1988). IQ and delinquency: A direct test of the differential detection hypothesis. *Journal of Abnormal Psychology, 97,* 330–333.

Morgan, A. B., & Lilienfeld, S. O. (2000). A meta-analytic review of the relation between antisocial behavior and neuropsychological measures of executive functioning. *Clinical Psychology Review, 20,* 113–136.

Nagin, D. S., Pogarsky, G., & Farrington, D. P. (1997). Adolescent mothers and the criminal behavior of their children. *Law and Society Review, 31,* 137–162.

Newman, T. K., Syagailo, Y. V., Barr, C. S., Wendland, J. R., Champoux, M., Graessle, M.,...Lesch, K-P. (2005). Monoamine oxidase A gene promoter variation and rearing experience influences aggressive behavior in rhesus monkeys. *Biological Psychiatry, 57,* 167–172.

Nilsson, K. W., Sjoberg, R. L., Damberg, M., Leppert, J., Ohrvik, J., Alm, P. O.,...Oreland, L. (2006). Role of monoamine oxidase A genotype and psychosocial factors in male adolescent criminal activity. *Biological Psychiatry, 59,* 121–127.

Nock, M. K. (2003). Progress review of the psychosocial treatment of child conduct problems. *Clinical Psychology: Science and Practice, 10,* 1–28.

Nottelmann, E. D., & Jensen, P. S. (1995). Comorbidity of disorders in children and adolescents: Developmental perspectives. In T. H. Ollendick & R. J. Prinz (Eds.), *Advances in clinical child psychology* (Vol. 17, pp. 109–155). New York, NY: Plenum.

Odgers, C. L., Moffitt, T. E., Broadbent, J. M., Dickson, N., Hancox, R. J., Harrington, H., & Caspi, A. (2008). Female and male antisocial trajectories: From childhood origins to adult outcomes. *Development and Psychopathology, 20,* 673–716.

Offord, D. R., Boyle, M. H., Szatmari, P., Rae-Grant, N., Links, P. S., Cadman, D. T.,...Woodward, C. A. (1987). Ontario child health study: II. Six-month prevalence of disorder and rates of service utilization. *Archives of General Psychiatry, 44,* 832–836.

Ortiz, J., & Raine, A. (2004). Heart rate level and antisocial behavior in children and adolescents: A meta-analysis. *Journal of the American Academy of Child and Adolescent Psychiatry, 43,* 154–162.

Patrick, C. J., Curtin, J. J., & Tellegen, A. (2002). Development and validation of a brief form of the Multidimensional Personality Questionnaire. *Psychological Assessment, 14,* 150–163.

Patterson, G. R., DeGarmo, D. S., & Knutson, N. (2000). Hyperactive and antisocial behaviors: Comorbid or two points in the same process? *Development and Psychopathology, 12,* 91–106.

Patterson, G. R., Reid, J. B., & Dishion, T. J. (1992). *Antisocial boys.* Eugene, OR: Castalia.

Patterson, G. R., & Stoolmiller, M. (1991). Replications of a dual failure model for boys' depressed mood. *Journal of Consulting and Clinical Psychology, 59,* 491–498.

Patterson, G. R., & Stouthamer-Loeber, M. (1984). The correlation of family management practices and delinquency. *Child Development, 55,* 1299–1307.

Petty, C. R., Monuteaux, M. C., Mick, E., Hughes, S., Small, J., Faraone, S. V., & Biederman, J. (2009). Parsing the familiality of oppositional defiant disorder from that of conduct disorder: A familial risk analysis. *Journal of Psychiatric Research, 43,* 345–352.

Piquero, A. R., Brame, R., & Moffitt, T. E. (2005). Extending the study of continuity and change: Gender differences in the linkage between adolescent and adult offending. *Journal of Quantitative Criminology, 21*, 219–243.

Plomin, R., DeFries, J. C., & Loehlin, J. C. (1977). Genotype-environment interaction and correlation in the analysis of human behavior. *Psychological Bulletin, 84*, 309–322.

Popma, A., Jansen, L. M. C., Vermeiren, R., Steiner, H., Raine, A., Van Goozen, S. H. M.,... Doreleijers, T. A. H. (2006). Hypothalamus pituitary adrenal axis and autonomic activity during stress in delinquent males adolescents and controls. *Psychoneuroendocrinology, 31*, 948–957.

Quay, H. C. (1965). Psychopathic personality as pathological stimulation-seeking. *American Journal of Psychiatry, 122*, 180–183.

Quay, H. C. (1987). Patterns of delinquent behavior. In H. C. Quay (Ed.), *Handbook of juvenile delinquency* (pp. 118–138). New York, NY: Wiley.

Quay, H. C. (1993). The psychobiology of undersocialized aggressive conduct disorder: A theoretical perspective. *Development and Psychopathology, 5*, 165–180.

Quay, H. C., & Love, C. T. (1977). The effect of a juvenile diversion program on rearrests. *Criminal Justice and Behavior, 4*, 377–396.

Raine, A. (2002). The role of prefrontal deficits, low autonomic arousal and early health factors in the development of antisocial and aggressive behavior in children. *Journal of Child Psychology and Psychiatry, 43*, 417–434.

Raine, A., Dodge, K., Loeber, R., Gatzke-Kopp, L., Lynam, D., Reynolds, C., & Liu, J. H. (2006). The reactive-proactive aggression questionnaire: Differential correlates of reactive and proactive aggression in adolescent boys. *Aggressive Behavior, 32*, 159–171.

Raine, A., Moffitt, T. E., Caspi, A., Loeber, R., Stouthamer-Loeber, M., & Lynam, D. (2005). Neurocognitive impairments in boys on the life-course persistent antisocial path. *Journal of Abnormal Psychology, 114*, 38–49.

Raine, A., Reynolds, C., Venables, P. H., Mednick, S. A., & Farrington, D. P. (1998). Fearlessness, stimulation-seeking, and large body size at age 3 years as early predispositions to childhood aggression at age 11 years. *Archives of General Psychiatry, 55*, 745–751.

Raine, A., Venables, P. H., & Williams, M. (1995). High autonomic arousal and electrodermal orienting at age 15 years as protective factors against criminal behavior at age 29 years. *American Journal of Psychiatry, 152*, 1595–1600.

Raz, S., Shah, F., & Sander, C. J. (1996). Differential effects of perinatal hypoxic risk on early developmental outcome: A twin study. *Neuropsychology, 10*, 429–436.

Rhee, S. H., & Waldman, I. D. (2002). Genetic and environmental influences on antisocial behavior: A meta-analysis of twin and adoption studies. *Psychological Bulletin, 128*, 490–529.

Robins, L. N. (1966). *Deviant children grown up*. Huntington, NY: Krieger.

Rowe, D. C., & Osgood, D. W. (1984). Heredity and sociology theories of delinquency: A reconsideration. *American Sociological Review, 49*, 526–540.

Rowe, R., Costello, E. J., Angold, A., Copeland, W. E., & Maughan, B. (2010). Developmental pathways in oppositional defiant disorder and conduct disorder. *Journal of Abnormal Psychology, 119,* 726–738.

Rowe, R., Maughan, B., Costello, E. J., & Angold, A. (2005). Defining oppositional defiant disorder. *Journal of Child Psychology and Psychiatry, 46,* 1309–1316.

Rowe, R., Maughan, B., & Eley, T. C. (2006). Links between antisocial behavior and depressed mood: The role of life events and attributional style. *Journal of Abnormal Child Psychology, 34,* 293–302.

Rowe, R., Maughan, B., Pickles, A., Costello, E. J., & Angold, A. (2002). The relationship between DSM-IV oppositional defiant disorder and conduct disorder: Findings from the Great Smoky Mountains study. *Journal of Child Psychology and Psychiatry, 43,* 365–373.

Rubia, K. (2011). "Cool" inferior frontostriatal dysfunction in attention-deficit/hyperactivity disorder versus "hot" ventromedial orbitofrontal-limbic dysfunction in conduct disorder: A review. *Biological Psychiatry, 69,* 69–87.

Rutter, M. (1997). Comorbidity: Concepts, claims and choices. *Criminal Behaviour and Mental Health, 7,* 265–285.

Rutter, M. (2006). *Genes and behavior: Nature-nurture interplay explained.* Malden, MA: Blackwell.

Rutter, M., & Giller, H. (1983). *Juvenile delinquency: Trends and perspectives.* Harmondsworth, United Kingdom: Penguin.

Rutter, M., Moffitt, T. E., & Caspi, A. (2006). Gene–environment interplay and psychopathology: Multiple varieties but real effects. *Journal of Child Psychopathology and Psychiatry, 47,* 226–261.

Rutter, M., Yule, B., Quinton, D., Rowlands, O., Yule, W., & Berger, M. (1975). Attainment and adjustment in two geographical areas: III—Some factors accounting for area differences. *British Journal of Psychiatry, 126,* 520–33.

Sampson, R. J., Raudenbush, S. W., & Earls, F. (1997). Neighborhoods and violent crime: A multilevel study of collective efficacy. *Science, 277,* 918–924.

Sanson, A., Pedlow, R., Cann, W., Prior, M., & Oberklaid, F. (1996). Shyness ratings: Stability and correlates in early childhood. *International Journal of Behavioral Development, 19,* 705–724.

Sanson, A., & Prior, M. (1999). Temperament and behavioral precursors to oppositional defiant disorder and conduct disorder. In H. Quay & A. Hogan (Eds.), *Handbook of the disruptive behavior disorders* (pp. 397–417). New York, NY: Kluwer Academic/Plenum.

Saudino, K. J. (2005). Behavioral genetics and child temperament. *Journal of Developmental and Behavioral Pediatrics, 26,* 214–223.

Scarr, S., & McCartney, K. (1983). How people make their own environments: A theory of genotype- environment effects. *Child Development, 54,* 424–435.

Seguin, J. R., Boulerice, B., Harden, P. W., Tremblay, R. E., & Pihl, R. O. (1999). Executive functions and physical aggression after controlling for attention deficit hyperactivity disorder, general memory and IQ. *Journal of Child Psychology and Psychiatry, 40,* 1197–1208.

Serbin, L. A., Cooperman, J. M., Peters, P. L., Lehoux, P. M., Stack, D. M., & Schwartzman, A. E. (1998). Intergenerational transfer of psychosocial risk in women with childhood histories of aggression, withdrawal, or aggression and withdrawal. *Developmental Psychology, 34*, 1246–1262.

Silverthorn, P., & Frick, P. J. (1999). Developmental pathways to antisocial behavior: The delayed-onset pathway in girls. *Development and Psychopathology, 11*, 101–126.

Shannon, K. E., Sauder, C., Beauchaine, T. P., & Gatzke-Kopp, L. (2009). Disrupted effective connectivity between the medial frontal cortex and the caudate in adolescent boys with externalizing behavior disorders. *Criminal Justice and Behavior, 36*, 1141–1157.

Simonoff, E. (2001). Gene-environment interplay in oppositional defiant and conduct disorder. *Child and Adolescent Psychiatric Clinics of North America, 10*, 351–374.

Sparks, R., Ganschow, L., & Thomas, A. (1996). Role of intelligence tests in speech/language referrals. *Perceptual and Motor Skills, 83*, 195–204.

Stattin, H., & Klackenberg-Larsson, I. (1993). Early language and intelligence development and their relationship to future criminal behavior. *Journal of Abnormal Psychology, 102*, 369–378.

Stringaris, A., & Goodman, R. (2009). Three dimensions of oppositionality in youth. *Journal of Child Psychology and Psychiatry, 50*, 216–223.

Tackett, J. L., Krueger, R. F., Iacono, W. G., & McGue, M. (2005). Symptom-based subfactors of DSM-defined conduct disorder: Evidence for etiologic distinctions. *Journal of Abnormal Psychology, 114*, 483–487.

Tackett, J. L., Waldman, I. D., & Lahey, B. B. (2009). Etiology and measurement of relational aggression: A multi-informant behavior genetic investigation. *Journal of Abnormal Psychology, 118*, 722–733.

Thapar, A., Langley, K., Fowler, T., Rice, F., Turic, D., Whittinger, N., . . . O'Donovan, M. (2005). Catechol-O-methyltransferase gene variant and birth weight predict early-onset antisocial behavior in children with attention-deficit/hyperactivity disorder. *Archives of General Psychiatry, 62*, 1275–1278.

Tuvblad, C., Grann, M., & Lichtenstein, P. (2006). Heritability for adolescent antisocial behavior differs with socioeconomic status: Gene-environment interaction. *Journal of Child Psychology and Psychiatry, 47*, 734–743.

van Os, J., Wichers, M., Danckaerts, M., Van Gestel, S., Derom, C., & Vlietinck, R. (2001). A prospective twin study of birth weight discordance and child problem behavior. *Biological Psychiatry, 501*, 593–599.

Viding, E., Blair, R. J. R., Moffitt, T. E., & Plomin, R. (2005). Evidence for substantial genetic risk for psychopathy in 7-year-olds. *Journal of Child Psychology and Psychiatry, 46*, 592–597.

Viding, E., Frick, P. J., & Plomin, R. (2007). Aetiology of the relationship between callous-unemotional traits and conduct problems in childhood. *British Journal of Psychiatry, 190*, S33–S38.

Viding, E., Jones, A. P., Frick, P. J., Moffitt, T. E., & Plomin, R. (2008). Heritability of antisocial behaviour at 9: Do callous unemotional traits matter? *Developmental Science, 11*, 17–22.

Wakschlag, L. S., Pickett, K. E., Cook, E., Benowitz, N. L., & Leventhal, B. L. (2002). Maternal smoking during pregnancy and severe antisocial behavior in offspring. Are they causally linked? *American Journal of Public Health, 92*, 966–974.

Waldman, I. D. (1996). Aggressive children's hostile perceptual and reponse biases: The role of attention and impulsivity. *Child Development, 67*, 1015–1033.

Waldman, I. D., Rhee, S. H., Levy, F., & Hay, D. A. (2001). Genetic and environmental influences on the covariation among symptoms of attention deficit hyperactivity disorder, oppositional defiant disorder, and conduct disorder. In D. A. Hay & F. Levy (Eds.), *Attention, genes and ADHD*. East Sussex, United Kingdom: Brunner-Routledge.

Waldman, I. D., Tackett, J. L., Van Hulle, C. A., Applegate, B., Pardini, D., Frick, P. J., & Lahey, B. B. (2011). Child and adolescent conduct disorder substantially shares genetic influences with three socioemotional dispositions. *Journal of Abnormal Psychology, 120*, 57–70.

Wichers, M. C., Purcell, S., Danckaerts, M., Derom, C., Derom, R., Vlietinck, R., & Van Os, J. (2002). Prenatal life and post-natal psychopathology: Evidence for negative gene-birth weight interaction. *Psychological Medicine, 32*, 1165–1174.

Wichström, L., Skogen, K., & Oia, T. (1996). Increased rate of conduct problems in urban areas: What is the mechanism? *Journal of the American Academy of Child and Adolescent Psychiatry, 35*, 471–479.

World Health Organization. (1993). *ICD-10 classification of mental and behavioural disorders: Diagnostic research criteria*. Geneva, Switzerland: World Health Organization.

Young, S., Smolen, A., Corley, R., Krauter, K., DeFries, J., Crowley, T. J., . . . Hewitt, J. K. (2002). Dopamine transporter polymorphism associated with externalizing behavior problems in children. *American Journal of Medical Genetics Part B: Neuropsychiatric Genetic, 114*, 144–149.

Young S. E., Smolen A., Hewitt, J. K., Haberstick, B., Stallings, M., Corley, R., . . . Crowley, T. J. (2006). Interaction between MAO-A genotype and maltreatment in the risk for conduct disorder: Failure to confirm in adolescent patients. *American Journal of Psychiatry, 163*, 1019–1025.

Zoccolillo, M. (1992). Co-occurrence of conduct disorder and its adult outcomes with depressive and anxiety disorders: A review. *Journal of the American Academy of Child and Adolescent Psychiatry, 31*, 547–556.

# CHAPTER 14

# Development of Adult Antisocial Behavior

THOMAS J. DISHION AND KRISTINA HIATT RACER

M ANY CHILDREN AND ADOLESCENTS show episodes of problem behavior at some point in their development that desist as they mature. Thus, many if not most of these children and adolescents eventually develop prosocial skills, suspend problem behaviors, and assume adult responsibilities. Unfortunately, some youth fail to make this transition and instead show a consistent pattern of impulsive, violent, and even criminal behaviors well into adulthood. In this chapter, we review current knowledge and understanding of the development of antisocial behavior that persists in adulthood, often referred to as *antisocial personality disorder* (ASPD).

## HISTORICAL CONTEXT

Throughout history, societies have been faced with individuals who routinely and persistently engage in behavior that violates societal norms and the rights of others. Across longitudinal studies of antisocial behavior, a small group of offenders typically commit approximately 50% of cohort crimes. Even a small number of these individuals can incur extremely large costs to society given their disproportionate involvement in crime and violence (e.g., Farrington, Barnes, & Lambert, 1996; Jacoby, Weiner, Thornberry, & Wolfgang, 1973; Le Blanc & Loeber, 1993: Loeber & Farrington, 1998). Individuals with a developmental history of antisocial behavior tend to accumulate a variety of health-risking behaviors, economic difficulties, and health-related problems (Odgers et al., 2008). When costs to victims, financial mismanagement, and health care needs are accounted for, persistent antisocial behavior may be the most costly of all personality disorders (Miller, 2004). Accordingly, virtually all communities struggle with prevention, management, and rehabilitation of severely antisocial individuals.

This work was supported by grants DA07031 to the first author, MH0822127 to the second author, and 018760 to Dr. Anthony Biglan, all from the National Institutes of Health.

Historically, there have been two predominant philosophical perspectives on the origins of antisocial behavior: antisocial qualities are either considered to be innate and characterological or acquired through poor socialization. Hobbes, in *Leviathan* (Rogers & Schulman, 1651/2003), argued that antisocial tendencies are innate, and consequently that prosocial behaviors conducive to group living require careful training and socialization. Socialization culls naturally occurring antisocial tendencies and thereby renders individuals more capable of living in groups harmoniously. John Locke (Anstey, 2003) took a more neutral position, proposing the *tabula rasa* perspective on human nature and behavior in which both sense of self and knowledge of good and evil are outcomes of experience and learning. In contrast, Rousseau, in *Emile* (Friedlander, 1762/2004), emphasized that prosocial behavior is a natural human trait and that children learn antisocial behavior in the context of misguided efforts of adults to socialize them. Rousseau's philosophical perspective was perhaps the most directly articulated with respect to practices of education and has influenced policies and practices intended to educate and socialize youth over generations.

It has been only in the past 100 years that an empirical approach to the study of antisocial behavior has dominated thinking about its developmental origins and affected policies of education and juvenile justice aimed at preventing and treating serious and persistent antisocial behavior (Dishion & Patterson, 2006). With the collection of data, the broad-brush philosophical views associated with nature and nurture blend (Rutter, 2006; Chapter 3), with an emphasis on understanding specific transactions between children and their environments that may result in extreme outcomes such as persistent antisocial behavior (Sameroff, 2009). Inherent in this transactional or diathesis–stress perspective is the idea that the same outcome (e.g., persistent antisocial behavior) may be due, across individuals, to a relatively greater contribution of either internal vulnerabilities or environmental risks (see Chapters 1, 2). Thus, an individual with relatively few vulnerabilities may require a severely maladaptive environment to become antisocial, whereas relatively minor environmental deficiencies may promote antisocial behavior in an individual with strong vulnerabilities. From this perspective, there are multiple pathways to persistent antisocial behavior (signifying equifinality) and divergent outcomes for youths who begin life with key risk factors for such behavior (signifying multifinality). Strategies for prevention and intervention should be tailored accordingly to address the specific risk factors that may be operating among individual youth.

Early approaches to antisocial behavior were concerned primarily with managing individuals who broke the law. Consequently, much of our knowledge of antisocial behavior comes from professional fields such as juvenile justice, corrections, social work, and criminology. The role of psychology is relatively recent. Healy (1926) published the first psychologically oriented treatise on the etiology and treatment of antisocial behavior. Influenced heavily by the psychodynamic theory of that time, his thinking emphasized internal, intraindividual factors in the development of crime, especially lack of cognitive abilities (e.g., "dull thinking") and problematic parenting.

Despite his focus on personality, Healy noted that peers are often a proximal factor in the commission of antisocial acts, and the influence of environmental factors was underscored by his publication of quasi-experimental findings, which showed that rates of recidivism vary as a function of the correctional strategy used (Healy & Bronner, 1936). In Chicago, where institutionalization was the dominant strategy, failure rates reached 70%, whereas in Boston, where foster care was the pervasive practice, the recidivism rate was only 27%. Aware of the limitations of quasi-experimental strategies, these researchers suggested tentatively that institutionalization may not be the ideal solution for diverting youths from a life of crime. This suggestion has gone largely unheeded, despite later studies using random assignment and solid measurement procedures that produced essentially the same results (Chamberlain & Reid, 1998; Eddy & Chamberlain, 2000).

Current approaches to studying adolescent and adult antisocial behavior are usually oriented toward identifying developmental processes through the use of longitudinal studies, a strategy that began to be applied in earnest to the domain of antisocial behavior in the late 1970s and early 1980s. Modern studies represent a fusion of the seminal works of Robins (1966), who demonstrated the continuity of antisocial behavior, with the life-course perspective of Elder (1985). Earlier work by S. Glueck and E. Glueck (1950), which emphasized the contribution of family and contextual factors, had been largely rejected by many sociologists. However, a new generation of sociologists (e.g., Sampson & Laub, 1993) resurrected the Glueck data set and reanalyzed the findings by using modern statistical techniques. The results suggest that family variables should be a central focus for theories about the development of antisocial behavior in children. A review of research from multiple longitudinal studies on the development of antisocial behavior by Loeber and Dishion (1983) also provided a strong empirical base for emphasizing family variables. The 1970s and 1980s also witnessed the emergence of improved methodologies for studying social interactions within close relationships, with direct observations of family and peer interactions suggesting specific patterns of relationship dynamics that amplify antisocial behavior at various stages of development (reviewed later).

In addition to the increased focus on relationship dynamics, modern statistical techniques enable us to examine the effects of broad social contexts (e.g., schools, neighborhoods) on the development of antisocial behavior. Furthermore, advances in neuroscience and genetics have allowed for greater specification of individual differences that may be critical for understanding the development of persistent antisocial behavior (see Viding, 2004).

## TERMINOLOGICAL, CONCEPTUAL, AND DIAGNOSTIC ISSUES

Broadly speaking, *antisocial behavior* refers to activities that violate societal norms, laws, and the rights of others. Such behaviors may include criminal acts (e.g., theft, fraud, assault, driving while intoxicated, illicit drug use) and noncriminal acts (e.g., deceitfulness, irresponsibility). In childhood and adolescence, violations of family rules and expectations through disobedience and defiance also fall under the rubric of antisocial behavior and are generally referred to as *conduct problems* or *disruptive behaviors* (milder forms may be termed *oppositional/defiant*). Antisocial behavior that leads to contact with the legal system is usually referred to as *delinquent behavior* in children and adolescents and as *criminal behavior* in adults.

When antisocial behavior persists across time and situations, it is often considered pathological and can result in the diagnosis of a disruptive behavior disorder. Among children and adolescents, persistent antisocial behavior may lead to a *Diagnostic and Statistical Manual of Mental Disorders* (*DSMV-IV*; American Psychiatric Association [APA], 2000) diagnosis of oppositional defiant disorder (ODD) or conduct disorder (CD; see Chapter 13). In individuals age 18 years or older, persistent antisocial behavior may lead to a diagnosis of ASPD. The development of ASPD is the main focus of this chapter.

Current *DSMV-IV* diagnostic criteria for ASPD include a pervasive pattern of disregard for and violation of the rights of others, as indicated by three or more of the following: (1) failure to conform to social norms regarding lawful behaviors, as indicated by repeatedly performing acts that are grounds for arrest; (2) deceitfulness, as indicated by repeated lying, use of aliases, or conning others for personal pleasure or profit; (3) impulsivity or failure to plan ahead; (4) irritability and aggressiveness, as indicated by repeated physical fights or assaults; (5) reckless disregard for the safety of self or others; (6) consistent irresponsibility, as indicated by repeated failure to sustain consistent work behavior or honor financial obligations; and (7) lack of remorse, as indicated by being indifferent to or rationalizing having hurt, mistreated, or stolen from another. As with all personality disorders, the individual must be at least 18 years of age (Criterion B). There must also be evidence of CD before age 15 years (Criterion C), and the antisocial behavior must not occur exclusively during the course of schizophrenia or mania.

ASPD is so common among criminal offenders that the terms *ASPD* and *criminal offending* are often used synonymously (Widiger & Corbitt, 1995). However, some adults who commit crimes are not characterized by ASPD in that they do not have a developmental history of antisocial behavior in childhood and adolescence. For example, individuals who commit isolated crimes (e.g., a single episode of theft, assault, drug use, or even murder) and who do not have a broader history of irresponsible or antisocial behavior would not meet criteria for ASPD. *Antisocial personality* refers specifically to individuals with a persistent pattern of antisocial behavior (criminal or not) over an extended period of time and beginning before age 15 years.

Moreover, aggressive and violent antisocial behavior is not necessarily a key indicator of ASPD, despite the salience of such behavior to communities and victims. Aggression has many contributing causes, and isolated acts of aggression or violence can occur without a significant history of antisocial behavior (e.g., crimes of passion). Furthermore, some persistently aggressive and violent individuals may not be considered to have an antisocial personality; for example, engagement in occasional fist fights at the local bar is not an indicator of ASPD if the individual does not cause serious harm and otherwise behaves lawfully and responsibly. On the other hand, both males and females with a history of antisocial behavior that persists into adulthood are indeed at more risk of aggression, and violence occurs more often among people with ASPD than among people without ASPD, perhaps because many individuals with ASPD also have personality traits that place them at greater risk for repeated aggression and violence.

Discussion of ASPD overlaps to some degree with the terms *dyssocial personality*, *sociopathy*, and *psychopathy*. Dyssocial personality disorder is the diagnostic term for persistent adult antisocial behavior used in the World Health Organization's International Classification of Diseases (ICD-10) diagnostic manual. Although similar to the *DSM-IV* diagnosis of ASPD in many respects, dissocial personality does not require a history of CD in childhood or adolescence.

*Sociopathy* is a frequently used term that has no defined diagnostic criteria and is not formally used in clinical psychology or psychiatry. The original *DSM* (APA, 1952) included diagnostic criteria for sociopathic personality disturbance, otherwise known as *antisocial reaction*, which was revised and renamed *antisocial personality disorder* in the second edition of the *DSM* (APA, 1968).

*Psychopathy* refers to a subtype of ASPD that is based on the clinical descriptions of Cleckley (1941) and emphasizes affective and interpersonal traits (e.g., callousness, shallow affect, lack of interpersonal connectedness, superficial charm) in addition to chronic antisocial behavior. Accordingly, many individuals who show psychopathic behavior also meet criteria for ASPD. However, the relation between ASPD and psychopathy is not transitive, because only a small subset of individuals with ASPD meets criteria for psychopathy.

Originally, the *DSM* construct of ASPD was rooted in personality, with diagnostic criteria drawn from the construct of psychopathy (Cleckley, 1941). In its earliest instantiation, a diagnosis of ASPD required not only the presence of persistent antisocial behavior but also specific personality features, such as lack of emotional depth, lack of remorse or guilt, and shallow interpersonal relationships. However, it became clear that practitioners were unable to reliably infer the personality traits described by Cleckley in the course of standard clinical assessments. As early versions of the *DSM* were revised to improve diagnostic reliability, there was an increased focus on observable behavioral criteria (i.e., antisocial acts) rather than inferred personality characteristics. This focus on greater reliability was most clearly evidenced in *DSM-III* (APA, 1980), which equated ASPD with persistent antisocial behavior, irrespective of personality traits. Personality characteristics returned to some extent in the *DSM-IV*; psychopathic personality features are specifically referenced in the "Associated Features and Disorders" section of the *DSM-IV* text, and current diagnostic criteria include some subjective features, such as lack of remorse. Nevertheless, current ASPD criteria can be (and often are) met on the basis of antisocial behavior alone.

There continues to be active debate about the *DSM* ASPD construct and whether it should remain behavioral and objective or include some or all of the personality characteristics of psychopathy. As defined by the *DSM*, ASPD is common in criminal populations, with as many as 80% of incarcerated individuals meeting criteria for the diagnosis (Widiger & Corbitt, 1995). Accordingly, those with the disorder are heterogeneous with respect to personality, attitudes, and motivations for engaging in criminal behavior, so a diagnosis of ASPD has limited utility for making differential predictions of institutional adjustment, response to treatment, or behavior following release from prison. In contrast, psychopathy is present in only a small subset of criminal offenders and has substantial predictive validity (e.g., institutional adjustment, recidivism rates) within forensic populations (e.g., Hare, Clark, Grann, & Thornton, 2000). Specifically, individuals with psychopathy have a particularly pernicious criminal course, and suggestions abound that they have a more homogeneous set of psychophysiological and biological risk factors (see later section about individual differences).

Although current *DSM-IV* criteria for ASPD identify a heterogeneous group of individuals with persistent antisocial behavior, there are some benefits to the present approach. First, diagnostic reliability in clinical settings has improved. Second, ASPD diagnoses may be informative and discriminating when used with community populations, despite the lack of discrimination among individuals in forensic settings. However, even in community samples, those who meet criteria for ASPD are heterogeneous in terms of etiologic and maintenance factors, suggesting that clinicians may need to further differentiate individuals using other diagnostic methods in order to determine the most appropriate treatments. In addition, research investigators and forensic psychologists must continue to use specialized diagnostic instruments (e.g., the Psychopathy Checklist-Revised [PCL-R]; Hare, 2003) to identify subgroups of particular interest within the ASPD category.

In the remainder of this chapter, we review current knowledge and theories regarding the development of persistent adult antisocial behavior. Most of the existing work defines adult antisocial behavior in ways that are compatible with *DSM-IV* ASPD diagnostic criteria, although the criteria used often vary across studies. This chapter follows the *DSM* model in emphasizing antisocial behavior as the outcome of interest, irrespective of personality or other individual differences. This approach allows an overview of the factors that have been associated with adult antisocial behavior across individuals while recognizing that different pathways may ultimately prove to be more or less relevant for particular subgroups within the broad ASPD category.

## PREVALENCE

The 2001 to 2002 National Epidemiologic Survey on Alcohol and Related Conditions ($N = 43,093$) indicated a lifetime prevalence rate of 3.6% for ASPD, with risk being 3 times greater among men than among women (Compton, Conway, Stinson, Colliver, & Grant, 2005; Grant et al., 2004). For comparison, the lifetime prevalence of adult antisocial behavior only (not meeting the childhood CD criterion) was 12.3%, and the prevalence of retrospectively reported CD in childhood without antisocial behavior in adulthood was 1.1% (Compton et al., 2005). Estimates of ASPD prevalence within incarcerated populations range from 49% to 80% (Widiger & Corbitt, 1995).

Longitudinal analyses of community samples of males and females can provide estimates of the prevalence and continuity of antisocial behavior from early childhood through adulthood. Using a mixture modeling approach to trajectory analyses, data from the Dunedin, New Zealand, study suggests the prevalence of early-onset and persistent antisocial behavior to be 8.2% in males and 7.5% in females (Odgers et al., 2008). These estimates show less sex disparity and higher prevalence estimates than do classic epidemiological studies in part because the overall developmental pattern is of concern rather than the actual diagnostic threshold. Of note, the adolescence-onset group was also quite large, revealing a prevalence rate of 19.6% and 17.4% for males and females, respectively. It is noteworthy that the average level of antisocial behavior in early adulthood for the adolescence-onset and the childhood-onset groups was by all practical purposes equivalent—although the incidence of violence is greater in the childhood-onset group, questioning the idea that adolescence-onset is a more temporary, episodic display of rebelliousness (see also Moffitt, 2006, for additional information on the persistence of adolescence-onset ASB). These estimates from the Dunedin study suggest that antisocial behavior in adulthood is not as rare as clinical studies suggest. Given the disruptiveness of antisocial behavior on adult roles such as parenting, working, and education, the relatively high rates of antisocial behavior in a community sample is of some concern.

## RISK FACTORS

Because of the marked continuity of childhood-onset and adolescent conduct problems and later antisocial behavior, many if not all of the risk factors for child and adolescent conduct problems are relevant to the development of adult ASPD. In behavioral genetics studies, estimates of environmental and genetic risk for CD and ASPD are roughly equivalent for males and for females (Meier, Slutske, Heath, & Martin, 2011). Thus, factors associated with childhood and adolescence CD, such as child vulnerabilities (e.g., negative emotionality, "difficult" temperament, prenatal or perinatal complications), family risk (e.g., large family size, antisocial parent), parenting risk (e.g., harsh and inconsistent discipline, poor monitoring), peer risk (e.g., peer rejection, deviant peers), and sociocultural risk (e.g., high-delinquency neighborhood or school), all contribute risk for ASPD (see also Chapters 6, 10). This overlap between CD and ASPD is due to both the natural continuity of antisocial behavior and the diagnostic requirement of CD prior to age 15.

Accordingly, childhood conduct problems are perhaps the best single predictor of adult ASPD. Lahey, Loeber, Burke, and Applegate (2005) followed a clinical sample of boys with behavior problems and found that 54% of those who received a CD diagnosis at the time they enrolled in the study (ages 7 to 12 years) met criteria for ASPD at age 18 or 19, compared with 27% of those who did not meet criteria for CD. Interestingly, these effects were moderated by family socioeconomic status (SES). Children with CD who were from higher SES families were far less likely to meet criteria for ASPD as young adults (20%) than were those from lower SES families (65%). Childhood aggression alone is also predictive of adult ASPD. Petras et al. (2004) found that 27% of boys with consistently high levels of teacher-rated aggression in elementary school met ASPD criteria at age 19 to 20, compared with 11% of boys with stable low aggression in elementary school. Boys with increasing levels of aggression from Grades 1 to 5 were also at risk for ASPD (25.6%).

In general, earlier onset of conduct problems is associated with greater risk of persistence into adulthood (Moffitt, 1993, 2006). Data from the NIMH Epidemiological Catchment Area (ECA) survey of more than 8,000 adults indicated a 12.4-fold increase in risk for adult antisocial behavior among those with childhood-onset (before age 13) conduct problems compared with a 5.5-fold increase among those with adolescence-onset (age 13 or later) conduct problems, relative to those with no history of conduct problems (Ridenour et al., 2002).

Although earlier onset is typically associated with poorer outcomes, these data and others (e.g., Moffitt, Caspi, Harrington, & Milne, 2002) also make clear that adolescence-onset conduct problems are themselves associated with increased risk of adult ASPD. In Moffitt and colleagues' longitudinal study of a New Zealand birth cohort, 34% of men with adolescence-onset conduct problems were convicted in adult criminal court by age 26, compared with 55% of men with childhood-onset conduct problems. Despite this difference in criminal conviction rates, comparable percentages from each group met criteria for ASPD at age 26 (Moffitt et al., 2002).

Studies have been conducted to statistically disentangle the prognostic value of frequency of antisocial behavior with the timing of onset for later ASPD. In analysis of twin data with assessments of children's behavior at ages 11, 14, and 17, the frequency of aggressive and rule-breaking behavior in early and later adolescence was a better predictor of adult antisocial behavior than nominal classification of early versus adolescence-onset (Burt, Donnellan, Iacono, & McGue, 2011). Analyses such as these underscore the value of a transactional perspective on the development and progression of antisocial behavior, with an emphasis on conditions that predict frequency, variety, and continuity in such behaviors over time (Dishion & Patterson, 2006; Patterson, DeBaryshe, & Ramsey, 1989; Sameroff, 2009).

As outlined earlier, it is important to note that not all youth with conduct problems continue to show antisocial behavior in adulthood. Data from multiple large-scale longitudinal studies reveal that only about 50% of boys with childhood conduct problems develop adult ASPD (Moffitt et al., 2002; Patterson & Yoerger, 1999; Robins, 1966). Although those who do not become antisocial adults remain at risk for other forms of psychopathology in adulthood (Moffitt, 2006; Robins, 1966; Wiesner, Kim, & Capaldi, 2005), their desistence from antisocial behavior emphasizes how important it is to identify (a) early risk factors that are differentially associated with persistent antisocial behavior, and (b) the developmental and transactional processes that maintain and promote antisocial behavior in adolescence and adulthood, as well as those that may promote desistence.

With regard to early risk factors, many researchers have proposed that childhood abuse and neglect may be particularly important in the etiology of antisocial personality styles and persistent adult antisocial behavior. Luntz and Widom (1994) found that 20% of boys who were abused or neglected before age 12 met criteria for

ASPD 20 years later, compared with only 10% of controls. Similarly, maltreatment in adolescence is associated with increased risk of adult antisocial behavior (Smith, Ireland, & Thornberry, 2005), and childhood abuse and neglect are associated with higher psychopathy scores among young adults (Weiler & Widom, 1996). Childhood physical abuse appears to be more strongly related to adult antisocial behavior than is childhood neglect or emotional abuse (Cohen, Brown, & Smailes, 2001). The effects of abuse and neglect may be mediated by other environmental risk factors, such as other stressful life events, rather than associated directly with later adjustment (Horwitz, Widon, McLaughlin, & White, 2001). Odgers et al. (2008) suggest that observed parent maltreatment in the research laboratory was associated with early-onset and persistent antisocial behavior into adulthood. It is noteworthy that early-onset but desisting children were also more likely to have experienced maltreatment than typically developing controls, thus, maltreatment apparently predicts childhood onset but not necessarily continuity and progression to more serious antisocial behavior in adulthood. In addition, Gene × Environment (G × E) interaction and gene-environment correlation (rGE) research reveals that early maltreatment and genetic vulnerabilities interact to account for adult violence (Caspi et al., 2002; see Chapter 3). To date, specific transactional dynamics that might account for G × E and rGE effects have only begun to be articulated (see Beauchaine, Klein, Crowell, Derbidge, & Gatzke-Kopp, 2009). Research discussed later in this chapter suggests that self-organization into peer groups that promote more serious forms of coercion and violence is crucial to this developmental progression.

It has been hypothesized that neurobiological risk factors may play a role in early-onset and persisting antisocial behavior (Moffitt, 1993). Minor physical anomalies (MPAs), such as low-seated ears, adherent ear lobes, and furrowed tongues, are associated with increased risk of antisocial behavior, perhaps because they are indictors of fetal maldevelopment or prenatal/perinatal trauma (e.g., anoxia, infection). When combined with an adverse home environment, MPAs are associated with increased risk of violence and aggression in adulthood (Brennan, Mednick, & Raine, 1997; Mednick & Kandel, 1988). Raine, Venables, and Williams (1995) found that physiological arousal and reactivity at age 14 years were related to persistence of antisocial behavior through age 29 years. Those who desisted between early adolescence and adulthood had higher electrodermal orienting at age 14 than did those who persisted, suggesting that normal autonomic arousal may serve as a protective factor against persistent antisocial behavior. Consistent with this conjecture, Shannon, Beauchaine, Brenner, Neuhaus, and Gatzke-Kopp (2007) reported that children with antisocial fathers were protected from developing conduct problems if they had normal autonomic arousal patterns. The developmental trajectory study of Odgers et al. (2008) revealed that low IQ, an undercontrolled temperament as rated in the laboratory setting, and diagnosis of ADHD were characteristic of early-onset and persistent patterns for both males and females, but low resting heart rate was prognostic for males only.

Antisocial behavior tends to run in families (e.g., Farrington et al., 1996). Although some of this familial transmission can be explained through behavioral or environmental learning (e.g., Dishion, Owen, & Bullock, 2004; Patterson & Dishion,

1988), genetic factors are also at play. Behavioral genetic studies suggest that anti-social behavior that persists from early adolescence through adulthood may have a stronger genetic basis than do other forms of antisocial behavior (see Moffitt, 2006). As with other behavioral traits (see Chapter 3), there is also evidence that the influence of genes increases from childhood to adulthood, whereas the influ-ence of environmental factors becomes weaker (Jacobson, Prescott, & Kendler, 2002), strongly suggestive of the operation of $r$GE. Most genetic risk for antisocial behavior appears to operate through general predisposing vulnerabilities, such as temperament (e.g., negative affectivity, impulsivity), that confer broad risk for psychopathology—especially externalizing behaviors—rather than specific risk for ASPD (e.g., Krueger et al., 2002). However, as discussed later, such vulnerability appears to be associated with exposure to both healthy and pathogenic environ-mental contexts, meaning that "environmental" interventions for such children are quite effective (e.g., Belsky, Bakermans-Kranenburg, & van Ijzendoorn, 2007; Petras et al., 2008; Chapter 8).

Susceptibility to environmental conditions is one form of G × E interaction. The work by Caspi et al. (2002) was the first to strongly suggest a G × E interaction in the development of antisocial behavior problems for males. Caspi and colleagues (Caspi et al., 2002) examined the interaction between exposure to maltreatment and polymorphisms in the monoamine oxidase-A (MAO-A) gene, which encodes an enzyme that metabolizes all monoamines, including dopamine, serotonin, and norepinephrine. Outcome measures were juvenile and adult antisocial behavior. Among males with the low MAO-A activity genotype, childhood maltreatment greatly increased the risk of antisocial behavior (85% showed some form of antisocial behavior). However, childhood maltreatment had relatively little impact on risk of adult antisocial behavior among those with the high MAO-A activity allele. This particular G × E interaction has been replicated (Kim-Cohen et al., 2006), suggesting that genetically vulnerable boys may be more reactive to coercive, harsh discipline practices characteristic of maltreating families, with important implications for prevention and treatment.

Beauchaine, Hinshaw, and Gatzke-Kopp (2008) offered a conceptual review of findings linking single nucleotide polymorphisms (SNPs) associated with the neurotransmission of dopamine with the development of antisocial behavior. The evidence suggests child impulsivity (i.e., low self-regulation in the presence of rewards) is an endophenotype that accounts for the G × E interaction associated with persistence of antisocial behavior into adulthood. A similar case can be made for the effortful attention control construct (Rothbart, Sheese, & Posner, 2007). What constitutes the specific environmental processes that amplify genetic influences is a question actively being pursued. Gamma-aminobutyric acid receptor alpha 2 (GABRA2) is a genetic polymorphism associated with the neurotransmission of dopamine. Perhaps the most provocative finding to date is the association between GABRA2 and the persistent problem behavior trajectory for adolescent males and females, which was moderated by parental monitoring practices (Dick et al., 2009). That is, genetic risk for problem behavior in adolescence and adulthood was significantly reduced by parental monitoring practices in adolescence. The inclusion of parenting practices in adolescence in the analysis of the persistent antisocial trajectory is a major theoretical breakthrough for understanding the progression from childhood antisocial behavior to more serious adult forms of problem behaviors, including substance use and violence. However, there remains room for further investigation. One relevant mechanism may be reduction of access to peer reward for deviance; as such, impulsivity in the presence of reward is the risk dynamic associated with persistent antisocial behavior.

Substance use and abuse also play an important role in the continuity of antisocial behavior from adolescence to adulthood. Although minor delinquent offenses typically precede the initiation of drug use (e.g., Moffitt, Caspi, Dickson, Silva, & Stanton, 1996; Taylor, Malone, Iacono, & McGue, 2002), substance use itself increases the frequency of delinquent and antisocial behaviors (e.g., Zhang, Wieczorek, & Welte, 1997). Furthermore, lack of drug or alcohol problems is associated with the desistence of childhood conduct problems (Moffitt et al., 1996; Zucker, Ellis, Fitzgerald, Bingham, & Sanford, 1996). As revealed in the work of Dick et al. (2009), antisocial behavior and substance use share common genetic and environmental risk factors. The genetic vulnerability has been recently extended to account for comorbid substance dependence and ASPD (Li et al., 2012).

## ETIOLOGY AND TRANSACTIONAL PROGRESSIONS

As discussed earlier, ASPD is an extremely heterogeneous diagnostic category. The diagnosis of ASPD is based primarily upon overt behaviors without regard to causes or context. As a result, seemingly different individuals can receive the same diagnosis, and a single etiological model is unlikely to account for all instances of ASPD. Accordingly, many researchers have sought to understand variation and progressions of adult antisocial behaviors that are functionally equivalent, such as violent offending, and moved away from core personality characteristics, such as narcissism.

For example, the longest standing and most empirically supported subtype of ASPD, psychopathy, refers to a personality type characterized by distinct affective, behavioral, and interpersonal traits (see previous discussion). As noted earlier, psychopathy accounts for a relatively small subset of individuals with ASPD—about 15% to 25% (Hare, 1991). Thus, given the low incidence of ASPD in the community, the number of psychopathic offenders is quite small. Compared with individuals with ASPD only, psychopathic individuals are at heightened risk for recidivism and violent offending (Hare et al., 2000). In addition to their unique clinical and prognostic correlates, individuals with psychopathy differ from other ASPD individuals with respect to physiology, neuropsychology, attention, emotion, and behavior (see Hiatt & Newman, 2006, for a review). Several well-established etiological theories and models of psychopathy include Newman's (e.g., Newman, 1998; Newman & Wallace, 1993) response-modulation hypothesis, Lykken's (1995) low-fear hypothesis, and Blair's (e.g., Blair, 2002) amygdala/orbital-frontal deficit model. Although these models are quite different in the specific processes implicated, they all suggest that the primary cause of psychopathy is biological or temperamental, is present at or near birth, and persists throughout the life course, driving the clinical symptoms.

## ONSET PATTERN

By far the most important etiological consideration is when the antisocial behavior emerged during development and the transactional factors that account for amplification of childhood antisocial behaviors through adolescence to more serious forms in adulthood. An enormous amount of research was stimulated by the nominal distinction raised in the field regarding early-onset antisocial behavior (Robins, 1966) and the distinction between it and adolescence onset (Moffitt, 1993; Patterson, 1993). As reviewed earlier, there is now less evidence that adolescence-onset antisocial behavior is temporary and trivial with respect to adult development (Odgers et al., 2008). Certainly there are adolescents who use substances and engage in minor antisocial acts that are largely undetected by police. However, those who are more serious offenders tend to persist with this behavior into adulthood and have a greater likelihood of meeting criteria for ASPD than do typically developing youth (Odgers et al., 2008).

Critical to etiological theory is understanding the series of transactions that occur at each stage of development that support antisocial behavior patterns and amplify risk for continuance of the behavior into later development. One of the best predictors of serious adolescent antisocial behavior in adolescence is teacher ratings of antisocial behavior in childhood (Loeber & Dishion, 1983). Research by Shaw and colleagues (2003) identified the Person × Environment transaction in early childhood that accounted for children being identified by teachers as antisocial in Grade 2. As would be expected by the person-centered risk factors described earlier (also see Beauchaine et al., 2008), 2-year-old boys identified as having low levels of fear and a depressed mother were those who were more likely to be on the early-onset and persistent antisocial trajectory from age 2 through 7. In subsequent randomized intervention studies, Shaw, Dishion, and colleagues found that brief support (i.e., the Family Check-Up) to caregivers to practice positive behavior support improved parenting and reduced antisocial behavior in children from age 2 to 4 (Shaw, Dishion, Supplee, Gardner, & Arnds, 2006); these effects of the Family Check-Up were extended to both males and females and were most pronounced in children with clinically elevated problem behavior at age 2 (Dishion et al., 2008). Yearly brief support for parenting practices was recently found to reduce parent-reported antisocial behavior from age 2 through 5 and significantly reduced teacher ratings of antisocial behavior at age 7 (Dishion et al., under review).

A core feature of antisocial behavior in adulthood, believed to be linked to psychopathy, is callousness/lack of remorse. Hyde, Shaw, and Moilanen (2010) found that parent reports of their child's deceitful and calloused behavior were reliable and stable from age 2 through 5. However, children showing these behaviors were not less responsive to the randomized parenting intervention. Later, Waller, Gardner, Hyde, Shaw, Dishion, and Wilson (2012) examined observed parenting characteristics as they related to parents' perceptions of young children's calloused and deceitful behavior and found observed harsh parenting to be among the strongest correlates. These data suggest that some features of antisocial behavior often thought of as *psychopathy* may in part be a reaction to troubled interpersonal relationships, beginning with the family in early childhood.

Experimental manipulation of parenting practices in the past 10 years has dramatically reduced the concern that parenting is simply a reaction to the child's "traits" and does not cause antisocial behavior. Without doubt, the transactional perspective would support a bidirectional effect between parenting and adjustment. Certainly, coercion theory continues to be a dominant framework for thinking about the etiology and progression of antisocial behavior to adulthood. Patterson's coercion model focuses specifically on contributions of parent–child interactions to child antisocial behavior (Patterson, 1982; Patterson, Reid, & Dishion, 1992: Snyder, Reid, & Patterson, 2003). According to this model, antisocial behavior often functions to reduce an aversive interpersonal experience. During childhood to adolescence, caregivers giving negative feedback reinforces the problem behavior. Coercive interactions between the parent and child consist of a cycle of intrusive demands, compliance refusals, escalating distress and negative affect, and finally, withdrawal of the demand. A high rate of coercive behavior between the parent and child sets the stage for more serious antisocial behavior. Furthermore, the impact of contextual variables, such as divorce, poverty, and neighborhood risk, on child outcomes is proposed to be mediated by their impact on parenting practices. According to this model, the individual with early-onset delinquency is trained by family members to engage in high rates of overt antisocial behavior at the expense of well-developed social and self-regulatory skills.

Patterson's coercion model has received considerable empirical support (see Dishion & Patterson, 2006; Snyder & Stoolmiller, 2002) with respect to child and adolescent antisocial behavior. Nevertheless, the effectiveness of interventions that reduce coercive interactions and improve family management with regard to reducing child and adolescent antisocial behavior suggests that parenting may contribute independently to the development of antisocial behavior (Beauchaine, Webster-Stratton, & Reid, 2005; Forgatch, Bullock, & Patterson, 2004; Martinez & Forgatch, 2002). In a review of empirically supported intervention strategies, studies on parent management training reveal mediation between reduction in parent–child coercive interactions and improvement in children's behavior in adolescence (Forgatch & Patterson, 2010).

As these intervention trials suggest, about half the children who develop antisocial behaviors in childhood desist by adolescence. Moreover, about 25% of those with no evidence of serious antisocial behaviors in middle childhood develop antisocial behavior in adolescence (Odgers et al., 2008). Over the years, one tension in the behavioral sciences has been the paradox between the effectiveness of interventions that target antisocial behavior in middle childhood and the high stabilities noted between childhood and adult antisocial behavior (Loeber, 1982; Olweus, 1980; Stattin & Magnusson, 1991). As prevention and developmental science merge, this tension seems to have been reduced and the transactional processes of stability and change have been clarified. For example, a randomized experiment reported by

Petras and colleagues (2008) suggests that systematically improving the classroom environment in the first year of elementary school can reduce the likelihood of children meeting the diagnosis of ASPD 10 years later. Moreover, the environmental intervention was most effective for those who at 6 years old were the most severely aggressive. The transactional framework is helpful for explaining how children's antisocial behavior in childhood can undermine a series of key adaptations that function to promote prosocial development and discourage progressions in antisocial behavior.

Considerable research suggests that childhood antisocial behavior leads to a developmental cascade that supports progression to more serious forms of antisocial behavior in adolescence and adulthood (Dishion, Véronneau, & Myers, 2010; Dodge, Greenberg, & Malone, 2008; Masten et al., 2005). The cascade models converge on the notion that childhood antisocial behavior is associated with poor academic learning and compromised relationships with peers and teachers—and that these experiences predict association with deviant peers, which in turn amplifies problem behaviors into adolescence and adulthood.

As children become adolescents, peer relationships increase in importance. In a series of studies discussed later in this chapter, we have tested the hypothesis that interactions with friends play a critical role in the persistence or desistance of antisocial behavior in later childhood and adolescence. We posited that peers are a major proximal cause of antisocial behavior, beginning in early childhood and accelerating in influence during early adolescence. Three pathways are relevant: (1) antisocial behavior interferes with positive peer relations, depriving children of the positive benefits of peer learning and confining them within marginal social niches; (2) children may act as models and a source of reinforcement for antisocial behavior; and (3) as children develop friendship networks, support for antisocial behavior is established by providing both reinforcement and opportunity for such behavior within networks of deviant peers. Monahan, Steinberg, and Cauffman (2009) suggest that in early adolescence, peer socialization accounts for increases in antisocial behavior, and in adulthood, peer effects are diminished generally. However, observation of friendship dynamics suggests that peer effects are pronounced through all three phases of development, but the specific behaviors that are affected vary by developmental stage.

Dishion and colleagues have found that well-organized interactions with adolescent friends on deviant topics are associated with increased levels of antisocial behavior at ages 18 (Piehler & Dishion, 2007) and 26 (Dishion, Nelson, Winter, & Bullock, 2004). The association between friendship patterns and persistent antisocial behavior fits the classic definition of a maladaptation within a developmental psychopathology framework. That is, youth adapt to failure in school and among peers by formulating their own social niches, which reinforce the very traits that led to failure and rejection. Not only are deviant peer relationships highly correlated with antisocial behavior, but randomized intervention trials that aggregate high-risk adolescents in treatment groups often show *increases* in problem behavior rather than the hoped-for decreases (Dishion, McCord, & Poulin, 1999; Dodge, Dishion, & Lansford, 2006).

Children's tendency to self-organize into deviant peer clusters may be an evolutionary-based adaptation (Dishion, Ha, & Véronneau, 2012) within the framework of a life-history strategy (Belsky, Steinberg, & Draper, 1991). Life-history theory describes a "fast" life-history strategy as an epigenetic response to harsh and stressful early child-rearing environments that promotes risky behavior in adolescence and early pubertal development (Ellis, Figuero, Brumbach, & Schlomer, 2009). A core feature of a fast life-history strategy is self-organization into deviant peer clusters in early to middle adolescence. We extend the concept of harsh environments to include a history of peer rejection, attenuated family ties, and low socioeconomic status. Not only do peer associations account for the age–crime curve, which reveals a peak prevalence of antisocial activity during adolescence (Hirschi & Gottfredson, 1991; Warr, 1993), but peer clustering is one of the best predictors of adolescent sexual activity (Boislard & Poulin, 2011; Capaldi, Crosby, & Stoolmiller, 1996; French & Dishion, 2003) and the number of offspring (Dishion et al., 2012).

When marginalized children self-organize into deviant peer clusters, the venue for connection and friendship is problem behavior in a process referred to as *peer contagion* (Dishion & Tipsord, 2011). Dishion, Nelson, Winter, et al., (2004) found that boys with a combination of well-organized peer interactions (low "entropy") and high levels of deviancy training (i.e., peer reinforcement of deviant talk and behaviors) at age 14 were most likely to engage in substance use and antisocial behavior in adulthood (age 26), suggesting that adolescents who organize their relationships around deviance are the most at risk for long-term maintenance of antisocial behavior. Similarly, Piehler and Dishion (2007) found that friendships that were both mutual and more deviant predicted high levels of antisocial behavior by age 18 as defined by arrests and self-report. Recently, we expanded the concept of deviancy training in friendships to reveal a dynamic of "coercive joining" in which adolescent friendships (male and female) are characterized by struggles for dominance, coercion, and aggression (see Figure 14.1). Direct observations of coercive joining in adolescent friendships were highly predictive of serious violence ($\beta = .52$, $p < .001$) by age 25 in both males and females (accounting for 45% of the variance), controlling for a multiagent and multimethod construct of antisocial behavior ($\beta = .25$, $p < .01$). Serious violence was defined by self-reported violent behavior, arrests for violence, and parent reports of violent acts in young adulthood.

The quality of the friendships at age 16 was associated negatively with progressions from antisocial behavior in adolescence to progressions to serious violence by adulthood. There was also a statistical interaction between friendship quality and coercive joining in friendships in which males and females with poor quality friendships and high levels of coercive joining were the most likely to escalate to more serious forms of violence. This finding suggests that ASPD is associated with a general tendency to fail to form mutually satisfying friendships, and this critical disability perhaps underlies the transactional view of the development of ASPD.

Van Ryzin and Dishion (2012) recently used a randomized intervention trial to test a model linking parent–child conflict from early to late adolescence with young adult antisocial behavior, which was mediated through association with deviant

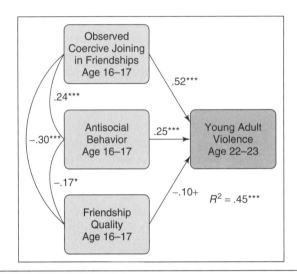

**Figure 14.1**  A model for the amplification of antisocial behavior to violence.

peers. The Family Check-Up in early adolescence reduced conflict and young adult antisocial behavior, according to youth report and observed interactions in the home (Van Ryzin & Dishion, 2012). Moreover, Patterson, DeGarmo, and Forgatch (2004) documented that randomized parent management training produced a cascade of positive effects that began with reduced parent–child coercion and segued to improvements in child compliance, reduction of involvement with deviant peer groups, and reduction of antisocial behavior, through adolescence. Developmental and intervention research converge on the perspective that transactions between family, peer, school, and individual vulnerabilities account for stability and change in antisocial behavior.

Numerous sociocultural variables correlate with improvement in adult antisocial behavior, including marriage (Farrington, 1995), good social integration (Reiss, Grubin, & Meux, 1996), parenthood and increased family responsibilities (Black, Baumgard, & Bell, 1995), academic success (Robins & Regier, 1991), and stable employment (Farrington, 1995; Robins, 1966). Still, it is difficult to know from correlational data whether certain individuals with antisocial behavior patterns "migrate" or self-select into these advantageous ecologies or whether these sociocultural influences independently predict desistence.

Although there is evidence that supportive romantic relationships are associated with transitioning away from deviant behavior in early adulthood (Quinton, Pickles, Maughan, & Rutter, 1993), this is not always the case. In some instances, antisocial individuals may partner with other antisocial individuals. Such assortative mating can lead to amplification of antisocial behavior (Caspi & Herbener, 1990; Quinton et al., 1993). Follow-up studies of adolescent males suggest that marriage and continued involvement in deviant peer groups can go hand in hand, contributing to the persistence, rather than desistence, of antisocial behavior (Shortt, Capaldi, Dishion, Bank, & Owen, 2003). Capaldi, Kim, and Owen (2008) documented that male selection of an antisocial partner was the strongest predictor of persistence to age 30 whereas a positive, healthy intimate relationship was a predictor of desistence. Similarly, as would be expected, selection of an antisocial partner was a key factor in predicting coercive discipline practices in the next-generation family (Capaldi, Pears, Kerr, & Owen, 2008). This finding is consistent with those of Odgers and colleagues (2008) that showed early-onset and persistent antisocial females are much more likely to engage in harsh coercive discipline than adolescence-onset individuals. Follow-up studies of females suggest that a history of antisocial behavior plays a key role in the cross-generation of familial antisocial behavior. Intervention trials are needed that target females with a history of problem behavior early to evaluate malleability with respect to their own subsequent parenting.

In general, symptoms of ASPD diminish with age in adulthood (Mulder, Wells, & Bushnell, 1994; Robins & Regier, 1991). Desistence is particularly pronounced between ages 45 and 64 (Black et al., 1995). In a community sample of women, Mulder et al. (1994) found that no one age 45 or older met ASPD criteria. The reasons for the decline in antisocial behavior with age have not been investigated systematically but are likely to include both social and biological factors, such as increased attachment to social institutions (marriage, employment; see Sampson & Laub, 1993) and decreased impulsivity and sensation seeking (see Giambra, Camp, & Grodsky, 1992; Reio & Choi, 2004). However, recent longitudinal research that has followed individuals to their 40s suggests that physical aggression continues and is predicted by peer reports of physical aggression in childhood and adolescence in both the United States and Finland (Kokko, Pulkkinen, & Mesiäinen, 2009).

Sampson and Laub (e.g., 2005) propose that attenuated societal bonds play a primary role in criminal risk. Their model emphasizes social connections throughout development, with different social institutions changing in importance over time (e.g., parenting and attachment in childhood, schooling and peers in adolescence, marital stability and employment in adulthood). An individual's degree of investment in and connection to each of these domains is seen as an important predictor of criminal persistence and desistence. Consistent with this model, Sampson and Laub (1990) found that job stability and marital attachment in adulthood were related to changes in antisocial behavior across a wide variety of outcomes, with stronger ties to work and family predicting lower rates of crime and deviance.

## COMORBIDITY

In child and adolescent samples, ADHD frequently co-occurs with conduct disorders and appears to increase risk for persistent antisocial and criminal behavior (e.g., Barkley, Fischer, Edelbrock, & Smallish, 1990; Biederman, Faraone, Milberger, & Guite, 1996; Mannuzza, Klein, Abikoff, & Moulton, 2004; see also Chapters 6, 12). Epidemiological studies indicate that 30% to 50% of children with ADHD also meet criteria for ODD and/or CD. However, the evidence is mixed as to whether ADHD alone (i.e., in the absence of conduct problems) places children at risk for later criminality (e.g., Langley & Thapar, 2006; Satterfield & Schell, 1997; Thapar, van den Bree, Fowler, Langley, & Whittinger, 2006).

In adulthood, substance abuse is the most prominent comorbid condition. Nearly all *DSM-IV* substance use disorders are highly comorbid with adult antisocial behavior, with odds ratios of 2.5 to 8.8 (Compton et al., 2005). Patterns of comorbidity are essentially the same for individuals with *full* ASPD and those who exhibit adult antisocial behavior only (no history of childhood CD; Compton et al., 2005). Similarly, Robins and Regier (1991) reported that men with ASPD are 3 times as likely to abuse alcohol and 5 times as likely to abuse drugs as those without ASPD. For women, those comorbidity rates are even higher. Women with ASPD show 10 to 13 times the risk for alcohol abuse (Mulder et al., 1994; Robins & Regier, 1991) and 12 times the risk for drug abuse (Robins & Regier, 1991) compared with women without ASPD. Substance use disorder may either precede (Martens, 2000) or follow (Ross, Glaser, & Germanson, 1988) the development of ASPD. Evidence indicates that the comorbidity between ASPD and substance use disorder emanates in large part from common genetic risk, although environmental factors also play a substantial role (Kendler, Prescott, Myers, & Neale, 2003; Krueger et al., 2002; Young, Rhee, Stallings, Corley, & Hewitt, 2006).

Although externalizing syndromes are the most common comorbid disorders, individuals with ASPD also have an increased risk of anxiety disorders (e.g., Goodwin & Hamilton, 2003; Grant et al., 2004) and depression (e.g., Grant et al., 2004).

## SEX DIFFERENCES

A prominent sex difference is found in the population prevalence of ASPD, with men being 2 to 3 times more likely to receive a diagnosis (APA, 2000; Flynn, Craddock, Luckey, Hubbard, & Dunteman, 1996; Hesselbrock, Meyer, & Keener, 1985; Mulder et al., 1994). Despite this difference in prevalence, the prognosis and correlates of ASPD appear to be similar for men and women (see Cale & Lilienfeld, 2002). Nevertheless, some studies have found sex differences in the correlates of persistent antisocial behavior. In a combined analysis of four different longitudinal samples, Broidy et al. (2003) found that childhood physical aggression predicted adolescent offending among boys but not among girls. Broidy et al. (2003). found that girls' delinquency was relatively difficult to predict from childhood risk factors.

## CULTURAL CONSIDERATIONS

As noted previously, sociocultural factors may contribute substantial risk for anti-social behavior. Family- and neighborhood-level risk factors, such as poverty, unemployment, single parenthood, and low income, often co-occur with ethnic minority status. Thus, ethnic and cultural differences in crime and antisocial behavior are amplified by socioeconomic and neighborhood risk factors.

In addition, risk factors for antisocial behavior may operate differently across ethnic groups. For example, Deater-Deckard, Dodge, Bates, and Pettit (1996) found that spanking correlated with higher rates of problem behavior among European American youth but not among African American youth. Dishion and Bullock (2002) found that observed relationship quality between parent and child was higher among high-risk African American boys than among successful African American boys. This paradoxical finding has yet to be explained by current etiological theories of ASPD. Nevertheless, family-management interventions appear to work equally well across ethnic groups (Connell, Dishion, & Deater-Deckard, 2006: Dishion, Nelson, & Kavanagh, 2003; Gross et al., 2003; Henggeler, Schoenwald, Borduin, Rowland, & Cunningham, 1998).

Inequalities in the perception of and interpretation of, as well as reactions to, antisocial behavior across ethnic groups may also have a substantial impact on the course of antisocial behavior. Studies suggest that African American children receive more negative feedback for their school behavior and performance than do European American children (Alexander & Entwisle, 1988), and they are more likely to be placed into special education classes for emotional disturbance (Wang, Reynolds, & Walberg, 1986). Perhaps most notable is the discrepancy between self-reported antisocial behavior and arrest and rearrest rates among African American and European American adolescents (Elliott, 1994). Although self-reported rates of antisocial behavior are similar for both ethnic groups, arrest and rearrest rates are dramatically higher among African Americans. These findings suggest that similar behaviors may evoke harsher responses from society toward African American youth than toward European American youth. Harsher societal responses (e.g., expulsion versus detention, juvenile detention versus probation) may further entrench minority youth in an antisocial lifestyle by limiting access to prosocial opportunities. There is a pressing need for further examination of cultural and ethnic contributions to antisocial behavior and greater understanding of the sociocultural factors that initiate and maintain criminal involvement in minority populations.

## THEORETICAL SYNTHESIS AND FUTURE DIRECTIONS

Although considerable progress has been made toward understanding the development of persistent and severe patterns of antisocial behavior, continued research is needed to clarify linkages across levels of analysis, from the genome to the community. Thankfully, some of this research is currently underway because of increasing appreciation and support for transactional models that examine concurrent influences and interactions. Figure 14.2 provides a summary of the existing literature on antisocial behavior from adolescence to adulthood. Rather than list all possible risk factors, we consider research on the broader domains with a known linkage to antisocial behavior.

### Relationship Dynamics

It is well established that parent–child and peer–child interactions are relevant to the development and progression of antisocial behavior. Historically, the majority of the research has focused on parental socialization processes in childhood and the later development of ASPD (e.g., Loeber & Dishion, 1983). Recent years have seen an increased focus on the parenting received by adolescents and the continuance of

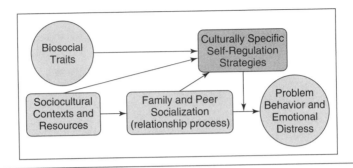

**Figure 14.2**   A model for self-regulation in the development of problem behavior.
Adapted from Dishion and Patterson, 2006.

problem behavior from adolescence to adulthood. Interventions that target parenting reduce problem behavior in children (e.g., Webster-Stratton & Taylor, 2001) and in adolescents (Connell, Dishion, Yasui, & Kavanagh, 2007).

As discussed previously, peer contagion dynamics are especially relevant to understanding the progression from adolescent antisocial behavior to adult ASPD (Dishion & Van Ryzin, 2011). As youth develop peer groups and romantic relationships, the extent to which these relationships are organized around deviance is a strong predictor of continued antisocial behavior across adolescence and early adulthood (Dishion, Nelson, & Bullock, 2004; Shortt et al., 2003). There is growing evidence that a combination of parental disengagement and youth involvement with deviant peers during adolescence greatly increases the risk of persistent antisocial behavior (Dishion, Nelson, & Bullock, 2004). Deviancy training among peers also has important implications for the design of interventions. Aggregating high-risk adolescents in treatment groups may be counterproductive in that peer reinforcement of antisocial behavior outweighs the effects of treatment (Dishion et al., 1999; Dishion & Tipsord, 2011; Dodge et al., 2006).

Given the importance of parent and peer relationships with respect to the persistence and escalation of antisocial behavior, examination of parent and peer relationship dynamics will be important for further specifying pathways to ASPD. For example, analyses that attempt to confirm the differential prognoses of early versus late starters may benefit from inclusion of parent and peer dynamics. We hypothesize that for many youth the risk for ASPD depends largely upon parent involvement and the quality of peer networks that evolve in adolescence. Compared with late starters, early starters may experience greater parental disengagement in adolescence and may develop peer groups that are more tightly organized around antisocial and deviant behaviors.

Recent methodological advances have created new opportunities for the analysis of parent and peer relationships. The dynamic systems framework may prove to be particularly useful. This approach enables examination of change and stability in systems (e.g., dyadic relationships) over time, and has been applied to parent–child and peer–peer interactions observed in the laboratory. Using dynamic systems methods, it is possible to examine relationship patterns in real time (e.g., moment-to-moment observations) and developmental time (e.g., days, weeks, years). The dynamic systems approach can produce measures such as stable relationship patterns (*attractors*), abrupt changes in the system (*phase transitions*), and the overall predictability of the system (*entropy*). Granic and Hollenstein (2003) provided an excellent review of dynamic systems strategies as they might be applied to understanding deviance and adjustment.

Relationship measures derived from a dynamic systems approach may be even more valuable when combined with measures of the content or valence of the interaction. For example, predictable relationship patterns (low entropy) may be associated with either positive or negative adjustment, depending on the content of the interaction. Dishion, Nelson, Winter, et al. (2004) found that low entropy predicted positive future adjustment when the content of the interaction was prosocial, but predicted negative future adjustment (antisocial behavior 10 years later) when the content of the interaction was antisocial. Furthermore, antisocial youth with well-organized relationships (low entropy) were at greater risk for future antisocial behavior than similarly deviant youth with poorly organized peer relationships (high entropy).

Identification of key relationship patterns may also be improved by "perturbing" the system. For example, rigid negativity in parent–child relationships is predictive of poor adjustment but may not be noticeable unless the system is challenged. Thus, it may be necessary to stress the dyad in order to observe patterns of interest (e.g., by asking the parent to resolve a dispute with the child during the interaction; Granic & Lamey, 2002).

These and other methodological and analytic innovations for examining relationship dynamics are invigorating social interaction research and may play a key role in differentiating patterns of antisocial behavior and creating a better understanding of the pathways that lead to persistent antisocial behavior and adult ASPD (Dishion & Snyder, 2004).

## Self-Regulation

Another promising direction for research is the study of intraindividual factors that moderate vulnerability or resilience to risks, such as deviant peers in adolescence. Self-regulation may be a critical moderator of relationship dynamics (see Chapter 11). Two studies of adolescents have shown that youth with good self-regulatory skills (i.e., high effortful control) are less vulnerable to deviant peer influences with respect to the continuity and maintenance of antisocial behavior in adolescence (Dishion & Connell, 2006; Goodnight, Bates, Newman, Dodge, & Pettit, 2006). Effortful control (Rothbart, Ellis, Rueda, & Posner, 2003) also seems to protect youth against the development of ASPD and major depression. Research into the genetic and neurobiological components of self-regulatory abilities is ongoing (e.g., Rothbart et al., 2003) and is revealing promising directions for future links across levels of analysis.

One relatively overlooked area of research in the domain of self-regulation involves cultural differences. Little attention has been given to cultural factors in the development of self-regulation in children and adolescents. Early cross-cultural work by Whiting and Edwards (1988) suggested that children in cultures that assigned chores to them and required supervised participation in the adult community were more prosocial. By extension, one might hypothesize that cultural rituals that involve daily routines within the context of the extended family and community function to promote high levels of self-regulation among adolescents, which in turn may protect against negative peer influences and help prevent the development of ASPD. Future research would do well to define and measure culturally specific self-regulatory factors that may account for why some risk factors promote antisocial behavior in some ethnic cultures and not in others (e.g., Deater-Deckard & Dodge, 1997). For example, self-regulatory skills may be embedded in beliefs and social cognitions, such as expectations of fairness and future events, and in the meaning of parent and peer relationships.

## Biosocial Factors

Informed, theoretically driven inclusion of genetic and neurobiological measurements (e.g., functional magnetic resonance imaging) in longitudinal research is likely to greatly advance our understanding of antisocial behavior development. Genetic factors, in particular, have shown remarkable Person × Environment interactions and require further investigation and inclusion in developmental and transactional models (see, e.g., Beauchaine et al., 2009). A critical further step is to link G × E interactions with behavioral and physiological measures, to better understand the mechanism and processes through which they lead to adaptive or maladaptive outcomes, and to identify targets for intervention (Lewis & Stieben, 2004; Rueda, Posner, & Rothbart, 2004; Steinberg et al., 2006; Tucker, Derryberry, & Luu, 2000). Interactions among risk factors is likely to be the rule rather than the exception with regard to explaining antisocial behavior. It has become increasingly clear that many risk factors have marginal effects in isolation but substantial effects in conjunction with particular environmental or individual characteristics.

## Sociocultural Factors

There is extensive evidence that disrupted neighborhoods, schools, and communities increase risk of antisocial behavior (e.g., Eamon & Mulder, 2005; Ingoldsby, Shaw, Winslow, Schonberg, & Gilliom, 2006; Lynam et al., 2000). However, much of this risk is mediated by parenting and peer factors. In addition, some individuals seem to be less negatively influenced by impoverished social environments. An exciting direction for future research would be to systematically apply and evaluate systems-level policies and interventions for improving sociocultural contexts and reducing antisocial behavior. Commonly held community standards for behavior can have a substantial impact on rates of antisocial behavior. One obvious setting for systems-level intervention is the public school system. Research by Kellam and colleagues suggests that systematic interventions that improve the behavior management practices of teachers in the first grade can have far-reaching effects on children up to adolescence (Ialongo, Poduska, Werthhamer, & Kellam, 2001; Kellam, Mayer, Rebok, & Hawkins, 1998). A school-wide approach to improving school behavior management and academic instruction has been designed and tested by Horner and colleagues (Crone & Horner, 2003; Horner, Day, & Day, 1997). However, there has yet to be an experiment done with random assignment of a large number of schools to school-wide (as opposed to classroom-specific) training in behavior management and academic instruction, to determine the impact on the reduction of antisocial behavior.

## DEFINING DISORDERS

Cutting across each of these future directions is the need to carefully define and measure the syndrome of interest with regard to adult antisocial behavior, and to improve our understanding of which risk and protective factors and which developmental pathways are most relevant for different forms of antisocial behavior (see Chapters 2, 3). The *DSM-IV* conceptualization of ASPD provides a starting point for research by identifying a broad group of individuals with a persistent pattern of antisocial behavior, but future research must build upon the ASPD construct to examine issues such as (a) whether ASPD differs in nature from less severe or persistent forms of antisocial behavior, and (b) whether the development (and treatment) of persistent antisocial behavior can be better understood by disaggregating ASPD into more homogenous groupings.

## Summary

The past several decades have seen great progress in understanding persistent antisocial behavior, due in large part to several large-scale, long-term longitudinal research projects that have documented the progression of antisocial behavior from childhood to adulthood. However, much work is yet to be done to separate correlates from causes, to illuminate the complex and interactive processes among risk and protective factors, to improve early identification of children at risk for long-term behavior problems, and to improve the efficacy of treatments and interventions. Progress in understanding antisocial behavior will come from research that becomes both more specific by improving diagnostic specificity and examining individual differences at the level of genetics and neurobiology, and more general by using increasingly sophisticated analytic techniques to examine complex interactions across multiple domains an developmental periods.

## REFERENCES

Alexander, K. L., & Entwisle, D. R. (1988). Achievement in the first 2 years of school: Patterns and processes. *Monographs of the Society for Research in Child Development, 53*, 157.

American Psychiatric Association. (1952). *Diagnostic and statistical manual of mental disorders*. Washington, DC: Author.

American Psychiatric Association. (1968). *Diagnostic and statistical manual of mental disorders*. Washington, DC: Author.

American Psychiatric Association. (1980). *Diagnostic and statistical manual of mental disorders*. Washington, DC: Author.

American Psychiatric Association. (2000). *Diagnostic and statistical manual of mental disorders*. Washington, DC: Author.

Anstey, P. (2003). *The philosophy of John Locke: New perspectives*. New York, NY: Routledge.

Barkley, R. A., Fischer, M., Edelbrock, C. S., & Smallish, I. (1990). The adolescent outcome of hyperactive children diagnosed by research criteria. *Journal of the American Academy of Child and Adolescent Psychiatry, 29*, 546–557.

Beauchaine, T. P., Hinshaw, S. P., & Gatzke-Kopp, L. (2008). Genetic and environmental influences on behavior. In T. P. Beauchaine & S. P. Hinshaw (Eds.), *Child and adolescent psychopathology* (pp. 58–90). Hoboken, NJ: Wiley.

Beauchaine, T. P., Klein, D. N., Crowell, S. E., Derbidge, C., & Gatzke-Kopp, L. M. (2009). Multifinality in the development of personality disorders: A Biology × Sex × Environment interaction model of antisocial and borderline traits. *Development and Psychopathology, 21*, 735–770.

Beauchaine, T. P., Webster-Stratton, C., & Reid, M. J. (2005). Mediators, moderators, and predictors of one-year outcomes among children treated for early-onset conduct problems: A latent growth curve analysis. *Journal of Consulting and Clinical Psychology, 73*, 371–388.

Belsky, J., Bakermans-Kranenburg, M. J., & van Ijzendoorn, M. H. (2007). For better and for worse: Differential susceptibility to environmental influences. *Current Directions in Psychological Science, 16*, 300–304.

Belsky, J., Steinberg, L., & Draper, P. (1991). Childhood experience, interpersonal development, and reproductive strategy: An evolutionary theory of socialization. *Child Development, 62*, 647–670.

Biederman, J., Faraone, S., Milberger, S., & Guite, J. (1996). A prospective 4-year follow-up study of attention-deficit hyperactivity and related disorders. *Archives of General Psychiatry, 53*, 437–446.

Black, D. W., Baumgard, C. H., & Bell, S. E. (1995). A 16- to 45-year follow-up of 71 men with antisocial personality disorder. *Comprehensive Psychiatry, 36*, 130–140.

Blair, R. J. R. (2002). Neuro-cognitive models of acquired sociopathy and developmental psychopathy. In J. Glicksohn (Ed.), *The neurobiology of criminal behavior* (pp. 157–186). Dordrecht, Netherlands: Kluwer.

Boislard, P. M.-A., & Poulin, F. (2011). Individual, familial, friends-related and contextual predictors of early sexual intercourse. *Journal of Adolescence, 34*, 289–300.

Brennan, P. A., Mednick, S. A., & Raine, A. (1997). Biosocial interactions and violence: A focus on perinatal factors. In A. Raine, P. Brenna, D. Farrington, & S. A. Mednick (Eds.), *Biosocial bases of violence* (pp. 163–174). New York, NY: Plenum.

Broidy, L. M., Tremblay, R. E., Brame, B., Fergusson, D., Horwood, J. L., Laird, R. D., . . . Vitaro, F. (2003). Developmental trajectories of childhood disruptive behaviors and adolescent delinquency: A six-site, cross-national study. *Developmental Psychology, 39*, 222–245.

Burt, S. A., Donnellan, M. B., Iacono, W. G., & McGue, M. (2011). Age-of-onset or behavioral sub-types? A prospective comparison of two approaches to characterizing the heterogeneity within antisocial behavior. *Journal of Abnormal Child Psychology, 39*, 633–644.

Cale, E. M., & Lilienfeld, S. O. (2002). Sex differences in psychopathy and antisocial personality disorder: A review and integration. *Clinical Psychology Review, 22*, 1179–1207.

Capaldi, D. M., Crosby, L., & Stoolmiller, M. (1996). Predicting the timing of first sexual intercourse for at-risk adolescent males. *Child Development, 67*, 344–359.

Capaldi, D. M., Kim, H. K., & Owen, L. D. (2008a). Romantic partners' influence on men's likelihood of arrest in early adulthood. *Criminology, 46*, 401–433.

Capaldi, D. M., Pears, K. C., Kerr, D. C. R., & Owen, L. D. (2008b). Intergenerational and partner influences on fathers' negative discipline. *Journal of Abnormal Child Psychology, 36*, 347–358.

Caspi, A., & Herbener, E. S. (1990). Continuity and change: Assortative marriage and the consistency of personality in adulthood. *Journal of Personality and Social Psychology, 58*, 250–258.

Caspi, A., McClay, J., Moffitt, T., Mill, J., Craig, I. W., & Poulton, R. (2002). Role of genotype in the cycle of violence in maltreated children. *Science, 297*, 851–854.

Chamberlain, P., & Reid, J. (1998). Comparison of two community alternatives to incarceration for chronic juvenile offenders. *Journal of Consulting and Clinical Psychology, 6*, 624–633.

Cleckley, H. (1941). *The mask of sanity*. Oxford, United Kingdom: Mosby.

Cohen, P., Brown, J., & Smailes, E. (2001). Child abuse and neglect and the development of mental disorders in the general population. *Development and Psychopathology, 13*, 981–999.

Compton, W. M., Conway, K. P., Stinson, F. S., Colliver, J. D., & Grant, B. F. (2005). Prevalence, correlates, and comorbidity of DSM–IV antisocial personality syndromes and alcohol and specific drug use disorders in the United States: Results from the National Epidemiologic Survey on Alcohol and Related Conditions. *Journal of Clinical Psychiatry, 66*, 677–685.

Connell, A. M., Dishion, T. J., & Deater-Deckard, K. (2006). Variable- and person-centered approaches to the analysis of early adolescent substance use: Linking peer, family, and intervention effects with developmental trajectories. [Special Issue]. *Merrill-Palmer Quarterly, 52*, 421–448.

Connell, A., Dishion, T. J., Yasui, M., & Kavanagh, K. (2007). An adaptive approach to family intervention: Linking engagement in family-centered intervention to reductions in adolescent problem behavior. *Journal of Consulting and Clinical Psychology, 75*, 568–579.

Crone, D. A., & Horner, R. H. (2003). *Building positive behavior support systems in schools: Functional behavioral assessment*. New York, NY: Guilford Press.

Deater-Deckard, K., & Dodge, K. A. (1997). Externalizing behavior problems and discipline revisited: Nonlinear effects in variation by culture, context, and gender. *Psychological Inquiry, 8*, 161–175.

Deater-Deckard, K., Dodge, K. A., Bates, J. E., & Pettit, G. S. (1996). Physical discipline among African American and European American mothers: Links to children's externalizing behaviors. *Developmental Psychology, 32,* 1065–1072.

Dick, D. M., Latendresse, S. J., Lansford, J. E., Budde, J. P., Goate, A., Dodge, K. A., & Bates, J. E. (2009). Role of GABRA2 in trajectories of externalizing behavior across development and evidence of moderation by parental monitoring. *Archives of General Psychiatry, 66,* 649–657.

Dishion, T. J., Brennan, L. M., Shaw, D. S., McEachern, A. D., Wilson, M. N., & Jo, B. (under review). Prevention of problem behavior through annual family check-ups in early childhood: Intervention effects from the home to the second grade of elementary school. *Journal of Consulting and Clinical Psychology.*

Dishion, T. J., & Bullock, B. M. (2002). Parenting and adolescent problem behavior: An ecological analysis of the nurturance hypothesis. In J. G. Borkowski, S. L. Ramey, & M. Bristol-Power (Eds.), *Parenting and the child's world: Influences on academic, intellectual, and social–emotional development* (pp. 231–249). Mahwah, NJ: Erlbaum.

Dishion, T. J., & Connell, A. (2006). Adolescents' resilience as a self-regulatory process: Promising themes for linking intervention with developmental science. In B. Lester, A. Masten, & B. McEwen (Eds.), *Resilience in children.* New York, NY: Academy of Sciences.

Dishion, T. J., Ha, T., & Véronneau, M.-H. (2012). An ecological analysis of the effects of deviant peer clustering on sexual promiscuity, problem behavior, and childbearing from early adolescence to adulthood: An enhancement of the life history framework. *Developmental Psychology,* 703–717.

Dishion, T. J., McCord, J., & Poulin, F. (1999). When interventions harm: Peer groups and problem behavior. *American Psychologist, 54,* 755–764.

Dishion, T. J., Nelson, S. E., & Bullock, B. M. (2004a). Premature adolescent autonomy: Parent disengagement and deviant peer process in the amplification of problem behavior [Special issue]. *Journal of Adolescence, 27,* 515–530.

Dishion, T. J., Nelson, S. E., & Kavanagh, K. (2003). The family check-up with high-risk young adolescents: Preventing early-onset substance use by parent monitoring [Special issue]. *Behavior Therapy, 34,* 553–571.

Dishion, T. J., Nelson, S. E., Winter, C. E., & Bullock, B. M. (2004b). Adolescent friendship as a dynamic system: Entropy and deviance in the etiology and course of male antisocial behavior. *Journal of Abnormal Child Psychology, 32,* 651–663.

Dishion, T. J., Owen L. D., & Bullock, B. M. (2004c). Like father, like son: Toward a developmental model for the transmission of male deviance across generations. *European Journal of Developmental Psychology, 1,* 105–126.

Dishion, T. J., & Patterson, G. R. (2006). The development and ecology of antisocial behavior. In D. Cicchetti & D. J. Cohen (Eds.), *Developmental psychopathology: Vol. 3. Risk, disorder, and adaptation* (2nd ed., pp. 503–541). Hoboken, NJ: Wiley.

Dishion, T. J., Shaw, D. S., Connell, A. M., Gardner, F., Weaver, C. M., & Wilson, M. N. (2008). The family check-up with high-risk indigent families: Preventing problem behavior by increasing parents' positive behavior support in early childhood. *Child Development, 79,* 1395–1414.

Dishion, T. J., & Snyder, J. (2004). An introduction to the special issue on advances in process and dynamic system analysis of social interaction and the development of antisocial behavior. *Journal of Abnormal Child Psychology, 32*, 575–578.

Dishion, T. J., & Tipsord, J. M. (2011). Peer contagion in child and adolescent social and emotional development. *Annual Review of Psychology, 62*, 189–214.

Dishion, T. J., & Van Ryzin, M. J. (2011). Peer contagion dynamics in problem behavior and violence: Implications for intervention and policy. *ISSBD Bulletin, 60*, 6–11.

Dishion, T. J., Véronneau, M.-H., & Myers, M. W. (2010). Cascading peer dynamics underlying the progression from problem behavior to violence in early to late adolescence. *Development and Psychopathology, 22*, 603–619.

Dodge, K. A., Dishion, T. J., & Lansford, J. E. (Eds.). (2006). *Deviant peer influences in programs for youth: Problems and solutions.* New York, NY: Guilford Press.

Dodge, K. A., Greenberg, M. T., & Malone, P. S. (2008). Testing an idealized dynamic cascade model of the development of serious violence in adolescence. *Child Development, 79*, 1907–1927.

Eamon, M. K., & Mulder, C. (2005). Predicting antisocial behavior among Latino young adolescents: An ecological systems analysis. *American Journal of Orthopsychiatry, 75*, 117–127.

Eddy, J. M., & Chamberlain, P. (2000). Family management and deviant peer association as mediators of the impact of treatment conditions on youth antisocial behavior. *Journal of Consulting and Clinical Psychology, 68*, 857–863.

Elder, G. H. Jr., (1985). *Life course dynamics: Trajectories and transitions, 1968–1980.* Ithaca, NY: Cornell University Press.

Elliott, D. S. (1994). Serious violent offenders: Onset, developmental course, and termination—The American Society of Criminology 1993 presidential address. *Criminology, 32*, 1–21.

Ellis, B. J., Figuero, A. J., Brumbach, B. H., & Schlomer, G. L. (2009). Fundamental dimensions of environmental risk: The impact of harsh versus unpredictable environments on the evolution and development of life history strategies. *Human Nature, 20*, 204–218.

Farrington, D. P. (1995). The twelfth Jack Tizard Memorial Lecture. The development of offending and antisocial behavior from childhood: Key findings from the Cambridge study in delinquent development. *Journal of Child Psychology and Psychiatry, 36*, 929–964.

Farrington, D. P., Barnes, G. C., & Lambert, S. (1996). The concentration of offending in families. *Legal and Criminological Psychology, 1*(Part 1), 47–63.

Flynn, P. M., Craddock, S. G., Luckey, J. W., Hubbard, R. L., & Dunteman, G. H. (1996). Comorbidity of antisocial personality and mood disorders among psychoactive substance-dependent treatment clients. *Journal of Personality Disorders, 10*, 56–67.

Forgatch, M. S., Bullock, B. M., & Patterson, G. R. (2004). From theory to practice: Increasing effective parenting through role-play. In H. Steiner (Ed.), *Handbook of mental health interventions in children and adolescents: An integrated developmental approach* (pp. 782–813). San Francisco, CA: Jossey–Bass.

Forgatch, M. S., & Patterson, G. R. (2010). Parent management training–Oregon model: An intervention for antisocial behavior in children and adolescents. In J. R. Weisz & A. E. Kazdin (Eds.), *Evidence-based psychotherapies for children and adolescents* (pp. 159–178). New York, NY: Guilford Press.

French, D., & Dishion, T. J. (2003). Predictors of early initiation of sexual intercourse among high-risk adolescents. *Journal of Early Adolescence, 23,* 295–315.

Friedlander, E. (2004). *J. J. Rousseau: An afterlife of words.* Cambridge, MA: Harvard University Press. (Original work published 1762)

Giambra, L. M., Camp, C. J., & Grodsky, A. (1992). Curiosity and stimulation seeking across the adult life span: Cross-sectional and 6- to 8-year longitudinal findings. *Psychology and Aging, 7,* 150–157.

Glueck, S., & Glueck, E. (1950). *Unraveling juvenile delinquency.* Oxford, United Kingdom: Commonwealth Fund.

Goodnight, J. A., Bates, J. E., Newman, J. P., Dodge, K. A., & Pettit, G. S. (2006). The interactive influences of friend deviance and reward dominance on the development of externalizing behavior during middle adolescence. *Journal of Abnormal Child Psychology, 34,* 573–583.

Goodwin, R. D., & Hamilton, S. P. (2003). Lifetime comorbidity of antisocial personality disorder and anxiety disorders among adults in the community. *Psychiatry Research, 177,* 159–166.

Granic, I., & Hollenstein, T. (2003). Dynamic systems methods for developmental psychopathology. *Development and Psychopathology, 15,* 641–669.

Granic, I., & Lamey, A. V. (2002). Combining dynamic systems and multivariate analyses to compare the mother–child interactions of externalizing subtypes. *Journal of Abnormal Child Psychology, 30,* 265–283.

Grant, B. F., Hasin, D. S., Stinson, F. S., Dawson, D. A., Chou, S. P., Ruan, W. J., & Pickering, R. P. (2004). Prevalence, correlates, and disability of personality disorders in the United States: Results from the national epidemiologic survey on alcohol and related conditions. *Journal of Clinical Psychiatry, 65,* 948–958.

Gross, D., Fogg, L., Webster-Stratton, C., Garvey, C., Julion, W., & Grady, J. (2003). Parent training of toddlers in day care in low-income urban communities. *Journal of Consulting and Clinical Psychology, 71,* 261–278.

Hare, R. D. (1991). *The Hare Psychopathy Checklist-Revised.* Toronto, Canada: Multi-Health Systems.

Hare, R. D. (2003). *The Hare PCL-R* (2nd ed.). Toronto, Canada: Multi-Health Systems.

Hare, R. D., Clark, D., Grann, M., & Thornton, D. (2000). Psychopathy and the predictive validity of the PCL-R: An international perspective. *Behavioral Sciences & the Law, 18,* 623–645.

Hare, R. D., Forth, A. E., Strachan, K. E. (1992). Psychopathy and crime across the life span. In R. D. Peters, R. J. McMahon, & V. L. Quinsey, *Aggression and violence throughout the life span.* (pp. 285–300). Newbury Park, CA: Sage.

Healy, W. (1926). Preventing delinquency among children. *Proceedings and addresses of the National Educational Association, 64,* 113–118.

Healy, W., & Bronner, A. F. (1936). *New light on delinquency and its treatment.* New Haven, CT: Yale University Press.

Henggeler, S. W., Schoenwald, S. K., Borduin, C. M., Rowland, M. D., & Cunningham, P. B. (1998). *Multisystemic treatment of antisocial behavior in children and adolescents*. New York, NY: Guilford Press.

Hesselbrock, M. N., Meyer, R. E., & Keener, J. J. (1985). Psychopathology in hospitalized alcoholics. *Archives of General Psychiatry, 42*, 1050–1055.

Hiatt, K. D., & Newman, J. P. (2006). Understanding psychopathy: The cognitive side. In C. J. Patrick (Ed.), *Handbook of psychopathy* (pp. 334–352). New York, NY: Guilford Press.

Hirschi, T., & Gottfredson, M. (1983). Age and the explanation of crime. *American Journal of Sociology, 89*, 552–583.

Horner, R. H., Day, H. M., & Day, J. R. (1997). Using neutralizing routines to reduce problem behaviors. *Journal of Applied Behavior Analysis, 30*, 601–614.

Horwitz, A. V., Widon, C. S., McLaughlin, J., & White, H. R. (2001). The impact of childhood abuse and neglect on adult mental health: A prospective study. *Journal of Health and Social Behavior, 42*, 184–201.

Hyde, L. W., Shaw, D. S., & Moilanen, K. L. (2010). Developmental precursors of moral disengagement and the role of moral disengagement in the development of antisocial behavior. *Journal of Abnormal Child Psychology, 38*, 197–209.

Ialongo, N., Poduska, J., Werthhamer, L., & Kellam, S. (2001). The distal impact of two first-grade preventive interventions on conduct problems and disorder in early adolescence. *Journal of Health and Social Behavior, 9*, 146–160.

Ingoldsby, E. M., Shaw, D. S., Winslow, E. B., Schonberg, M., & Gilliom, M. (2006). Neighborhood disadvantage, parent–child conflict, neighborhood peer relationships, and early antisocial behavior problem trajectories. *Journal of Abnormal Psychology, 34*, 303–319.

Jacobson, K. C., Prescott, C. A., & Kendler, K. S. (2002). Sex differences in the genetic and environmental influences on the development of antisocial behavior. *Development and Psychopathology, 14*, 395–416.

Jacoby, J. E., Weiner, N., Thornberry, T. P., & Wolfgang, M. E. (1973). Drug use and criminality in a birth cohort. In *National Commission on Marijuana and Drug Use in America*, Appendix 1: Patterns and consequences of drug use (pp. 300–345). Washington, DC: U.S. Government Printing Office.

Kellam, S. G., Mayer, L. S., Rebok, G. W., & Hawkins, W. E. (1998). Effects of improving achievement on aggressive behavior and of improving aggressive behavior on achievement through two preventive interventions: An investigation of causal paths. In B. P. Dohrenwend (Ed.), *Adversity, stress and psychopathology* (pp. 486–505). New York, NY: Oxford University Press.

Kendler, K. S., Prescott, C. A., Myers, J., & Neale, M. C. (2003). The structure of genetic and environmental risk factors for common psychiatric and substance use disorders in men and women. *Archives of General Psychiatry, 60*, 929–937.

Kim-Cohen, J., Caspi, A., Taylor, A., Williams, B., Newcombe, R., Craig, I. W., & Moffitt, T. E. (2006). MAOA, maltreatment, and gene–environment interaction predicting children's mental health: New evidence and a meta-analysis. *Molecular Psychiatry, 11*, 903–913.

Kokko, K., Pulkkinen, L., & Mesiäinen, P. (2009). Timing of parenthood in relation to other life transitions and adult social functioning. *International Journal of Behavioral Development, 33*, 356–365.

Krueger, R. F., Hicks, B. M., Patrick, C. J., Carlson, S. R., Iacono, W. G., & McGue, M. (2002). Etiologic connections among substance dependence, antisocial behavior and personality: Modeling the externalizing spectrum. *Journal of Abnormal Psychology, 111*, 411–424.

Lahey, B. B., Loeber, R., Burke, J. D., & Applegate, B. (2005). Predicting future antisocial personality disorder in males from a clinical assessment in childhood. *Journal of Consulting and Clinical Psychology, 73*, 389–399.

Langley, K., & Thapar, A. (2006). COMT gene variant and birth weight predict early-onset antisocial behavior in children with attention deficit hyperactivity disorder. *Directions in Psychiatry, 26*, 219–225.

Le Blanc, M., & Loeber, R. (1993). Precursors, causes and the development of criminal offending. In D. F. Hay & A. Angold (Eds.), *Wiley series on studies in child psychiatry: Precursors and causes in development and psychopathology* (pp. 233–263). Oxford, United Kingdom: Wiley.

Lewis, M. D., & Stieben, J. (2004). Emotion regulation in the brain: Conceptual issues and directions for developmental research. *Child Development, 75*, 371–376.

Li, D., Zhao, H., Kranzler, H. R., Oslin, D., Anton, R. F., Farrer, L. A., & Gelernter, J. (2012). Association of COL25A1 with comorbid antisocial personality disorder and substance dependence. *Biological Psychiatry*, 733–740.

Loeber, R. (1982). The stability of antisocial and delinquent child behavior: A review. *Child Development, 53*, 1431–1446.

Loeber, R., & Dishion, T. J. (1983). Early predictors of male delinquency: A review. *Psychological Bulletin, 94*, 68–99.

Loeber, R., & Farrington, D. P. (Eds.). (1998). *Serious & violent juvenile offenders. Risk factors and successful interventions.* Thousand Oaks, CA: Sage.

Luntz, B. K., & Widom, C. S. (1994). Antisocial personality disorder in abused and neglected children grown up. *American Journal of Psychiatry, 151*, 670–674.

Lykken, D. T. (1995). *The antisocial personalities.* Hillsdale, NJ: Erlbaum.

Lynam, D. R., Caspi, A., Moffit, T. E., Wilstrom, P. O., Loeber, R., & Novak, S. (2000). The interaction between impulsivity and neighborhood context on offending: The effects of impulsivity are stronger in poorer neighborhoods. *Journal of Abnormal Psychology, 109*, 563–574.

Mannuzza, S., Klein, R. G., Abikoff, H., & Moulton, J. L. III. (2004). Significance of childhood conduct problems to later development of conduct disorder among children with ADHD: A prospective follow-up study. *Journal of Abnormal Child Psychology, 32*, 565–573.

Martens, W. H. J. (2000). Antisocial and psychopathic personality disorders: Causes, course, and remission—A review article. *International Journal of Offender Therapy and Comparative Criminology, 44*, 406–430.

Martinez, C. R., & Forgatch, M. S. (2002). Adjusting to change: Linking family structure transitions with parenting and boys' adjustment. *Journal of Family Psychology, 16*, 107–117.

Masten, A. S., Roisman, G. I., Long, J. D., Burt, K. B., Obradović, J., Riley, J. R., & Tellegen, A. (2005). Developmental cascades: Linking academic achievement and externalizing and internalizing symptoms over 20 years. *Developmental Psychology, 41*, 733–749.

Mednick, S. A., & Kandel, E. S. (1988). Congenital determinants of violence. *Bulletin of the American Academy of Psychiatry and the Law, 16*, 101–109.

Meier, M. H., Slutske, W. S., Heath, A. C., & Martin, N. G. (2011). Sex differences in the genetic and environmental influences on childhood conduct disorder and adult antisocial behavior. *Journal of Abnormal Psychology, 120*, 377–388.

Miller, T. R. (2004). The social costs of adolescent problem behavior. In A. Biglan, P. A. Brennan, S. L. Foster, & H. D. Holder (Eds.), *Helping adolescents at risk: Prevention of multiple problem behaviors* (pp. 31–56). New York, NY: Guilford Press.

Moffitt, T. E. (1993). Adolescence-limited and life course persistent antisocial behavior: Developmental taxonomy. *Psychological Review, 100*, 674–701.

Moffitt, T. E. (2006). Life-course-persistent versus adolescence-limited antisocial behavior. In D. Cicchetti & D. J. Cohen (Eds.), *Developmental psychopathology: Vol. 3. Risk, disorder, and adaptation* (2nd ed., pp. 570–598). Hoboken, NJ: Wiley.

Moffitt, T. E., Caspi, A., Dickson, N., Silva, P., & Stanton, W. (1996). Childhood-onset versus adolescent-onset antisocial conduct problems in males: Natural history from ages 3 to 18 years. *Development and Psychopathology, 8*, 399–424.

Moffitt, T. E., Caspi, A., Harrington, H., & Milne, B. J. (2002). Males on the life-course-persistent and adolescence-limited antisocial pathways: Follow-up at age 26 years. *Development and Psychopathology, 14*, 179–207.

Monahan, K. C., Steinberg, L., & Cauffman, E. (2009). Affiliation with antisocial peers: Susceptibility to peer influence, and antisocial behavior during the transition to adulthood. *Developmental Psychology, 45*, 1520–1530.

Mulder, R. T., Wells, J. E., & Bushnell, J. A. (1994). Antisocial women. *Journal of Personality Disorders, 8*, 279–287.

Nelson, S. E., & Dishion, T. J. (2004). From boys to men: Predicting adult adaptation from middle childhood sociometric status. *Development and Psychopathology, 16*, 441–459.

Newman, J. P. (1998). Psychopathic behavior: An information processing perspective. In D. J. Cooke, R. D. Hare, & A. Forth (Eds.), *Psychopathy: Theory, research, and implications for society* (pp. 81–104). Dordrecht, Netherlands: Kluwer.

Newman, J. P., & Wallace, J. F. (1993). Diverse pathways to deficient self-regulation: Implications for disinhibitory psychopathology in children. *Clinical Psychology Review, 13*, 699–720.

Odgers, C. L., Moffitt, T. E., Broadbent, J. M., Dickson, N., Hancox, R. J., Harrington, H., & Caspi, A. (2008). Female and male antisocial trajectories: From childhood origins to adult outcomes. *Development and Psychopathology, 20*, 673–716.

Olweus, D. (1980). Familial and temperamental determinants of aggressive behavior in adolescent boys: A causal analysis. *Developmental Psychology, 16*, 644–660.

Patterson, G. R. (1982). *A social learning approach: III. Coercive family process.* Eugene, OR: Castalia.

Patterson, G. R. (1993). Orderly change in a stable world: The antisocial trait as a chimera. *Journal of Consulting and Clinical Psychology, 61,* 911–919.

Patterson, G. R., DeBaryshe, B. D., & Ramsey, E. (1989). A developmental perspective on antisocial behavior. *American Psychologist, 44,* 329–335.

Patterson, G. R., DeGarmo, D. S., & Forgatch, M. S. (2004). Systematic changes in families following prevention trials. *Journal of Abnormal Child Psychology, 32,* 621–633.

Patterson, G. R., & Dishion, T. J. (1988). Multilevel family process models: Traits, interactions, and relationships. In R. Hinde & J. Stevenson-Hinde (Eds.), *Relationships and families: Mutual influences* (pp. 283–310). Oxford, United Kingdom: Clarendon.

Patterson, G. R., Reid, J. B., & Dishion, T. J. (1992). *Antisocial boys.* Eugene, OR: Castalia.

Patterson, G. R., & Yoerger, K. (1999). Intraindividual growth in covert antisocial behavior: A necessary precursor to chronic juvenile and adult arrests? *Criminal Behaviour & Mental Health, 9,* 24–38.

Petras, H., Kellam, S. G., Brown, C. H., Muthén, B. O., Ialongo, N. S., & Poduska, J. M. (2008). Developmental epidemiological courses leading to antisocial personality disorder and violent and criminal behavior: Effects by young adulthood of a universal preventive intervention in first- and second-grade classrooms. *Drug and Alcohol Dependence, 95*(S1), S45–S59.

Petras, H., Schaeffer, C. M., Ialongo, N., Hubbard, S., Muthén, B. O., Lambert, S., & Kellam, S. (2004). When the course of aggressive behavior in childhood does not predict antisocial outcomes in adolescence and young adulthood: An examination of potential explanatory variable. *Development and Psychopathology, 16,* 919–941.

Piehler, T. F., & Dishion, T. J. (2007). Interpersonal dynamics within adolescent friendship: Dyadic mutuality, deviant talk, and patterns of antisocial behavior. *Child Development, 78,* 1611–1624.

Quinton, D., Pickles, A., Maughan, B., & Rutter, M. (1993). Partners, peers, and pathways: Assortative pairing and continuities in conduct disorder. *Development and Psychopathology, 5,* 763–783.

Raine, A., Venables, P. H., & Williams, M. (1995). High autonomic arousal and electrodermal orienting at age 15 years as protective factors against criminal behavior at age 29 years. *American Journal of Psychiatry, 152,* 1595–1600.

Reio, T. G. Jr., & Choi, N. (2004). Novelty seeking in adulthood: Increases accompany decline. *Journal of Genetic Psychology, 165,* 119–133.

Reiss, D., Grubin, D., & Meux, C. (1996). Young "psychopaths" in special hospital: Treatment and outcome. *British Journal of Psychiatry, 168,* 99–104.

Ridenour, T. A., Cottier, L. B., Robins, L. N., Compton, W. M., Spitznagel, E. L., & Cunningham-Williams, R. M. (2002). Test of the plausibility of adolescent substance use playing a causal role in developing adulthood antisocial behavior. *Journal of Abnormal Psychology, 111,* 144–155.

Robins, L. N. (1966). *Deviant children grow up: A sociological and psychiatric study of sociopathic personality.* Baltimore, MD: Williams & Wilkins.

Robins, L. N., & Regier, D. A. (1991). *Psychiatric disorders in America: The epidemiologic catchment area study*. New York, NY: Free Press.

Rogers, G., & Schulman, K. (2003). *Leviathan/Thomas Hobbes: A critical edition*. Bristol, United Kingdom: Thoemmes Continuum. (Original work published 1651)

Ross, H. E., Glaser, F. B., & Germanson, T. (1998). The prevalence of psychiatric disorders in patients with alcohol and other drug problems. *Archives of General Psychiatry, 45,* 1023–1031.

Rothbart, M. K., Ellis, L. K., Rueda, M. R., & Posner, M. I. (2003). Developing mechanisms of temperamental effortful control. *Journal of Personality, 71,* 1113–1143.

Rothbart, M. K., Sheese, M. B., & Posner, M. I. (2007). Executive attention and effortful control: Linking temperament, brain networks and genes. *Child Development Perspectives, 1,* 2–7.

Rueda, M. R., Posner, M. I., & Rothbart, M. K. (2004). Attentional control and self-regulation. In R. F. Baumeister & K. D. Vohs (Eds.), *Handbook of self-regulation: Research, theory, and applications* (pp. 283–300). New York, NY: Guilford Press.

Rutter, M. (2006). *Genes and behavior: Nature–nurture interplay explained*. Malden, NJ: Blackwell.

Sameroff, A. (Ed.). (2009). *The transactional model of development: How children and contexts shape each other*. Washington, DC: American Psychological Association.

Sampson, R. J., & Laub, J. H. (1990). Crime and deviance over the life course: The salience of adult social bonds. *American Sociological Review, 55,* 609–627.

Sampson, R. J., & Laub, J. H. (1993). *Crime in the making: Pathways and turning points through life*. Cambridge, MA: Harvard University Press.

Sampson, R. J., & Laub, J. H. (2005). A life-course view of the development of crime. *Annals of the American Academy of Political and Social Science, 602,* 12–45.

Satterfield, J. H., & Schell, A. (1997). A prospective study of hyperactive boys with conduct problems and normal boys: Adolescent and adult criminality. *Journal of the American Academy of Child and Adolescent Psychiatry, 36,* 1726–1735.

Shannon, K. E., Beauchaine, T. P., Brenner, S. L., Neuhaus, E., & Gatzke-Kopp, L. (2007). Familial and temperamental predictors of resilience in children at risk for conduct disorder and depression. *Development and Psychopathology, 19,* 701–727.

Shaw, D. S., Dishion, T. J., Supplee, L., Gardner, F., & Arnds, K. (2006). Randomized trial of a family-centered approach to the prevention of early conduct problems: Two-year effects of a randomized trial of the family check-up in early childhood. *Journal of Consulting and Clinical Psychology, 74,* 1–9.

Shaw, D. S., Gilliom, M., Ingoldsby, E. M., & Nagin, D. (2003). Trajectories leading to school-age conduct problems. *Developmental Psychology, 39,* 189–200.

Shortt, J. W., Capaldi, D. M., Dishion, T. J., Bank, L., & Owen, L. D. (2003). The role of adolescent friends, romantic partners, and siblings in the emergence of the adult antisocial lifestyle. *Journal of Family Psychology, 17,* 521–533.

Smith, C. A., Ireland, T. O., & Thornberry, T. P. (2005). Adolescent maltreatment and its impact on young adult antisocial behavior. *Child Abuse and Neglect, 29,* 1099–1119.

Snyder, J., Reid, J. B., & Patterson, G. R. (2003). A social learning model of child and adolescent antisocial behavior. In B. B. Lahey, T. E. Moffitt, & A. Caspi (Eds.),

*Causes of conduct disorder and juvenile delinquency* (pp. 27–48). New York, NY: Guilford Press.

Snyder, J., & Stoolmiller, M. (2002). Reinforcement and coercion mechanisms in the development of antisocial behavior: The family. In J. B. Reid, G. R. Patterson, & J. Snyder (Eds.), *Antisocial behavior in children and adolescents: A developmental analysis and model for intervention* (pp. 65–100). Washington, DC: American Psychological Association.

Stattin, H., & Magnusson, D. (1991). Stability and change in criminal behavior up to age 30. *British Journal of Criminology, 31,* 327–346.

Steinberg, L., Dahl, R., Keating, D., Kupfer, D. J., Masten, A. S., & Pine, D. S. (2006). The study of developmental psychopathology in adolescence: Integrating affective neuroscience with the study of context. In D. Cicchetti & D. J. Cohen (Eds.), *Developmental psychopathology: Vol. 2. Developmental neuroscience* (2nd ed., pp. 710–741). Hoboken, NJ: Wiley.

Taylor, L., Malone, S., Iacono, W. G., & McGue, M. (2002). Development of substance dependence in two delinquency subgroups and nondelinquents from a male twin sample. *Journal of the American Academy of Child & Adolescent Psychiatry, 41,* 386–393.

Thapar, A., van den Bree, M., Fowler, T., Langley, K., & Whittinger, N. (2006). Predictors of antisocial behavior in children with attention deficit hyperactivity disorder. *European Child & Adolescent Psychiatry, 15,* 118–125.

Tucker, D. M., Derryberry, D., & Luu, P. (2000). Anatomy and physiology of human emotion: Vertical integration of brainstem, limbic, and cortical systems. In J. C. Borod (Ed.), *The neuropsychology of emotion* (pp. 56–79). New York, NY: Oxford University Press.

Van Ryzin, M. J., & Dishion, T. J. (2012). The impact of a family-centered intervention on the ecology of adolescent antisocial behavior: Modeling developmental sequelae and trajectories during adolescence. *Development and Psychopathology, 24,* 1139–1155.

Viding, E. (2004). On the nature and nurture of antisocial behavior and violence. In J. Devine, J. Gilligan, K. Miczek, R. Sahikh, & K. Pfaff (Eds.), *Youth violence: Scientific approaches to prevention.* New York, NY: New York Academy of Sciences.

Waller, R., Gardner, F., Dishion, T. J., Shaw, D. S., & Wilson, M. N. (2012). Validity of a brief measure of parental effective attitudes in high-risk preschoolers. *Journal of Abnormal Child Psychology, 40*(6), 945–995.

Wang, M. C., Reynolds, M. C., & Walberg, H. J. (1986). Rethinking special education. *Educational Leadership, 44,* 26–31.

Warr, M. (1993). Age, peers, & delinquency. *Criminology, 31,* 17–40.

Webster-Stratton, C., & Taylor, T. (2001). Nipping early risk factors in the bud: Preventing substance abuse, delinquency, and violence in adolescence through interventions targeted at young children (0 to 8 years). *Prevention Science, 2,* 165–192.

Weiler, B. L., & Widom, C. S. (1996). Psychopathy and violent behavior in abused and neglected young adults. *Criminal Behaviour and Mental Health, 6,* 253–271.

Whiting, B. B., & Edwards, C. P. (1998). *Children of different worlds: The formation of social behavior*. Cambridge, MA: Harvard University Press.

Widiger, T. A., & Corbitt, E. (1995). Antisocial personality disorder. In W. J. Livesley (Ed.), *The DSM–IV personality disorders* (pp. 103–134). New York, NY: Guilford Press.

Wiesner, M., Kim, H. K., & Capaldi, D. M. (2005). Developmental trajectories of offending: Validation and prediction to young adult alcohol use, drug use, and depressive symptoms. *Development and Psychopathology, 17,* 251–270.

Young, S. E., Rhee, S. H., Stallings, M. C., Corley, R. P., & Hewitt, J. K. (2006). Genetic and environmental vulnerabilities underlying adolescent substance use and problem use: General or specific? *Behavior Genetics, 36,* 603–615.

Zhang, L., Wieczorek, W. F., & Welte, J. W. (1997). The impact of onset of substance use on delinquency. *Journal of Research in Crime and Delinquency, 34,* 253–268.

Zucker, R. A., Ellis, D. A., Fitzgerald, H. E., Bingham, C. R., & Sanford, D. P. (1996). Other evidence for at least two alcoholisms. Vol II: Life course variation in antisociality and heterogeneity of alcoholic outcome. *Development and Psychopathology, 8,* 831–848.

# CHAPTER 15

# Substance Use Disorders in Adolescence

SANDRA A. BROWN, KRISTIN TOMLINSON, AND JENNIFER WINWARD

## SUBSTANCE USE DISORDERS IN ADOLESCENCE

ALCOHOL AND DRUG USE is a salient concern during adolescence. National surveys in the United States indicate that alcohol is consistently the drug of choice for teens, and increasingly, youth consume alcohol in a particularly hazardous fashion (Brown et al., 2008). The greatest escalation in alcohol involvement occurs between 12 and 15 years of age. Results of the Monitoring the Future study (MTF; Johnston, O'Malley, Bachman, & Schulenberg, 2010) indicate that 20% of 8th graders and 42% of 10th graders report being drunk on at least one occasion in their lifetime. As youth progress into middle and late adolescence, alcohol and other drug involvement continues to escalate, as does intensity of use. By 12th grade (modal age = 18 years), almost 80% of youth report having ingested alcohol at least once and nearly three fifths have been drunk at least once (Johnston et al., 2010). Among high school seniors, half report using alcohol in the past 30 days, 31% report being drunk in that time frame, and 28% report 5 or more drinks per occasion during the prior 2 weeks. By contrast, rates of daily drinking remain low (3%), highlighting the heavy, episodic nature of youth involvement with alcohol and other substances. According to the National Epidemiological Survey of Alcohol and Related Conditions (NESARC; Grant & Dawson, 1997), adolescents drink alcohol half as often as adults but consume 4.9 drinks per occasion, whereas the mean consumption of adults is 2.6 drinks.

The second most commonly used drug among adolescents is nicotine, with more than 60% of high school seniors reporting any lifetime use. Approximately one third of seniors indicate smoking cigarettes in the past month. Cigarette use among adults has decreased over the past decade, yet nicotine use among adolescents has been more resistant to reductions in prevalence.

Rates of illicit substance use have shown a gradual rise in recent years, related primarily to marijuana. Approximately half of high school seniors report lifetime use of a drug other than alcohol or cigarettes (Johnston et al., 2010) and one quarter report use in the prior month. Marijuana is the most widely used illicit substance by adolescents, with half of high school seniors reporting use at some time in the past, 1 in 5 indicating use in the prior month, and 7% using almost daily. The greatest increase in use of any substance among adolescents over the past decade has been MDMA (Ecstasy). Seven percent of high school seniors reported use of ecstasy in 1997; by 2001, that number had increased to 11.7%. Currently, 5.3% of seniors indicate use in the past year. Over the past decade, greater access and availability and changes in the perception of risk have been linked to trends of increased use of hard drugs (e.g., opiates, cocaine, crack), while hallucinogens and inhalants displayed decreases in prevalence rates, and prescription drug use rates appear stable.

These reported rates in national school-based samples may underestimate actual prevalence. Indeed, adolescents with problematic substance involvement have higher rates of truancy, suspensions, and expulsions (Brown, McGue, Maggs, et al., 2008), meaning that the youth most at risk for substance use may not be fully represented in school surveys. Furthermore, among adolescents involved in substance abuse treatment programs, more than half report not attending school in the months immediately preceding admission to treatment (e.g., Brown, Myers, Mott, & Vik, 1994). Youth in treatment programs are also more likely to use multiple substances in significantly greater quantities than in community-based samples, and to meet criteria for dependence on multiple substances (Brown, McGue, Maggs, et al., 2008).

## ABUSE AND DEPENDENCE: CRITERIA AND DIAGNOSTIC ISSUES

Substance use disorders (SUDs) in adolescence involve the self-administration of any substance that induces long-term changes in mood, perception, or brain functioning (Bukstein & Lutka-Fedor, 2007). In general, substances are used initially by youth in social settings to produce a positive affective state or change in consciousness. Almost all abused substances can lead to psychological dependence or the subjective feeling of needing the substance to function adequately. Some substances also produce physical dependence, when physiological and psychological adaptations to the substance occur. Tolerance—the need to ingest larger amounts of a substance for an effect once obtained at a lower dose—exemplifies such a physical adaptation. Another aspect of physical dependence involves the experience of withdrawal symptoms or a syndrome when consumption of an abused substance is ended (or the dose is lowered) abruptly.

Indicators of SUDs among adolescents often involve physical, socioemotional, and health changes. Such changes may include deterioration in appearance (e.g., rapid weight loss, unusual breath and body odors, cuts and bruises); bloodshot eyes, very large or small pupils, and watery or blank stares; increased energy or lethargy, insomnia or excessive sleep; clinically significant levels of depression or anxiety; deviant behaviors that were not evident in childhood; decreases in school grades;

changes in social activities or peer groups; chronic coughing or sniffing; skin boils or sores; nasal bleeding; and evidence of intravenous drug use (needle tracks) or inhalation (perforated nasal septum) (Brown & Abrantes, 2005).

Diagnostic criteria for alcohol and other substance use disorders appear in the *Diagnostic and Statistical Manual of Mental Disorders—IV* (American Psychiatric Association, 2000). Two types of substance use disorders (abuse and dependence) are characterized by a maladaptive pattern of use and symptoms that result in clinical impairment or distress. These diagnoses are mutually exclusive, with abuse typically considered less severe and less chronic than dependence. Substance dependence diagnoses are also characterized by presence vs. absence of physiological dependence occurs—that is, whether or not tolerance or withdrawal are experienced.

According to the National Household Survey on Drug Abuse, 7.8% of adolescents ages 12 to 17 meet criteria for substance abuse or dependence, with prevalence rates increasing from early to late adolescence (Substance Abuse and Mental Health Services Administration, 1999). The largest increase in dependence is in the age range of 18 to 20. The prevalence of SUDs among youth ages 13 to 18 has been examined in multiple sectors of public service care including mental health, alcohol and drug, child welfare, juvenile justice, and severely emotionally disturbed groups in schools (Aarons, Brown, Hough, Garland, & Wood, 2001). Using *DSM-IV* lifetime rates of SUDs, 35% of adolescents within these systems of care meet diagnostic criteria for either substance abuse or substance dependence. Alcohol and marijuana use disorders are the most prevalent, with the highest rates reported in mental health settings. Other illicit SUDs are more prevalent in juvenile justice settings.

As these figures indicate, alcohol and drug involvement progresses to the level of a SUD for a significant number of youth. Among adolescents, this progression occurs more rapidly than among adults. Adolescent SUDs are associated with a variety of developmentally significant impairments such as poor academic functioning, family problems (e.g., Dakof, 2000), health problems (Brown & Tapert, 2004), morphological and functional neuroanatomical abnormalities (Tapert et al., 2004), and psychiatric comorbidity (Abrantes, Brown, & Tomlinson, 2003). Moreover, emerging evidence from developmentally focused longitudinal studies indicates that SUDs during adolescence predict a wide range of adverse outcomes in adulthood (Anderson, et al., 2010).

## HISTORICAL CONTEXT AND ETIOLOGICAL FORMULATIONS

Considerable research has been devoted to understanding the onset of SUDs and the progression to abuse and dependence among youth. Early etiological theories of substance use among adolescents focused on the interplay of person and environment and include the theory of planned behavior (TPB), social learning theory (SLT), problem behavior theory (PBT), and the domain model. More recent models incorporate genetic, neurobiological, neurophysiological, and neuropsychological factors.

## ENVIRONMENTAL MODELS

*Theory of planned behavior (TPB).* This theory, based on a model of reasoned action (Ajzen & Fishbein, 1980), has been used to explain why youth engage in addictive behaviors. Attitudes about using substances, perceived social norms of alcohol/drug use, and self-efficacy for coping in potential use situations influence youths' intentions to use substances. Behavioral intentions influence substance use decisions and behavior. Substance-specific attitudes result from underlying expectations about personal consequences associated with substance use and the value placed on these consequences (Ajzen & Fishbein, 1980; Goldman, Brown, Christiansen, & Smith, 1991; Petraitis, Flay, & Miller, 1995). Normative beliefs about substance use are determined by perceived use rates of others, the perception that others prefer the adolescent in question to use a substance, and personal motivation to please others. Self-efficacy about substance use refers to whether the adolescent feels control over his or her own behaviors in use situations. Two types of self-efficacy related to substance use intentions are described in this model: substance use self-efficacy, or the ability to successfully obtain and use substances, and refusal self-efficacy, or the ability to resist perceived pressures to use (Ajzen, 1988, 2001). Although support for TPB has been demonstrated for experimental substance use, causal links between substance-specific beliefs and substance uses may be more bidirectional, as proposed in other cognitively-oriented models (e.g., expectancy theory; see later).

*Social learning theory (SLT).* Initially developed by Akers (1977) and subsequently refined by Bandura (1986), SLT focuses on relations between perceived contingencies and substance use. From this perspective, adolescents develop outcome expectations about the effects of substance use by observing parents, peers, and/or the media, or by learning about the effects of substance use (e.g., discussions of use effects). SLT posits that positive social, personal, and physiological expectations, which result from attending to influential social role models, are predictive of adolescent substance use. Aspects of this model are salient in broader decision-making models of deviant youth (Brown, McGue, Maggs, et al., 2008).

*Problem behavior theory (PBT).* Problem behavior theory is a generalist model that considers substance involvement to be one of a number of deviant behaviors that typically co-occur among adolescents (R. Jessor & S. Jessor, 1977). From this perspective, adolescent deviant behavior reflects unconventionality. Thus, if an adolescent is prone to engage in one deviant behavior, he or she is likely to engage in others (Beauchaine, Neuhaus, Brenner, & Gatzke-Kopp, 2008). Numerous studies support the high co-occurrence of multiple problems or delinquent behaviors, including marijuana and alcohol use, early and high-risk sexual behavior, illegal activity, truancy, and aggression. Compared to those low on this risk-taking characteristic, individuals high on it are less likely to engage in health-promoting behaviors, more detached from their parents, and more influenced by their peers. They are also less responsive to punishment and show distinct neuroanatomical response patterns reflective of poorer executive functioning skills (e.g., R. Jessor & S. Jessor, 1977; Zucker et al., 2006).

*Domain model.* Huba and colleagues (Huba, Wingard, & Bentler, 1980) extended these models to focus on the interaction of biological, intrapersonal, interpersonal, and sociocultural factors in jointly influencing adolescent substance use behavior. Biological mechanisms include genetic susceptibility, physiological reactions to substance use, and general health. Psychological state, cognitive style, personality traits, and personal values comprise the intrapersonal domain; interpersonal factors of social support, modeling, social reinforcement, personal identity, and belonging also contribute to use decisions. Finally, sociocultural and environmental factors include social sanctions of substance use, degree of availability of substances, social expectations, and environmental stressors.

## BEHAVIORAL GENETIC, NEUROBIOLOGICAL, AND INTEGRATED PERSPECTIVES

Behavioral genetics studies (see Chapter 3) have consistently linked parental alcohol and drug dependence to risk for alcohol and drug dependence in offspring (e.g., Schuckit, 1988). Although associated risks (e.g., conduct disorder) may influence outcomes, differences in behavioral, cognitive, and neurological measures have been observed between offspring of alcoholics (family history positive, FHP) and offspring of nonalcoholics (family history negative, FHN). For example, when FHP adolescents are compared to FHN teens, even predating drug or alcohol exposure, they demonstrate greater impulsivity and rebelliousness (Knop, Teasdale, Schulsinger, & Goodwin, 1985), poorer response inhibition (Nigg et al., 2006), poorer neuropsychological performance (Tapert & Brown, 2002; Tarter & Edwards, 1988), and fewer physiological and subjective effects of alcohol (Newlin, 1994). These preexisting vulnerabilities, which predispose FHP adolescents to problematic substance use, are consistent with behavioral genetics studies indicating that a substantial portion of risk for SUDs is heritable, and over half of this risk is nondrug specific (e.g., Kendler, Prescott, Myers, & Neale, 2003; Tsuang et al., 1998).

Multiple genetic pathways that are influenced by environmental risk factors and life experiences have been proposed. Early research of Cadoret and colleagues (Cadoret, Yates, Troughton, Woodworth, & Stewart, 1995) found support for a direct pathway from parental alcoholism to drug abuse and dependency in male offspring, and for an indirect pathway from parental antisocial personality disorder to externalizing behaviors and eventually drug abuse and dependence. A prospective study by Schuckit and colleagues (Schuckit, Smith, Anderson, & Brown, 2004) indicated that perceptions of lower response to alcohol among children who are offspring of alcoholics predate personal exposure, and identified a pathway of genetic risk in which the effect of family history is mediated through low physiological responding, which in turn predicts higher use per drinking episode, developing eventually into patterns of alcohol dependence 20 years later (Schuckit et al., 2005).

In addition, molecular genetics research has identified a number of candidate liability genes affecting liver enzyme activity (e.g., Wall, Shea, Chan, & Carr, 2001), serotonin neurotransmission (e.g., Schuckit et al., 1999) and dopamine neurotransmission in the mesolimbic reward system (e.g., Koob & LeMoal, 2008; Limosin, Loze, Rouillon, Adès, & Gorwood, 2003). These findings are consistent with prominent animal models of abuse and dependence that implicate primary reward pathways (see, e.g., Robinson & Berridge, 2003).

*Maturation theory.* Maturation theory (Tarter et al., 1999) is a recent heuristic model of the development of early-onset SUDs. According to this model, deviations in somatic and neurological maturation, along with stressful and adverse environments, predispose children to difficulties in regulating affect and behavior. Children with difficult temperaments in infancy are predisposed to oppositional behaviors. Family conflict then leads to conduct problems and, in turn, to SUDs. Maturation theory incorporates an epigenetic perspective whereby from the moment of conception, genetic and environmental interactions result in developmental sequences of events leading to increased risk for substance use disorders. Thus, no single genetic or nongenetic factor dominates risk for addictive disorders. Instead, clusters of vulnerabilities interact with environmental experiences to culminate in one of many phenotypic patterns of addiction.

*Expectancy theory.* Expectancy theory (Goldman et al., 1991; Goldman et al., 2010) has emerged as an alcohol/drug-specific integrative model of youth substance involvement because it considers multiple system levels of potential influence on youth substance use as well as processes through which these systems interact over time in the context of development. Expectancies of the effects of alcohol and drugs are understood to reflect both content of cognitions (e.g., immediate and distal consequences of use), memories of prior use (that influence access to perceived consequences), and motivation (e.g., neural activation patterns).

Expectancies, which are influenced by both genetic and environmental factors including learning experiences, are proximal to youth substance use decisions and are continually modified via acquisition of updated cognitive content, as well as adapted physiological and neuroanatomical responses (Anderson, Schweinsburg, Paulus, Brown, & Tapert, 2005). Such modifications occur with each use experience or substance-related exposure to increase the likelihood of use in future high-risk situations. Thus, vulnerabilities present in childhood (e.g., genetic predispositions, temperament) affect learning processes by (a) influencing self-selection of environments, (b) directing attention to specific rewards, and (c) magnifying the subjective experience of the reward itself. In concert, this unfolding process builds a network of alcohol and drug expectancies, which dominate adolescent use decisions.

## ENVIRONMENTAL AND GENETIC RISK FACTORS

Given widespread use of alcohol over the course of adolescence and exposure to diverse substances during this period, there is great interest in discovering factors that increase risk for early-onset use and predict escalation to frequent use or involvement with other substances, high-dose drinking, and/or emergence of associated problems. A broad range of risk factors has been identified, yet few are specific to alcohol/drugs. Clusters of co-occurring risk factors appear to facilitate progression of certain use trajectories (Tarter et al., 1999). These developmental trajectories may be viewed as a succession of intermediary phenotypes which, depending on the severity of alcohol/drug consequences, may reach threshold for a SUD diagnosis. A diagnosis of dependence (the endpoint phenotype) is multidimensional and developmentally variable. Because the phenotype varies across development, the significance of individual risk and protective factors changes as youth traverse changing demands during adolescence.

The following summarizes alcohol/drug-specific risk and protective factors for children and adolescents. Risk factors range from biogenetic (e.g., liver enzyme activity) to intraindividual (e.g., personality), interpersonal (family, peers), and environmental (community, cultural). Multiple risk factors often co-occur or are nested in certain contexts (families with alcohol/drug dependent parents). Certain risks are dynamic in that they provoke other risks that shape developmental experiences. For example, youth with genetically influenced sensation-seeking tendencies seek out risky environments, which provide exposure to substance use and reinforcement for use, as well as involvement in other problematic behaviors. This exemplifies an evocative Gene × Environment correlation (see Chapter 3).

*Temperament*, construed as neurobiological-influenced biases in certain behaviors (see Chapter 7), is present early in life, and may directly and indirectly influence substance involvement among adolescents. Several heritable temperamental traits have been associated with increased risk for adolescent substance use and substance use problems. In particular, high sensation-seeking (Zuckerman, 1994), behavioral disinhibition (McGue, Iacono, Legrand, Malone, & Elkins, 2001), impulsivity (Baker & Yardley, 2002), aggression (Kuo, Yang, Soong, & Chen, 2002), and behavioral undercontrol (Colder & Chassin, 1993) have been associated with early-onset of substance use and SUDs throughout adolescence. Temperament may set the stage for developmental psychopathology as well as predisposing to adolescent substance abuse through a cascade of inattention, disruptive behavior, and early substance involvement in the context of less than fully developed self-regulatory skills (Brown et al., 2008; Martel et al., 2009). These developing risks result in lower inhibitory control over behavior via neurochemical and neurophysiological substrates that influence decision making in both positive social situations where teens have initial alcohol/drug exposure, and in more distressing contexts such as high-risk relapse situations (Cyders et al., 2007; Smith et al., 2007). Other temperamental features such as trait anxiety and anxiety sensitivity influence youth motivation for alcohol, cigarette, and marijuana use (Comeau, Stewart, & Loba, 2001). Furthermore, genetically influenced individual differences in alcohol metabolism influence motivation-related expectancies and drinking behavior (McCarthy, Brown, Carr, & Wall, 2001).

*Childhood behavior problems.* Substance use disorders and concomitant mental health problems may develop independently, one may cause or exacerbate the other, or common mechanisms may underlie both. Prospective studies demonstrate that disruptive behavior at early ages (e.g., hyperactivity, aggression, symptoms of conduct disorder) predicts early onset of substance involvement and more rapid progression to substance-related problems (Dobkin, Tremblay, Masse, & Vitaro, 1995; Johnson, Arria, Borges, Ialongo, & Anthony, 1995). High rates of comorbid mental health disorders with adolescent SUDs are present in both community and clinical samples. In a large community sample of 14- to 18-year-olds, two thirds of adolescents who met diagnostic criteria for an SUD also met lifetime criteria for at least one other Axis I disorder (Lewinsohn, Rohde, & Seeley, 1995). The Methods for the Epidemiology of Child and Adolescent Mental Disorders (MECA) study obtained similar rates of comorbidity in a stratified community sample of youth, ages 9 to 18 (Kandel et al., 1997). Among weekly drinkers, two thirds met criteria for a *DSM-IV* psychiatric disorder. Furthermore, among those who used illicit drugs 3 or more times in the past year, 85% of girls and 58% of boys met criteria for a nonalcohol-, nondrug-related Axis I disorder. In their review of community based samples, Armstrong and Costello (2002) found that 60% of adolescent substance users evidenced a comorbid disorder.

Rates of psychiatric disorders are even higher among substance-abusing adolescents who are in treatment (Abrantes et al., 2003; Greenbaum, Foster-Johnson, & Petrila, 1996). Adolescents in inpatient substance abuse treatment report rates of Axis I mental health disorders ranging from 68% (Novins, Beals, Shore, & Manson, 1996) to 82% (Stowell & Estroff, 1992). Conversely, one third to one half of adolescents admitted to acute care psychiatric settings meet criteria for one of more SUDs (Grilo et al., 1995).

Recent reviews addressing comorbid SUDs and psychiatric disorders (e.g., Bukstein & Lutka-Fedor, 2007) are consistent in identifying both externalizing disorders (conduct disorder, attention deficit/hyperactivity disorder, and oppositional defiant disorder) and internalizing disorders (depression, anxiety) among youth with SUDs. In addition, a history of physical and/or sexual abuse is also prevalent among adolescents with SUDs. For example, in a large multisite study of adolescents in drug treatment, 59% of girls and 39% of boys reported a history of physical and/or sexual abuse (Grella & Joshi, 2003).

*Alcohol and drug expectancies.* Alcohol and drug outcome expectancies—the anticipated effects of using a specific substance (Brown, 1993; Goldman et al., 1991)—develop through both direct and vicarious learning experiences with substances, including peer and parental modeling, and media exposure. Expectancies (e.g., more global positive effects, increased social facilitation, and enhancement of cognitive and motor performance) partially mediate the relationship between family histories of substance problems and substance involvement in offspring (Goldman & Rather, 1993; Sher, 1994; Zucker et al., 2006). Furthermore, expectancies predict both (a) the progression from initiation of use to problematic use (Brown, 1993; Smith, Goldman, Greenbaum, & Christiansen, 1995) and (b) especially poor outcomes among adolescents (Vik, Brown, & Myers, 1997). Furthermore, higher positive expectancies and lower negative expectancies are associated with extraversion (Anderson et al., 2005; Brown & Munson, 1987) and neuroanatomical activation patterns that indicate low response inhibition. Specifically, lower activation levels in the right inferior parietal, right middle frontal, and left superior and temporal regions as measured by functional magnetic resonance imaging (fMRI) during inhibition tasks predict more positive and lower negative expectancies (Anderson et al., 2005). These regions are implicated in sustained and selective attention, inhibitory control, and risk-taking decision making. In general, positive expectancies are related to accelerated substance involvement and substance-related problems, whereas negative outcome expectancies operate as a protective factor against the initiation of use (Brown, 1993).

*Age of onset.* The age at which involvement with psychoactive substances is initiated has important epidemiological and developmental implications. Clearly, not all youth with exposure to psychoactive substances develop substance use disorders. However, age of first use is a reliable risk factor for the onset of substance use problems and later disorders. Early-onset of alcohol and marijuana use is also predictive of binge drinking in adolescence (D'Amico et al., 2001). According to the National Longitudinal Survey of Youth (NLSY), the odds of developing alcohol dependence decrease by 9% for each year that the onset of drinking is delayed (Grant, Stinson, & Harford, 2001).

*Family influences.* Both disruptions in family relations and functioning, and parental psychopathology are precursors, correlates, and consequences of adolescent SUDs. A family history (FH) of alcohol or drug dependence is associated with a four-to-ninefold risk of SUDs in male offspring, and a two-to-threefold risk in female offspring. This transmission appears to be nonspecific to SUDs, extending to delayed or deficient behavioral, emotional, and cognitive regulation (Tarter et al., 1999). A positive FH is also associated with elevated rates of comorbid mental health disorders and SUDs during adolescence and with altered neurocognitive and neurophysiological functioning during childhood and adolescence. For example, children with FH show (a) altered neural responses—as measured using electroencephalography—in response to novel stimuli, (b) different neural activation responses to memory tests, (c) blunted inferior parietal responses to inhibition tasks, and (c) lower executive functioning on neurocognitive tests (Brown & Tapert, 2004; Tapert et al., 2004) compared to youth without such a family history. Parental deviance and psychopathology may also confer risk for SUDs through lack of parental involvement and/or low levels of parent–child affection (Baer & Bray, 1999; Loukas, Zucker, Fitzgerald, & Krull, 2003; Zucker et al., 2006). Inconsistent parental discipline, lower monitoring of behavior, excessive punishment, and permissiveness are all risk factors for SUDs among adolescents (Brody & Forehand, 1993; Chilcoat & Anthony, 1996; Gilvarry, 2000; Williams & Hine, 2002). In addition, family conflict is predictive of more disruptive behavior in children, which elevates risk for SUDs during adolescence (Loukas et al., 2003; Zucker et al., 2000). The extent to which parents monitor youth activities also influences the selection of peers (Chassin, Pillow, Curran, Molina, & Barrera, 1993) and, consequently, future risk.

*Peers.* Peer influences have long been identified as one of the most significant and consistent risk factors for adolescent substance involvement (e.g., Bates & Labouvie, 1995; Fergusson, Horwood, & Lynskey, 1995). Higher perceptions of peer use and more friends who engage in substance use and deviant behaviors (Barnes, Farrell, & Banerjee, 1994; Epstein & Botvin, 2002; Vik, Grizzle, & Brown, 1992) create greater access to substances and lead to the adoption of beliefs and values consistent with a drug use lifestyle (Tapert & Brown, 1999). Furthermore, associations with substance abusing and deviant peers mediate the relationship between parental alcoholism, low socioeconomic status and family conflict on the one hand, and substance abuse during adolescence on the other.

*Stress.* Stressful life experiences increase substantially during early and middle adolescence, as does heightened reactivity to stress, especially for girls (Arnett, 1999). Stressful life events are correlated with substance use, and when occurring in the context of economic adversity, predict progression of substance involvement over the course of adolescence (e.g., Pandina & Schuele, 1983; Wills, Vaccaro, & McNamara, 1992). Youth from alcohol abusing families experience more life stress and rate stressful life events as more negative than youth from families with no parental alcohol or substance abuse (Tate, Patterson, Nagel, Anderson, & Brown, 2007). Consistent with a developmental framework, the stress-substance involvement association is bidirectional, as adolescent alcohol and drug use provokes substantial stress in the form of subsequent physical, academic, legal, family, peer, and emotional problems (Tate et al., 2007).

*Neurocognitive functioning.* Evidence is emerging that processes underlying poor executive functions may predispose youth to SUDs. Executive functions mediate thinking, affect, motivation, and social judgment (Luna, Padmanabhan, & O'Hearn, 2010). Delayed or poorly developed executive functioning is observed among youth at greater risk of developing SUDs, including children of alcoholics (Hill, Steinhauer, Park, & Zubin, 1990), children with conduct disorder and ADHD (Martel et al., 2009), and adolescents with attentional disorders (Pogge, Stokes, & Harvey, 1992; Sullivan & Rudnik-Levin, 2001). Executive functioning also negatively predicts age at first drink (Deckel, Bauer, & Hesselbrock, 1995), and among FH youth executive functioning predicts the number of drinks used per occasion (Deckel & Hesselbrock, 1996; Luna et al., 2010). Finally, poor executive functioning is associated with reduced ability to appreciate abuse consequences (Blume, Marlatt, & Schmaling, 2000). It should be noted that deficiencies in executive functioning are not specific to SUDs. Rather, they increase risk for all externalizing behaviors.

## PROTECTIVE FACTORS

Protective factors are not simply the absence of risk characteristics. Rather, they are distinctive characteristics or circumstances associated with decreased likelihood of engaging in health-damaging behaviors, despite the presence of one or more significant risk factors (Jessor, Van Den Bos, Vanderryn, Costa, & Turbin, 1995). Protective factors for substance use and associated problems among adolescents include certain temperamental traits, high intelligence, social support, involvement with conventional peers, religiosity, and low-risk taking (Brown et al., 2008; Gilvarry, 2000). Competence skills (e.g., decision making and self-efficacy) and psychological wellness are also protective agents against alcohol involvement across adolescence (Epstein & Botvin, 2002). A genetic deficiency in the Km aldehyde dehydronase (ALDH2) isoenzyme is associated with adverse reactions to alcohol. This genetic polymorphism is more prevalent in northern Asians (Chinese, Japanese, and Koreans) than in Caucasians, African Americans, and Native Americans, and results in adverse physiological response to alcohol including flushing, tachycardia, hypotension, nausea, and vomiting (Luczak, Glatt, & Wall, 2006). These physiological responses act as a protective factor against the development of heavy drinking patterns by lowering the positive reinforcement value of alcohol. By disrupting both regular use and binge onset, ALDH2 polymorphisms and related expectancies may also act to deter progression to other drugs, although this remains to be examined.

## DEVELOPMENTAL PATHWAYS TO ABUSE AND DEPENDENCE

Over the course of adolescence in industrialized countries, autonomy and independence from parents becomes an increasingly salient feature. Across species, increases in exploration, risk taking, and independence emerge during adolescence (Arnett, 2000; Brown et al., 2008). It is therefore not surprising that middle school and high school students explore new activities, often shift friendships, and may begin to experiment with substance use (Schinke, Botvin, & Orlandi, 1991). In the United States, initiation of substance use typically occurs in early to middle adolescence, with cigarettes, alcohol, and or marijuana. Exposure to other illicit substances most typically follows use of one or more of these substances in middle to late adolescence. This sequence varies across ethnic groups and among multiethnic adolescents (Chen et al., 2002). Binge drinking and more diversified substance involvement peaks during late adolescence and early adulthood (Chen & Kandel, 1995). Transitions out of the family of origin to independent and less restrictive living situations tend to result in greater access to and acceptance of use of alcohol and other substances (Chassin & Ritter, 2001; Kypri, McCarthy, Coe, & Brown, 2004). National and international epidemiological studies indicate that prevalence of substance use as well as substance dependence rates diminish in the mid-twenties. This change in prevalence is consistent with transition to adult roles including work, marriage, and parenthood, which have been concurrently and prospectively associated with a decline in substance involvement and abuse/dependence symptoms (Arnett, 2000; Gotham, Sher, & Wood, 1997; Zucker et al., 2006). Additionally, although personality is understood to be relatively stable over time, recent evidence suggests that young adult shifts in personality characteristics identified as early risk factors for substance involvement and other behavior problems are also linked to decrements in use and problematic use (Littlefield, Sher, & Wood, 2009). Thus, a portion of substance-abusing youth transition out of problematic use when anticipating or transitioning into adult responsibilities, with changing environments or with shifts in personality features which reflect risk level changes.

Biological, individual, and environmental factors operate in concert to predict SUDs in adolescence. Although certain factors predict substance involvement during adolescence directly, mediators and moderators at multiple system levels influence the initiation and progression of adolescent substance involvement and appear to vary in salience with age, gender, and cultural context (Brown et al., 2008). A number of studies have investigated the predominant longitudinal trajectories for use of alcohol, marijuana, nicotine, and other substances as well as more hazardous use (e.g., binge drinking, dependence criteria) among community, high-risk, and clinical samples of youth. Although the majority of these studies have focused on a single substance, youth substance involvement more typically involves exposure to multiple substances and only a limited number of longitudinal projects have considered simultaneously the onset, accelerations, and desistence of multiple substances extending over the full time course of adolescence (Anderson et al., 2010). Nonetheless, these longitudinal investigations shed light on the topography of substance involvement for subgroups of youth. Across studies it is clear there are subgroups of youth who have little or no engagement with alcohol or other drugs, early onset of involvement, late onset, and persistent higher intensity use (e.g., Chassin, Flora, & King, 2004; Jackson, Sher, & Schulenberg, 2008). Although there are grounds to be concerned about statistical features of this approach, developmentally focused research has identified time-limited patterns of involvement or excess, which are distinct from more chronic involvement over adolescence and into youth adulthood (e.g., Anderson et al., 2010; Schulenberg, Wadsworth, O'Malley, Bachman, & Johnston, 1996). This more fine-grained approach allows for articulation of mediators and moderators in relation to the timing of onset of use, escalation to excess or problems, and transitions out of problems/use. For example, Chassin and colleagues found that higher family history of dependence and negative emotionality, and lower constraint were associated with more rapid rise of polysubstance use and dependence relative to other patterns of use (Chassin et al., 2004).

*Deviance prone pathway.* Zucker and colleagues (2000) have described a parental alcoholism/deviance proneness pathway that operates as a risk factor for behavioral difficulties among offspring. Behavior problems including conduct disorder elevate risk for early substance involvement and persistent deviant behaviors in adolescence. Because parental SUDs and psychopathology are associated with ineffective parenting, risk for behavioral and cognitive problems is elevated in offspring. These result in emotional distress and affiliation with substance using, deviant peers, and eventually the offspring's own substance involvement and problematic behaviors (Sher, 1994). A key feature of this model involves the child's reduced ability to self-regulate emotional distress and inhibit behaviors, which elevates risk for the development of substance use problems in adolescence. Difficulties in self-regulation are reflected in higher-order executive functioning deficits that have been demonstrated in neuropsychological and neuroimaging studies of adolescent substance abusers (e.g., Anderson et al., 2005; De Bellis et al., 2000; Giancola & Parker, 2001). Although the primary emphasis among substance abuse researchers has been on environmental mechanisms operating within high-risk families, genetic factors also contribute to heterotypic continuity among adolescents on the deviance-prone trajectory (e.g., see Chapter 3). Furthermore, genetic and environmental risk are likely to interact to reinforce one another in affecting SUD outcomes, reflecting a passive Gene × Environment correlation (Rutter, 2007; Chapter 3).

*Negative affectivity pathway.* A second developmental pathway to SUDs relates to deficient regulation of negative affect. This pathway appears to be associated with both exposure to environmental stressors and temperamental negative emotionality (Colder & Chassin, 1993; Cooper, Frone, Russell, & Mudar, 1995). Research suggests that substance use among those on this trajectory is also mediated by peer use and/or adolescent-onset deviant behavior, and is associated with an elevated incidence of comorbid internalizing disorders (Abrantes et al., 2003). Although the negative affectivity pathway has received support in both cross-sectional and cross-cultural research (e.g., Rose et al., 1997), associations between negative affectivity and substance involvement have been modest in prospective high risk studies (Chassin & Ritter, 2001). Only about one quarter of those who evidence negative affectivity as children and who possess poor self-regulation and coping skills exemplify this trajectory (Colder & Chassin, 1993; Cooper et al., 1995).

*Enhanced reinforcement pathway.* Some youth are less sensitive to the effects of substances and consequently use substances more frequently and/or in greater quantities (e.g., Schuckit et al., 2004). This low response to alcohol is associated with higher positive reinforcement expectancies. The pathway appears to be genetically influenced and based on physiological response differences to the pharmacological effects of substances (e.g., Conrod, Peterson, & Pihl, 1997; Schuckit et al., 2004). Genetically influenced physiological and subjective responses appear to affect use decisions via expectancies, which develop in part as a result of individual reactions to alcohol (McCarthy et al., 2001). Thus, in addition to the physiological effects of substances, positive cognitions and outcome expectancies develop based on personal use of a substance and continued drinking. In turn, escalation to abuse occurs via the impact of both expectancies and continued use on decision making.

## FUTURE DIRECTIONS FOR PREVENTION

Alcohol and drug prevention programs for youth are varied and extensive. These programs range from education-based school approaches, to risk reduction and skill development programs all the way to community-wide application. Among these, overall effectiveness is mixed, with some programs demonstrating modest improvements (e.g., Botvin's Life Skills Training; Botvin, 2000), while others appear to actually accelerate onset and use rates in high-risk populations (e.g., DARE; see, e.g., Lilienfeld, 2007). Those with the largest, positive effect sizes typically operate across multiple reinforcement system (e.g., individual, school, family, community/public policy). Primary and early intervention effects involving peer leaders, motivational enhancement, improved accuracy of perceived social norms, challenges to outcome expectancies, and social practice appear most promising, particularly if including a Motivational Interviewing approach (Brown et al., 2008; Winters & Leitten, 2007).

There is growing appreciation for considering developmental factors in the timing (e.g., primary prevention prior to typical onset of use), content (e.g., common social contextual features of initial and early use episodes), and process (e.g. consideration of cognitive development) of effective interventions. The application of neuroscience findings to interventions is a relatively new but particularly promising endeavor (Brown et al., 2008).

Because the initiation or refusal to use alcohol and other drugs typically involves a social decision, prevention programs may target components of the decision-making process, including accuracy of information available for consideration, consequences of use and perceived social pressures to use (Ellickson, Bell, & McGuigan, 1993), as well as generation of behavioral alternatives and problem solving skills practice (Brown et al., 2001). Although prevention research is in its infancy regarding identification of specific cognitive functions that support high-level processes such as decision making, executive functions may be a particularly fruitful focus. By creating concrete interventions to facilitate goal generation, negotiation of social contexts, increased variability in responses, and regulation of response initiation and inhibition, adolescents should have more intrapersonal resources for dealing with the risks they will face.

## REFERENCES

Aarons, G. A., Brown, S. A., Hough, R. L., Garland, A. F., & Wood, P. A. (2001). Prevalence of adolescent substance use disorders across five sectors of care. *Journal of the American Academy of Child and Adolescent Psychiatry, 40*, 419–426.

Abrantes, A. M., Brown, S. A., & Tomlinson, K. L. (2003). Psychiatric comorbidity among inpatient substance abusing adolescents. *Journal of Child and Adolescent Substance Abuse, 13*, 83–101.

Ajzen, I. (1988). *Attitudes, personality, and behavior:* Homewood, IL: Dorsey Press.

Ajzen, I. (2001). Nature and operation of attitudes. *Annual Review Psychology, 52*, 27–58.

Ajzen, I., & Fishbein, M. (1980). *Understanding attitudes and predicting social behavior.* Englewood Cliffs, NJ: Prentice Hall.

Akers, R. L. (1977). *Deviant behavior: A social learning approach* (2nd ed.). Belmont, CA: Wadsworth.

American Psychiatric Association. (2000). *Diagnostic and statistical manual of mental disorders* (4th ed., text rev.). Washington, DC: Author.

Anderson, K. G., Ramo, D. E., Cummins, K., & Brown, S. A. (2010). Alcohol and drug involvement after adolescent treatment and functioning during emerging adulthood. *Drug and Alcohol Dependence, 107*, 171–181.

Anderson, K. G., Schweinsburg, A., Paulus, M. P., Brown, S. A., & Tapert, S. F. (2005). Examining personality and alcohol expectancies using fMRI with adolescents. *Journal of Studies on Alcohol, 66*, 323–332.

Armstrong, T. D., & Costello, E. J. (2002). Community studies on adolescent substance use, abuse, or dependence and psychiatric comorbidity. *Journal of Consulting and Clinical Psychology, 70*, 1224–1239.

Arnett, J. J. (1999). Adolescent storm and stress, reconsidered. *American Psychologist, 54*, 317–326.

Arnett, J. J. (2000). Emergent adulthood: A theory of development from the late teens through the twenties. *American Psychologist, 55*, 469–480.

Baer, P. E., & Bray, J. H. (1999). Adolescent individuation and alcohol use. *Journal of Studies on Alcohol Supplement, 13*, 52–62.

Baker, J. R., & Yardley, J. K. (2002). Moderating effect of gender on the relationship between sensation seeking-impulsivity and substance use in adolescents. *Journal of Child and Adolescent Substance Abuse, 12*, 27–43.

Bandura, A. (1986). *Social foundations of thought and action: A social cognitive theory.* Englewood Cliffs, NJ: Prentice Hall.

Barnes, G. M., Farrell, M. P., & Banerjee, S. (1994). Family influence on alcohol abuse and other problem behaviors among black and white adolescents in a general population sample. *Journal of Research on Adolescence, 4*, 183–201.

Bates, M. E., & Labouvie, E. W. (1995). Personality-environment constellation and alcohol use: A process-oriented study of intraindividual change during adolescence. *Psychology of Addictive Behaviors, 9*, 23–35.

Beauchaine, T. P., Neuhaus, E., Brenner, S. L., & Gatzke-Kopp, L. (2008). Ten good reasons to consider biological variables in prevention and intervention research. *Development and Psychopathology, 20*, 745–774.

Bekman, N. M., Diulio, A. R., Anderson, K. G., Metrik, J., Trim, R. S., Myers, M. G., Brown, S. A., (2010). The role of alcohol-related cognitions in various stages of adolescent alcohol use. *Alcoholism: Clinical & Experimental Research, 34*(6), 108A.

Blume, A. W., Marlatt, G. A., & Schmaling, K. B. (2000). Executive cognitive function and heavy drinking behavior among college students. *Psychology of Addictive Behaviors, 14*, 299–302.

Botvin, G. J. (2000). Preventing drug abuse in schools: Social and competence enhancement approaches targeting individual-level etiologic factors. *Addictive Behaviors, 25*, 887–897.

Brody, G. H., & Forehand, R. (1993). Prospective associations among family form, family process, and adolescents' alcohol and drug use. *Behaviour Research, and Therapy, 31*, 587–593.

Brown, S. A. (1989). Life events of adolescents in relation to personal and parental substance abuse. *American Journal of Psychiatry, 146*, 484–489.

Brown, S. A. (1993). Drug effect expectancies and addictive behavior change. *Experimental and Clinical Psychopharmacology, 1*, 55–67.

Brown, S. A., Aarons, G. A., & Abrantes, A. M. (2001). Adolescent alcohol and drug abuse. In C. E. Walker & M. C. Roberts (Eds.), *Handbook of clinical child psychology* (3rd ed., pp. 757–775). New York, NY: Wiley.

Brown, S. A., & Abrantes, A. M. (2005). Substance use disorders. In D. A. Wolfe & E. J. Mash (Eds.), *Behavioral and emotional disorders in adolescents* (pp. 226–258). New York, NY: Guilford Press.

Brown, S. A., McGue, M. K., Maggs, J., Schulenberg, J. E., Hingson, R., Swartzwelder, H. S., ... Murphy, S. (2008). A developmental perspective on alcohol and youth ages 16–20. *Pediatrics, 121*(Suppl 4), 290–310.

Brown, S. A., & Munson, E. (1987). Extroversion, anxiety and the perceived effects of alcohol. *Journal of Studies on Alcohol, 48*, 272–276.

Brown, S. A., Myers, M., Mott, M. A., & Vik, P. W. (1994). Correlates of success following treatment for adolescent substance abuse. *Applied and Preventive Psychology, 3*, 61–73.

Brown, S. A., & Tapert, S. F. (2004). Adolescence and the trajectory of alcohol use: Basic to clinical studies. In R. E. Dahl & L. P. Spear (Eds.), *Adolescent brain development: Vulnerabilities and opportunities. Annals of the New York Academy of Sciences, 1021*, 234–244.

Bukstein, O. G., & Lutka-Fedor, T. (2007). Principles of assessment for adolescents with substance use disorders. In E. Gilvarry & P. McArdle (Eds.), *Alcohol, drugs and young people* (pp. 127–135). Newcastle Upon Tyne, United Kingdom: Mac Keith Press.

Cadoret, R. J., Yates, W. R., Troughton, E., Woodworth, G., & Stewart, M. A. (1995). Adoption study demonstrating two genetic pathways to drug abuse. *Archives of General Psychiatry, 52,* 42–52.

Chassin, L., Pillow, D. R., Curran, P. J., Molina, B. S., & Barrera, M. (1993). Relation of parental alcoholism to early adolescent substance use: A test of three mediating mechanisms. *Journal of Abnormal Psychology, 102,* 3–19.

Chassin, L., & Ritter, J. (2001). Vulnerability to substance use disorders in childhood and adolescence. In R. E. Ingram & J. M. Price (Eds.), *Vulnerability to psychopathology* (pp. 107–134). New York: Guilford.

Chassin, L., Flora, D. B., & King, K. M. (2004). Trajectories of alcohol and drug use and dependence from adolescence to adulthood: The effects of familial alcoholism and personality. *Journal of Abnormal Psychology, 113*(4), 483–498.

Chatlos, J. C. (1997). Substance use and abuse and the impact on academic difficulties. *Journal of the American Academy of Child and Adolescent Psychiatry, 6,* 545–568.

Chen, K., & Kandel, D. B. (1995). The natural history of drug use from adolescence to the mid-thirties in a general population sample. *American Journal of Public Health, 85,* 41–47.

Chen, X., Unger, J. B., Palmer, P., Weiner, M. D., Johnson, C. A., Wong, M. A., & Austin, G. (2002). Prior cigarette smoking initiation predicting current alcohol use: Evidence for a gateway drug effect among California adolescents from eleven ethnic groups. *Addictive Behaviors, 27,* 799–817.

Chilcoat, H. D., & Anthony, J. C. (1996). Impact of parent monitoring on initiation of drug use through late childhood. *Journal of the American Academy of Child and Adolescent Psychiatry, 35,* 91–100.

Chilcoat, H., & Breslau, N. (1996). Alcohol disorders in young adulthood: Effects of transitions into adult roles. *Journal of Health and Social Behavior, 37,* 339–349.

Cloninger, C. R., Sigvardsson, S., & Bohman, M. (1988). Childhood personality predicts alcohol abuse in young adults. *Alcoholism: Clinical and Experimental Research, 12,* 494–505.

Colder, C., & Chassin, L. (1993). The stress and negative affect model of adolescent alcohol use and the moderating effects of behavioral undercontrol. *Journal of Studies on Alcohol, 54,* 326–333.

Comeau, N., Stewart, S. H., & Loba, P. (2001). The relations of trait anxiety, anxiety sensitivity and sensation seeking to adolescents' motivations for alcohol, cigarette, and marijuana use. *Addictive Behaviors, 26,* 803–825.

Conrod, P. J., Peterson, J. B., & Pihl, R. O. (1997). Disinhibited personality and sensitivity to alcohol reinforcement: Independent correlates of drinking behavior in sons of alcoholics. *Alcoholism Clinical and Experimental Research, 21,* 1320–1332.

Cooper, M. L., Frone, M. R., Russell, M., & Mudar, P. (1995). Drinking to regulate positive and negative emotions: A motivational model of alcohol use. *Journal of Personality and Social Psychology, 69,* 990–1005.

Cyders, M. A., Smith, G. T., Spillane, N. S., Fischer, S., Annus, A. M., & Peterson, C. (2007). Integration of impulsivity and positive mood to predict risky behavior: Development and validation of a measure of positive urgency. *Psychological Assessment, 19,* 107–118.

D'Amico, E. J., Metrik, J., McCarthy, D. M., Appelbaum, M., Frissell, K. C., & Brown, S. A. (2001). Progression into and out of binge drinking among high school students. *Psychology of Addictive Behaviors, 15,* 341–349.

Dakof, G. A. (2000). Understanding gender differences in adolescent drug abuse: Issues of comorbidity and family functioning. *Journal of Psychoactive Drugs, 32,* 25–32.

De Bellis, M. D., Clark, D. B., Beers, S. R., Soloff, P. H., Boring, A. M., Hall, J., . . . Keshavan, M. S. (2000). Hippocampal volume in adolescent-onset alcohol use disorders. *American Journal Psychiatry, 157,* 737–744.

Deckel, A. W., Bauer, L., & Hesselbrock, V. (1995). Anterior brain dysfunctioning as a risk factor in alcoholic behaviors. *Addiction, 90,* 1323–1334.

Deckel, A. W., & Hesselbrock, V. (1996). Behavioral and cognitive measurements predict scores on the MAST: A 3-year prospective study. *Alcoholism: Clinical Experimental Research, 20,* 1173–1178.

Dobkin, P. L., Tremblay, R. E., Masse, L. C., & Vitaro, F. (1995). Individual and peer characteristics in predicting boys' early onset of substance abuse: A seven-year longitudinal study. *Child Development, 66,* 1198–1214.

Ellickson, P. L., Bell, R. M., & McGuigan, K. (1993). Preventing adolescent drug use: Long-term results of a junior high program. *American Journal of Public Health, 83,* 856–861.

Epstein, J. A., & Botvin, G. J. (2002). The moderating role of risk-taking tendency and refusal assertiveness on social influences in alcohol use among inner-city adolescents. *Journal of Studies on Alcohol, 63,* 456–459.

Fergusson, D., Horwood, J., & Lynskey, M. (1995). The prevalence and risk factors associated with abusive or hazardous alcohol consumption in 16-year-olds. *Addiction, 90,* 935–946.

Giancola, P. R., & Parker, A. M. (2001). A six-year prospective study of pathways toward drug use in adolescent boys with and without a family history of a substance use disorder. *Journal of Studies on Alcohol, 62,* 166–178.

Gilvarry, E. (2000). Substance abuse in young people. *Journal of Child Psychology and Psychiatry, 41,* 55–80.

Goldman, M. S., Brown, S. A., Christiansen, B. A., & Smith, G. T. (1991). Alcoholism and memory broadening the scope of alcohol-expectancy research. *Psychological Bulletin, 110,* 137–146.

Goldman, M. S., Darkes, J., Reich, R. R., & Broandon, K. O. (2010). From DNA to conscious thought: Anticipatory processing as a transdisciplinary bridge in addiction. In D. Ross, H. Kincaid, D. Spurrett, & P. Collins (Eds.), *What is addiction?* (pp. 291–334). Cambridge, MA: MIT Press.

Goldman, M. S., & Rather, B. C. (1993). Substance use disorders: Cognitive models and architecture. In P. C. Kendall & K. Dobson (Eds.), *Psychopathology and cognition* (pp. 245–292). New York: Academic Press.

Gotham, H., Sher, K., & Wood, P. (1997). Predicting stability and change in frequency of intoxication from the college years to beyond: Individual difference and role transition variables. *Journal of Abnormal Psychology, 106,* 619–629.

Grant, B. F., & Dawson, D. A. (1997). Age at onset of alcohol use and its association with DSM-IV alcohol abuse and dependence: Results from the national longitudinal alcohol epidemiologic survey. *Journal of Substance Abuse, 9,* 103–110.

Grant, B. F., Stinson, F. S., & Harford, T. C. (2001). Age of onset of alcohol use and DSM-IV alcohol abuse and dependence: A 12-year follow-up. *Journal of Substance Abuse, 13,* 493–504.

Greenbaum, P. E., Foster-Johnson, L., & Petrila, A. (1996). Co-occurring addictive and mental disorders among adolescents: Prevalence research and future directions. *American Journal of Orthopsychiatry, 66,* 52–60.

Grella, C. E., & Joshi, V. (2003). Treatment processes and outcomes among adolescents with a history of abuse who are in drug treatment. *Child Maltreatment: Journal of the American Professional Society on the Abuse of Children, 8,* 7–18.

Grilo, C. M., Becker, D. F., Walker, M. L., Levy, K. N., Edell, W. S., & McGlashan, T. H. (1995). Psychiatric comorbidity in adolescent inpatients with substance use disorder. *Journal of the American Academy of Child and Adolescent Psychiatry, 34,* 1085–1091.

Hill, S. Y., Steinhauer, S., Park, J., & Zubin, J. (1990). Event-related potential characteristics in children of alcoholics from high density families. *Alcoholism: Clinical and Experimental Research, 14,* 6–16.

Huba, G. J., Wingard, J. A., & Bentler, P. M. (1980). Framework for an interactive theory of drug use. *NIDA Research Monograph, 30,* 95–101.

Jackson, K. M., Sher, K. J., & Schulenberg, J. E. (2008). Conjoint developmental trajectories of young adult substance use. *Alcoholism: Clinical and Experimental Research, 32,* 723–737.

Jessor, R., & Jessor, S. L. (1977). *Problem behavior and psychosocial development:* New York, NY: Academic Press.

Jessor, R., Van Den Bos, J., Vanderryn, J., Costa, F. M., & Turbin, M. (1995). Protective factors in adolescent problem behavior: Moderator effects and developmental change. *Developmental Psychology, 31,* 923–933.

Johnson, E. O., Arria, A. M., Borges, G., Ialongo, N., & Anthony, J. C. (1995). The growth of conduct problem behaviors from middle childhood to early adolescence: Sex differences and the suspected influence of early alcohol use. *Journal of Studies on Alcohol, 56,* 661–671.

Johnston, L. D., O'Malley, P. M., Bachman, J. G., & Schulenberg, J. E. (2010). *Monitoring the future national survey results on drug use, 1975–2005: Vol. I. Secondary school students (NIH Publication No. 06–5883).* Bethesda, MD: National Institute on Drug Abuse.

Kandel, D. B., Johnson, J. G., Bird, H. R., Canino, G., Goodman, S. H., Lahey, B. B., . . . Schwab-Stone, M. (1997). Psychiatric disorders associated with substance use among children and adolescents: Findings from the methods for the epidemiology of child and adolescent mental disorders (MECA) study. *Journal of Abnormal Child Psychology, 25,* 121–132.

Kendler, K. S., Prescott, C. A., Myers, J., & Neale, M. C. (2003). The structure of genetic and environmental risk factors for common psychiatric and substance use disorders in men and women. *Archives of General Psychiatry, 60,* 929–937.

Knop, J., Teasdale, T. W., Schulsinger, F., & Goodwin, D. W. (1985). A prospective study of young men at high risk for alcoholism: School behavior and achievement. *Journal of Studies on Alcohol, 46,* 273–278.

Koob, G. F., & Le Moal, M. (2008). Neurobiological mechanisms for opponent motivational processes in addiction. *Philosophical Transactions of the Royal Society: Biological Sciences, 363,* 3113–3123.

Kuo, P. H., Yang, H. J., Soong, W. T., & Chen, W. J. (2002). Substance use among adolescents in Taiwan: Associated personality traits, incompetence, and behavioral/emotional problems. *Drug and Alcohol Dependence, 67,* 27–39.

Kypri, K., McCarthy, D. M., Coe, M. T., & Brown, S. A. (2004). Transition to independent living and substance involvement of treated and high-risk youth. *Journal of Child and Adolescent Substance Abuse, 13,* 85–100.

Lewinsohn, P. M., Rohde, P., & Seeley, J. R. (1995). Adolescent psychopathology: III. The clinical consequences of comorbidity. *Journal of the American Academy of Child and Adolescent Psychiatry, 34,* 510–519.

Lewinsohn, P. M., Solomon, A., Seeley, J. R., & Zeiss, A. (2000). Clinical implications of "subthreshold" depressive symptoms. *Journal of Abnormal Psychology, 109,* 345–351.

Lilienfeld, S. O. (2007). Psychological treatments that cause harm. *Perspectives on Psychological Science, 2,* 53–70.

Limosin, F., Loze, J. Y., Rouillon, F., Adès, J., & Gorwood, P. (2003). Association between dopamine receptor D1 gene DdeI polymorphism and sensation seeking in alcohol-dependent men. *Alcoholism: Clinical and Experimental Research, 27,* 1226–1228.

Littlefield, A. K., Sher, K. J., & Wood, P. K. (2009). Is "maturing out" of problematic alcohol involvement related to personality change?

Loukas, A., Zucker, R. A., Fitzgerald, H. E., & Krull, J. L. (2003). Developmental trajectories of disruptive behavior problems among sons of alcoholics: Effects of parent psychopathology, family conflict, and child undercontrol. *Journal of Abnormal Psychology, 112,* 119–131.

Luczak, S. E., Glatt, S. J., & Wall, T. L. (2006). Meta-analyses of ALDH2 and ADH1B with alcohol dependence in Asians. *Psychological Bulletin, 132,* 607–621.

Luna, B., Padmanabhan, A., & O'Hearn K. (2010). What has fMRI told us about the development of cognitive control through adolescence? *Brain and Cognition, 72,* 101–113.

Martel, M. M., Pierce, L., Nigg, J. T., Jester, J. M., Adams, K., Putter, L., . . . Zucker, R. A. (2009). Temperament pathways to childhood disruptive behavior and adolescent substance abuse: Testing a cascade model. *Journal of Abnormal Child Psyhcology, 37,* 363–373.

McCarthy, D. M., Brown, S. A., Carr, L. G., & Wall, T. L. (2001). ALDH2 Status, alcohol expectancies and alcohol response: Preliminary evidence for a mediation model. *Alcoholism Clinical and Experimental Research, 25,* 1558–1563.

McGue, M., Iacono, W. G., Legrand, L. N., Malone, S., & Elkins, I. (2001). Origins and consequences of age at first drink. I. Associations with substance-use disorders, disinhibitory behavior and psychopathology, and P3 amplitude. *Alcoholism: Clinical and Experimental Research, 25,* 1156–1165.

Newlin, D. B. (1994). Alcohol challenge in high-risk individuals. In R. Zucker, G. Boyd, & J. Howard (Eds.), *The development of alcohol problems: Exploring the biopsychosocial matrix of risk* (DHHS Publication No. ADM 94–3495, pp. 47–68). Washington, DC: U.S. Government Printing Office.

Nigg, J. T., Wong, M. M., Martel, M. M., Jester, J. M., Puttler, L. I., Glass, J. M., . . . Zucker, R. A. (2006). Poor response inhibition as a predictor of problem drinking and illicit drug use in adolescents at risk for alcoholism and other substance use disorders. *Journal of the American Academy of Child & Adolescent Psychiatry, 45,* 468–475.

Novins, D. K., Beals, J., Shore, J. H., & Manson, S. M. (1996). Substance abuse treatment of American Indian adolescents: Comorbid symptomatology, gender differences, and treatment patterns. *Journal of the American Academy of Child and Adolescent Psychiatry, 35,* 1593–1601.

Pandina, R. J., & Schuele, J. A. (1983). Psychosocial correlates of alcohol and drug use of adolescent students and adolescents in treatment. *Journal of Studies on Alcohol, 44,* 950–973.

Petraitis, J., Flay, B. R., & Miller, T. Q. (1995). Reviewing theories of adolescent substance use: Organizing pieces of the puzzle. *Psychological Bulletin, 117,* 67–86.

Pogge, D. L., Stokes, J., & Harvey, P. D. (1992). Psychometric vs. attentional correlates of early onset alcohol and substance-abuse. *Journal of Abnormal Child Psychology, 20,* 151–162.

Robinson, T. E., & Berridge, K. C. (2003). Addiction. *Annual Review of Psychology, 54,* 25–53.

Rose, R. J., Kaprio, J., Pulkkinen, L., Koskenvuo, M., Viken, R. J., & Bates, J. E. (1997). FinnTwin 12 and FinnTwin 16: Longitudinal twin-family studies in Finland. *Behavioral Genetics, 27,* 603–604.

Rutter, M. (2007). Gene-environment interdependence. *Developmental Science, 10,* 12–18.

Schinke, S. P., Botvin, G. J., & Orlandi, M. A. (1991). *Substance abuse in children and adolescents: Evaluation and intervention.* Newbury Park, CA: Sage.

Schuckit, M. (1988). Reactions to alcohol in sons of alcoholics and controls. *Alcoholism: Clinical and Experimental Research, 12,* 465–470.

Schuckit, M. A., Mazzanti, C., Smith, T. L., Ahmed, U., Radel, M., Iwata, N., & Goldman, D. (1999). Selective genotyping for the role of 5HT2A, 5HT2C, and GABAα6 receptors and the serotonin transporter in level of response to alcohol. *Biological Psychiatry, 45,* 647–651.

Schuckit, M. A., Smith, T. L., Anderson, K. G., & Brown, S. A. (2004). Testing the level of response to alcohol-social information processing model of the alcoholism risk: A 20-year prospective study. *Alcoholism: Clinical and Experimental Research, 28,* 1881–1889.

Schuckit, M. A., Smith, T. L., Danko, G. P., Anderson, K. G., Brown, S. A., Kuperman, S., . . . Bucholz, K. (2005). Evaluation of a "level of response to alcohol based" structural equation model in adolescents. *Journal of Studies on Alcohol, 66,* 174–185.

Schulenberg, J., Wadsworth, K. N., O'Malley, P. M., Bachman, J. G., & Johnston, L. D. (1996). Adolescent risk factors for binge drinking during the transition to young adulthood: Variable- and pattern-centered approaches to change. *Developmental Psychology, 32,* 659–679.

Sher, K. J. (1994). Individual-level risk factors. In R. Zucker, G. Boyd, & J. Howard (Eds.), *The development of alcohol problems: Exploring the biopsychosocial matrix of risk* (DHHS Publication No. ADM 94–2495, pp. 77–108). Washington, DC: U.S. Government Printing Office.

Smith, G. T., Fischer, S., Cyders, M. A., Annus, A. M., Spillane, N. S., & McCarthy, D. M. (2007). On the validity and utility of discriminating among impulsivity-like traits. *Assessment,14,* 155–170.

Smith, G. T., Goldman, M. S., Greenbaum, P. E., & Christiansen, B. A. (1995). Expectancy for social facilitation from drinking: The divergent paths of high-expectancy and low-expectancy adolescents. *Journal of Abnormal Psychology, 104,* 32–40.

Stowell, R. J., & Estroff, T. W. (1992). Psychiatric disorders in substance-abusing adolescent inpatients: A pilot study. *Journal of the American Academy of Child and Adolescent Psychiatry, 31,* 1036–1040.

Substance Abuse and Mental Health Services Administration. (1999). *Treatment of adolescents with substance use disorders: Treatment improvement protocol (TIP), Series 32.* Rockville, MD: Department of Health and Human Services.

Sullivan, M. A., & Rudnik-Levin, F. (2001). Attention deficit/hyperactivity disorder and substance abuse: Diagnostic and therapeutic considerations. *Annals of the New York Academy of Sciences, 931,* 251–270.

Tapert, S. F., & Brown, S. A. (1999). Neuropsychological correlates of adolescent substance abuse: Four year outcomes. *Journal of the International Neuropsychological Society, 5,* 475–487.

Tapert, S. F., Schweinsburg, A. D., Barlett, V. C., Brown, S. A., Frank, L. R., Brown, G. G., & Meloy, M. J. (2004). Blood oxygen level dependent response and spatial working memory in adolescents with alcohol use disorders. *Alcoholism: Clinical and Experimental Research, 28,* 1577–1586.

Tarter, R., Vanyukov, M., Giancola, P., Dawes, M., Blackson, T., Mezzich, A., & Clark, D. B. (1999). Etiology of early age onset substance use disorder: A maturational perspective. *Development and Psychopathology, 11,* 657–683.

Tarter, R. E., & Edwards, K. (1988). Psychological factors associated with the risk for alcoholism. *Alcoholism: Clinical and Experimental Research, 12,* 471–480.

Tate, S. R., Patterson, K. A., Nagel, B. J., Anderson, K. G., & Brown, S. A. (2007). Addiction and stress in adolescents. In M. al'Absi (Ed.), *Stress and addiction: Biological and psychological mechanisms* (pp. 249–262). New York, NY: Elsevier.

Tsuang, M. T., Lyons, M. J., Meyer, J. M., Doyle, T., Eisen, S. A., Goldberg, J., . . . Eaves, L. (1998). Co-occurrence of abuse of different drugs in men: The role of drug-specific and shared vulnerabilities. *Archives of General Psychiatry, 55,* 967–972.

Vik, P. W., Brown, S. A., & Myers, M. G. (1997). Adolescent substance abuse problems: In E. J. Mash & L. G. Terdal (Eds.), *Assessment of childhood disorders* (3rd ed., pp. 717–748). New York, NY: Guilford Press.

Vik, P. W., Grizzle, K., & Brown, S.A (1992). Social resource characteristics and adolescent substance abuse relapse. *Journal of Adolescent Chemical Dependency, 2,* 59–74.

Wall, T. L., Shea, S. H., Chan, K. K., & Carr, L. G. (2001). A genetic association with the development of alcohol and other substance use behavior in Asian Americans. *Journal of Abnormal Psychology, 110,* 173–178.

Williams, P. S., & Hine, D. W. (2002). Parental behaviour and alcohol misuse among adolescents: A path analysis of mediating influences. *Australian Journal of Psychology, 54,* 17–24.

Wills, T. A., Vaccaro, D., & McNamara, G. (1992). The role of life events, family support, and competence in adolescent substance use: A test of vulnerability and protective factors. *American Journal of Community Psychology, 20,* 349–374.

Windle, M. (1990). Temperament and personality attributes of children of alcoholics. In M. Windle & J. S. Searles (Eds.), *Children of alcoholics: Critical perspectives* (pp. 129–167). New York, NY: Guilford Press.

Winters, K. C., & Leitten, W. (2007). Brief interventions for moderate drug abusing adolescents. *Psychology of Addictive Behaviors, 21,* 151–156.

Zucker, R. A., Wong, M. M., Clark, D. B., Leonard, K. E., Schulenberg, J. E., Cornelius, J. R., . . . Puttler, L. I. (2006). Predicting risky drinking outcomes longitudinally: What kind of advance notice can we get? *Alcoholism: Clinical and Experimental Research, 30,* 243–252.

Zuckerman, M. (1994). *Behavioral expressions and biosocial bases of sensation seeking:* New York, NY: Cambridge University Press.

# PART IV

# INTERNALIZING BEHAVIOR DISORDERS

# CHAPTER 16

# Anxiety Disorders

CARL F. WEEMS AND WENDY K. SILVERMAN

## HISTORICAL CONTEXT

LTHOUGH THE *OXFORD ENGLISH Dictionary* reports evidence for the noun "anxiety" as early as the 1500s, interest in childhood anxiety problems can be traced as far back as the writings of Hippocrates in ancient Greece (Silverman & Field, 2011). Descriptions of child anxiety and phobias also can be found in writings from early America (e.g., Benjamin Rush), and in many famous case reports (e.g., Freud's Little Hans; Watson's Little Albert; see Silverman & Field, 2011, for review). In the second edition of the *Diagnostic and Statistical Manual of Mental Disorders* (*DSM-II*; American Psychiatric Association [APA], 1968) there was only one specific childhood anxiety category: overanxious reaction. The *DSM-III* (APA, 1980) then introduced—and the *DSM-III-R* (APA, 1987) retained—a new broad category termed *anxiety disorders* of childhood and adolescence. Within this broad category three specific anxiety disorders were introduced: (1) separation anxiety disorder, (2) overanxious disorder, and (3) avoidant disorder. Children could also receive diagnoses of other anxiety/phobic disorders classified among adults, with identical criteria to the adult depictions.

Claims were soon made that the majority of new *DSM-III* categories and subcategories, including those relating to anxiety, were overrefined, untested, and excessive in number (see Silverman, 1992). It was also contended that the use of similar diagnostic criteria in children and adults was inconsistent with developmental changes in the expression of psychopathology across the life span. These were serious issues, and the research community was faced with the challenge of providing empirical evidence to either support or refute the validity of each new diagnostic category. Hence, a great deal of time and energy was devoted toward establishing basic requirements of a useful taxonomic scheme, including reliability, coverage, descriptive validity, and predictive validity (Blashfield, 1989). This work spurred concentrated efforts toward developing and evaluating structured interviewing procedures as a way to yield improved reliability of diagnoses (e.g., Silverman & Rabian, 1994; Silverman, Saavedra, & Pina, 2001; see Silverman & Ollendick, 2005).

The fourth version of the *DSM* (APA, 1994) witnessed major changes. The broad category of anxiety disorders of childhood and adolescence (and its subcategories: overanxious disorder, avoidant disorder) from the *DSM-III* and *DSM-III-R* were abandoned. Only separation anxiety disorder was retained as a distinct child anxiety disorder under "other disorders of infancy, childhood or adolescence." Thus, in the *DSM-IV* the same basic definitions of anxiety disorders apply to children, adolescents, and adults, with the exception of separation anxiety disorder which requires onset before age 18 although this requirement has been questioned (Manicavasagar, Silove, Curtis, & Wagner, 2000). For specific phobia, social phobia, obsessive compulsive disorder, posttraumatic stress disorder, and generalized anxiety disorder there are notes in the diagnostic criteria delineating child specific considerations (e.g., for specific phobia, Criterion C indicates that children may not recognize that the fear is unreasonable).

## TERMINOLOGICAL AND CONCEPTUAL ISSUES

Anxiety is viewed as a higher-order feeling state produced by specific brain mechanisms responsible for basic emotion (Damasio, 2003). We define anxiety in this chapter as the product of a multicomplex response system, involving affective, behavioral, physiological, and cognitive components (e.g., Barlow, 2002; Lang, 1977). Worry, for example, is one component of anxiety that can be viewed as a cognitive process preparing the individual to anticipate future danger. Fear, in contrast, is part of the response system that fosters preparation for either freezing to avoid impending punishment or escaping as part of the fight/flight response (Barlow, 2002; Gray & McNaughton, 2000; Mathews, 1990).

A core defining feature of anxiety is emotion dysregulation of the anxiety response system (Weems, 2008). Such dysregulation may involve intense and disabling worry that does not help anticipate true future danger, or intense fear reactions in the absence of true threat. Distress/impairment may also result from dysregulation in corresponding negative emotional states (e.g., being upset or overconcerned). For convenience we refer to these *primary* features of anxiety problems as anxious emotion. These core features of anxiety may be expressed behaviorally (e.g., avoidance), cognitively (e.g., concentration difficulties), physiologically (e.g., dizziness, racing heart), or interpersonally (e.g., difficulty making friends). These features cut across all of the anxiety disorders in the *DSM-IV*. In contrast, *secondary* features of anxiety are aspects that differentiate specific categories of anxiety disorder (Weems, 2008). For example, worry about separation from parents is specific to separation anxiety disorder, being embarrassed in public is specific to social anxiety disorder, and uncued panic attacks are specific to panic disorder (APA, 1994).

## DIAGNOSTIC ISSUES AND *DSM-IV* CRITERIA

The conceptualization and classification of the anxiety disorders in the *DSM-IV* (1994, 2000) currently dominate the field. The fifth edition of the *DSM* is anticipated for release in May 2013. Several changes to the classification scheme for anxiety disorders have been proposed. At the time of the writing of this chapter, no final decisions had been made. However, it does appear that anxiety disorders included in *DSM-IV* will continue to be included in *DSM-5*. These include (1) specific phobias, (2) social anxiety disorder, (3) generalized anxiety disorder, (4) separation anxiety disorder, (5) obsessive compulsive disorder, (6) panic disorder, and (7) posttraumatic stress disorder (PTSD). These disorders can appear at any age, with the exception of separation anxiety disorder, which is diagnosed only if it emerges before age 18.

According to the *DSM-IV* (APA, 1994, 2000), specific phobias are characterized by extreme and unreasonable fears of a specific object or situation such as dogs, loud noises, or the dark; social anxiety disorder is characterized by an extreme and unreasonable fear of being embarrassed or humiliated in front of other youths or adults. Next, generalized anxiety disorder is characterized by persistent and excessive worry about a number of events or activities, whereas separation anxiety disorder is characterized by excessive worry concerning separation from home or loved ones. Obsessive compulsive disorder (OCD) is characterized by recurrent thoughts or behavior patterns that are severe enough to be time consuming, distressful, and highly interfering, including repeated thoughts about contamination, repeated doubts, having things in a particular order, and aggressive or horrible impulses. Panic disorder is characterized by sudden and severe attacks of anxiety.

In addition, a child or adolescent who experiences a catastrophic or otherwise traumatic event may develop posttraumatic stress disorder (PTSD; APA, 1994, 2000). The traumatic event must involve a situation in which someone's life has been threatened or severe injury has occurred. Following exposure to the trauma, the youth may exhibit agitated or confused behavior as well as intense fear, helplessness, anger, sadness, horror, and/or denial. Youth with PTSD usually avoid situations or places that remind them of the trauma. They also may become depressed, withdrawn, emotionally unresponsive, and detached from their feelings.

The *DSM* anxiety disorders exhibit high rates of comorbidity with one another (Costello, Egger, & Angold, 2004; Curry, March, & Hervey, 2004). In fact, only secondary features outlined above, such as social concerns in social anxiety disorder and worries about separation in separation anxiety disorder, distinguish the anxiety disorders from one another. Moreover, genetic risk for anxiety disorders is nonspecific (Gregory & Eley, 2011). With the exceptions of OCD and possibly PTSD, there is little evidence that anxiety disorders are related differentially to treatment outcomes, although it is recognized that such null findings may be attributed in part to insufficient sample sizes (see Berman, Weems, Silverman, & Kurtines, 2000; see also Dadds, James, Barrett & Verhulst, 2004; Saavedra & Silverman, 2001). Finally, longitudinal research on the stability of child and adolescent anxiety disorders has produced inconsistent results (e.g., Last, Perrin, Hersen, & Kazdin, 1996; Newman et al., 1996).

## PREVALENCE

Anxiety disorders are one of the most common emotional problems in childhood and adolescence. In a recent meta-analysis, Costello, Egger, Copeland, and Angold

(2011) reported that the mean estimate for any anxiety disorder is 12.3% for children between ages 6 and 12, with the following disorders being most prevalent: specific phobia (6.7%), separation anxiety disorder (3.9%), social phobia (2.2%), and generalized anxiety disorder (1.7%). For adolescents, the prevalence estimate for any anxiety disorder was 11.0%. The following specific disorders were most prevalent: specific phobia (6.6%), social phobia (5.0%), separation anxiety disorder (2.3%), generalized anxiety disorder (1.9%), and panic disorder (1.1%).

## RISK FACTORS AND ETIOLOGICAL FORMULATIONS

To understand the development of anxiety problems, a number of biological, cognitive, behavioral, and social risk factors are salient. Some of these may be part of "normal" developmental processes (e.g., biological maturation) or may be atypical experiences (e.g., traumatic event). Symptoms of anxiety and phobic disorders can be understood as stemming from transactions among biological vulnerabilities (e.g., genetic, neural) and environmental risk factors (e.g., parenting, exposure to trauma) that produce emotion dysregulation, distress, and impairment. These factors give rise to undifferentiated anxious emotion. Specific anxiety disorders are then shaped by biological, cognitive, behavioral, and social processes (Vasey & Dadds, 2001; Weems & Stickle, 2005). For example, genetic predispositions and early experiences may render a child vulnerable to elevated levels of anxiety and distress, sometimes termed trait anxiety (or behavioral inhibition). More specific experiences such as being excluded or teased by peers upon school entry may foster the development of social anxiety; a frightening experience with a dog may result in an animal phobia; and biological vulnerability such as the experience of uncued physiological arousal may lead to panic disorder.

In understanding the etiology of childhood anxiety we use a developmental perspective that emphasizes complex transactions among various vulnerabilities and factors (Weems, 2008; Weems & Silverman, 2006). From this perspective, behavior patterns among individuals have varying trajectories over time (Baltes, Reese, & Lipsitt, 1980; Baltes, Reese, & Nesselroade, 1988), resulting in both equifinality and multifinality (see Chapter 1).

Specific etiological influences on the development of problematic anxiety span genetics, temperament, and physiology (biology); operant, observational, and respondent learning (associative learning); information processing and stimulus/event interpretation (cognition); attachment relations and sociability (socialization), and interactions among these processes in diverse contexts (e.g., parent–child relationships, family, home, school, community).

### Biological Processes

*Genetic influences.* Twin studies suggest that about a third of the variance in childhood anxiety symptoms is accounted for by heritable influences (see Eley, 2001; Gregory & Eley, 2011). Heritability may help to account for children's early anxious styles, including physiological reactivity and avoidance behaviors. It is important to note, however, that genes do not act directly on behavior. Genes code for proteins, which in turn affect brain structures and regulative processes, such as neurotransmitter receptors. The heritability of anxiety also depends on many other factors including the type of anxiety assessed, the age and sex of the population, the specific assessment method, and whether anxiety is viewed as a personality trait or a clinical disorder (Gregory & Eley, 2011). It is also important to note that the heritability of anxiety increases considerably in adolescence and young adulthood, a phenomenon seen for many psychiatric disorders (Bergen, Gardner, & Kendler, 2007). This pattern suggests that genetic vulnerabilities unfold across development as environmental risks mount (see Chapter 3).

Molecular genetics studies of anxiety have also grown rapidly. Such investigations have focused on genes encoding components of the 5-HT and GABA systems. Results have been mixed, but the strongest findings have linked genes to anxiety-related traits such as behavioral inhibition and not to specific disorders. Such findings point to the importance of differentiating between primary and secondary features of anxiety (see earlier). For example, the gene encoding the GABA-synthetic enzyme GAD65 has been associated with behavioral inhibition, a risk factor for anxiety disorders such as panic disorder, yet no genes encoding GABA receptors have been linked directly to panic disorder (see Gordon & Hen, 2004). One of the most promising lines of research suggests that polymorphisms in the promoter region of the gene for the 5-HT transporter (5-HTT) may also be associated with behavioral inhibition, particularly among individuals exposed to environmental risk (Fox et al., 2005). However, the particular polymorphisms in genes identified (e.g., the 5-HTT) may not simply lead to increased risk under negative environments but rather may be associated with malleability to both positive and negative environmental influences (Belsky & Beaver, 2011; Belsky, & Pluess, 2009).

Temperament theorists have drawn from genetic models, suggesting that anxiety problems stem from biological predispositions to react negatively to novelty (Biederman et al., 1990, 1993; Kagan et al., 1988; Kagan, Reznick, & Gibbons, 1989; Kagan, Reznick, & Snidman, 1987; see Lonigan, Phillips, Wilson, & Allan, 2011, for review). Temperamentally inhibited children display many of the same behavioral, affective, and physiological characteristics as children with anxiety disorders, including avoidance and withdrawal from novelty, clinging or dependence on parents, fearfulness, and autonomic hyperarousal (Kagan et al., 1987). Such children are more likely than their peers to respond to potentially fearful situations (e.g., interactions with a stranger, separations from mother) with heightened physiological reactivity, which may result from a lower threshold of amygdalar and hypothalamic activity.

*Central nervous system.* The concept of a behavioral inhibition system (BIS) is a good starting point for understanding central nervous system structures involved in the anxiety response (Gray, 1982). The BIS comprises the septohippocampal system, including the amygdala, noradrenergic projections of the locus coeruleus, and serotonergic projections of the median raphe (Gray 1982; Gray & McNaughton, 2000). Important for this discussion, the BIS is activated under conditions of perceived threat, helping us avoid exposure to punishment and danger. Overactivation of the BIS is associated with excessive fear, hyperarousal, and negative emotionality.

Among septo-hippocampal structures, the amygdala has received particular attention in theories of the pathogenesis of anxiety (e.g., Davis, 1998; LeDoux, 2000). The amygdala is a collection of nuclei found in the anterior portion of the temporal lobes. It functions to evaluate the emotional significance of incoming stimuli after receiving input from the cortex, hippocampus, and thalamus. The amygdala projects to other brain structures in the frontal cortex (choice), the hippocampus (memory consolidation), the striatum (approach/avoidance), and the hypothalamus and brain stem (autonomic responses, startle, corticosteroid response) (see Gordon & Hen, 2004; LeDoux, 2000). Importantly, no single structure, neurotransmitter, or gene controls the experience of anxiety or any other complex behavioral trait (see Pine, 2011; Chapter 3).

As noted, negative affect is an important component of anxiety. Functional brain studies suggest normal threat assessment and emotional learning may involve differential hemispheric activation. Electroencephalography (EEG) research has demonstrated increased right prefrontal and anterior temporal region activation during the experience of negative emotion and increased left prefrontal activation during the experience of positive emotion (Davidson, 1998). Furthermore, increased left prefrontal activation is associated with the ability to suppress startle responses to negative stimuli (Davidson, 1998; Davidson, Marshall, Tomarken, & Henriques, 2000). Davidson et al. (2000) have also demonstrated greater relative right versus left prefrontal activation among adults with social anxiety and depression. These findings have been replicated in infants (Davidson & Fox, 1989) and school-age children (8 to 11 years) with diagnosable anxiety disorders (Baving, Laucht, & Schmidt, 2002). Similar findings have emerged in anxious youth using functional magnetic resonance imaging (fMRI) techniques, with research implicating frontal regions in anxiety disorders in youth (Carrión, Garrett, Menon, Weems, & Reiss, 2008). The greater spatial resolution of fMRI has recently shown sensitized amygdala and hippocampal activation to facial expressions in youth with PTSD symptoms. For example, youth with PTSD symptoms (ages 11 to 17) showed faster right amygdala activation in response to angry faces than age and gender matched controls (Garrett et al., 2012). In addition, a number of specific neurotransmitters and neurotransmitter systems have been implicated in anxiety and anxiety-related behavior. Both gamma-aminobutyric acid (GABA) and serotonin (5-HT) have been the foci of research. This interest follows from findings that anti-anxiety (anxiolytic) medications such as benzodiazepines and selective serotonin reuptake inhibitors (SSRIs) modulate GABA and 5-HT neurotransmission. The noradrenergic system also has been implicated in the expression of anxiety disorders (Gordon & Hen, 2004).

Another theoretically important system is the hypothalamic-pituitary-adrenal (HPA) axis. Activation of the HPA axis often follows from fight/flight reactions in response to stress and fear, although its time course is considerably longer, spanning minutes to hours. Fear reactions are associated with elevations in the secretion of cortisol, a corticosteroid hormone produced by the adrenal cortex (see Gunnar, 2001). The release of cortisol is controlled by the hypothalamus, where corticotropin-releasing hormone (CRH) is secreted. CRH then stimulates the pituitary gland, resulting in the release of adrenocorticotrophic hormone (ACTH), which in turn causes the adrenal cortex to release cortisol. Cortisol helps to regulate behavioral and emotional responding through a feedback loop to the pituitary and hypothalamus.

Cortisol secretion may underlie protective mechanisms on exposure to danger; however, prolonged exposure to glucocorticoids such as cortisol may also be neurotoxic and related to anxiety problems. For example, animal studies demonstrate hippocampal atrophy in rats and primates exposed to either psychological stress or elevated levels of glucocorticoids (see Sapolsky, 2000). Maltreated children with PTSD symptoms and those diagnosed with PTSD demonstrate dysregulation in diurnal cortisol rhythms (Carrión et al., 2002; De Bellis et al., 1999a), and symptoms of social anxiety disorder are associated with heightened cortisol reactivity among clinic referred youth (Granger, Weisz, & Kauneckis, 1994; see Gunnar, 2001, for a review). Moreover, youth who have experienced severe stress are more likely to display reductions in cerebral volume and frontal lobe asymmetry, possibly due to effects of prolonged cortisol secretion (Carrión et al., 2001; De Bellis et al., 1999b). Carrión, Weems, and Reiss (2007) found that cortisol levels were associated with changes in the volume of the hippocampus in a sample of youth ages 8 to 14 who were exposed to traumatic stressors. Higher cortisol levels were related to decreases in hippocampal volume over a 1-year period. Finally, research on behavioral inhibition, a risk factor for later childhood anxiety disorders (see Kagan, this volume), has linked the construct with increased cortisol levels in very young children (e.g., Kagan et al., 1987, 1988). Carrión, Weems, Richert, Hoffman, and Reiss (2010) have also found decreased prefrontal cortical volume associated with increased bedtime cortisol in traumatized youth.

*Peripheral nervous system.* A growing body of research suggests that youth with anxiety disorders are marked by excessive sympathetic nervous system (SNS) activity, expressed by increased heart rate, blood pressure, and electrodermal responding (e.g., Beidel, 1991; Carrión et al., 2002). Behavioral inhibition is also associated longitudinally with elevated heart rates in community samples of youth (Kagan et al., 1987, 1988). Data available from youth with elevated anxiety scores also suggest different physiological responses to anxiety provoking stimuli. For example, in a community sample of children with and without test-taking anxiety, Beidel (1991) found significant group differences in pulse rate and systolic blood pressure during social evaluative tasks. Scheeringa, Zeanah, Myers, and Putnam (2004) found that young children with symptoms of PTSD exhibited higher heart rates during recall of their trauma memories than matched controls.

In a community-recruited sample, Weems, Zakem, Costa, Cannon, and Watts (2005) examined skin conductance and heart rate responses among youth exposed to a fear-eliciting stimulus (video of a large dog), and their relation to youth- and parent-rated anxiety symptoms and cognitive bias. Heart rate and skin conductance were associated with youth ratings of anxiety disorder symptoms. These responses were associated uniquely with youth-rated symptoms of anxiety but not depression.

There are also individual differences in absolute levels of arousal that individuals comfortably tolerate. Indeed, research on anxiety sensitivity shows that absolute levels of arousal are not crucial for anxiety problems to develop (Schmidt, Lerew, & Jackson, 1997). Anxiety sensitivity involves the belief that anxiety sensations (e.g., heart beat awareness, increased heart rate, trembling, shortness of breath) have negative social, psychological, and/or physical consequences (Reiss, 1991). One's interpretation of arousal symptoms appears to be especially important in influencing his or her experience of anxiety (Reiss, 1991; Weems, Hammond-Laurence, Silverman, & Ginsburg, 1998). In other words, some individuals experience considerable negative affect and distress with relatively little physiological arousal.

## ASSOCIATIVE LEARNING PROCESSES

Behavioral conceptualizations of anxiety disorders propose respondent (classical or Pavlovian conditioning), vicarious (social modeling), and operant (Skinnerian conditioning) mechanisms of the acquisition of fear. Limitations of early classical conditioning accounts involving the direct pairing of stimuli with aversive events (e.g., a large dog bites a child, resulting in fear of dogs) have prompted theorists to posit multiple learning pathways to anxiety and phobic disorders (Bouton, Mineka, & Barlow, 2001). Although the following focuses on specific conditioning events, it is important to realize that many individuals with phobias and anxiety disorders do not develop these problems following a single exposure to a feared stimulus (Bouton et al., 2001), bespeaking the role of preexisting vulnerabilities and additional risk factors in the generation of clinical-level problems. Although recent conceptualizations highlight the complexities involved in learning processes with respect to fear and anxiety development and maintenance, we focus here on three pathways posited by Rachman (1977).

One pathway is through classical aversive conditioning (Wolpe & Rachman, 1960). A large body of research suggests that exposure to traumatic events is associated with increased risk for anxiety disorders, particularly PTSD (indeed, the diagnostic criteria for PTSD mandate exposure to life-threatening trauma). Events that have been researched extensively as traumatic during childhood include experiences of child abuse, maltreatment, and exposure to community violence. Between 25% and 55% of youth with past histories of physical and sexual abuse meet criteria for PTSD (Ackerman, Newton, McPherson, Jones, & Dykman, 1998; Kiser, Heston, Millsap, & Pruitt, 1991). Exposure to natural disasters, such as earthquake and hurricanes, is also associated with PTSD symptoms in youth (e.g., La Greca, Silverman, Vernberg, & Prinstein, 1996). Furthermore, the level of PTSD symptoms a child or adolescent experiences is related to the number of disaster exposure events (La Greca, Silverman, & Wasserstein, 1998). Importantly, preexisting vulnerabilities such as trait anxiety confer susceptibility to postdisaster PTSD and predict symptoms beyond exposure to the stressful event (La Greca et al., 1998).

The second of Rachman's pathways is vicarious acquisition through observational learning or modeling. Via this pathway, children may acquire fears by observing the actions of salient others such as parents, caregivers, siblings, or friends (Bandura, 1982). For example, a child who sees his or her mother react fearfully to a dog may begin to model this reaction.

The third pathway is through verbal transmission of information. Through this mechanism, children may acquire fears by talking about fearful things with parents, caregivers, siblings, or friends. For example, the type of information (positive versus negative) youth receive about a potential fear stimulus (e.g., an animal) changes the valence of fear beliefs (Field, 2006; Field, Argyris, & Knowles, 2001; Field & Lawson, 2003).

Ollendick, Vasey, and King (2001) have suggested a fourth pathway to anxiety problems through negative reinforcement, also called *escape conditioning*. This account suggests that if a child learns to cope with normative anxiety and fear responses through avoidance of the anxiety or fear-provoking stimulus, then normal anxiety responses may be maintained at high levels and may eventually turn into problematic anxiety. Withdrawal from the stimulus may be negatively reinforced by reduction in anxiety after withdrawing; in addition, avoidance may be positively reinforced by caregivers through approval of avoidance behaviors. Exposure to feared stimuli fails to occur, maintaining anxious and avoidant responses. Considerable evidence exists to support these learning pathways in anxiety disorders generally (Craske et al., 2009) and in childhood anxiety in particular (see Ollendick, Vasey, & King, 2001, for a review).

## COGNITIVE PROCESSES

Proponents of cognitive and information processing models propose that various cognitive processes, such as encoding, interpretation, and recall, may contribute to the etiology and maintenance of anxiety disorders (see Field, Hadwin, & Lester, 2011; Vasey, Dalgleish, & Silverman, 2003). According to these models, anxious children have biased interpretations, judgments, and memories, as well as attentional selectivity (Vasey & MacLeod, 2001). These biases are hypothesized to work together to foster and maintain heightened anxiety. Weems and Watts (2005) developed a model of the cognitive influences on childhood anxiety, which suggests that attentional biases may foster selective encoding of threat information into memory, and such selective attention could increase negatively biased threat memories. Memory biases, in turn, may become internalized in cognitive working models or cognitive schemas, fostering interpretive and judgment biases. For example, existing threat memories may bias attention toward only the threatening part of the situation and away from mitigating aspects of the situation (such as safety signals), thereby fostering anxiety provoking interpretations. Existing threat memories may then bias the new interpretation of the event and help to consolidate existing interpretation and judgment biases.

In conjunction with biological and learning accounts, cognitive factors may foster or hamper learning acquisition, exacerbate biological predispositions, and maintain anxiety disorder symptoms. Selective attention, memory biases, interpretation biases (e.g., negative cognitive errors) and judgment biases are four broad forms of cognitive processes that have begun to garner attention in relation to youth anxiety symptoms.

Selective attention involves focusing attention toward a category of stimuli (e.g., threatening stimuli) when such stimuli are placed in a context with other categories of stimuli (e.g., neutral or other nonthreatening stimuli). A predisposition for attending to and processing potentially threatening stimuli is thought to characterize anxious individuals and may maintain anxiety by overallocating intellectual resources toward threat (Mathews, 1990). Studies demonstrate a link between childhood anxiety problems and selective attention (e.g., Dalgleish et al., 2003; Vasey, Daleiden, Williams, & Brown, 1995). Using a dot-probe detection task, Vasey et al. (1995) demonstrated that youth with anxiety disorders show shorter detection latencies for threat words than do controls. Similar results have been found among test-anxious youth (Vasey, El-Hag, & Daleiden, 1996) and among youth with generalized anxiety disorder (Dalgleish et al., 2003). It is important to note that such studies do not inform us about causal or directional associations between such cognitive biases and anxiety. However, an exciting line of research using the modification of attentional biases has suggested causal linkages. When attentional biases toward threat are trained in nonanxious individuals, anxiety symptoms increase (e.g., Mathews & Mackintosh, 2000; Mathews & MacLeod, 2002; Salemink, van den Hout, & Kindt, 2010). Moreover, training anxious individuals toward neutral or away from threat improves anxiety disorder symptoms (e.g., Amir, Beard, Burns, & Bomyea, 2009) with evidence for a similar effect in youth samples (Bar-Haim, Morag, & Glickman, 2011).

Memory biases refer to a predisposition to recall threatening information (see Vasey & MacLeod, 2001). Similar to research on selective attention, evidence supports a link between memory biases and anxiety problems in children (Daleiden, 1998; Moradi, Taghavi, Neshat-Doost, Yule, & Dalgleish, 2000). More research is needed to examine associations between both selective attention and memory biases and youth anxiety symptoms to determine whether these differences exist only in extremely impaired individuals. Most past research on youth anxiety compared groups that represent the extremes of anxious psychopathology (e.g., those with diagnosed disorders compared to groups with no history of psychiatric diagnosis).

Interpretive bias involves predisposition toward negative or erroneous interpretations of neutral, ambiguous, or potentially threatening stimuli. Negatively biased cognitions have long been implicated in both anxiety and depression (e.g., Beck, 1976). Clinically anxious youth presented with ambiguous vignettes and asked to explain what is happening are more likely to provide interpretations indicating threat than nonanxious controls (Barrett, Rapee, Dadds, & Ryan, 1996). A well-validated measure for assessing negative interpretive biases is the Children's Negative Cognitive Error Questionnaire (CNCEQ; Leitenberg, Yost, & Carroll-Wilson, 1986). Research using the CNCEQ suggests that cognitive biases are associated with symptoms of anxiety and can be assessed validly in both children and adolescents (Epkins, 1996; Leitenberg et al., 1986; Leung & Wong, 1998; Weems, Berman, Silverman, & Saavedra, 2001). Research has also implicated anxiety sensitivity as a risk factor for panic attacks, panic disorder, and other anxiety problems (e.g., Maller & Reiss, 1992; Schmidt et al., 1997, 1999; Weems et al., 1998, 2001; Weems, Hammond-Laurence, Silverman, & Ferguson, 1997). Anxiety sensitivity involves the belief that anxiety sensations have negative social, psychological, and/or physical consequences (Reiss, 1991) and so involves a negative interpretation of anxiety related sensations. Anxiety sensitivity differentiates youth with panic disorder from youth with other anxiety disorders (Kearney, Albano, Eisen, Allan, & Barlow, 1997) and predicts the onset of panic attacks in adolescents (Hayward, Killen, Kraemer, & Taylor, 2000; Weems, Hayward, Killen, & Taylor, 2002).

Judgment bias involves negative and/or lowered estimates of the individual's coping ability or style. Several investigators have emphasized a key role for the construct of *control* in anxiety and anxiety disorders in youth (e.g., Capps, Sigman, Sena, Henker, & Whalen, 1996; Cortez & Bugental, 1995; Granger et al., 1994; Muris, Schouten, Meesters, & Gijsbers, 2003; see Chorpita & Barlow, 1998; Weems & Silverman, 2006, for reviews). For example, Chorpita and Barlow (1998) described how early childhood experiences with diminished control may result in a cognitive style that increases the probability of interpreting events as out of one's control. Based on these findings, Chorpita and Barlow proposed a model in which perceived control (or lack thereof) may represent a psychological vulnerability for anxiety problems. Barlow's (2002) model of anxiety suggests that a perceived lack of control over "external" threats (events, objects, situations that are fear producing) and/or negative "internal" emotional and bodily reactions are central to the experience of anxiety problems. Nonpathological anxiety is differentiated from pathological anxiety both by subjective anxiety responses to the experience and by the belief that the event is uncontrollable. Empirical support exists for the importance of control cognitions in youth (Ginsburg, Lambert, & Drake, 2004; Muris et al., 2003; Weems, Silverman, Rapee, & Pina, 2003).

Watts and Weems (2006) examined links among selective attention, memory bias, cognitive errors, and anxiety problems in a community sample of youth ages 9 to 17. Selective attention, memory bias, and cognitive errors were each independently associated with childhood anxiety symptoms. Cannon and Weems (2010) found that both interpretive biases (CNCEQ) and judgment biases (ACQ-C) each provided incremental discrimination of youth meeting *DSM-IV* criteria for anxiety disorders from matched comparison youth. Furthermore, Weems, Costa, Watts, Taylor, and Cannon (2007) found that each was independently associated with anxiety symptoms in a community sample.

Models integrating the affective, cognitive, and physiological components of anxiety suggest that cognitive biases may exert their effect by exacerbating negative feelings that heightened physiological responding elicit. Thus, negative cognitive biases may not be correlated with physiological reactivity but should interact with physiological responses to produce negative affective states that characterize anxiety disorders (see Alfano, Beidel, & Turner, 2002; Vasey & Dadds, 2001.) As noted above, Weems et al. (2005) examined the physiological responses of youth exposed to a mildly phobic stimulus. Heart rate response to threat interacted with cognitive biases (CNCEQ scores) in predicting anxiety disorder symptoms indicating that those with high cognitive errors and a high heart rate reaction had the greatest anxiety disorder symptoms. Studies integrating the affective, cognitive, and physiological components of anxiety while simultaneously placing them in a broader developmental context are needed (Muris, Vermeer, & Horselenberg, 2008; Weems & Pina, 2010).

## SOCIAL AND INTERPERSONAL PROCESSES

Interpersonal theories focus on children's relationships with others. Research suggests important peer (Bell-Dolan, Foster, & Christopher, 1995) and parenting (Berg, 1976; Bögels & Phares, 2008; Creveling, Varela, Weems, & Corey, 2010; Dadds, Barrett, Rapee, & Ryan, 1996) influences on childhood anxiety. Moreover, social contextual approaches suggest that factors such as poverty, parental psychopathology, exposure to trauma, and exposure to violence can exacerbate vulnerability to anxiety disorders. According to attachment theory, for example, a child's interactions with the environment are influenced by the underlying quality of the parent–child relationship, and a number of factors influence the quality of that relationship (e.g., poverty, parental psychopathology). Attachment theory suggests that human infants form enduring emotional bonds with their caretakers (Bowlby, 1977; Cassidy, 1999). When the child's caretakers are responsive, the resultant emotional bonds can provide a lasting sense of security that continues even when the caretaker is not present. However, an inconsistently responsive caretaker, a neglectful caretaker, or some other disruption in the parent–child bond may be associated with insecure attachment. Children with insecure attachments have particular difficulty during separations from their parents (Ainsworth, Blehar, Waters, & Wall, 1978).

The reactions of children with anxiety disorders such as separation anxiety disorder (SAD) can be similar to those reported of insecurely attached children in the Strange Situation (Ainsworth et al., 1978). For example, children with SAD protest desperately when separation is imminent, cry and become agitated during separation, and may act angrily or aggressively toward the parent on return. Warren, Huston, Egeland, and Sroufe (1997) found that children classified as anxious/resistant in their attachment (assessed at 12 months of age) were more likely than children with other types of attachment to have anxiety disorders at age 17, even when controlling for measures of temperament and maternal anxiety.

Overcontrolling parenting may also influence childhood anxiety, although it is not clear if such patterns are maintaining factors or truly causal. For example, anxiety in either member of the mother-child dyad tends to elicit maternal overcontrol during interactions (Whaley, Pinto, & Sigman, 1999; Woodruff-Borden, Morrow, Bourland, & Cambron, 2002), and higher levels of maternal control are observed in anxious mother-child dyads than in control dyads (e.g., Siqueland, Kendall, & Steinberg, 1996). Costa and Weems (2005) tested a model of the association between maternal and child anxiety that included mother and child attachment beliefs and children's perceptions of maternal control as mediators. Maternal anxiety was associated with child anxiety and maternal anxious attachment beliefs, whereas child anxiety was associated with maternal anxious attachment beliefs, child insecure attachment beliefs, and children's perceptions of maternal control. Maternal anxious attachment beliefs also mediated the association between maternal and child anxiety. Taken together, research suggests that parents who exhibit overcontrolling, overinvolved, dependent, or intrusive behavior may (a) prevent youth from facing fear-provoking events, a developmentally important task that allows children to face fear; and/or (b) send the message that particular stimuli are threatening, which may reinforce a child's or adolescent's anxiety (Rapee, 1997, 2009; Rapee, Wignall, Hudson, & Schniering, 2000; Vasey & Ollendick, 2000).

Social-interpersonal models emphasize experiences in which behaviors of parents are learned by children. These models are consistent with research showing associations between children's and mothers' interpretation biases (Creswell & O'Connor, 2006; Creswell, O'Connor, & Brewin, 2006). In discussing mediation in this section, we have focused on possible behaviors of the parent or parent–child relationship that foster children's learning of anxious behaviors. However, some of these processes may be influenced by genes. For example, in the Fox et al. (2005) study noted earlier, neither genotype (i.e., the short allele for serotonin transporter) nor low social support predicted behavioral inhibition alone. However, their interaction was predictive. Thus, only among children with relatively low social support was the short allele associated with behavioral inhibition. Such findings point to the importance of considering Gene × Environment interactions in developmental psychopathology research on childhood anxiety (see Chapter 3). Moreover, the literature implicates parenting behaviors as unique predictors, moderators of other predictors (e.g., Costa, Weems, & Pina, 2009), mediators of other influences (Costa & Weems, 2005), with possible bi-directional influences over time (Silverman, Kurtines, Jaccard, & Pina, 2009). Integrative theories and research studies are needed to elucidate the specific parenting variables involved in childhood anxiety and also parenting's role in the context of other predictors.

## DEVELOPMENTAL PROGRESSION

Childhood anxiety disorders are associated with adult anxiety and depressive disorders (Pine, Cohen, Gurley, Brook, & Ma, 1998). As noted earlier, however, results from prospective longitudinal studies of childhood anxiety disorders have reported widely varying stabilities, ranging from 4% to 80% (e.g., Keller et al., 1992; Last et al., 1996; March, Leonard, & Swedo, 1995; Newman et al., 1996). Such wide-ranging stability estimates may exist for several reasons, including the type of disorder, the informant, the sample, and the amount of time between evaluations. Interestingly, studies show similarly wide estimates even for the same anxiety disorder across similar time frames. For example, Last et al. (1996) found that 13.6% of youth with social phobia retained the diagnosis after 3 to 4 years, whereas Newman et al. (1996) found that 79.3% of youth with social phobia retained the diagnosis after 0 to 3 years. The main difference between these studies was the age of participants (5 to 18 in Last et al., 1996; 11 to 21 in Newman et al., 1996). As already noted, genetic influences on anxiety increase with age, which could account for some of the discrepancy. Other possible sources of inconsistency include the types of assessment instruments used, sample variations, different definitions of impairment, and limited understanding and use of empirically derived developmental information in the classification of anxiety disorders (see Curry et al., 2004; Scheeringa, Peebles, Cook, & Zeanah, 2001).

Some authors have also posited specific age differences in the onset and expression of phobic and anxiety disorders in youth (Warren & Sroufe, 2004; Weems, 2008;

Westenberg, Siebelink, & Treffers, 2001). Drawing on stage theories (e.g., Loevinger, 1976), Westenberg et al. (2001) suggested that the predominant expression of fear and anxiety symptoms may be tied in part to sequential developmental challenges. For example, children ages 6 to 9 years have begun the process of individuation and are expressing autonomy from their parents. The developmental challenge is self-reliance, but this challenge is likely to give rise to concerns about separation from or loss of parents. In contrast, youth ages 10 to 13 years are gaining insight into mortality and broader world concerns. Finally, emerging social understanding and comprehension in adolescence may lead to a predominance of social and evaluative concerns in older youth (see Warren & Sroufe, 2004; Westenberg et al., 2001).

According to both Westenberg et al. (2001) and Warren and Sroufe (2004), separation anxiety symptoms and animal fears are the predominant expression of anxiety in children ages 6 to 9, compared with generalized anxiety symptoms and fears concerning danger and death in children ages 10 to 13, and social anxiety symptoms and social/performance related fears in adolescents around ages 14 to 17. Epidemiological data from community samples are fairly consistent with these assertions (see Costello et al., 2004), providing empirical evidence that the predominant expression of phobic and anxiety symptoms is tied to normative developmental milestones. Research in clinical samples also suggests that separation anxiety disorder is more common in children whereas social phobia is more common in adolescents (Weems et al., 1998; Weems, Silverman, Saavedra, Pina, & Lumpkin, 1999). Research examining specific fear and anxiety symptoms dimensionally across age ranges also supports the notion of sequential developmental differences in the expression of symptoms (Chorpita, Yim, Moffitt, Umemoto, & Francis, 2000; Ollendick, Matson, & Helsel, 1985; Ollendick, King, & Frary, 1989).

In terms of a priori tests of the developmental hypothesis, Westenberg, Siebelink, Warmenhoven, and Treffers (1999) reported that separation anxiety disorder precedes overanxious disorder (using *DSM-III-R* criteria). Moreover, Westenberg, Drewes, Siebelink, and Treffers (2004) found that child self-rated fears of physical danger and punishment decrease with age and self-rated fears of social and achievement evaluation increase with age, controlling for overall fears. Weems and Costa (2005) tested this developmental theory and found that specific symptoms dominated at certain ages, specifically separation anxiety in children 6 to 9 years, death and danger fears in youth 10 to 13 years, and social anxiety and fears of criticism in youth 14 to 17 years (see also Westenberg, Gullone, Bokhorst, Heyne, & King, 2007). These findings suggest that models of the etiology of childhood anxiety should consider differences across childhood and adolescence in developmental expression. This concept has been termed *heterotypic continuity* (e.g., Moffitt, 1993).

## COMORBIDITY

As noted earlier, comorbidity among anxiety disorders (i.e., homotypic comorbidity) in youth is substantial, with estimates as high as 50% in population studies (see Costello et al., 2004) and as high as 70% in clinical samples (Weems et al., 1998). Furthermore, across studies, comorbidity of anxiety disorders with ADHD (heterotypic comorbidity) range from 0% to 21%, with conduct disorder and oppositional defiant disorder from 3% to 13%, and with depression from 1% to 20% (Costello et al., 2004). In general, there is a high degree of association between depression and anxiety. Similar findings in community samples suggest that comorbidity is not just a function of referral biases. Rates of comorbidity exceed those predicted by intersecting base rates (see Costello et al., 2011; Curry et al., 2004).

## CULTURAL CONSIDERATIONS

A growing body of literature indicates cultural and ethnic differences in the expression of anxious symptoms (see Cooley & Boyce, 2004; Varela & Hensley-Maloney, 2009). For example, Latino children often report higher levels of internalizing symptoms than white non-Latino children, both in terms of anxious and somatic complaints (Ginsburg & Silverman, 1996; Pina & Silverman, 2004; Varela & Hensley-Maloney, 2009; Varela et al., 2004a, 2004b). Little is known about the mechanisms underlying this cultural variability. Researchers have focused on the effects that culture-specific socialization practices and family variables may have on emotion expression. Some have speculated that because Latino culture is characterized by a collectivistic ideal, emotions and willingness to express emotions will tend to be consistent with cultural norms (Triandis, Leung, Villareal, & Clack, 1985). In a collectivistic society, interdependence and subordination to the group are cultivated through strict social norms and expectations of conformity, self-restraint, and social inhibition.

Thus, symptom elevations in anxiety reflect the societal emphasis on those particular mood states and behaviors (Weisz, Suwanlert, Chaiyasit, & Walter, 1987). From this perspective, individualistic cultures such as the United States, which emphasize autonomous, outgoing, self-promoting behaviors, should have more children with disruptive behavior problems because this type of expression is supported (Weisz et al., 1987). An alternative explanation for an association between collectivistic cultures and internalizing symptoms is that an emphasis on the control of emotions may stifle children's understanding and managing of their internal states (Varela et al., 2004a, 2004b). From this perspective, the social constraints on expressing emotions may lead to a failure to develop emotion regulation skills, which predicts greater emotional difficulties.

## SEX DIFFERENCES

Girls and women experience higher levels of anxiety and related symptoms than boys and men (Silverman & Carter, 2006), at a roughly 2:1 girl:boy ratio (Costello et al., 2004). These findings are consistent with research on youth self-reports of fear, which show that girls report more fears than boys (Ginsburg & Silverman, 2000; Ollendick et al., 1985; Ollendick et al., 1989; Ollendick, Langley, Jones, & Kephart, 2001). Although these findings are consistent, the mechanisms responsible for the observed sex differences remain obscure. Twin studies suggest there may be a genetic basis for the sex difference, as the genetic contribution to individual differences in anxiety appears to be greater for females (Eley, 2001).

Genetic influences do not rule out socialization processes in the expression of symptoms or in girls' increased willingness to report certain types of symptoms (Ginsburg & Silverman, 2000; Rutter, Caspi, & Moffitt, 2003). Recent research also has broadened the theoretical frame for understanding observed sex differences. For example, Carter, Silverman, and Jaccard (2011) recently found in a sample of clinic-referred anxious youth that early pubertal development and self-reported gender role orientation were significant contributors to levels of youth anxiety.

## THEORETICAL SYNTHESIS AND FUTURE DIRECTIONS

In this chapter, we have provided a developmental psychopathology approach to describing continuity and change in childhood anxiety disorders. Such an approach suggests that a comprehensive theory of anxiety disorders requires differentiation between primary and secondary features. Primary features of problematic anxiety are (a) dysregulation of the anxiety response system, and (b) negative affect and distress/impairment that result from physiological arousal. Secondary features are aspects that distinguish the *DSM-IV* (APA, 1994) anxiety disorders from one another (e.g., interpersonal concerns in social anxiety disorder, uncued panic attacks in panic disorder). Significant advances have been made in understanding the developmental psychopathology of childhood anxiety disorders: research has identified biological, behavioral, cognitive, interpersonal, and contextual processes important to understanding the origins of childhood anxiety.

The developmental psychopathology view can be summarized via a hypothetical child's emotional development from childhood through adulthood. This child may be behaviorally inhibited early in his or her life. This behavioral inhibition is likely to be the product of genetic risk factors (e.g., short 5HTT allele), which may interact with environmental risks (e.g., low social support, parental reinforcement of avoidance). A child exposed to this combination of genetic vulnerability and environmental risk is likely to experience elevated anxiety (i.e., dysregulation of anxious emotion and corresponding distress), which is in turn shaped by normative developmental processes and individual experiences. For example, a child with a propensity for elevated arousal and avoidance may live with parents who are not skilled in reducing the child's anxious responding or who model withdrawn or anxious behaviors in social contexts. Such parents may themselves be anxious. The child may also be exposed repeatedly to socially challenging events that he or she is allowed to avoid. This avoidance may result in a failure to develop cognitive, social, and behavioral skills for facing social situations. Vulnerability to developing an anxiety disorder is high for this child, and the specific set of risk factors may potentiate social anxiety. Early in the child's life, the resultant emotion dysregulation may manifest as separation anxiety disorder; later, especially in adolescence, social anxiety disorder may be the predominant expression of this child's anxious emotion.

We encourage research that tests the hypothesized factors of influence on shaping continuity and change in both the primary and secondary features of anxiety. Our view emphasizes trajectories (versus purely categorical approaches) throughout the period of childhood and adolescence, to determine common and unique pathways in anxious emotion. We also encourage research aimed at clarifying the role of the factors that are hypothesized to shape these pathways. We suggest that taking an approach emphasizing the distinction between core and secondary features of anxious emotion will facilitate understanding the basic developmental psychopathology of anxiety and also individual variation in expression of anxious emotion.

In closing it is important to note that the research literature indicates that interventions, such as cognitive behavioral therapy, are efficacious in reducing anxiety disorders in youth (see Silverman, Pina, & Viswesvaran, 2008; Silverman & Motoca, 2011). Results suggest that cognitive behavior therapy is efficacious across various types of childhood anxiety disorders and age groups (Berman, Weems, Silverman, & Kurtines, 2000; Kendall, 1994; Scheeringa, Weems, Cohen, Amaya-Jackson, & Guthrie, 2011), can serve preventative functions (Dadds, Holland, Barrett, Laurens, & Spence, 1999), and is associated with long-term positive outcomes (Saavedra, Silverman, Morgan-Lopez, & Kurtines, 2010). We encourage the use of intervention research to further the understanding the mechanisms involved in anxiety disorder development as well as the use of the empirical literature on the developmental psychopathy of anxiety to inform the next generation of intervention research.

# REFERENCES

Ackerman, P. T., Newton, J. E. O., McPherson, W. B., Jones, J. G., & Dykman, R. A. (1998). Prevalence of posttraumatic stress disorder and other psychiatric diagnoses in three groups of abused children (sexual, physical, and both). *Child Abuse and Neglect, 22*, 759–794.

Ainsworth, M. D., Blehar, M. C., Waters, E., & Wall, S. (1978). *Patterns of attachment: A psychological study of the strange situation.* Hillsdale, NJ: Erlbaum.

Alfano, C. A., Beidel, D. C., & Turner, S. C. (2002). Cognition in childhood anxiety: Conceptual methodological and developmental issues. *Clinical Psychology Review, 22*, 1208–1238.

American Psychiatric Association. (1968). *Diagnostic and statistical manual of mental disorders* (2nd ed.). Washington, DC: Author.

American Psychiatric Association. (1980). *Diagnostic and statistical manual of mental disorders* (3rd ed.). Washington, DC: Author.

American Psychiatric Association. (1987). *Diagnostic and statistical manual of mental disorders* (3rd ed., rev.). Washington, DC: Author.

American Psychiatric Association. (1994). *Diagnostic and statistical manual of mental disorders* (4th ed.). Washington, DC: Author.

American Psychiatric Association. (2000). *Diagnostic and statistical manual of mental disorders* (4th ed., text rev.). Washington, DC: Author.

Amir, N., Beard, C., Burns, M., & Bomyea, J. (2009). Attention modification program in individuals with generalized anxiety disorder. *Journal of Abnormal Psychology, 118*, 28–33.

Bandura, A. (1982). Self-efficacy mechanism in human agency. *American Psychologist, 37*, 122–147.

Bar-Haim, Y., Morag, I., & Glickman, S. (2011). Training anxious children to disengage attention from threat: A randomized controlled trail. *Journal of Child Psychology and Psychiatry, 52*, 861–869.

Barlow, D. H. (2002). *Anxiety and its disorders: The nature and treatment of anxiety and panic* (2nd ed.). New York, NY: Guilford Press.

Baltes, P. B., Reese, H. W., & Lipsitt, L. P. (1980). Life-span developmental psychology. *Annual Review of Psychology, 31*, 65–110.

Baltes, P. B., Reese, H. W., & Nesselroade, J. R. (1988). *Life-span developmental psychology: An introduction to research methods*. Hillsdale, NJ: Erlbaum.

Barrett, P. M., Rapee, R. M., Dadds, M. M., & Ryan, S. M. (1996). Family enhancement of cognitive style in anxious and aggressive children. *Journal of Abnormal Child Psychology, 24*, 187–203.

Baving, L., Laucht, M., & Schmidt, M. H. (2002). Frontal brain activation in anxious school children. *Journal of Child Psychology and Psychiatry, 43*, 265–274.

Beck, A. T. (1976). *Cognitive therapy and the emotional disorders*. New York, NY: International Universities Press.

Beidel, D. C. (1991). Determining the reliability of psychophysiological assessment in childhood anxiety. *Journal of Anxiety Disorders, 5*, 139–150.

Bell-Dolan, D. J., Foster, S. L., & Christopher, J. S. (1995). Girls' peer relations and internalizing problems: Are socially neglected, rejected, and withdrawn girls at risk? *Journal of Clinical Child Psychology, 24*, 463–473.

Belsky, J., & Beaver, K. M. (2011). Cumulative-genetic plasticity, parenting and adolescent self regulation. *Journal of Child Psychology and Psychiatry, 52*, 619–626.

Belsky, J., & Pluess, M. (2009). Beyond diathesis-stress: Differential susceptibility to environmental influences. *Psychological Bulletin, 135*, 885–908.

Berg, I. (1976). School phobia in the children of agoraphobic women. *British Journal of Psychiatry, 128*, 86–89.

Bergen, S. E., Gardner, C. O., & Kendler, K. S. (2007). Age-related changes in heritability of behavioral phenotypes over adolescence and young adulthood: A meta-analysis. *Twin Research and Human Genetics, 10*, 423–433.

Berman, S. L., Weems, C. F., Silverman, W. K., & Kurtines, W. M. (2000). Predictors of outcome in exposure based cognitive and behavioral interventions for phobic and anxiety disorders. *Behavior Therapy, 31*, 713–731.

Biederman, J., Rosenbaum, J. F., Bolduc-Murphy, E. A., Faraone, S. V., Chaloff, J., Hirshfeld, D. R., & Kagan, J. (1993). Behavioral inhibition as a temperamental risk factor for anxiety disorders. *Child and Adolescent Psychiatric Clinics of North America, 2*, 667–684.

Biederman, J., Rosenbaum, J. F., Hirshfeld, D., Faraone, V., Bolduc, E., Gersten, M., . . . Reznick, S. (1990). Psychiatric correlates of behavioral inhibition in young children of parents with and without psychiatric disorders. *Archives of General Psychiatry, 47*, 21–26.

Blashfield, R. K. (1989). Alternative taxonomic models of psychiatric classification. In L. N. Robins & J. E. Barrett (Eds.), *The validity of psychiatric diagnosis* (pp. 19–31). New York, NY: Raven Press.

Bögels, S. M., & Phares, V. (2008). Fathers' role in the etiology, prevention and treatment of child anxiety: A review and new model. *Clinical Psychology Review, 28,* 539–528.

Bouton, M. E., Mineka, S., & Barlow, D. H. (2001). A modern learning theory perspective on the etiology of panic disorder. *Psychological Review, 108,* 4–32.

Bowlby, J. (1977). The making and breaking of affectional bonds: Aetiology and psycho-pathology in the light of attachment theory. *British Journal of Psychiatry, 130,* 201–210.

Capps, L., Sigman, M., Sena R., Henker, B., & Whalen, C. (1996). Fear, anxiety, and perceived control in children of agoraphobic parents. *Journal of Child Psychology and Psychiatry, 37,* 445–452.

Cannon, M. F., & Weems, C. F. (2010). Cognitive biases in childhood anxiety disorders: Do interpretive and judgment biases distinguish anxious youth from their non-anxious peers? *Journal of Anxiety Disorders, 24,* 751–758.

Carrión, V. G., Garrett, A., Menon, V., Weems, C. F., & Reiss, A. L. (2008). Posttraumatic stress symptoms and brain function during a response-inhibition task: An fMRI study in youth. *Depression and Anxiety, 25,* 514–526.

Carrión, V. G., Weems, C. F., Eliez, S., Patwardhan, A., Brown, W., Ray R., & Reiss, A. L. (2001). Attenuation of frontal lobe asymmetry in pediatric PTSD. *Biological Psychiatry, 50,* 943–951.

Carrión, V. G., Weems, C. F., Ray, R., Glasser, B., Hessl, D., & Reiss, A. (2002). Diurnal salivary cortisol in pediatric Posttraumatic Stress Disorder. *Biological Psychiatry, 51,* 575–582.

Carrión, V. G., Weems, C. F., & Reiss, A. L. (2007). Stress predicts brain changes in children: A pilot longitudinal study on youth stress, PTSD, and the hippocampus. *Pediatrics, 119,* 509–516.

Carrión, V. G., Weems, C. F., Richert, K., Hoffman, B., & Reiss, A. L. (2010). Decreased prefrontal cortical volume associated with increased bedtime cortisol in traumatized youth. *Biological Psychiatry, 68,* 491–493.

Carter, R., Silverman, W. K., & Jaccard, J. (2011). Sex variations in youth anxiety symptoms: Effects of pubertal development and gender role orientation. *Journal of Clinical Child and Adolescent Psychology, 40,* 730–741.

Cassidy, J. (1999). The nature of the child's ties. In J. Cassidy & P. R. Shaver (Eds.), *Handbook of attachment: Theory, research, and clinical applications* (pp. 3–20). New York, NY: Guilford Press.

Chorpita, B. F., & Barlow, D. H. (1998). The development of anxiety: The role of control in the early environment. *Psychological Bulletin, 124,* 3–21.

Chorpita, B. F., Yim, L., Moffitt, C., Umemoto, L. A., & Francis, S. E. (2000). Assessment of symptoms of DSM-IV anxiety and depression in children: A revised child anxiety and depression scale. *Behaviour Research and Therapy, 38,* 835–855.

Cooley, M. R., & Boyce, C. A. (2004). An introduction to assessing anxiety in child and adolescent multiethnic populations: Challenges and opportunities for enhancing knowledge and practice. *Journal of Clinical Child & Adolescent Psychology, 33,* 210–215.

Cortez, V. L., & Bugental, D. B. (1995). Priming of perceived control in young children as a buffer against fear-inducing events. *Child Development, 66*, 687–696.

Costa, N. M., & Weems, C. F. (2005). Maternal and child anxiety: Do attachment beliefs or children's perceptions of maternal control mediate their association? *Social Development, 14*, 574–590.

Costa, N. M., Weems, C. F., & Pina, A. A. (2009). Hurricane Katrina and youth anxiety: The role of perceived attachment beliefs and parenting behaviors. *Journal of Anxiety Disorders, 23*, 935–941.

Costello, E. J., Egger, H. L., & Angold, A. (2004). Developmental epidemiology of anxiety disorders. In T. H. Ollendick & J. S. March (Eds.), *Phobic and anxiety disorders in children and adolescents: A clinician's guide to effective psychosocial and pharmacological interventions* (pp. 61–91). New York, NY: Oxford University Press.

Costello, E. J., Egger, H. L., Copeland, W., Erkanli, A., & Angold, A. (2011). The developmental epidemiology of anxiety disorders, phenomenology, prevalence, and comorbidity. In W. K. Silverman & A. Fields (Eds.), *Anxiety disorders in children and adolescents: Research, assessment, and intervention* (2nd ed.). Cambridge, United Kingdom: Cambridge University Press.

Craske, M. G., Rauch, S. L., Ursano, R., Prenoveau, J., Pine, D. S., & Zinbarg, R. E. (2009). What is an anxiety disorder. *Depression and Anxiety, 26*, 1066–1085.

Creswell, C., & O'Connor, T. G. (2006). "Anxious cognitions" in children: An exploration of associations and mediators. *British Journal of Developmental Psychology, 24*, 761–766.

Creswell, C., O'Connor, T. G., & Brewin, C. R. (2006). A longitudinal investigation of maternal and child 'anxious cognitions'. *Cognitive Therapy and Research, 30*, 135–147.

Creveling, C. C., Varela, R. E., Weems, C. F., & Corey, D. M. (2010). Maternal control, cognitive style, and childhood anxiety: A test of a theoretical model in a multi-ethnic sample. *Journal of Family Psychology, 24*, 439–448.

Curry, J. F., March, J. S., & Hervey, A. S. (2004). Comorbidity of childhood and adolescent anxiety disorders. In T. H. Ollendick & J. S. March (Eds.), *Phobic and anxiety disorders in children and adolescents: A clinician's guide to effective psychosocial and pharmacological interventions* (pp. 116–140). New York, NY: Oxford University Press.

Dadds, M. R., Barrett, P. M., Rapee, R. M., & Ryan, S. (1996). Family process and child psychopathology: An observational analysis. *Journal of Abnormal Child Psychology, 24*, 715–734.

Dadds, M. R., Holland, D., Barrett, P. M., Laurens, K., & Spence, S. (1999). Early intervention and prevention of anxiety disorders in children: Results at 2-year follow-up. *Journal of Consulting and Clinical Psychology, 67*, 145–150.

Dadds, M. R., James, R. C., Barrett, P. M., & Verhulst (2004). Diagnostic issues (pp. 3–33). In T. H. Ollendick & J. S. March (Eds.), *Phobic and anxiety disorders in children and adolescents: A clinician's guide to effective psychosocial and pharmacological interventions*. London, United Kingdom: Oxford University Press.

Daleiden, E. L. (1998). Childhood anxiety and memory functioning: A comparison of systemic and processing accounts. *Journal of Experimental Child Psychology, 68,* 216–235.

Dalgleish, T., Taghavi, M. R., Neshat-Doost, H. T., Moradi, A. R., Canterbury, R., & Yule, W. (2003). Patterns of processing bias for emotional information across clinical disorders: A comparison of attention, memory, and prospective cognition in children and adolescents with depression, generalized anxiety, and posttraumatic stress disorder. *Journal of Clinical Child and Adolescent Psychology, 32,* 10–21.

Damasio, A. (2003). *Looking for Spinoza: Joy, sorrow, and the feeling brain.* Orlando, FL: Harcourt.

Davidson, R. J. (1998). Affective style and affective disorders: Perspectives from affective neuroscience. *Cognition and Emotion, 12,* 307–320.

Davidson, R. J., & Fox, N. A. (1989). Frontal brain asymmetry predicts infants' response to maternal separation. *Journal of Abnormal Psychology, 98,* 127–131.

Davidson, R. J., Marshall, J. R., Tomarken, A. J., & Henriques, J. B. (2000). While a phobic waits: Regional brain electrical and autonomic activity in social phobics during anticipation of public speaking. *Biological Psychiatry, 47,* 85–95.

Davis, M. (1998). Are different parts of the amygdala involved in fear versus anxiety? *Biological Psychiatry, 48,* 51–57.

De Bellis, M. D., Baum, A. S., Birmaher, B., Keshavan, M. S., Eccard, C. H., Boring, A. M.,. . .Ryan N. D. (1999a). Developmental traumatology: I. Biological stress systems. *Biological Psychiatry, 45,* 1259–1270.

De Bellis, M. D., Keshavan, M. S., Clark, D. B., Casey, B. J., Giedd, J. N., Boring, A. M.,. . .Ryan N. D. (1999b). Developmental traumatology: II. Brain development. *Biological Psychiatry, 45,* 1271–1284.

Eley, T. C. (2001). Contributions of behavioral genetics research: Quantifying genetic, shared environmental and nonshared environmental influences. In M. W. Vasey & M. R. Dadds (Eds.), *The developmental psychopathology of anxiety* (pp. 45–59). London, United Kingdom: Oxford University Press.

Epkins, C. C. (1996). Cognitive specificity and affective confounding in social anxiety and dysphoria in children. *Journal of Psychopathology and Behavioral Assessment, 18,* 83–101.

Field, A. P. (2006). Watch out for the beast: Fear information and attentional bias in children. *Journal of Clinical Child & Adolescent Psychology, 35,* 431–439.

Field, A. P., Argyris, N. G., & Knowles, K. A. (2001). Who's afraid of the big bad wolf: A prospective paradigm to test Rachman's indirect pathways in children. *Behaviour Research and Therapy, 39,* 1259–1276.

Field, A. P., Hadwin, J. A., & Lester, K. J. (2011). Information processing biases in child and adolescent anxiety: A developmental perspective. In W. K. Silverman & A. Fields (Eds.), *Anxiety disorders in children and adolescents: Research, assessment, and intervention* (2nd ed.). Cambridge, United Kingdom: Cambridge University Press.

Field, A. P., & Lawson, J. (2003). Fear information and the development of fears during childhood: Effects on implicit fear responses and behavioural avoidance. *Behaviour Research and Therapy, 41,* 1277–1293.

Fox, N. A., Nichols, K. E., Henderson, H. A., Rubin, K., Schmidt, L., Hamer, D., . . . Pine, D. S. (2005). Evidence for a gene-environment interaction in predicting behavioral inhibition in middle childhood. *Psychological Science, 16,* 921–926.

Garrett, A. S., Carrión, V. G., Kletter, H., Karchemskiy, A., Weems, C. F., & Reiss, A. L. (2012). Brain activation to facial expressions in youth with PTSD symptoms. *Depression and Anxiety, 29,* 449–459.

Ginsburg, G. S., Lambert, S. F., & Drake, K. L. (2004). Attributions of control, anxiety sensitivity, and panic symptoms among adolescents. *Cognitive Therapy and Research, 28,* 745–763.

Ginsburg, G. S., & Silverman, W. K. (1996). Phobic and anxiety disorders in Hispanic and Caucasian youth. *Journal of Anxiety Disorders, 10,* 517–528.

Ginsburg, G. S., & Silverman, W. K. (2000). Gender role orientation and fearfulness in children with anxiety disorders. *Journal of Anxiety Disorders, 14,* 57–68.

Gordon, J. A., & Hen, R. (2004). Genetic approaches to the study of anxiety. *Annual Review of Neuroscience, 27,* 193–222.

Granger, D. A., Weisz, J. R., & Kauneckis, D. (1994). Neuroendocrine reactivity, internalizing behavior problems, and control related cognitions in clinic-referred children and adolescents. *Journal of Abnormal Psychology, 103,* 267–276.

Gray, J. A. (1982). *Neuropsychological theory of anxiety: An investigation of the septo-hippocampal system.* Cambridge, United Kingdom: Cambridge University Press.

Gray, J. A., & McNaughton, N. (2000). *The neuropsychology of anxiety* (2nd ed.). New York, NY: Oxford University Press.

Gregory, A. M., & Eley, T. C. (2011). The genetic basis of child and adolescent anxiety. In W. K. Silverman & A. Fields (Eds.), *Anxiety disorders in children and adolescents: Research, assessment, and intervention* (2nd ed.). Cambridge, United Kingdom: Cambridge University Press.

Gunnar, M. (2001). Cortisol and anxiety. In M. W. Vasey & M. R. Dadds (Eds.), *The developmental psychopathology of anxiety.* London, United Kingdom: Oxford University Press.

Hayward, C., Killen, J. D., Kraemer, H. C., & Taylor, C. (2000). Predictors of panic attacks in adolescents. *Journal of the American Academy Child and Adolescent Psychiatry, 39,* 207–214.

Kagan, J., Reznick, J. S., & Gibbons, J. (1989). Inhibited and uninhibited types of children. *Child Development, 60,* 838–845.

Kagan, J., Reznick, J. S., & Snidman, N. (1987). The physiology and psychology of behavioral inhibition. *Child Development, 58,* 1459–1473.

Kagan, J., Reznick, J. S., & Snidman, N. (1988). Biological bases of childhood shyness. *Science, 240,* 167–171.

Kearney, C. A., Albano, A. M., Eisen, A. R., Allan, W. D., & Barlow, D. H. (1997). The phenomenology of panic disorder in youngsters: An empirical study of a clinical sample. *Journal of Anxiety Disorders, 11,* 49–62.

Keller, M. B., Lavori, P. W., Wunder, J., Beardslee, W. R., Schwartz, C. E., & Roth, J. (1992). Chronic course of anxiety disorders in children and adolescents. *Journal of the American Academy of Child and Adolescent Psychiatry, 31*, 595–599.

Kendall, P. C. (1994). Treating anxiety disorders in children: Results of a randomized clinical trial. *Journal of Consulting and Clinical Psychology, 62*, 200–210.

Kiser, L. J., Heston, J., Millsap, P. A., & Pruitt, D. B. (1991). Physical and sexual abuse in childhood: Relationship with posttraumatic stress disorder. *Journal of the American Academy of Child and Adolescent Psychiatry, 30*, 776–783.

La Greca, A. M., Silverman, W. K., Vernberg, E. M., & Prinstein, M. (1996). Symptoms of posttraumatic stress after Hurricane Andrew: A prospective study. *Journal of Consulting and Clinical Psychology, 64*, 712–723.

La Greca, A. M., Silverman, W. K., & Wasserstein, S. B. (1998). Children's predisaster functioning as a predictor of posttraumatic stress following Hurricane Andrew. *Journal of Consulting and Clinical Psychology, 66*, 883–892.

Lang, P. J. (1977). Imagery in therapy: An information processing analysis of fear. *Behavior Therapy, 8*, 862–886.

Last, C. G., Perrin, S., Hersen, M., & Kazdin, A. E. (1996). A prospective study of childhood anxiety disorders. *Journal of the American Academy of Child and Adolescent Psychiatry, 35*, 1502–1510.

LeDoux, J. (2000). Emotion circuits in the brain. *Annual Review of Neuroscience, 23*, 155–184.

Leitenberg, H., Yost, L. W., & Carroll-Wilson, M. (1986). Negative cognitive errors in children: Questionnaire development, normative data, and comparisons between children with and without self-reported symptoms of depression, low self-esteem, and evaluation anxiety. *Journal of Consulting and Clinical Psychology, 54*, 528–536.

Leung, P. W. L., & Wong, M. M. T. (1998). Can cognitive errors differentiate between internalizing and externalizing problems? *Journal of Child Psychology Psychiatry and Allied Disciplines, 39*, 263–269.

Loevinger, J. (1976). *Ego development: Conceptions and theories*. San Francisco, CA: Jossey-Bass.

Lonigan, C. J., Phillips, B. M., Wilson, S. B., & Allan, N. P. (2011). Temperament and anxiety in children and adolescents. In W. K. Silverman & A. Fields, *Anxiety disorders in children and adolescents: Research, assessment, and intervention* (2nd ed.). Cambridge, United Kingdom: Cambridge University Press.

March, J. S., Leonard, H. L., & Swedo, S. E. (1995). Obsessive-compulsive disorder. In J. S. March (Ed.), *Anxiety disorders in children and adolescents* (pp. 251–275). New York, NY: Guilford Press.

Maller, R. G., & Reiss, S. (1992). Anxiety sensitivity in 1984 and panic attacks in 1987. *Journal of Anxiety Disorders, 6*, 241–247.

Manicavasagar, V., Silove, D., Curtis, J., & Wagner, R. (2000). Continuities of separation anxiety from early life into adulthood. *Journal of Anxiety Disorders, 14*, 1–18.

Mathews, A. (1990). Why worry? The cognitive function of anxiety. *Behaviour Research and Therapy, 28*, 455–468.

Mathews, A., & Mackintosh, B. (2000). Induced emotional interpretation bias and anxiety. *Journal of Abnormal Psychology, 109,* 602–615.

Mathews, A., & MacLeod, C. (2002). Induced processing biases have causal effects on anxiety. *Cognition & Emotion, 16,* 331–354.

Moffitt, T. E. (1993). Adolescence–limited and life–course–persistent antisocial behavior: A developmental taxonomy. *Psychological Review, 100,* 674–701.

Moradi, A. R., Taghavi, M. R., Neshat-Doost, H. T., Yule, W., & Dalgleish, T. (2000). Memory bias for emotional information in children and adolescents with posttraumatic stress disorder: A preliminary study. *Journal of Anxiety Disorders, 14,* 521–532.

Muris, P., Schouten, E., Meesters, C., & Gijsbers, H. (2003). Contingency-competence-control-related beliefs and symptoms of anxiety and depression in a young adolescent sample. *Child Psychiatry and Human Development, 33,* 325–339.

Muris, P., Vermeer, E., & Horselenberg, R. (2008). Cognitive development and the interpretation of anxiety-related physical symptoms in 4- to 12-year-old non-clinical children. *Journal of Behavior Therapy and Experimental Psychiatry, 39,* 73–86.

Newman, D. L., Moffitt, T. E., Caspi, A., Magdol, L., Silva, P. A., & Stanton, W. R. (1996). Psychiatric disorder in a birth cohort of young adults: Prevalence, comorbidity, clinical significance, and new case incidence from ages 11–21. *Journal of Consulting and Clinical Psychology, 64,* 552–562.

Ollendick, T. H., King, N. J., & Frary, R. B. (1989). Fears in children and adolescents: Reliability and generalizability across gender, age, and nationality. *Behaviour Research and Therapy, 27,* 19–26.

Ollendick, T. H., Langley, A. K., Jones, R. T., & Kephart, C. (2001). Fear in children and adolescents: Relations with negative life events, attributional style, and avoidant coping. *Journal of Child Psychology and Psychiatry, 42,* 1029–1034.

Ollendick, T. H., Matson, J. L., & Helsel, W. J. (1985). Fears in children and adolescents: Normative data. *Behaviour Research and Therapy, 23,* 465–467.

Ollendick, T. H., Vasey, M. W., & King, N. J. (2001). Operant conditioning influences in childhood anxiety. In M. W. Vasey & M. R. Dadds (Eds.), *The developmental psychopathology of anxiety* (pp. 231–252). London, United Kingdom: Oxford University Press.

Pina, A. A., & Silverman, W. K. (2004). Clinical phenomenology, somatic symptoms, and distress in Hispanic/Latino and Euro-American youths with anxiety disorders. *Journal of Clinical Child and Adolescent Psychology, 33,* 227–236.

Pine, D. F. (2011). The brain and behavior in childhood and adolescent anxiety disorders. In W. K. Silverman & A. Field (Eds.), *Anxiety disorders in children and adolescents: Research, assessment and intervention* (2nd ed.). Cambridge, United Kingdom: Cambridge University Press.

Pine, D. S., Cohen, P., Gurley, D., Brook, J., & Ma, Y. (1998). The risk for early-adulthood anxiety and depressive disorders in adolescents with anxiety and depressive disorders. *Archives of General Psychiatry, 55,* 56–64.

Rachman, S. (1977). The conditioning theory of fear-acquisition: A critical examination. *Behaviour Research and Therapy, 15,* 375–387.

Rapee, R. M. (1997). Potential role of childrearing practices in the development of anxiety and depression. *Clinical Psychology Review, 17,* 47–67.

Rapee, R., (2009). Early adolescents' perceptions of their mother's anxious parenting as a predictor of anxiety symptoms 12 months later. *Journal of Abnormal Child Psychology, 37,* 103–1112.

Rapee, R. M., Wignall, A., Hudson, J. L., & Schniering, C. A. (2000). *Treating anxious children and adolescents.* Oakland, CA: New Harbinger.

Reiss, S. (1991). Expectancy model of fear, anxiety, and panic. *Clinical Psychology Review, 11,* 141–153.

Rutter, M., Caspi, A., & Moffitt, T. E. (2003). Using sex differences in psychopathology to study causal mechanisms: Unifying issues and research strategies. *Journal of Child Psychology & Psychiatry and Allied Disciplines, 44,* 1092–1115.

Saavedra, L. M., & Silverman, W. K. (2001). What a difference two decades make: Classification of anxiety disorders in children. *International Journal of Psychiatry, 14,* 87–101.

Saavedra, L. M., Silverman, W. K., Morgan-Lopez, A. A., & Kurtines, W. M. (2010). Cognitive behavioral treatment for childhood anxiety disorders: Long-term effects on anxiety and secondary disorders in young adulthood. *Journal of Child Psychology and Psychiatry and Allied Disciplines, 51,* 924–934.

Salemink, E., van den Hout, M., & Kindt, M. (2010). How does cognitive bias modification affect anxiety? Mediation analyses and experimental data. *Behavioural and Cognitive Psychotherapy, 38,* 59–66.

Sapolsky, R. M. (2000). Glucocorticoids and hippocampal atrophy in neuropsychiatric disorders. *Archives of General Psychiatry, 57,* 925–935.

Schmidt, N. B., Lerew, D. R., & Jackson, R. J. (1997). The role of anxiety sensitivity in the pathogenesis of panic: Prospective evaluation of spontaneous panic attacks during acute stress. *Journal of Abnormal Psychology, 106,* 355–364.

Schmidt, N. B., Lerew, D. R., & Jackson, R. J. (1999). Prospective evaluation of anxiety sensitivity in the pathogenesis of panic: Replication and extension. *Journal of Abnormal Psychology, 108,* 532–537.

Scheeringa, M. S., Peebles, C. D., Cook, C. A., & Zeanah, C. H. (2001). Toward establishing procedural, criterion, and discriminant validity for PTSD in early childhood. *Journal of the American Academy of Child and Adolescent Psychiatry, 40,* 52–60.

Scheeringa, M. S., Weems, C. F., Cohen, J., Amaya-Jackson, L., & Guthrie, D. (2011). Trauma-focused cognitive-behavioral therapy for posttraumatic stress disorder in three- through six-year-old children: A randomized clinical trial. *Journal of Child Psychology and Psychiatry, 52,* 853–860.

Scheeringa, M. S., Zeanah, C. H., Myers, L., & Putnam, F. (2004). Heart period and variability findings in preschool children with post traumatic stress symptoms. *Biological Psychiatry, 55,* 685–691.

Silverman, W. K. (1992). Taxonomy of anxiety disorders in children. In G. D. Burrows, R. Noyes, & S. M. Roth (Eds.), *Handbook of anxiety* (Vol. 5, pp. 281–308). Amsterdam, Netherlands: Elsevier.

Silverman, W. K., & Carter, R. (2006). Anxiety disturbance in girls and women. In J. Worell & C. Goodheart (Eds.), *Handbook of girls' and women's psychological health* (pp. 60–68). New York, NY: Oxford University Press.

Silverman, W. K., & Field, A. (Eds.). (2011). *Anxiety disorders in children and adolescents: Research, assessment and intervention* (2nd ed.). Cambridge, United Kingdom: Cambridge University Press.

Silverman, W. K., Kurtines, W. M., Jaccard, J., & Pina, A. A. (2009). Directionality of change in youth anxiety treatment involving parents: An initial examination. *Journal of Consulting and Clinical Psychology, 77,* 474–485.

Silverman, W. K., & Motoca, L. (2011). Psychosocial interventions for anxiety disorders in children: An update and future directions. In W. K. Silverman & A. Fields (Eds.), *Anxiety disorders in children and adolescents: Research, assessment and intervention* (2nd ed.). Cambridge, United Kingdom: Cambridge University Press.

Silverman, W. K., Pina, A. A., & Viswesvaran, C. (2008). Evidence-based psychosocial treatments for phobic and anxiety disorders in children and adolescents. *Journal of Clinical Child & Adolescent Psychology, 37,* 105–130.

Silverman, W. K., & Ollendick, T. H. (2005). Evidence-based assessment of anxiety and its disorders in children and adolescents. *Journal of Clinical Child & Adolescent Psychology, 34,* 380–411.

Silverman, W. K., & Rabian, B. (1995). Test-retest reliability of the DSM-III-R anxiety disorders symptoms using the anxiety disorders interview schedule for children. *Journal of Anxiety Disorders, 9,* 139–150.

Silverman, W. K., Saavedra, L. M., & Pina, A. A. (2001). Test-retest reliability of anxiety symptoms and disorders with the anxiety disorders interview schedule for DSM-IV: Child and parent versions. *Journal of the American Academy of Child and Adolescent Psychiatry, 40,* 937–943.

Siqueland, L., Kendall, P. C., & Steinberg, L. (1996). Anxiety in children: Perceived family environments and observed family interaction. *Journal of Clinical Child Psychology, 25,* 225–237.

Triandis, H. C., Leung, K., Villareal, M. J., & Clark, F. L. (1985). Allocentric versus idiocentric tendencies: Convergent discriminant validation. *Journal of Research in Personality, 19,* 395–415.

Varela, R. E., & Hensley-Maloney, L. (2009). The influence of culture on anxiety in Latino youth: A review. *Clinical Child and Family Psychology Review, 12,* 217–233.

Varela, R. E., Vernberg, E. M., Sanchez-Sosa, J. J., Riveros, A., Mitchell, M., & Mashunkashey, J. (2004a). Anxiety reporting and culturally associated interpretation biases and cognitive schemas: A comparison of Mexican, Mexican American, and European American families. *Journal of Clinical Child and Adolescent Psychology, 33,* 237–247.

Varela, R. E., Vernberg, E. M., Sanchez-Sosa, J. J., Riveros, A., Mashunkashey, J., & Mitchell, M. (2004b). Parenting practices of Mexican, Mexican American, and

European American families: Social context and cultural influences. *Journal of Family Psychology, 18*, 651–657.

Vasey, M. W., & Dadds, M. R. (2001). (Eds.). *The developmental psychopathology of anxiety*. London, United Kingdom: Oxford University Press.

Vasey M. W., Daleiden E. L., Williams L. L., & Brown L. M. (1995). Biased attention in childhood anxiety disorders: A preliminary study. *Journal of Abnormal Child Psychology, 23*, 267–279.

Vasey, M. W., Dalgleish, T., & Silverman, W. K. (2003). Research on information processing factors in child and adolescent psychopathology: A critical commentary. *Journal of Clinical Child and Adolescent Psychology, 32*, 81–93.

Vasey, M. W., El-Hag, N., & Daleiden, E. L. (1996). Anxiety and the processing of emotionally-threatening stimuli: Distinctive patterns of selective attention among high- and low-test anxious children. *Child Development, 67*, 1173–1185.

Vasey, M. W., & MacLeod, C. (2001). Information-processing factors in childhood anxiety: A review and developmental perspective. In M. W. Vasey & M. R. Dadds (Eds.), *The developmental psychopathology of anxiety* (pp. 253–277). London, United Kingdom: Oxford University Press.

Vasey, M. W., & Ollendick, T. H. (2000). Anxiety. In M. Lewis & A. Sameroff (Eds.), *Cognitive interference: Theory, methods, and findings* (pp. 117–138). Hillsdale, NJ: Erlbaum.

Warren S. L., Huston L., Egeland B., & Sroufe L. A. (1997). Child and adolescent anxiety disorders and early attachment. *Journal of the American Academy of Child and Adolescent Psychiatry, 36*, 637–644.

Warren, S. L., & Sroufe, L. A. (2004). Developmental issues. In T. H. Ollendick & J. S. March (Eds), *Phobic and anxiety disorders in children and adolescents: A clinician's guide to effective psychosocial and pharmacological interventions* (pp. 92–115). New York, NY: Oxford University Press.

Watts, S. E., & Weems, C. F. (2006). Associations among selective attention, memory bias, cognitive errors and symptoms of anxiety in youth. *Journal of Abnormal Child Psychology, 34*, 838–849.

Weems, C. F. (2008). Developmental trajectories of childhood anxiety: Identifying continuity and change in anxious emotion. *Developmental Review, 28*, 488–502.

Weems, C. F., Berman, S. L., Silverman, W. K., & Saavedra, L. S. (2001). Cognitive errors in youth with anxiety disorders: The linkages between negative cognitive errors and anxious symptoms. *Cognitive Therapy and Research, 25*, 559–575.

Weems, C. F., & Costa, N. M. (2005). Developmental differences in the expression of childhood anxiety symptoms and fears. *Journal of the American Academy of Child and Adolescent Psychiatry, 44*, 656–663.

Weems, C. F., Costa, N. M., Watts, S. E., Taylor, L. K., & Cannon, M. F. (2007). Cognitive errors, anxiety sensitivity and anxiety control beliefs: Their unique and specific associations with childhood anxiety symptoms. *Behavior Modification, 31*, 174–201.

Weems, C. F., Hammond-Laurence, K., Silverman, W. K., & Ferguson, C. (1997). The relation between anxiety sensitivity and depression in children referred for anxiety. *Behaviour Research and Therapy, 35*, 961–966.

Weems, C. F., Hammond-Laurence, K., Silverman, W. K., & Ginsburg, G. S. (1998). Testing the utility of the anxiety sensitivity construct in children and adolescents referred for anxiety disorders. *Journal of Clinical Child Psychology, 27*, 69–77.

Weems, C. F., Hayward, C., Killen, J. D., & Taylor, C. B. (2002). A longitudinal investigation of anxiety sensitivity in adolescence. *Journal of Abnormal Psychology, 111*, 471–477.

Weems, C. F., & Pina, A. A. (2010). The assessment of emotion regulation: Improving construct validity in research on psychopathology in youth—An introduction to the special section. *Journal of Psychopathology and Behavioral Assessment, 32*, 1–7.

Weems, C. F., & Silverman, W. K. (2006). An integrative model of control: Implications for understanding emotion regulation and dysregulation in childhood anxiety. *Journal of Affective Disorders, 91*, 113–124.

Weems, C. F., Silverman W. K., Rapee, R., & Pina, A. A. (2003). The role of control in childhood anxiety disorders. *Cognitive Therapy and Research, 27*, 557–568.

Weems, C. F., Silverman, W. K., Saavedra, L. S., Pina, A. A., & Lumpkin, P. W. (1999). The discrimination of children's phobias using the revised fear survey schedule for children. *Journal of Child Psychology and Psychiatry and Allied Disciplines, 35*, 941–952.

Weems, C. F., & Stickle, T. R. (2005). Anxiety disorders in childhood: Casting a nomological net. *Clinical Child and Family Psychology Review, 8*, 107–134.

Weems, C. F., & Watts, S. E. (2005). Cognitive models of childhood anxiety. In C. M. Velotis (Ed.), *Anxiety disorder research* (pp. 205–232). Nova Science Publishers, Inc.: Hauppauge, NY.

Weems, C. F., Zakem, A., Costa, N. M., Cannon M. F., & Watts, S. E. (2005). Physiological response and childhood anxiety: Association with symptoms of anxiety disorders and cognitive bias. *Journal of Clinical Child and Adolescent Psychology, 34*, 712–723.

Weisz, J., Suwanlert, S., Chaiyasit, W., & Walter, B. (1987). Over- and under-controlled referral problems among children and adolescents from Thailand and the United States: The *Wat* and *Wai* of cultural differences. *Journal of Consulting and Clinical Psychology, 55*, 719–726.

Westenberg, P. M., Drewes, M. J., Siebelink, B. M., & Treffers, P. D. A. (2004). A developmental analysis of self-reported fears in late childhood through mid-adolescence: Social-evaluative fears on the rise? *Journal of Child Psychology and Psychiatry, 45*, 481–496.

Westenberg, P. M., Gullone, E., Bokhorst, C. L., Heyne, D. A., & King, N. J. (2007). Social evaluation fear in childhood and adolescence: Normative developmental course and continuity of individual differences. *British Journal of Developmental Psychology, 25*, 471–483.

Westenberg, P. M., Siebelink, B. M., & Treffers, P. D. A. (2001). Psychosocial developmental theory in relation to anxiety and its disorders. In W. K. Silverman & P. D. A. Treffers (Eds.), *Anxiety disorders in children and adolescents: Research, assessment and intervention* (pp. 72–89). Cambridge, United Kingdom: Cambridge University Press.

Westenberg, P. M., Siebelink, B. M., Warmenhoven, N. J., & Treffers, P. D. A. (1999). Separation anxiety and overanxious disorders: Relations to age and level of psychosocial maturity. *Journal of the American Academy of Child and Adolescent Psychiatry, 38,* 1000–1007.

Whaley, S. E., Pinto, A., & Sigman, M. (1999). Characterizing interactions between anxious mothers and their children. *Journal of Consulting and Clinical Psychology, 67,* 826–836.

Wolpe, J., & Rachman, S. (1960). Psychoanalytic "evidence": A critique based on Freud's case of little Hans. *Journal of Nervous & Mental Disease, 131,* 135–148.

Woodruff-Borden, J., Morrow, C., Bourland, S., & Cambron, S. (2002). The behavior of anxious parents: Examining mechanisms of transmission of anxiety from parent to child. *Journal of Clinical Child and Adolescent Psychology, 31,* 364–374.

# CHAPTER 17

# Depressive Disorders

DANIEL N. KLEIN, AUTUMN J. KUJAWA,
SARAH R. BLACK, AND ALLISON T. PENNOCK

## HISTORICAL CONTEXT

RECOGNITION OF CHILD AND adolescent depressive disorders did not emerge until the late 1970s. Before then, depression was thought to be rare in childhood because children had not yet developed the cognitive capacity to experience symptoms such as guilt and hopelessness. In addition, many clinicians believed that to the extent that children did experience depression, it was expressed in behavioral disturbances such as behavior problems, enuresis, and somatic concerns (i.e., "depressive equivalents" or "masked depression"). However, in the late 1970s, Puig-Antich, Blau, Marx, Greenhill, and Chambers (1978), Carlson and Cantwell (1980), and several other groups of investigators demonstrated that many children and adolescents met full adult criteria for major depressive disorder (MDD).

## TERMINOLOGICAL AND CONCEPTUAL ISSUES

Depressive disorders in youth constitute a significant social and public health problem. Depressed children and adolescents often exhibit significant impairment in family, school, and peer functioning, and this impairment may persist after recovery from the depressive episode. Depressed adolescents are also at risk for school dropout and unplanned pregnancy. Moreover, depression is the leading risk factor for youth suicide, and as discussed below, may be a risk factor for other psychiatric disorders (Garber, Gallerani, & Frankel, 2009; Rudolph, 2009).

Depression is a complex phenomenon, for a number of reasons. First, the term can encompass (1) a mood *state*; (2) a clinical *syndrome* that can be caused by a variety of nonpsychiatric factors such as neuroendocrine disorders and psychoactive drug use; and (3) a psychiatric *disorder*. In this chapter, we emphasize depressive disorders, particularly MDD, although we also consider dimensional measures of depressive symptoms.

Second, many of the processes responsible for the pathogenesis of MDD and other depressive disorders remain unknown, although we discuss a number of biological vulnerabilities and environmental risk factors that may contribute to etiology, at least for some individuals. As this statement suggests, it is likely that the depressive disorders are *multifactorial* conditions—caused by combinations of many etiological factors. Moreover, depressive disorders are probably *etiologically heterogeneous*, meaning that there are different subtypes of depression that are caused by different sets of etiological processes. As a result, depressive disorders are characterized by both *equifinality* and *multifinality*. Consistent with the idea of etiological heterogeneity, depression exhibits equifinality in that a variety of different developmental pathways may lead to the same clinical syndrome. At the same time, depression is also characterized by multifinality in that it is unlikely that any set of etiological factors is entirely specific to depression. Rather, the same etiological factor may contribute to a variety of outcomes depending on other moderating variables (e.g., other risk and protective factors).

In this chapter, we (1) discuss the diagnosis and classification of depressive disorders in children and adolescents, (2) review briefly their prevalence in community samples, (3) summarize data on the course of juvenile depression and its comorbidity with other psychiatric disorders, and (4) discuss genetic, neurobiological, cognitive, interpersonal, and socioenvironmental factors that may contribute to the pathogenesis of depression in youth.

## DIAGNOSIS AND CLASSIFICATION

The fourth edition of the *Diagnostic and Statistical Manual of Mental Disorders*—text revision (*DSM-IV-TR*; American Psychiatric Association, 2000) defines MDD in children and adolescents as a period of persisting depressed or irritable mood or loss of interest or pleasure that lasts at least two weeks and is accompanied by a variety of other symptoms, including low energy and fatigue; inappropriate feelings of guilt or worthlessness; difficulty thinking, concentrating, or making decisions; sleep disturbance (insomnia or hypersomia); appetite disturbance (eating too little or too much or significant weight loss or gain); psychomotor disturbance (either retardation [extreme slowing in movement and speech], or agitation [extreme restlessness]); and thoughts of death or suicidal thoughts or behavior. Dysthymic disorder (DD) is a milder but more chronic condition, characterized by a period of depressed or irritable mood that is present for at least half the time for at least one year and is accompanied by several other depressive symptoms. The definition of MDD is unlikely to change significantly in *DSM-5*, which is scheduled for release in 2013 (see also Chapter 2). However, dysthymic disorder will probably be folded into a broader category of chronic depressive disorder that includes other persistent forms of depression (e.g., chronic major depressive episode).

There are a number of controversies in the diagnosis and classification of depression in general, and in children and adolescents in particular. These include continuity between child, adolescent, and adult depression; whether depression has discrete boundaries or shades continuously into normal mood states; identification of more homogeneous subtypes; whether there are age-specific expressions of depression; and whether depression exists in very young children and if so, how it might be manifested. We discuss each of these in turn below.

*Homotypic continuity.* Two forms of continuity can be distinguished. Homotypic continuity refers to a disorder that has similar clinical manifestations across development; heterotypic continuity refers to situations in which the clinical expressions of a single disorder differ at different points in development.

Most studies have reported significant homotypic continuity between adolescent and adult depression, but there is less evidence for homotypic continuity of prepubertal with adolescent and adult depression. Three lines of research that inform the issue of continuity include studies of clinical presentation, longitudinal course, and familial aggregation.

Depressed children, adolescents, and adults tend to exhibit similar symptoms, although as discussed later, there may be some developmental variations. Most follow-up studies indicate that adolescents with MDD are at elevated risk for developing major depressive episodes as adults (Fergusson & Woodward, 2002; Lewinsohn, Rohde, Klein, & Seeley, 1999; Pine, Cohen, Gurley, Brook, & Ma, 1998; Weissman, Wolk, Goldstein et al., 1999). In a notable exception, Copeland, Shanahan, Costello, and Angold (2009) reported that the association between depression in adolescence and young adulthood disappeared when comorbid anxiety and externalizing disorders in adolescence were controlled. Because other studies have not controlled for comorbidity, they argued that previous evidence for homotypic continuity reflected heterotypic continuity of adolescent anxiety and externalizing disorders with young adult depression. However, it is important to note that rather than focusing on MDD, Copeland et al. (2009) combined all depressive disorders, including depressive disorder not otherwise specified (D-NOS), which is likely to be a particularly unstable diagnosis. Moreover, when Lewinsohn et al.'s (1999) data were reanalyzed controlling for comorbidity, there continued to be significant homotypic continuity of MDD (John R. Seeley, personal communication, November 2009). It is also important to note, as Miller and Chapman (2001) articulated, that statistically partialing the effects of anxiety from depression may make little sense in practice if both disorders share a common etiology, which many models suggest (e.g., Krueger & Markon, 2006).

There have been fewer follow-up studies of prepubertal children, and the results have been inconsistent. Some studies have found that depressed children are at increased risk for depression in adulthood, but other studies failed to find evidence of increased risk (Copeland et al., 2009; Geller, Zimmerman, Williams, Bolhofner, & Craney, 2001; Harrington, Fudge, Rutter, Pickles, & Hill, 1990; Weissman, Wolk, Wickramaratne et al., 1999).

Finally, family studies have found significantly higher rates of MDD in the first-degree relatives of depressed adolescents than adolescents with other forms of psychopathology and adolescents with no history of psychiatric disorder (e.g., Klein, Lewinsohn, Seeley, & Rohde, 2001). Family studies have also found higher rates of MDD in the relatives of depressed children than in the relatives of healthy children, but there is less evidence for differences from relatives of children with other psychiatric disorders (Kovacs, Devlin, Pollock, Richards and Mukerji, 1997; Puig-Antich et al., 1989). The likelihood that there is at least partial discontinuity between prepubertal and postpubertal depression is further reinforced by differences in the ratio of males to females and in the heritability of childhood-onset versus adult-onset depression (see later).

*Discreteness and Boundaries.* The question of whether mood disorders are discrete entities versus regions on a continuum has been long debated. This issue has implications for defining disorders and subtypes, identifying etiological factors, and selecting assessment approaches and statistical models. Several studies have applied taxometric procedures to child and adolescent depression, with both negative (Hankin, Fraley, Lahey, & Waldman, 2005) and positive (Richey et al., 2009; Solomon, Ruscio, Seeley, & Lewinsohn, 2006) findings.

A few studies have also examined the discreteness of some subtypes of depression, such as melancholia. Melancholia is a subtype that is characterized by severe anhedonia, lack of reactivity to positive events, and vegetative (or physical) symptoms such as severe loss of appetite. It is hypothesized to be characterized by more severe biological abnormalities (e.g., hypothalamus-pituitary-adrenal axis dysregulation), less likely to be precipitated by life stress, and more responsive to pharmacotherapy than psychotherapy compared to nonmelancholic depression, although evidence for these claims is weak (Klein, Shankman, & McFarland, 2006). Ambrosini and colleagues reported that melancholic depression in youth is taxonic (Ambrosini, Bennett, Cleland, & Haslam, 2002). On balance, however, the weight of the evidence suggests that most forms of youth depression are not discrete entities. Even if they were discrete, however, it does not mean that the current diagnostic criteria identify the boundaries correctly. Moreover, if depression is dimensional, it would still be useful to establish cut-offs to indicate the point at which clinical attention is warranted, as is done for hypertension.

Unfortunately, distinctions among mood disorders, nonpathological dysphoria, and responses to major stressors are difficult to make, and can be influenced by a variety of sociocultural factors. Some investigators believe that boundaries in the *DSM-IV* definition of depression are too broad and thereby include many individuals with demoralization and transient responses to stress. Given the major developmental transitions and emotional intensity that characterize adolescence, it may be particularly difficult to distinguish mood disorders from normal variations in mood. Consistent with this notion, Wickramaratne and Weissman (1998) reported that rates of depression in offspring of depressed versus nondepressed parents differed in childhood and again in young adulthood, yet there were no differences during adolescence, a period marked by significant increases in depression regardless of parental diagnosis.

Conversely, there is also reason to believe that the current boundaries for depressive disorders are too strict, as subthreshold depressive symptoms are common in youth and adults and are frequently associated with significant functional impairment (e.g., Lewinsohn, Solomon, Seeley, & Zeiss, 2000). Regardless of whether subthreshold depressive symptoms are conceptualized as a form of disorder or a precursor to it, they should be taken seriously because they are the strongest predictor of later MDD (Kovacs & Lopez-Duran, 2010). For example, Klein, Shankman, Lewinsohn, and Seeley (2009) found that approximately two thirds of adolescents with subthreshold depressive symptoms but no history of depressive disorders developed MDD by age 30.

## Subtypes

Because depression is so heterogeneous, there has been considerable effort spent in trying to delineate more homogeneous subtypes of mood disorders in adults. In addition to the unipolar-bipolar distinction (see Chapter 19), subtypes have been proposed on the basis of differential symptom presentation (e.g., psychotic, melancholic [described earlier], atypical) and course (e.g., age of onset, recurrent, chronic, and seasonal pattern). Unfortunately, subtyping has largely been ignored in child and adolescent depression. Despite some intriguing findings for melancholia discussed above (e.g., Ambrosini et al., 2002; Luby, Mrakotosky, & Heffelfinger, 2004), the validity of distinct subtypes of depression in children and adolescents remains to be established.

*Age-specific manifestations.* The question of whether the clinical presentations of MDD and DD differ as a function of developmental level is complex and remains unresolved. The available literature suggests that the symptoms of MDD are fairly similar in school-aged children, adolescents, and adults, although hopelessness and some vegetative (e.g., disturbances in sleep and appetite) and motivational symptoms (e.g., loss of interest or pleasure) may be somewhat more frequent in adolescents than children (Weiss & Garber, 2003). Nonetheless, manifestations of particular symptoms vary as a function of children's levels of cognitive and social development. For example, younger children may appear sad but have difficulty reporting their mood, and prepubertal children may lose interest in play but do not experience decreased libido. There have also been several studies exploring whether there are developmental differences in the structure of the depressive syndrome, but findings are inconsistent (Weiss & Garber, 2003).

## Depression in Very Young Children

There has been little systematic research on depression in infants and preschool-aged children. However, in an important series of papers, Luby and colleagues (e.g., Luby et al., 2002, 2003) reported that MDD can be identified in preschool-aged children using modified *DSM-IV* criteria with a shorter duration requirement, arguing that these children exhibit substantial impairment and neurobiological abnormalities that are similar to those in adolescents and adults with melancholic MDD. Moreover, preschoolers meeting modified criteria for MDD had an 11-fold greater risk of exhibiting MDD 12 to 24 months later compared to healthy children (Luby, Si, Belden, Tandon, & Spitznagel, 2009).

## EPIDEMIOLOGY

In this section, we review the prevalence of depressive disorders in youth, sex difference in rates of depression, and comorbidity with other mental disorders.

### PREVALENCE

To estimate the prevalence of depressive (and any other) disorders, it is important to examine representative community samples, as treatment-seeking samples are biased in a number of respects, including greater severity and higher comorbidity rates. Studies of community samples indicate that depression is rare in early childhood, increases somewhat in middle/late childhood, and rises sharply in adolescence. The 3-month prevalence of depression in preschoolers is approximately 1% to 2% (Bufferd, Dougherty, Carlson, & Klein, 2011; Egger & Angold, 2006). In a meta-analysis of 26 studies, Costello, Erkanli, and Angold (2006) estimated that the point prevalence of MDD was 2.8% in school-age children and 5.7% in adolescents. Consistent with these estimates, in the only study available using a nationally representative sample, Merikangas et al. (2010) reported that the 12-month prevalence of MDD and dysthymic disorder was 2.5% in children ages 8 to 11 and 4.8% in adolescents ages 12 to 15.

By mid- to late adolescence, the lifetime prevalence of depression approaches adult rates (Rudolph, 2009). For example, Lewinsohn, Hops, Roberts, Seeley, and Andrews (1993) reported that in a large, representative sample of high school students, the lifetime prevalence of MDD and dysthymic disorder were 18.5% and 3.2%, respectively. Studies examining ethnic/racial differences in the prevalence of depression in youth have yielded inconsistent findings (e.g., Merikangas et al., 2010; Wight, Aneshensel, Botticello, & Sepulveda, 2005).

### SEX DIFFERENCES

One of the best-established findings in the depression literature is that rates of depressive symptoms and diagnoses in males and females are similar in child-hood but between the ages of 12 and 15 rates among females increase markedly (Hyde, Mezulis, & Abramson, 2008; Nolen-Hoeksema & Hilt, 2009). A variety of explanations for the increased vulnerability to depression in adolescent girls have been considered, with most focusing on sex differences in the many biological, psychological, and social changes and challenges that occur during this period.

There has been some support for the role of hormones and pubertal timing. For example, in a longitudinal study of adolescent females, Angold, Costello, Erkanli, and Worthman (1999) found that increases in estrogen and testosterone levels were associated with the onset of depressive disorders. Such biological changes at the time of puberty appear to interact with broader social and environmental factors. For example, physical changes associated with puberty may lead to greater dissatisfaction with one's body among girls than boys, which may predict onset of depression (Stice, Hayward, Cameron, Killen, & Taylor, 2000). In fact, early-maturing girls are at particularly high risk for depression compared to their peers (e.g., Copeland et al., 2010), perhaps because they are faced with expectations, pressures, and reactions that they are not ready for, or because they lack the support of peers who are dealing with the same issues. Indeed, recent work suggests that the effect of early puberty is moderated by peer relationships, as only unpopular early maturing youth exhibit increased depressive symptoms (Teunissen et al., 2011).

Another set of explanations suggests that increased rates of depression in adolescent females may relate to girls' experiencing more stress than boys during the transition to adolescence. Although boys and girls both report more stressors from childhood to adolescence, the increase may be greater for females, particularly for interpersonal stressors (Hankin, Mermelstein, & Roesch, 2007; Shih, Eberhart, Hammen, & Brennan, 2006). Moreover, females are more sensitive to the effects of stress, experiencing more depression than males at similar levels of stress (Hankin et al., 2007; Shih et al., 2006).

This last finding suggests that stress may activate preexisting differences in susceptibility. Thus, a third set of explanations posits that females have greater vulnerabilities than males even prior to adolescence, and these vulnerabilities interact with the stressors and challenges of adolescence to produce the higher rates of depression (Hyde et al., 2008; Nolen-Hoeksema & Hilt, 2009). A number of vulnerabilities have been hypothesized. For example, related to a combination of biological and socialization processes, girls may have greater affiliative needs than boys, rendering them more vulnerable to interpersonal stressors (Cyranowski, Frank, Young, & Shear, 2000; Rudolph, Flynn, & Abaied, 2008). There is also evidence that females are more prone to cope with adversity and dysphoric moods in a passive, ruminative fashion—a style associated with depression (Nolen-Hoeksema & Hilt, 2009). Indeed, Hankin (2009) found that the interaction between rumination and stress explained much of the sex difference in increasing levels of depressive symptoms in adolescents, such that girls who experienced more stress and were more prone to ruminate exhibited the largest increases in depressive symptoms.

There is growing evidence that sex differences in vulnerability to depression may be present at an early age. Levels of some temperamental traits that are associated with depression (see later) are higher in girls than boys in early childhood (Else-Quest, Hyde, Goldsmith, & van Hulle, 2006). In addition, Kujawa et al. (2011) found that attention biases for emotional stimuli were evident in 6-year old girls—but not boys—who were at risk for depression.

## Comorbidity

The majority of children and adolescents with MDD or DD also meet criteria for other psychiatric disorders. Although rates of comorbidity are high among adults, they are even higher in children and adolescents (Rohde, Lewinsohn, & Seeley, 1991). In a meta-analysis of studies using community samples, Angold, Costello, and Erkanli (1999) reported that depressed children and adolescents were 8.2 times more likely than nondepressed youths to meet criteria for an anxiety disorder, 6.6 times more likely to meet criteria for conduct disorder, and 5.5 times more likely to meet criteria for attention-deficit/hyperactivity disorder. Juvenile depression also frequently co-occurs with oppositional-defiant, substance use, eating, and developmental disorders (Angold et al., 1999). Comorbidity is even greater in clinical samples (Kovacs, 1996).

There are a number of potential explanations for the rates of high comorbidity (Klein & Riso, 1993). For example, anxiety may predispose to the development of depression (Garber & Weersing, 2010). Consistent with this idea, many studies have indicated that anxiety disorders/symptoms in children and adolescents predict subsequent depressive disorders/symptoms (e.g., Orvaschel, Lewinsohn, & Seeley, 1995). However, other studies have reported that the temporal relationship between anxiety and depression runs in both directions, raising the possibility of reciprocal influences (e.g., Costello, Mustillo, Erkanli, Keeler, & Angold et al., 2003; Pine et al., 1998).

Alternatively, comorbidity may be due to shared etiological factors. Clark and Watson (1991) hypothesized that depressive and anxiety disorders have both common and unique etiological influences. In their tripartite model, they propose that the temperament trait of negative emotionality (NE) predisposes to both depression and anxiety, increasing the likelihood that the two disorders will co-occur. NE refers to the propensity to experience sad, fearful, anxious, and/or irritable affect, particularly in response to stress. Both cross-sectional and longitudinal studies have confirmed that NE is associated with both depressive and anxious symptoms and disorders in youth (Anderson & Hope, 2008). Other shared etiological influences may also play a role (Garber & Weersing, 2010). For example, depressive and anxiety disorders have overlapping genetic influences (Lahey, Van Hulle, Singh, Waldman, & Rathouz, 2011), and these shared genes may be responsible for least part of the association of NE with both disorders (Kendler, Gardner, Gatz, & Pederson, 2007).

Explanations for comorbidity may not be mutually exclusive, as multiple processes are likely to be involved. For example, in a longitudinal twin study, Eaves and Silberg (2003) reported that childhood anxiety influences the development of depression in adolescence through three distinct pathways: one in which the same genes influence early anxiety and later depression (an example of heterotypic continuity); a second in which the genes that affect early anxiety increase sensitivity to adverse life events, indirectly increasing risk for depression (an example of gene-environment interaction, as discussed later); and a third in which genes that increase risk for early anxiety increase exposure to depressogenic environmental influences (an example of gene-environment correlation, also discussed later).

Comorbidity between depression and disruptive behavior disorders is also complex. There is growing evidence of overlapping genetic influences between child conduct disorder and both children (Lahey et al., 2011) and their parents (Silberg, Maes, & Eaves, 2010; Singh et al., 2011). Moreover, at least part of the association between depression and conduct disorder is due to shared relations with oppositional defiant disorder (ODD), which often precedes both conditions (Boylan, Georgiades, & Szatmari, 2010; Burke & Loeber, 2010). Interestingly, the negative affective symptoms in ODD (e.g., angry and resentful, touchy and easily annoyed) are a much stronger predictor of later depression than the oppositional behavior features per se (e.g., defiant and refuses to comply, argues with adults). This pattern is consistent with the possibility that temperamental NE is a final common pathway to depression. In conclusion, recent research on comorbidity indicates that, in accordance with the concept of equifinality, there are multiple etiological pathways to youth depression.

## COURSE AND OUTCOME

Almost all children and adolescents with an episode of MDD recover from that episode, although many continue to experience subsyndromal (i.e., residual) symptoms. However, length of episodes varies widely. In clinical samples, the mean duration of MDD episodes is approximately 7 to 8 months, and episodes of DD last an average of 48 months (Birmaher, Arbelaez, & Brent, 2002; Kovacs, 1996). However, episodes are much shorter in community samples. The majority of youth with DD experience superimposed episodes of MDD (a phenomenon referred to as "double depression"). A number of naturalistic follow-up studies have reported high rates of relapse and recurrence, with a substantial proportion of depressed juveniles experiencing another episode within several years (Birmaher et al., 2002; Kovacs, 1996). However, as noted earlier, these findings are more consistent for adolescents than children. Long-term follow-up studies indicate that 40% to 70% of adolescents with MDD experience a recurrence in adulthood (Fombonne, Wostear, Cooper, Harrington, & Rutter, 2001; Lewinsohn et al., 1999; Weissman, Wolk, Goldstein et al., 1999). In contrast, studies examining whether there is an increased risk of recurrence in children with MDD have reported conflicting findings (Harrington et al., 1990; Weissman, Wolk, Wickramaratne et al., 1999).

A number of predictors of duration of MDD episodes and probability of recurrence have been identified. Variables associated with a longer time to recovery include early age of onset, greater severity, suicidality, double depression, comorbid anxiety disorders or disruptive behavior disorders, depressotypic cognitions, and adverse family environments (Birmaher et al., 2002). Predictors of increased risk of recurrence include greater severity, psychotic symptoms, suicidality, prior history of recurrent MDD, double depression, subthreshold symptoms after recovery, depressotypic cognitions, recent stressful life events, adverse family environments, and a family history of MDD (particularly if it is recurrent) (Birmaher et al., 2002).

It is difficult to determine the relative importance of these prognostic factors, because there are few instances in which most of these variables have been included in the same study. However, in a community sample of depressed adolescents, Lewinsohn, Rohde, Seeley, Klein, and Gotlib (2000) examined several of these variables as predictors of recurrence in young adulthood. Prior history of recurrent MDD, family history of recurrent MDD, personality disorder traits, and for females, greater conflict with parents, independently predicted recurrence.

Children and adolescents with MDD and DD are also at risk for developing manic and hypomanic episodes (Geller et al., 2001; Kovacs, 1996). The probability of "switching" to bipolar disorder is higher in patients with psychotic symptoms, psychomotor retardation, a family history of bipolar disorder, and/or a high familial loading for mood disorders (Geller, Fox, & Clark, 1994). Here it is important to note that genetic risk for unipolar and bipolar depressive disorders is only partially overlapping, and that bipolar disorder is highly heritable, far more so than unipolar depression (see Chapter 19). Thus, cases of switching presumably occur among those with bipolar disorder whose first presentation of mood disturbance is depression.

## RISK FACTORS

In this section, we consider a number of risk factors for depressive disorders in children and adolescents, including genetics, temperament, maladaptive parenting and abuse, biological factors, cognitive factors, peer relationships, and life stress.

### GENETICS

We know from reviews of behavior genetic investigations of adult depression that there is modest heritability of major depression in men (nearly 30%) but somewhat stronger heritability in women, on the order of 40% (Sullivan, Neale, & Kendler, 2000). Thus, overall, genes play a role in contributing to individual differences in liability to depression, but environments play an even stronger role, particularly in childhood and adolescence (e.g., Bergen, Gardner, & Kendler, 2007; see also Chapter 3).

Relevant to the subject matter of this chapter, juvenile depression aggregates in families. Family studies indicate that there are elevated rates of MDD in the first-degree relatives (parents and siblings) of children and adolescents with MDD (Klein et al., 2001; Kovacs et al., 1997). Similarly, high-risk studies have documented increased rates of MDD in the offspring of parents with MDD (e.g., Klein, Lewinsohn, Seeley, Rohde, & Olino, 2005; Weissman et al., 2006). However, genetically informative designs (see Chapter 3) are required to determine whether familial aggregation is due to genetic or environmental factors.

Until recently, most studies examining genetic and environmental contributions to youth depression have used twins. Twin studies use sophisticated data analytic strategies (e.g., structural equation modeling) to partition the variance in twin resemblance into additive genetic factors, shared environmental factors (those aspects of the environment that make twins similar to one another), and unique environmental factors (aspects of the environment that make twins different from one another). Most of these studies have focused on depressive (or depressive and anxiety) symptoms, rather than diagnoses, and results vary somewhat as a function of the child's age and sex and the data source (parent versus child report; Franić, Middeldorp, Dolan, Ligthart, & Boomsma, 2010; Lau & Eley, 2008). Nonetheless, most twin studies indicate that additive genetic factors contribute to youth depression. Genes play a greater role in adolescent than childhood depression, whereas shared environmental factors play a greater role in child than adolescent depression (Franić et al., 2010; Lau & Eley, 2008). This is a common pattern in the behavioral genetics of psychopathology, whereby heritabilities for most human behavioral traits, including problem behaviors, increase over time (Bergen et al., 2007).

In addition to quantitative differences in the role of genes over the course of development, there is growing evidence from longitudinal twin studies of qualitative differences as well. Although genes are largely responsible for the moderate stability of depressive symptoms over time, new genetic influences on depression emerge as children grow older, whereas some genetic influences that were evident in younger children diminish with age (Franić et al., 2010; Kendler, Gardner, & Lichtenstein, 2008). These findings are consistent with the possibility, discussed above, of qualitative differences between prepubertal, adolescent, and adult depression. In addition, they suggest that genotype-phenotype associations may differ as a function of development: similar phenotypes may reflect different genetic and environmental influences at different ages, and the same genetic and environmental factors may be expressed as different phenotypes in different developmental periods (i.e., heterotypic continuity).

Recent studies using three other types of designs have further highlighted the role of environmental factors in the etiology of youth depression. In an adoption study, Tully, Iacono, and McGue (2008) found that adolescents who were raised by adoptive mothers with MDD had a significantly higher rate of MDD than adolescents who were raised by nondepressed adoptive mothers. In two studies examining the *children* of twins, the offspring of the depressed twins had higher rates/levels of depression than the offspring of the nondepressed co-twins, despite similar genetic relationships (Silberg et al., 2010; Singh et al., 2011). Finally, Lewis, Rice, Harold, Collishaw, and Thapar (2011) examined the transmission of depressive symptoms in parents who used assisted conception (i.e., in vitro fertilization). They found significant associations between parent and child depressive symptoms. Importantly, however, the magnitude of the correlations was similar for the genetically related and genetically unrelated parent–child pairs.

These studies provide important information on the role of genetic and environmental factors in depression, but they cannot identify the particular genes and/or environmental processes involved. The two major approaches to identifying specific genes are linkage and association studies (see Chapter 3). Linkage studies examine the relationships between genetic markers with known chromosomal locations and the occurrence of disorder within families. "Linkage" between a genetic marker and a disorder suggests that the marker, or a gene that is in close proximity to it, contributes to the etiology of the disorder. This approach has been successful in disorders that are caused by a single gene with large effects (e.g., Huntington's disease), but may be less useful for disorders that are caused by many genes, none of which have major effects. Indeed, genome-wide linkage studies on adult depression have yielded few consistent findings (Levinson, 2009).

Association studies compare the frequencies of common gene variants (polymorphisms) between groups of depressed and nondepressed individuals. This approach is more powerful than linkage studies in detecting genes with small effects. Specific polymorphisms (candidate genes) may be selected due to a hypothesized role in the pathophysiology of the disorder (e.g., genes involved in the regulation of neurotransmitters, such as serotonin [5-HT], or brain plasticity and response to stress, such as brain-derived neurotrophic factor [BDNF]). Alternatively, in genome-wide association studies, large numbers of polymorphisms across the genome are examined.

Most genetic association studies of depression have focused on adults. Thus far, association studies have produced few well-replicated findings for depressive (or other) psychiatric disorders (Levinson, 2009; McClellan & King, 2010). The reason for this lack of progress is not clear. One possibility is that rather than being caused by many common genetic variants, each with small effects, common disorders may be due to rare genetic mutations, each of which may have a large effect on a small number of cases (McClellan & King, 2010). This would represent an extreme example of equifinality, in that what we regard as a single disorder would actually consist of hundreds, if not thousands, of subgroups, each associated with a different genetic abnormality. If many of these abnormalities influence the same neural system, it could help elucidate the pathophysiology of the disorder and identify novel targets (the common pathway) for intervention. The search for rare genetic mutations is underway in autism and schizophrenia, but so far there have been few applications to MDD.

A second explanation for the difficulty in identifying genes for depression is that, consistent with diathesis-stress models of psychopathology, individuals with a genetic predisposition may not develop the disorder unless they experience significant environmental stress (a Gene × Environment interaction; Rutter, Moffitt, & Caspi, 2006). Thus, it may be crucial to take environment into account in studying the role of genes in depression (and vice versa).

The relationship between genetic and environmental risk factors is complex, with the possibility of both gene-environment correlations and gene-environment interactions (Rutter et al., 2006; see also Chapter 3). Gene-environment correlation refers to situations in which certain genotypes increase the risk of exposure to high-risk environments. There are three broad types of gene-environment correlations. Passive gene-environment correlations refer to the fact that children usually inherit their genes from the same people who raise them, so their genotypes and childrearing environments are correlated. For example, depressed parents are less engaged with and more hostile and critical of their children than nondepressed parents (Lovejoy, Graczyk, O'Hare, & Neuman, 2000). Parental maltreatment, in turn, is a risk factor for later depression (Widom, DuMont, & Czaja, 2007).

Evocative gene-environment correlations refer to the possibility that the child's genes may be expressed in ways that evoke certain reactions from others. For example, a child who is temperamentally inhibited and socially withdrawn may be more likely to be ignored by his or her peers, leading to loneliness and low self-esteem, limiting opportunities to develop social skills, all of which might increase risk for depression (Klein, Dyson, Kujawa, & Kotov, in press). Finally, active gene-environment correlations refer to the fact that as children grow older, they have more opportunity to choose their environments, such as activities and peers (i.e., "niche-picking"). Some of the same genes that predispose to depression may increase the likelihood that adolescents will experience higher rates of dependent life events (stressors that they help create), which in turn increase levels of depression (Silberg et al., 1999).

Genes may also interact with the environment by increasing susceptibility to environmental stress. A number of studies have reported gene-environment inter-actions for depression at both the aggregate and molecular levels (Franić et al., 2010; Lau & Eley, 2008). As an example of the latter, Caspi and colleagues (2003) reported that young adults with a short allele in the promoter region of the serotonin transporter gene (5-HTTLPR) had an increased rate of depressive disorders, but only when exposed to stressful life events. Similar findings have been reported for depressive symptoms in children and adolescents (Franić et al., 2010; Lau & Eley, 2008). Although there have been a number of failures to replicate this work, a recent meta-analysis found that when only studies using methodologically adequate assessments of life stress are considered, the data support the moderating role of life stress on 5-HTTLPR in predicting depression (Karg, Burmeister, Sjeddem, & Sen, 2011). Moreover, findings are strongest for early and chronic stressors, such as childhood maltreatment (Karg et al., 2011) and in females (Uher & McGuffin, 2010). Interestingly, some of these studies have suggested that not only does the short allele predispose to depression in the presence of stress, but it is also associated with lower than expected levels of depression in positive environments. This pattern is consistent with Belsky and Pluess's (2009) hypothesis regarding "plasticity genes" that confer differential sensitivity to both positive and negative environments.

Growing evidence that genes influence sensitivity to the environment has been paralleled by recent findings indicating that the environment also influences the expression and regulation of genes (epigenetics). For example, studies of rodents and primates have demonstrated that maternal behavior and separation can have lasting effects on neuroendocrine stress responses and neurotransmitter systems that are also dysregulated in depression (see later). Moreover, these effects are mediated by changes in gene expression. For example, maternal behavior in rats influences the methylation of binding sites on the pup's glucocorticoid receptor gene that regulates expression of that receptor, thereby influencing long-term neuroendocrine stress reactivity (Zhang & Meaney, 2010). Although early experience does not alter DNA sequence and is therefore not passed directly across generations, it does alter DNA structure and can have significant and persisting effects on regulation and expression of genes (see Chapter 3). Epigenetic processes may explain how different genes influence depression at different stages of development (Kendler et al., 2008).

## Temperament

Pathways from genes to disorders include a number of intermediate biological and behavioral processes, often termed intermediate phenotypes. One pathway from genes to depression may be mediated by child temperament. Two temperamental traits that have been linked to depression are high NE (discussed above) and low positive emotionality (PE), with the latter referring to a propensity to low levels of positive affect and exuberance, low appetitive drive/approach behavior, and high levels of social introversion. In addition to cross-sectional associations of these traits with depression, there is growing evidence linking them to risk for later depression (Klein et al., in press). For example, high-risk studies indicate that the young offspring of depressed parents have lower levels of PE and/or higher levels of NE than the offspring of nondepressed parents (Olino, Klein, Dyson, Rose, & Durbin, 2010). As noted above, this may in part reflect shared genetic influences between NE and MDD. In addition, longitudinal studies indicate that low PE and/or high NE in children predict subsequent depressive symptoms. Finally, there is growing evidence that low PE and high NE predict depressotypic cognitive biases, neuroendocrine dysregulation, and interpersonal problems that may mediate associations between early temperament and later depression (for review, see Klein et al., in press).

## MALADAPTIVE PARENTING AND ABUSE

A number of studies indicate modest but consistent associations between maladaptive parenting, including abuse, and child and adolescent depression (e.g., McLeod, Weisz, & Wood, 2007). In both clinical and community samples, depressed adolescents and their parents report lower levels of parental warmth and communication and higher levels of parental intrusiveness and maltreatment than psychiatric and healthy comparison groups (Hipwell et al., 2008; Patton, Coffey, Posterino, Carlin, & Wolfe, 2001). These problems often continue after depressive symptoms have remitted (Dietz et al., 2008).

These findings have been confirmed by observational data (McLeod et al., 2007). For example, parents of depressed children exhibit higher levels of expressed emotion (EE), characterized by criticism and emotional overinvolvement, when discussing their child, than do parents of nonaffectively ill children (Tompson et al., 2010). Although many of these data are cross-sectional or retrospective, longitudinal studies show that maladaptive parenting predicts later increases in depressive symptoms (Duggal, Carlson, Sroufe, & Egeland, 2001; Stice, Ragan, & Randall, 2004; Widom et al., 2007).

It is likely that the effects of maladaptive parenting and abuse on depression are indirect, influencing other processes that in turn increase risk. For example, adverse parenting and maltreatment are associated with dysregulated neurobiological and behavioral responses to stress (Dougherty, Klein, Rose, & Laptook, 2011), cognitive vulnerabilities (Alloy, Abramson, Smith, Gibb, & Neeren, 2006), interpersonal deficits (Rudolph et al., 2008), and later life stressors (Hazel, Hammen, Brennan, & Najman, 2008). In addition, early adversity may sensitize children to effects of subsequent life stressors, so depressive symptoms are provoked at lower levels of stress in children with versus without a history of adversity (Harkness, Bruce, & Lumley, 2006).

## BIOLOGICAL FACTORS

In this section, we discuss neuroendocrine and structural and functional brain imaging studies of youth depression. Other biological factors, such as neurotransmitters and sleep architecture, are reviewed elsewhere (Kaufman & Charney, 2003).

*Neuroendocrinology.* Adult depression is often characterized by dysregulation of the hypothalamic pituitary adrenal (HPA) axis, a key stress response system that controls the production of cortisol. There is mounting evidence that depressed children and adolescents also exhibit HPA axis abnormalities. Depressed youth often exhibit higher basal cortisol levels than their healthy peers and are more likely to fail to suppress cortisol production after ingesting the synthetic corticosteroid dexamethasone (Lopez-Duran, Kovacs, & George, 2009). In addition, several studies have reported that depressed youth have greater and more prolonged cortisol responses to laboratory stressors than non-depressed youth (Lopez-Duran et al., 2009; Luby et al., 2003). Abnormalities in cortisol reactivity to stress are also evident in children at risk for depression, although this link appears to be moderated by other factors. For example, Dougherty et al. (2011) found that preschoolers who had a depressed parent and were also exposed to hostile parenting behavior exhibited a greater and more sustained cortisol response to laboratory stress than other children. Developmental stage may also be an important moderator. Hankin, Badanes, Abela, and Watamura (2010) reported that among prepubertal youth, subclinical depression was associated with blunted cortisol responding to laboratory stressors, whereas in post-pubertal youth, subthreshold depression was associated with heightened cortisol reactivity.

There is also growing evidence that elevated levels of morning cortisol are associated with risk for developing MDD. Several studies have reported that young children of depressed parents exhibit elevated levels of morning cortisol (e.g., Dougherty et al., 2009). Moreover, other studies have reported that morning cortisol levels predict later onset of MDD in adolescents (e.g., Adam et al., 2010). Finally, HPA axis dysregulation may also influence the course of depression, as elevated basal cortisol levels in depressed adolescents are associated with a longer duration of depressive episodes (Rao, Hammen, & Poland, 2010).

Depressed youth also differ from healthy controls in their hyposecretion of growth hormone (GH) in response to GH-releasing hormone (Dahl et al., 2000). This may reflect vulnerability to depression, as it is evident following remission of symptoms (Dahl et al., 2000) and in children of depressed parents (Birmaher et al., 2000).

*Brain structure.* Many studies of depressed adults have reported structural brain abnormalities, particularly in areas that are involved in emotional reactivity and regulation, such as the prefrontal cortex (PFC), amygdala, and hippocampus. More recently magnetic resonance imaging (MRI) has been used to examine structural abnormalities in these areas among depressed children and adolescents. Consistent with adult studies, adolescent depression is associated with smaller white matter volumes, particularly in frontal brain regions (Medina, Nagel, Park, McQueeny, & Tapert, 2007; Steingard et al., 2002; but not Nolan et al., 2002).

MRI studies of amygdala and hippocampal volumes have yielded mixed results. In one study, smaller right amygdala volumes were associated with depressive symptoms in adolescent boys—an association that was moderated by maternal aggression (Yap et al., 2008). Although reduced hippocampal volumes have been observed in adult depression, many studies examining hippocampal volumes in children and adolescents have failed to find differences between depressed and nondepressed youth (MacMillan et al., 2003; Rosso et al., 2005; Yap et al., 2008). However, in a study of healthy adolescent daughters of mothers with and without a history of depression, Chen, Hamilton, and Gotlib (2010) found that at-risk youth exhibited reduced hippocampal volumes. There is also evidence that *greater* hippocampal volumes interact with environmental factors to increase risk for depression. In a sample of adolescent girls, Whittle and colleagues (2011) found that larger hippocampal volumes and higher levels of maternal aggression predicted a greater number of depressive symptoms. Thus, structural brain abnormalities may increase risk for youth depression, but the relations appear to be complex and may interact with other factors.

*Brain function.* A growing number of studies use functional MRI (fMRI) to examine brain function in depressed youth. This work suggests that there may be functional abnormalities in brain circuits involved in emotion and reward processing, as well as attention and cognitive control. With regard to emotional reactivity, some studies find increased neural reactivity to emotional stimuli in depressed youth, whereas other studies find reduced reactivity. Although task parameters and demands may account for some of these discrepancies, the nature of the contexts required to elicit specific patterns of reactivity is not well understood. For example, Thomas et al. (2001) found that compared to healthy controls, youth with MDD exhibited decreased left amygdala activation to fearful faces, and Beesdo et al. (2009) found that adolescents with MDD showed decreased amygdala activation to fearful faces during passive viewing but increased activation when participants were asked to focus on their own fear. On the other hand, in a high-risk sample of healthy children and adolescents with depressed parents, Monk et al. (2008) found increased amygdala activation to fearful faces compared to controls in a passive view paradigm. Other studies of emotional processing have examined the anterior cingulate cortex (ACC), and suggest that abnormalities in ACC function may precede the development of depression. For example, Masten et al. (2011) found that among adolescents, increased subgenual ACC activation during a peer rejection paradigm predicted higher levels of depressive symptoms a year later.

In addition, several studies have identified abnormalities in the neural circuitry underlying reward processing in youth depression. In two studies, Forbes et al. (2009, 2010) found that adolescents with MDD and adolescents with depressive symptoms showed reduced striatal responses and increased prefrontal activation to monetary reward, suggesting that depression in adolescence is associated with underresponsive reward circuits. There is also evidence that high-risk samples consisting of adolescent offspring of depressed parents exhibit abnormalities in neural processing of reward in both fMRI and event-related potential (ERP) paradigms (Foti, Kotov, Klein, & Hajcak, in press; Gotlib et al., 2010).

Finally, researchers have begun to examine neural correlates of attention, cognitive control, and decision making in youth depression. For example, on a battery of tasks requiring selective attention, attentional shifting, response inhibition, and error detection, depressed adolescents exhibited reduced activation in inferior and dorsolateral PFC, anterior cingulate gyrus, and striatal regions compared to controls (Halari et al., 2009). Similar abnormalities have been observed in adult depression. In addition, Shad, Bidesi, Chen, Ernst, and Rao (2011) recently examined decision making in the context of rewards. When making risky decisions, depressed adolescents engaged the caudal ACC, which is linked to conflict monitoring, whereas nondepressed youth engaged the right lateral orbitofrontal cortex, which is linked to inhibitory control, among other functions. This study illustrates how functional differences in brain regions activated in youth depression may be relatively subtle, contributing to inconsistent findings across studies. More work is needed to better understand the functional brain correlates of depression in children and adolescents, their relations to the structural abnormalities reviewed above, and the extent to which abnormalities precede (and may therefore play a causal role in) the onset of depression.

## Cognitive Factors

A range of cognitive factors have been hypothesized to predispose to depression, including negative self-concept, rumination, dysfunctional attitudes, negative attributional styles, and attention and memory biases. Although many of these hypotheses are extensions from the adult literature, a number of studies have confirmed the association between depressive cognitions and depressive symptoms in children and adolescents (Jacobs, Reinecke, Gollan, & Kane, 2008). At least some cognitive factors precede the onset of youth depression and may increase vulnerability to depressive episodes, whereas others appear to co-occur with, or be the result of, depressive symptoms (LaGrange et al., 2011). There also may be reciprocal relations between depressive symptoms and at least some cognitive factors (Jacobs et al., 2008). In addition, relations between depressive cognitions and symptoms change over the course of development, as cognitive styles become more stable and the strength of their associations with symptoms increase with age (Hankin, 2008; LaGrange et al., 2011).

Many investigators have examined the role of self-esteem, self-efficacy, and self-perceived competence in youth depression. For example, Cole (1991) reported that depressive symptoms are associated with low perceived competence in multiple domains (i.e., academic, social, sports, physical attractiveness, and behavioral conduct). However, longitudinal data indicate that there is a reciprocal relation between self-concept and depression, in that children's underestimation of their competence (compared to others' ratings) predicts depressive symptoms over time, and previous depression also predicts underestimation of competence (Hoffman, Cole, Martin, Tram, & Seroczynski, 2000).

Dysfunctional attitudes, such as believing that one must be perfect in order to be loved, and negative attributional styles, in which negative events are viewed as having internal, global and stable causes, may also be vulnerability factors for youth depression (Jacobs et al., 2008). Cole et al. (2008) reported that attributional style interacted with negative life events to predict depressive symptoms in adolescents. Interestingly, this effect did not emerge until eighth grade, suggesting that the relation between attributional style and depression changes from childhood to adolescence. Longitudinal studies have also reported reciprocal effects, as negative attributional style both precedes and follows depressive symptoms in adolescents (Lau & Eley, 2008).

Rumination, the tendency to respond to distress by focusing on the causes and consequences of one's problems rather than engaging in more active coping, may be a vulnerability factor for depression in children and adolescents. Abela and Hankin (2011) reported that it prospectively predicted later depression in adolescents. Ruminative response styles also appear to interact with negative life events to increase risk of depressive symptoms, and they may partially mediate sex differences in rates of depressive symptoms in adolescents as well as the association of temperament traits, such as negative emotionality, and depression (Hankin, 2009; Verstraeten, Vasey, Raes, & Bijttebier, 2009). The association between depressive symptoms and rumination appears to be reciprocal, as depressive symptoms predict increases in rumination (Nolen-Hoeksema, Stice, Wade, & Bohon, 2007). In addition, co-rumination, continually discussing problems with peers, prospectively predicts depression onset, as well as greater severity and longer duration of episodes (Stone, Hankin, Gibb, & Abela, 2011).

Finally, attentional and memory biases are additional cognitive factors linked to youth depression. There is evidence that depressed children and adolescents exhibit attentional biases toward sad faces, and similar patterns have been observed among girls of depressed mothers (Gotlib et al., 2010; Hankin, Gibb, Abela, & Flory, 2010; Kujawa et al., 2011). In one study, a high-risk sample showed avoidance of sad faces (Gibb, Benas, Grassia, & McGeary, 2009). With regard to memory, several studies have indicated that depressed children and adolescents and offspring of depressed mothers recall fewer positive and more negative self-descriptive words than nondepressed youth (Neshat-Doost, Taghavi, Moradi, Yule, & Dalgleish, 1998; Taylor & Ingram, 1999). Finally, overgeneral autobiographical memory, characterized by difficulties recalling specific past events, has also been linked to depressive symptoms in children and adolescents (Raes, Verstraeten, Bijttebier, Vasey, & Dalgleish, 2010). Moreover, overgeneral memory for positive cues predicts later depressive symptoms in adolescents (Hipwell, Sapotichne, Klostermann, Battista, & Keenan, 2011).

## PEER RELATIONSHIPS

A number of studies have documented that depressed children and adolescents have difficulties with peer (and for adolescents, romantic) relationships (Garber et al., 2009; Rudolph, 2009). Depressed children report poorer friendships and greater peer rejection than nondepressed children. In part, this reflects depressed youngsters' negative self-perceptions and low self-esteem. However, peer and teacher reports also indicate that depressed children have deficits in social skills and difficulties with interpersonal relationships, and observational studies indicate that depressed children are more withdrawn and isolated, and more hostile and aggressive than their peers (Rudolph et al., 2008).

The association between peer relationships and depression appears to be reciprocal and transactional (Prinstein, Borelli, Cheah, Simon, & Aikins, 2005). Difficulties with peer relationships prospectively predict increases in depression (Allen et al., 2006; Witvliet, Brendgen, Van Lier, Koot, & Vitaro, 2010). For example, Schrepferman, Eby, Snyder, and Stropes (2006) found that low peer sociometric ratings in kindergarten and first grade are associated with increased depressive symptoms in third and fourth grade, and observer ratings of disengagement from peers on the playground predict later depression. On the other hand, depression is also associated with subsequent reductions in peer support (Oppenheimer & Hankin, 2011; Stice et al., 2004).

### LIFE STRESS

Cross-sectional studies indicate that stressful life events are associated with depressive symptoms/disorders in young children, school-age children, and adolescents (Grant et al., 2006). In addition, prospective studies reveal that life stressors predict the onset of depressive episodes and increases in depressive symptoms in youth (Cole, Nolen-Hoeksema, Girgus, & Paul, 2006; Monroe, Rohde, Seeley, & Lewinsohn, 1999; Patton, Coffey, Posterino, Carlin, & Bowes, 2003).

Consistent with diathesis-stress models of psychopathology and with studies of gene-environment interactions discussed earlier, youth with preexisting vulnerabilities/risk factors, such as parental MDD (Morris, Ciesla, & Garber, 2010), temperamental high NE and low PE (Klein et al., in press) and depressotypic cognitive styles (Abela & Hankin, 2011; Cole et al., 2008) are more likely to experience depressive episodes or increased symptoms following life stressors than less vulnerable youth. In addition, depressed youth become increasingly sensitized to life stress with a greater number of episodes. Thus, associations between stress and depression appear to be weaker and higher levels of stress are required for a first depressive episode, whereas stress-depression associations become stronger and lower levels of stress are necessary for subsequent episodes (Morris et al., 2010; Stroud, Davila, Hammen, & Vrshek-Schallhorn, 2011).

In some cases, depressed individuals contribute to the occurrence of the stressors that they experience. The stress generation model (Hammen, 1991) suggests that depression and related features lead to impaired functioning, which increases the likelihood of self-generated stressful events. In turn, these "dependent" events can exacerbate depressive symptoms. Indeed, longitudinal studies indicate that depressive symptoms/disorders in youth are associated with subsequent dependent life events (Cole et al., 2006; Patton et al., 2003). Moreover, Rudolph, Flynn, Abaied, Groot, and Thompson (2009) found that among adolescent girls, depressive symptoms predict subsequent dependent life events, which predict increased depression. These findings are consistent with evidence for gene-environment correlations discussed earlier, and may explain why a genetic predisposition for depression is associated with an increased rate of dependent negative life events (Silberg et al., 1999).

## PROTECTIVE FACTORS

Protective factors are variables that reduce risk for psychopathology in high-risk contexts. Thus, the protective factor alters (or moderates) the association between a high-risk environmental or biological context and an adverse outcome (Luthar, Cicchetti, & Becker, 2000). Identifying such factors could have important implications for prevention. Unfortunately, there has been little research on protective factors in youth depression. Instead, most of this work focuses on variables that appear to be the absence or opposite of established risk factors, such as high self-esteem and self-efficacy, an "easy" temperament, and family and peer support. Demonstrating that a caring, involved parent is associated with lower risk provides little incremental information over and above existing evidence that parental rejection and neglect are associated with increased risk. To be useful, "protective factors" should be more than just the absence or opposite of established risk factors. For example, a protective factor might be a variable the presence of which shifts a high risk trajectory in a more positive direction but the absence of which has no influence on the risk trajectory.

## CONCLUSIONS AND FUTURE DIRECTIONS

Child and adolescent depression is multifactorial and etiologically heterogeneous—an outcome of multiple developmental pathways (equifinality). Few risk factors are specific to depression (multifinality). Indeed, etiological overlap with other psychiatric disorders contributes to the comorbidity that is ubiquitous in youth depression.

Genetic factors play a role in youth depression, but the strength of their influence varies as a function of development, given that genetic effects increase with age. Conversely, parental and family influences play a greater role at younger ages, although early adversity can have effects on depression that persist into adulthood. The nature of the genetic effects is poorly understood. There may be multiple common gene variants each with small effects, rare mutations with large effects on only a small number of cases, or some combination of both. In addition, due to developmentally mediated changes in gene expression, the relation between genotype and phenotype may vary over time, with the same set of genetic influences producing different phenotypes at various points in development and different genetic factors producing similar phenotypes at different ages.

Genetic influences are likely to operate through intermediate phenotypes such as temperament and susceptibility to stress. They are also mediated and/or moderated by a number of other risk factors including early adversity, dysregulation in key neural and hormonal systems, cognitive biases, interpersonal problems, and life stress. These risk factors may also have independent effects on depression, and they may be exacerbated by depressive symptoms.

We are still a long way from being able to formulate a comprehensive model of depression in children and adolescents. For heuristic purposes, however, we briefly outline one plausible, but undoubtedly oversimplified, model of the etiopathogenesis of youth depression.

The two major sets of distal causes include genetic susceptibilities and early adversities. These two sets of distal causes often co-occur (i.e., passive gene-environment correlation), and may have additive or interactive effects, but in some cases they can also comprise independent pathways to depression. Genetic susceptibilities may be expressed in the form of temperamental vulnerabilities that, at the behavioral level, are reflected by low PE and/or high NE, and are accompanied by dysregulation in key neurobiological systems. These temperamental vulnerabilities may also be influenced by environmental adversity, which can have lasting effects on neurobiological stress response systems. As the child enters the early school-age years, these temperamental vulnerabilities are elaborated cognitively, leading to the emergence of depressotypic cognitive styles/biases. At the same time, the temperamental, and eventually cognitive, vulnerabilities can lead to interpersonal deficits that in turn reinforce cognitive styles/biases and generate dependent stressors that may sensitize neurobiological stress response systems. When these emotional/neurobiological/cognitive vulnerabilities and environmental stressors combine, either additively or interactively, to exceed a critical threshold, the emotional and cognitive precursors of depression escalate to the point of a diagnosable disorder. This can occur at virtually any point during the life span. However, because of developmental effects on gene expression, the development of critical neurobiological and cognitive systems, and the developmental challenges and transitions that emerge at this time, this escalation is particularly likely to occur in adolescence. Moreover, it is much more likely to occur in females, related to sex differences in preexisting vulnerability factors and a greater increase in depression-relevant (e.g., interpersonal) stressors during this period.

To further our understanding of child and adolescent depression, research is needed to clarify the relations between depressive phenotypes at different developmental stages, as well the relations between depressive and nondepressive phenotypes across development. Genetically informative designs and prospective longitudinal studies of high risk and community samples of infants and young children prior to the onset of depressive disorders are necessary to elucidate the processes and mechanisms involved in the etiopathogenesis of youth depression. It is particularly important to continue the search for intermediate phenotypes and the attempt to trace the complex pathways among genes, neurobiology, and behavior. This search includes elucidating the role of early adversity on neurobiological and psychosocial sources of risk, and discovering the interactions between specific genes and specific environmental contexts. Finally, it is critical to understand the reasons for the increase in depression among females in early adolescence.

Knowledge of genetics and neurobiology is growing rapidly and is increasingly being applied within a developmental perspective. This progress provides grounds for guarded optimism for progress in understanding the etiopathogenesis of child and adolescent depression.

## REFERENCES

Abela, J. R. Z., & Hankin, B. L. (2011). Rumination as a vulnerability factor to depression during the transition from early to middle adolescence: A multiwave longitudinal study. *Journal of Abnormal Psychology, 120*, 259–271.

Adam, E. K., Doane, L. D., Zinbarg, R. E., Mineka, S., Craske, M. G., & Griffith, J. W. (2010). Prospective prediction of major depressive disorder from cortisol awakening responses in adolescence. *Psychoneuroendocrinology, 35*, 921–931.

Allen, J. P., Insabella, G., Porter, M. R., Smith, F. D., Land, D., & Phillips, N. (2006). A social-interactional model for the development of depressive symptoms in adolescents. *Journal of Consulting and Clinical Psychology, 74,* 55–65.

Alloy, L. B., Abramson, L. Y., Smith, J. M., Gibb, B. E., & Neeren, A. M. (2006). Role of parenting and maltreatment histories in unipolar and bipolar mood disorders: Mediation by cognitive vulnerability to depression. *Clinical Child and Family Psychology, Review, 9,* 23–64.

Ambrosini, P., Bennett, D. S., Cleland, C. M., & Haslam, N. (2002). Taxonicity of adolescent melancholia: A caterorical or dimensional construct? *Journal of Psychiatric Research 36,* 247–256.

American Psychological Association. (2000). *Diagnostic and statistical manual of mental disorders* (4th ed., text rev.). Washington, DC: American Psychological Association.

Anderson, E., & Hope, D. A. (2008). A review of the tripartite model for understanding the link between anxiety and depression in youth. *Clinical Psychology Review, 28,* 275–287.

Angold, A., Costello, E. J., & Erkanli, A. (1999). Comorbidity. *Journal of Child Psychology & Psychiatry & Allied Disciplines, 40,* 57–87.

Angold, A., Costello, E. J., Erkanli, A., & Worthman, C. M. (1999). Pubertal changes in hormone levels and depression in girls. *Psychological Medicine, 29,* 1043–1053.

Beesdo, K., Lau, J. Y. F., Guyer, A. E., McClure-Tone, E. B., Monk, C. S., Nelson, E. E., & Pine, D. S. (2009). Common and distinct amygdala-function perturbations in depressed vs anxious adolescents. *Archives of General Psychiatry,66,* 275–285.

Belsky, J., & Pluess, M. (2009). Beyond diathesis stress: Differential susceptibility to environmental influences. *Psychological Bulletin, 135,* 885–908.

Bergen, S. E., Gardner, C. O., & Kendler, K. S. (2007). Age-related changes in heritability of behavioral phenotypes over adolescence and young adulthood: A meta-analysis. *Twin Research and Human Genetics, 10,* 423–433.

Birmaher, B., Arbelaez, C., & Brent, D. (2002). Course and outcome of child and adolescent major depressive disorder. *Child and Adolescent Clinics of North America, 11,* 619–638.

Birmaher, B., Dahl, R. E., Williamson, D. E., Perel, J. M., Brent, D. A., Axelson, D. A., & Ryan, N. D. (2000). Growth hormone secretion in children and adolescents at high risk for major depressive disorder. *Archives of General Psychiatry, 57,* 867–872.

Boylan, K., Georgiades, K., & Szatmari, P. (2010). The longitudinal association between oppositional and depressive symptoms across childhood. *Journal of the American Academy of Child and Adolescent Psychiatry, 49,* 152–161.

Bufferd, S. J., Dougherty, L. R., Carlson, G. A., & Klein, D. N. (2011). Parent-reported DSM-IV disorders in a community sample of preschoolers. *Comprehensive Psychiatry, 52,* 359–369.

Burke, R., & Loeber, R. (2010). Oppositional defiant disorder and the explanation of the comorbidity between behavioral disorders and depression. *Clinical Psychology: Science and Practice, 17,* 319–326.

Carlson, G. A., & Cantwell, D. P. (1980). Unmasking masked depression in children and adolescents. *American Journal of Psychiatry, 137,* 445–449.

Caspi, A., Sugden, K., Moffitt, T. E., Taylor, A., Craig, I., Harrington, H. L., & Poulton, R. (2003). Influence of life stress on depression: Moderation by a polymorphism on the 5-HTT gene. *Science, 301,* 386–389.

Chen, M. C., Hamilton, J. P., & Gotlib, I. H. (2010). Decreased hippocampal volume in healthy girls at risk of depression. *Archives of General Psychiatry, 67,* 270–276.

Clark, L. A., & Watson, D. (1991). Tripartite model of anxiety and depression: Evidence and taxonomic implications. *Journal of Abnormal Psychology, 100,* 316–336.

Cole, D. A. (1991). Preliminary support for a competency-based model of depression in children. *Journal of Abnormal Psychology, 100,* 181–190.

Cole, D. A., Ciesla, J. A., Dallaire, D. H., Jacquez, F. M., Pineda, A. Q., LaGrange, B., & Felton, J. W.(2008). Emergence of attributional style and its relation to depressive symptoms. *Journal of Abnormal Psychology, 117,* 16–31.

Cole, D. A., Nolen-Hoeksema, S., Girgus, J., & Paul, G. (2006). Stress exposure and stress generation in child and adolescent depression: A latent trait-state-error approach to longitudinal analyses. *Journal of Abnormal Psychology, 115,* 40–51.

Copeland, W. E., Shanahan, L., Costello, J., & Angold, A. (2009). Child and adolescent psychiatric disorders as predictors of young adult disorders. *Archives of General Psychiatry, 66,* 764–772.

Copeland, W., Shanahan, L., Miller, S., Costello, E. J., Angold, A., & Maughan, B. (2010). Outcomes of early pubertal timing in young women: A prospective population-based study. *American Journal of Psychiatry, 167,* 1218–1225.

Costello, E. J., Erkanli, A., & Angold, A. (2006). Is there an epidemic of child or adolescent depression? *Journal of Child Psychology and Psychiatry, 47,* 1263–1271.

Costello, E. J., Mustillo, S., Erkanli, A., Keeler, G., & Angold, A. (2003). Prevalence and development of psychiatric disorders in childhood and adolescence. *Archives of General Psychiatry, 60,* 837–844.

Cyranowski, J. M., Frank, E., Young, E., & Shear, M. K. (2000). Adolescent onset of the gender difference in lifetime rates of major depression: A theoretical model. *Archives of General Psychiatry, 57,* 21–27.

Dahl, R. E., Birmaher, B., Williamson, D. E., Dorn, L., Perel, J., Kaufman, J., & Ryan, N. D.(2000). Low growth hormone response to growth hormone-releasing hormone in child depression. *Biological Psychiatry, 48,* 981–988.

Dietz, L. J., Birmaher, B., Williamson, D. E., Silk, J. S., Dahl, R. E., Axelson, D. A., & Ryan, N. D. (2008). Mother-child interactions in depressed children and children at high risk and low risk for future depression. *Journal of the American Academy of Child & Adolescent Psychiatry, 47,* 574–582.

Dougherty, L. R., Klein, D. N., Congdon, E., Olino, T. M., Dyson, M., Rose, S., & Canli, T. (2009). Increased waking salivary cortisol levels and depression risk in preschoolers: The role of maternal history of melancholic depression and early child temperament. *Journal of Child Psychology and Psychiatry, 50,* 1495–1503.

Dougherty, L. R., Klein, D. N., Rose, S., & Laptook, R. S. (2011). Hypothalamic-pituitary-adrenal axis reactivity in the preschool-aged offspring of depressed parents: Moderation by early parenting. *Psychological Science, 22,* 650–658.

Duggal, S., Carlson, E. A., Sroufe, L. A., & Egeland, B. (2001). Depressive symptomatology in childhood and adolescence. *Development and Psychopathology, 13,* 143–164.

Eaves, L., & Silberg, J. (2003). Resolving multiple epigenetic pathways to adolescent depression. *Journal of Child Psychology and Psychiatry and Allied Disciplines, 44,* 1006–1014.

Egger, H. L., & Angold, A. (2006). Common emotional and behavioral disorders in preschool children: Presentation, nosology, and epidemiology. *Journal of Child Psychology and Psychiatry, 47,* 313–337.

Else-Quest, N., Hyde, J., Goldsmith, H., & Van Hulle, C. (2006). Gender differences in temperament: A meta-analysis. *Psychological Bulletin, 132,* 33–72.

Fergusson, D. M., & Woodward, L. J. (2002). Mental health, educational, and social role outcomes of adolescents with depression. *Archives of General Psychiatry, 59,* 225–231.

Fombonne, E., Wostear, G., Cooper, V., Harrington, R., & Rutter, M. (2001). The Maudsley long-term follow-up of child and adolescent depression: 1. Psychiatric outcomes in adulthood. *British Journal of Psychiatry, 179,* 210–217.

Forbes, E. E., Hariri, A. R., Martin, S. L., Silk, J. S., Moyles, D. L., Fisher, P. M., & Dahl, R. E. (2009). Altered striatal activation predicting real-world positive affect in adolescent major depressive disorder. *American Journal of Psychiatry, 166,* 64–73.

Forbes, E. E., Ryan, N. D., Phillips, M. L., Manuck, S. B., Worthman, C. M., Moyles, D. L., & Dahl, R. E. (2010). Healthy adolescents' neural response to reward: Associations with puberty, positive affect, and depressive symptoms. *Journal of the American Academy of Child & Adolescent Psychiatry, 49,* 162–172.

Foti, D., Kotov, R., Klein, D., & Hajcak, G. (in press). Abnormal neural sensitivity to monetary gains versus losses among adolescents at risk for depression. *Journal of Abnormal Child Psychology.*

Franić, S., Middeldorp, C. M., Dolan, C. V., Ligthart, L., & Boomsma, D. I. (2010). Childhood and adolescent anxiety and depression: Beyond heritability. *Journal of the American Academy of Child and Adolescent Psychiatry, 49,* 820–829.

Garber, J., Gallerani, C. M., & Frankel, S. A. (2009). Depression in children. In I. H. Gotlib & C. L. Hammen (Eds.), *Handbook of depression* (2nd ed., pp. 405–443). New York, NY: Guilford Press.

Garber, J., & Weersing, V. R. (2010). Comorbidity of anxiety and depression in youth: Implications for treatment and prevention. *Clinical Psychology: Science & Practice, 17,* 293–306.

Geller, B., Fox, L. W., & Clark, K. A. (1994). Rate and predictors of prepubertal bipolarity during follow-up of 6- to 12-year-old depressed children. *Journal of the American Academy of Child and Adolescent Psychiatry, 33,* 461–468.

Geller, B., Zimmerman, B., Williams, M., Bolhofner, K., & Craney, J. L. (2001). Bipolar disorder at prospective follow-up of adults who had prepubertal major depressive disorder. *American Journal of Psychiatry, 158,* 135–127.

Gibb, B. E., Benas, J. S., Grassia, M., & McGeary, J. (2009). Children's attentional biases and 5-HTTLPR genotype: Potential mechanisms linking mother and child depression. *Journal of Clinical Child & Adolescent Psychology, 38,* 415–426.

Gotlib, I. H., Hamilton, J. P., Cooney, R. E., Singh, M. K., Henry, M. L., & Joormann, J. (2010). Neural processing of reward and loss in girls at risk for major depression. *Archives of General Psychiatry, 67*, 380–387.

Grant, K. E., Compas, B. E., Thurm, A. E., McMahon, S. D., Gipson, P. Y., Campbell, A. J., & Westerholm, R. I. (2006). Stressors and child and adolescent psychopathology: Evidence of moderating and mediating effects. *Clinical Psychology Review, 26*, 257–283.

Halari, R., Simic, M., Pariante, C. M., Papadopoulos, A., Cleare, A., Brammer, M., & Rubia, K. (2009). Reduced activation in lateral prefrontal cortex and anterior cingulate during attention and cognitive control functions in medication-naïve adolescents with depression compared to controls. *Journal of Child Psychology and Psychiatry, 50*, 307–316.

Hammen, C. (1991). Generation of stress in the course of unipolar depression. *Journal of Abnormal Psychology, 100*, 555–561.

Hankin, B. L. (2008). Stability of cognitive vulnerabilities to depression: A short-term prospective multiwave study. *Journal of Abnormal Psychology, 117*, 324–333.

Hankin, B. L. (2009). Development of sex differences in depressive and co-occurring anxious symptoms during adolescence: Descriptive trajectories and potential explanations in a multi-wave prospective study. *Journal of Clinical Child and Adolescent Psychology, 38*, 460–472.

Hankin, B. L., Badanes, L. S., Abela, J. R. Z., & Watamura, S. A. (2010). Hypothalamic-pituitary-adrenal axis dysregulation in dysphoric children and adolescents: Cortisol reactivity to psychosocial stress from preschool to middle adolescence. *Biological Psychiatry, 68*, 484–490.

Hankin, B. L., Fraley, R. C., Lahey, B. B., & Waldman, I. D. (2005). Is depression best viewed as a continuum or discrete category? A taxometric analysis of childhood and adolescent depression in a population-based sample. *Journal of Abnormal Psychology, 114*, 96–110.

Hankin, B. L., Gibb, B. E., Abela, J. R. Z., & Flory, K. (2010). Selective attention to affective stimuli and clinical depression among youths: Role of anxiety and specificity of emotion. *Journal of Abnormal Psychology, 119*, 491–501.

Hankin, B. L., Mermelstein, R., & Roesch, L. (2007). Sex differences in adolescent depression: Stress exposure and reactivity models. *Child Development, 78*, 279–295.

Harkness, K. L., Bruce, A. E., & Lumley, M. N. (2006). The role of childhood abuse and neglect in the sensitization to stressful life events in adolescent depression. *Journal of Abnormal Psychology, 115*, 730–741.

Harrington, R. C., Fudge, H., Rutter, M., Pickles, A., & Hill, J. (1990). Adult outcomes of childhood and adolescent depression, I. Psychiatric status. *Archives of General Psychiatry, 47*, 465–473.

Hazel, N. A., Hammen, C., Brennan, P. A., & Najman, J. (2008). Early childhood adversity and adolescent depression: The mediating role of continued stress. *Psychological Medicine, 38*, 581–589.

Hipwell, A., Keenan, K., Kasza, K., Loeber, R., Stouthamer-Loeber, M., & Bean, T. (2008). Reciprocal influences between girls' conduct problems and depression, and parental punishment and warmth: A six year prospective analysis. *Journal of Abnormal Child Psychology, 36,* 663–677.

Hipwell, A. E., Sapotichne, B., Klostermann, S., Battista, D., & Keenan, K. (2011). Autobiographical memory as a predictor of depression vulnerability in girls. *Journal of Clinical Child & Adolescent Psychology, 40,* 254–265.

Hoffman, K. B., Cole, D. A., Martin, J. M., Tram, J., & Seroczynski, A. D. (2000). Are the discrepancies between self- and others' appraisals of competence predictive or reflective of depressive symptoms in children and adolescents?: A longitudinal study, Part II. *Journal of Abnormal Psychology, 109,* 651–662.

Hyde, J. S., Mezulis, A. H., & Abramson, L. Y. (2008). The ABCs of depression: Integrating affective, biological, and cognitive models to explain the emergence of the gender difference in depression. *Psychological Review, 115,* 291–313.

Jacobs, R. H., Reinecke, M. A., Gollan, J. K., & Kane, P. (2008). Empirical evidence of cognitive vulnerability for depression among children and adolescents: A cognitive science and developmental perspective. *Clinical Psychology Review, 28,* 759–782.

Karg, K., Burmeister, M., Sjeddem, K., & Sen, S. (2011). The serotonin transporter promoter variant (5-HTTLPR), stress, and depression meta-analysis revisited: Evidence of genetic moderation. *Archives of General Psychiatry, 68,* 444–454.

Kaufman, J., & Charney, D. (2003). The neurobiology of child and adolescent depression. In D. Cicchetti & E. Walker (Eds.), *Neurodevelopmental mechanisms in psychopathology* (pp. 461–490). Cambridge, United Kingdom: Cambridge University Press.

Kendler, K. S., Gardner, C. O., Gatz, M., & Pedersen, N. L. (2007). The sources of comorbidity between major depression and generalized anxiety disorder in a Swedish national twin sample. *Psychological Medicine, 37,* 453–462.

Kendler, K. S., Gardner, C. O., & Lichtenstein, P. (2008). A developmental twin study of symptoms of anxiety and depression: Evidence for genetic innovation and attenuation. *Psychological Medicine, 38,* 1567–1575.

Klein, D. N., Dyson, M. W., Kujawa, A. J., & Kotov, R. (in press). Temperament and internalizing disorders. In M. Zentner & R. Shiner (Eds.), *Handbook of temperament.* New York, NY: Guilford Press.

Klein, D. N., Lewinsohn, P. M., Rohde, P., Seeley, J. R., & Olino, T. M. (2005). Psychopathology in the adolescent and young adult offspring of a community sample of mothers and fathers with major depression. *Psychological Medicine, 35,* 353–365.

Klein, D. N., Lewinsohn, P. M., Seeley, J. R., & Rohde, P. (2001). Family study of major depressive disorder in a community sample of adolescents. *Archives of General Psychiatry, 58,* 13–20.

Klein, D. N., & Riso, L. P. (1993). Psychiatric diagnoses: Problems of boundaries and co-occurrences. In C. G. Costello (Ed.), *Basic issues in psychopathology* (pp. 19–66). New York, NY: Guilford Press.

Klein, D. N., Shankman, S. A., Lewinsohn, P. M., & Seeley, J. R. (2009). Subthreshold depressive disorder in adolescents: Predictors of escalation to full syndrome depressive disorders. *Journal of the American Academy of Child and Adolescent Psychiatry, 48,* 703–710.

Klein, D. N., Shankman, S. A., & McFarland, B. (2006). Classification of mood disorders. In D. J. Stein, D. J. Kupfer, & A. F. Schatzberg (Eds.), *The American psychiatric publishing textbook of mood disorders* (pp. 17–32). Washington, DC: American Psychiatric.

Kovacs, M. (1996). Presentation and course of major depressive disorder during childhood and later years of the life span. *Journal of the American Academy of Child and Adolescent Psychiatry, 35,* 705–715.

Kovacs, M., Devlin, B., Pollock, M., Richards, C., & Mukerji, P. (1997). A controlled family history study of childhood-onset depressive disorder. *Archives of General Psychiatry, 54,* 613–623.

Kovacs, M., & Lopez-Duran, N. (2010). Prodromal symptoms and atypical affectivity as predictors of major depression in juveniles: Implications for prevention. *Journal of Child Psychology and Psychiatry, 51,* 472–496.

Krueger, R. F., & Markon, K. E. (2006). Understanding psychopathology: Melding behavior genetics, personality, and quantitative psychology to develop an empirically based model. *Current Directions in Psychological Science, 15,* 113–117.

Kujawa, A., Torpey, D., Kim, J., Hajcak, G., Rose, S., Gotlib, I., & Klein, D. N. (2011). Attentional biases for emotional faces in young children of mothers with chronic or recurrent depression. *Journal of Abnormal Child Psychology, 39,* 125–135.

LaGrange, B., Cole, D. A., Jacquea, F., Ciesla, J., Dallaire, D., Pineda, A., & Felton, J. (2011). Disentangling the prospective relations between maladaptive cognitions and depressive symptoms. *Journal of Abnormal Psychology, 120,* 511–527.

Lahey, B. B., Van Hulle, C. A., Singh, A. L., Waldman, I. D., & Rathouz, P. J. (2011). Higher order genetic and environmental structure of prevalent forms of child and adolescent psychopathology. *Archives of General Psychiatry, 68,* 181–189.

Lau, J. Y. F., & Eley, T. C. (2008). Attributional style as a risk marker of genetic effects for adolescent depressive symptoms. *Journal of Abnormal Psychology, 117,* 849–859.

Lau, J. Y. F., & Eley, T. C. (2008). New behavioral genetic approaches to depression in childhood and adolescence. In J. R. Z. Abela & B. L. Hankin (Eds.), *Handbook of depression in children and adolescents* (pp. 124–148). New York, NY: Guilford Press.

Levinson, D. F. (2009). Genetics of major depression. In I. H. Gotlib & C. L. Hammen (Eds.), *Handbook of depression* (2nd ed., pp. 165–186). New York, NY: Guilford Press.

Lewinsohn, P. M., Hops H., Roberts, R. E., Seeley, J. R., & Andrews, J. A. (1993). Adolescent psychopathology: I. Prevalence and incidence of depression and other DSM-III-R disorders in high school students. *Journal of Abnormal Psychology, 102,* 133–144.

Lewinsohn, P. M., Rohde, P., Klein, D. N., & Seeley, J. R. (1999). The natural course of adolescent major depressive disorder: I. Continuity into young adulthood. *Journal of the American Academy of Child and Adolescent Psychiatry, 38,* 56–63.

Lewinsohn, P. M., Rohde, P., Seeley, J. R., Klein, D. N., & Gotlib, I. H. (2000). The natural course of adolescent major depressive disorder: II. Predictors of depression recurrence in young adults. *American Journal of Psychiatry, 157*, 1584–1591.

Lewinsohn, P. M., Solomon, A., Seeley, J. R., & Zeiss, A. (2000). Clinical implications of "subthreshold" depressive symptoms. *Journal of Abnormal Psychology, 109*, 345–351.

Lewis, G., Rice, F., Harold, G. T., Collishaw, S., & Thapar, A. (2011). Investigating environmental links between parent depression and child anxiety/depressive symptoms using an assisted conception design. *Journal of the American Academy of Child and Adolescent Psychiatry, 50*, 451–459.

Lopez-Duran, N. L., Kovacs, M., & George, C. J. (2009). Hypothalamic-pituitary-adrenal axis dysregulation in depressed children and adolescents: A meta-analysis. *Psychoneuroendocrinology, 34*, 1271–1283.

Lovejoy, M. C., Graczyk, P. A., O'Hare, E., & Neuman, G. (2000). Maternal depression and parenting behavior: A meta-analytic review. *Clinical Psychology Review, 20*, 561–592.

Luby, J. L., Heffelfinger, A., Mrakotsky, C., Brown, K., Hessler, M., & Spitznagel, E. (2003). Alterations in stress cortisol reactivity in depressed preschoolers relative to psychiatric and no-disorder comparison groups. *Archives of General Psychiatry, 60*, 1248–1255.

Luby, J. L., Heffelfinger, A., Mrakotsky, C., Hessler, M. J., Brown, K. M., & Hildebrand, T. (2002). Preschool major depressive disorder: Preliminary validation for developmentally modified DSM-IV criteria. *Journal of the American Academy of Child and Adolescent Psychiatry, 41*, 928–937.

Luby, J. L., Mrakotsky, C., & Heffelfinger, A. (2004). Characteristics of depressed preschoolers with and without melancholia: Evidence for a melancholic depressive subtype in young children. *American Journal of Psychiatry, 161*, 1998–2004.

Luby, J. L., Si, X., Belden, A. C., Tandon, M., & Spitznagel, E. (2009). Preschool depression: Homotypic continuity and course over 24 months. *Archives of General Psychiatry, 66*, 897–905.

Luthar, S. S., Cicchetti, D., & Becker, B. (2000). The construct of resilience: A critical evaluation and guidelines for future work. *Child Development, 71*, 543–562.

MacMillan, S., Szeszko, P. R., Moore, G. J., Madden, R., Lorch, E., Ivey, J., & Rosenberg, D. R. (2003). Increased amygdala: Hippocampal volume ratios associated with severity of anxiety in pediatric major depression. *Journal of Child & Adolescent Psychopharmacology, 13*, 65–73.

Masten, C. L., Eisenberger, N. I., Borofsky, L. A., McNealy, K., Pfeifer, J. H., & Dapretto, M. (2011). Subgenual anterior cingulate responses to peer rejection: A marker of adolescents' risk for depression. *Development and Psychopathology, 23*, 283–292.

McLeod, B. D., Weisz, J. R., & Wood, J. J. (2007). Examining the association between parenting and childhood depression: A meta-analysis. *Clinical Psychology Review, 27*, 986–1003.

McClellan, J., & King, M.-C. (2010). Genetic heterogeneity in human disease. *Cell, 141*, 210–217.

Medina, K. L., Nagel, B. J., Park, A., McQueeny, T., & Tapert, S. F. (2007). Depressive symptoms in adolescents: Associations with white matter volume and marijuana use. *Journal of Child Psychology and Psychiatry, 48,* 592–600.

Merikangas, K. R., He, J.-P., Brody, D., Fisher, P. W., Bourdon, K., & Koretz, D. S. (2010). Prevalence and treatment of mental disorders among U.S. children in the 2001–2004 NHANES. *Pediatrics, 125,* 75–81.

Miller, G. E., & Chapman, J. P. (2001). Misunderstanding analysis of covariance. *Journal of Abnormal Psychology, 110,* 40–48.

Monk, C. S., Klein, R. G., Telzer, E. H., Schroth, E. A., Mannuzza, S., Moulton, J. L., III., & Ernst, M. (2008). Amygdala and nucleus accumbens activation to emotional facial expressions in children and adolescents at risk for major depression. *American Journal of Psychiatry, 165,* 90–98.

Monroe, S. M., Rohde, P., Seeley, J. R., & Lewinsohn, P. M. (1999). Life events and depression in adolescence: Relationship loss as a prospective risk factor for first onset of major depressive disorder. *Journal of Abnormal Psychology, 108,* 606–614.

Morris, M. C., Ciesla, J. A., & Garber, J. (2010). A prospective study of stress autonomy versus stress sensitization in adolescents at varied risk for depression. *Journal of Abnormal Psychology, 119,* 341–354.

Neshat-Doost, H. T., Taghavi, M. R., Moradi, A. R., Yule, W., & Dalgleish, T. (1998). Memory for emotional trait adjectives in clinically depressed youth. *Journal of Abnormal Psychology, 107,* 642–650.

Nolan, C. L., Moore, G. J., Madden, R., Farchione, T., Bartoi, M., Lorch, E., & Rosenberg, D. R. (2002). Prefrontal cortical volume in childhood-onset major depression. *Archives of General Psychiatry, 59,* 173–179.

Nolen-Hoeksema, S., & Hilt, L. M. (2009). Gender differences in depression. In I. Gotlib & C. Hammen (Eds.), *Handbook of depression* (2nd ed., pp. 386–404). New York, NY: Guilford Press.

Nolen-Hoeksema, S., Stice, E., Wade, E., & Bohon, C. (2007). Reciprocal relations between rumination and bulimic, substance abuse, and depressive symptoms in female adolescents. *Journal of Abnormal Psychology, 116,* 198–207.

Olino, T. M., Klein, D. N., Dyson, M. W., Rose, S. A., & Durbin, C. E. (2010). Temperamental emotionality in preschool-aged children and depressive disorders in parents: Associations in a large community sample. *Journal of Abnormal Psychology, 119,* 468–478.

Oppenheimer, C. W., & Hankin, B. L. (2011). Relationship quality and depressive symptoms among adolescents: A short-term multiwave investigation of longitudinal, reciprocal associations. *Journal of Clinical Child and Adolescent Psychology, 40,* 486–493.

Orvaschel, H., Lewinsohn, P. M., & Seeley, J. R. (1995). Continuity of psychopathology in a community sample of adolescents. *Journal of the American Academy of Child and Adolescent Psychiatry, 32,* 1155–1163.

Patton, G. C., Coffey, C., Posterino, M., Carlin, J. B., & Bowes, G. (2003). Life events and early onset depression: Cause or consequence? *Psychological Medicine, 33,* 1203–1210.

Patton, G. C., Coffey, C., Posterino, M., Carlin, J. B., & Wolfe, R. (2001). Parental "affectionless control" in adolescent depressive disorder. *Social Psychiatry and Psychiatric Epidemiology, 36*, 475–480.

Pine, D. S., Cohen, P., Gurley, D., Brook, J., & Ma, Y. (1998). The risk for early-adulthood anxiety and depressive disorders in adolescents with anxiety and depressive disorders. *Archives of General Psychiatry, 55*, 56–64.

Prinstein, M. J., Borelli, J. L., Cheah, C. S. L., Simon, V. A., & Aikins, J. W. (2005). Adolescent girls' interpersonal vulnerability to depressive symptoms: A longitudinal examination of reassurance-seeking and peer relationships. *Journal of Abnormal Psychology, 114*, 676–688.

Puig-Antich, J., Blau, S., Marx, J., Greenhill, L. L., & Chambers, W. (1978). Pre-pubertal major depressive disorder: A pilot study. *Journal of the American Academy of Child Psychiatry, 17*, 696–707.

Puig-Antich, J., Goetz, D., Davies, M., Kaplan, T., Davies, S., & Klepper, T. (1989). A controlled family history study of prepubertal major depressive disorder. *Archives of General Psychiatry, 46*, 406–418.

Raes, F., Verstraeten, K., Bijttebier, P., Vasey, M. W., & Dalgleish, T. (2010). Inhibitory control mediates the relationship between depressed mood and overgeneral memory recall in children. *Journal of Clinical Child & Adolescent Psychology, 39*, 276–281.

Rao, U., Hammen, C. L., & Poland, R. E. (2010). Longitudinal course of adolescent depression: Neuroendocrine and psychosocial predictors. *Journal of the American Academy of Child and Adolescent Psychiatry, 49*, 141–151.

Richey, J. A., Schmidt, N. B., Lonigan, C. J., Phillips, B. M., Catanzaro, S. J., Laurent, J., & Kotov, R. (2009). The latent structure of child depression: A taxometric analysis. *Journal of Child Psychology and Psychiatry, 50*, 1147–1155.

Rohde, P., Lewinsohn, P. M., & Seeley, J. R. (1991). Comorbidity of unipolar depression: II. Comorbidity with other mental disorders in adolescents and adults. *Journal of Abnormal Psychology, 100*, 214–222.

Rosso, I. M., Cintron, C. M., Steingard, R. J., Renshaw, P. F., Young, A. D., & Yurgelun-Todd, D. A. (2005). Amygdala and hippocampus volumes in pediatric major depression. *Biological Psychiatry, 57*, 21–26.

Rudolph, K. D. (2009). Adolescent depression. In I. H. Gotlib & C. L. Hammen (Eds.), *Handbook of depression* (2nd ed., pp. 444–466). New York, NY: Guilford Press.

Rudolph, K. D., Flynn, M., & Abaied, J. L. (2008). A developmental perspective on interpersonal theories of youth depression. In J. R. Z. Abela & B. L. Hankin (Eds.), *Child and adolescent depression: Causes, treatment, and prevention.* New York, NY: Guilford Press.

Rudolph, K. D., Flynn, M., Abaied, J., Groot, A., & Thompson, R. (2009). Why is past depression the best predictor of future depression? Stress generation as a mechanism of depression continuity in girls. *Journal of Clinical Child and Adolescent Psychology, 38*, 473–485.

Rutter, M., Moffitt, T. E., & Caspi, A. (2006). Gene-environment interplay and psychopathology: Multiple varieties but real effects. *Journal of Child Psychology and Psychiatry, 47*, 226–261.

Schrepferman, L. M., Eby, J., Snyder, J., & Stropes, J. (2006). Early affiliation and social engagement with peers: Prospective risk and protective factors for childhood depressive behaviors. *Journal of Emotional and Behavioral Disorders, 14,* 50–61.

Shad, M. U., Bidesi, A. P., Chen, L.-A., Ernst, M., & Rao, U. (2011). Neurobiology of decision making in depressed adolescents: A functional magnetic resonance imaging study. *Journal of the American Academy of Child & Adolescent Psychiatry, 50,* 612–621.

Shih, J. H., Eberhart, N. K., Hammen, C. L., & Brennan, P. A. (2006). Differential exposure and reactivity to interpersonal stress predict sex differences in adolescent depression. *Journal of Clinical Child and Adolescent Psychology, 35,* 103–115.

Silberg, J. L., Maes, H., & Eaves, L. J. (2010). Genetic and environmental influences on the transmission of parental depression to children's depression and conduct disturbance: An extended children of twins study. *Journal of Child Psychology and Psychiatry, 51,* 734–744.

Silberg, J., Pickles, A., Rutter, M., Hewitt, J., Simonoff, E., Maes, H., & Eaves, L. (1999). The influence of genetic factors and life stress on depression among adolescent girls. *Archives of General Psychiatry, 56,* 225–232.

Singh, A. L., D'Onofrio, B. M., Slutske, W. S., Turkheimer, E., Emery, R. E., Harden, K. P., & Martin, N. G. (2011). Parental depression and offspring psychopathology: A children of twins study. *Psychological Medicine, 41,* 1385–1395.

Solomon, A., Ruscio, J., Seeley Jr., & Lewinsohn, P. M. (2006). A taxometric investigation of unipolar depression in a large community sample. *Psychological Medicine, 36,* 973–985.

Steingard, R. J., Renshaw, P. F., Hennen, J., Lenox, M., Cintron, C. B., Young, A. D., & Yurgelun-Todd, D. A. (2002). Smaller frontal lobe white matter volumes in depressed adolescents. *Biological Psychiatry, 52,* 413–417.

Stice, E., Hayward, C., Cameron, R. P., Killen, J. D., & Taylor, C. B. (2000). Body-image and eating disturbances predict onset of depression among female adolescents: A longitudinal study. *Journal of Abnormal Psychology, 109,* 438–444.

Stice, E., Ragan, J., & Randall, P. (2004). Prospective relations between social support and depression: Differential direction of effects for parent and peer support? *Journal of Abnormal Psychology, 113,* 155–159.

Stone, L. B., Hankin, B. L., Gibb, B. E., & Abela, J. R. Z. (2011). Co-rumination predicts the onset of depressive disorders during adolescence. *Journal of Abnormal Psychology, 120,* 752–757.

Stroud, C. B., Davila, J., Hammen, C., & Vrshek-Schallhorn, S. (2011). Severe and non-severe events in first onsets versus recurrences of depression: Evidence for stress sensitization. *Journal of Abnormal Psychology, 120,* 142–154.

Sullivan, P. F., Neale, M. C., & Kendler, K. S. (2000). Genetic epidemiology of major depression: Review and meta-analysis. *American Journal of Psychiatry, 157,* 1552–1562.

Taylor, L., & Ingram, R. E. (1999). Cognitive reactivity and depressotypic information processing in children of depressed mothers. *Journal of Abnormal Psychology, 108,* 202–210.

Teunissen, H. A., Adelman, C. B., Prinstein, M. J., Spijkerman, R., Poelen, E. A. P., Engels, R. C. M. E., & Scholte, R. H. J. (2011). The interaction between pubertal timing and peer popularity for boys and girls: An integration of biological and interpersonal perspectives on adolescent depression. *Journal of Abnormal Child Psychology, 39,* 413–423.

Thomas, K. M., Drevets, W. C., Dahl, R. E., Ryan, N. D., Birmaher, B., Eccard, C. H., & Casey, B. J. (2001). Amygdala response to fearful faces in anxious and depressed children. *Archives of General Psychiatry, 58,* 1057–1063.

Tompson, M. C., Pierre, C. B., Boger, K. D., McKowen, J. W., Chan, P. T., & Freed, R. D. (2010). Maternal depression, maternal expressed emotion, and youth psychopathology. *Journal of Abnormal Child Psychology, 38,* 105–117.

Tully, E. C., Iacono, W. G., & McGue, M. (2008). An adoption study of parental depression as an environmental liability for adolescent depression and childhood disruptive disorders. *American Journal of Psychiatry, 165,* 1148–1154.

Uher, R., & McGuffin, P. (2010). The moderation by the serotonin transporter gene of environmental adversity in the etiology of depression: 2009 update. *Molecular Psychiatry, 15,* 18–22.

Verstraeten, K., Vasey, M., Raes, F., & Bijttebier, P. (2009). Temperament and risk for depressive symptoms in adolescence: Mediation by rumination and moderation by effortful control. *Journal of Abnormal Child Psychology, 37,* 349–361.

Weiss, B., & Garber, G. (2003). Developmental differences in the phenomenology of depression. *Development and Psychopathology, 15,* 403–430.

Weissman, M. M., Wolk, S., Goldstein, R. B., Moreau, D., Adams, P., Greenwald, S., & Wickramaratne, P. (1999). Depressed adolescents grown up. *Journal of the American Medical Association, 281,* 1707–1713.

Weissman, M. M., Wolk, S., Wickramaratne, P., Goldstein, R. B., Adams, P., Greenwald, S., & Steinberg, D. (1999). Children with prepubertal-onset major depressive disorder and anxiety grown up. *Archives of General Psychiatry, 56,* 794–801.

Weissman, M. M., Wickramaratne, P., Nomura, Y., Warner, V., Pilowsky, D., & Verdeli, H. (2006). Offspring of depressed parents: 20 years later. *American Journal of Psychiatry, 163,* 1001–1008.

Whittle, S., Yap, M. B. H., Sheeber, L., Dudgeon, P., Yücel, M., Pantelis, C., & Allen, N. B. (2011). Hippocampal volume and sensitivity to maternal aggressive behavior: A prospective study of adolescent depressive symptoms. *Development and Psychopathology, 23,* 115–129.

Wickramaratne, P., & Weissman, M. M (1998). Onset of psychopathology in offspring by developmental phase and parental depression. *Journal of the American Academy of Child and Adolescent Psychiatry, 37,* 933–942.

Widom, C. S., DuMont, K., & Czaja, S. J. (2007). A prospective investigation of major depressive disorder and comorbidity in abused and neglected children grown up. *Archives of General Psychiatry, 64,* 49–56.

Wight, R. G., Aneshensel, C. S., Botticello, A. L., & Sepulveda, J. E. (2005). A multilevel analysis of ethnic variation in depressive symptoms among adolescents in the United States. *Social Science & Medicine, 60,* 2073–2084.

Witvliet, M., Brendgen, M., Van Lier, P. A. C., Koot, H. M., & Vitaro, F. (2010). Early adolescent depressive symptoms: Predictions from clique isolation, loneliness, and perceived social acceptance. *Journal of Abnormal Child Psychology, 38*, 1045–1056.

Yap, M. B. H., Whittle, S., Yucel, M., Sheeber, L., Pantelis, C., Simmons, J. G., & Allen, N. B. (2008). Interaction of parenting experiences and brain structure in the prediction of depressive symptoms in adolescents. *Archives of General Psychiatry, 65*(12), 1377–1385.

Zhang, T.-Y., & Meaney, M. J. (2010). Epigenetics and the environmental regulation of the genome and its function. *Annual Review of Psychology, 61*, 439–466.

# CHAPTER 18

# The Development of Borderline Personality and Self-Inflicted Injury

SHEILA E. CROWELL, ERIN A. KAUFMAN, AND MARK F. LENZENWEGER

## INTRODUCTION

BORDERLINE PERSONALITY DISORDER (BPD) and self-inflicted injury (SII) are distinct yet related clinical problems (Crowell, Beauchaine, & Lenzenweger, 2008). Both are associated with significant psychiatric comorbidity, high rates of treatment utilization, and elevated risk for suicide (De La Fuente & Bobes, 2009; Gunderson, 2010). Epidemiological surveys suggest that BPD affects between 1.2% to 5.9% of community adults, with most studies converging on a prevalence rate just under 2% (Grant et al., 2008; Lenzenweger, Lane, Loranger, & Kessler, 2007; Trull, Jahng, Tomko, Wood, & Sher, 2010). Within clinical samples, however, up to 10% of outpatients and 20% of inpatients receive a BPD diagnosis (Widiger & Trull, 1993).

Epidemiological surveys with adolescents are only beginning to appear. Findings suggest that approximately 3% of adolescents meet criteria for BPD, although further research is needed (Zanarini et al., 2011). SII is far more prevalent than BPD. Each year, approximately 4,400 youth aged 10 to 24 die by suicide (Centers for Disease Control and Prevention [CDC], 2009). Furthermore, approximately 15% to 29% of 14- to 17-year-olds report suicidal ideation, 12% to 19% form a suicide plan, and 7% to 10% attempt suicide (Nock et al., 2008). Rates of nonsuicidal self-injury (NSSI) affect between 15% and 20% of community adolescents (see Heath, Baxter, Toste, & McLouth, 2010), although some researchers have found rates as high as 56% (Hilt, Cha, & Nolen-Hoeksema, 2008). Variation in definitions of self-inflicted injury, as well as sampling differences, may underlie such discrepant findings.

Self-injury is only one among nine diagnostic criteria for BPD (American Psychiatric Association [APA], 2000). However, the two conditions have a number of common features. As we review in this chapter, BPD and SII share many biological vulnerabilities, contextual risk factors, personality traits, and acquired coping

We would like to acknowledge Theodore P. Beauchaine for his contribution to the prior version of this chapter.

strategies. Thus, SII and BPD appear to derive from a common etiology, in spite of phenotypic differences. However, because SII is neither required nor sufficient for a BPD diagnosis, the two conditions are often studied separately. This disconnect has obscured much of the overlap between SII and BPD. More recently, psychopathology researchers have taken a trait-based approach to understanding psychiatric disorders (Clark, 2005; Crowell, Derbidge, & Beauchaine, in press; Depue & Lenzenweger, 2005; Krueger, Markon, Patrick, Benning, & Kramer, 2007). From this perspective, overlap across what have been conceptualized as distinct diagnostic categories may reflect shared etiologies. Thus, identifying etiological precursors to BPD and SII is critical. Indeed, each is a severely impairing and costly mental health problem that results in intense suffering for affected individuals and family members. Consistent with our theoretical model (Beauchaine, Klein, Crowell, Derbidge, & Gatzke-Kopp, 2009; Crowell et al., 2009), we highlight areas of overlap between BPD and SII, while acknowledging that multifinality and diagnostic heterogeneity shape important distinctions between the two conditions.

Although self-injury and BPD have identifiable developmental precursors, there have been relatively few attempts to articulate testable developmental hypotheses. As we review later, biological vulnerabilities for BPD are present early in life and are exacerbated within specific, high-risk environmental contexts. Many vulnerable individuals—even those exposed to significant environmental adversity—desist from a pathway leading to borderline pathology. Still others develop different disorders (e.g., Beauchaine et al., 2009). Such multifinality is common to nearly all developmental models of psychopathology (Cicchetti & Rogosch, 1996). Furthermore, much of the literature reviewed later may apply to conditions that share traits with and are often comorbid with BPD and SII (e.g., substance use, posttraumatic stress disorder, antisocial personality disorder, eating disorders).

In this chapter, we review evidence suggesting that (1) there are reliable etiological precursors to BPD and (2) identifying these early markers of risk could improve intervention and prevention. One behavioral marker is SII, which appears to be a developmental precursor to BPD for many individuals (Crowell, Beauchaine, & Linehan, 2009; Lamph, 2011). Nonetheless, there is increasing evidence to suggest that both prevention and intervention benefit from an etiological perspective in which common vulnerabilities and risk factors are identified and targeted clinically (Beauchaine, Neuhaus, Brenner, & Gatzke-Kopp, 2008; Cicchetti & Rogosch, 2002). Early identification and prevention are of the utmost importance.

## HISTORICAL CONTEXT

As noted earlier, the literatures on SII and BPD have independent traditions. Most studies of SII have been conducted by suicide researchers, and important distinctions between suicidal and nonsuicidal self-injury have only been acknowledged recently (Linehan, 1997; Muehlenkamp & Gurierrez, 2004). At the same time, researchers studying BPD have often viewed SII as a characteristic of underlying personality pathology (i.e., a behavioral manifestation of negative emotionality and lack of constraint) and, therefore, have accorded it less status in the literature (Muehlenkamp,

Ertelt, Miller, & Claes, 2011; Niedtfeld et al., 2010). This perspective shifted as behavioral conceptualizations of BPD and SII became more prominent and as research on both conditions increased. However, because SII and BPD have distinct research histories and current directions, we review each separately.

## SELF-INFLICTED INJURY

Broadly defined, self-inflicted injury (SII) includes all volitional acts of self-harm, ranging from repetitive self-mutilation to completed suicide. At the broadest level, SII can be divided into SII with and without suicidal intent (e.g., Zlotnick, Mattia, & Zimmerman, 1999), and most research has fallen into one of these two categories. Historically, both suicidal and nonsuicidal self-injury (NSSI) were considered to result from the same unconscious mechanisms and drives (Zilboorg, 1936). This perspective was summarized in an important review by Simpson (1950), who identified suicide as displaced desire to kill.

In this same review, Simpson (1950) highlighted significant methodological barriers to conducting suicide research. These included challenges of obtaining reliable statistics with regard to death by suicide, problems inherent in collecting data post mortem, and difficulties identifying those at risk for suicidal behavior prospectively given an unknown etiology and the infrequent occurrence of the behavior. Despite Simpson's efforts to identify variables predictive of suicide risk (e.g., family, religion, neighborhood, income, sex, age, race), there were several decades during which the literature consisted primarily of descriptive, single case studies (Flood & Seager, 1968; Mason, 1954). In contrast, Offer and Barglow (1960) identified a relatively large subgroup of hospitalized youth who harmed themselves without suicidal intent. These authors were among the first to conclude that nonsuicidal self-injury is learned and that the act of self-harm can serve both instrumental and emotional functions.

Following this report, the literatures on suicidal and nonsuicidal SII began to diverge. However, researchers in these areas often inferred suicidal intent from lethality of behavior. Thus, studies of NSSI were conducted primarily with individuals who engaged in lower lethality behaviors, such as repetitive cutting, burning, or bruising (e.g., Simpson, 1975), whereas research on suicidal self-injury focused more on high-lethality behaviors such as hanging, gun injuries, and asphyxiation (e.g., Seiden, 1978). Unfortunately, as these two bodies of work evolved independently, researchers often neglected to identify important similarities and differences between the two populations.

Furthermore, much of the research on SII has been conducted within, rather than across, diagnostic groups and age ranges. For example, researchers studying personality, mood, and psychotic disorders often examine risk for suicide and self-injury within their respective samples (e.g., Heisel, Conwell, Pisani, & Duberstein, 2011; Reutfors et al., 2010). There are also separate literatures examining SII within adolescents, young adults, and aging adults (e.g., Crowell et al., 2008; Thombs & Bresnick, 2008). Unfortunately, convergent findings across these literatures often go undetected and there have been few attempts to articulate life span theories of self-injury and suicide (however, see Crowell, Derbidge, et al., in press; Shneidman, 1991). Current research on adolescent suicide and nonsuicidal SII is focused on (a) understanding the etiology of SII, (b) placing adolescent SII within a theoretical context, (c) determining how to represent SII within the *DSM*, and (d) developing a standard of care for adolescents who engage in SII (e.g., Berman, Jobes, & Silverman, 2006; Gratz, 2003; Van Orden, Witte, Holm-Denoma, Gordon, & Joiner, 2011; Zlotnick, Donaldson, Spirito, & Pearlstein, 1997).

## BORDERLINE PERSONALITY DISORDER

Historically, the term *borderline* resulted from difficulties diagnosing those who did not fit into the psychiatric nomenclature of the early to mid-20th century. Because these individuals were not clearly "psychotic" or "neurotic," they were described as being on "the borderline of psychosis and neurosis" (Stern, 1938, p. 467). Thus, early practitioners were uncertain as to whether so-called borderline individuals would (1) develop psychotic disorders such as schizophrenia, (2) develop neurotic disorders such as anxiety and depression, or (3) vacillate between the two states (Knight, 1953). Following this initial description of borderline pathology, researchers began to delineate concrete diagnostic criteria for BPD. Kernberg (1967) was among the first to identify borderline personality organization as a specific and stable personality pattern that could be differentiated from both psychotic and neurotic conditions. Soon thereafter, two important reviews (Gunderson & Singer, 1975; Spitzer, Endicott, & Gibbon, 1979) established diagnostic criteria for BPD that would eventually be used in the *DSM-III* (APA, 1980).

Once BPD criteria were established, researchers focused increasingly on their assessment and validity. Several diagnostic measures were created, including the International Personality Disorders Examination (IPDE; Loranger, 1999; Loranger, Susman, Oldham, & Russakoff, 1988), and the Millon Clinical Multiaxial Inventory (MCMI; Millon, 1983). In addition, investigators sought to address patterns of comorbidity, the validity of the BPD diagnosis, correlates of BPD, and behavioral and pharmacological treatments for the disorder (e.g., Linehan, 1993; Loranger, Oldham, & Tulis, 1982; Soloff, 2000; Zanarini et al., 1998). More recently, theory-driven experimental studies have focused on dysfunctional psychosocial and biological underpinnings of BPD (e.g., Koenigsberg et al., 2009; Paris et al., 2004). There is also a push to reduce heterogeneity within the BPD diagnosis and identify clearer, more homogeneous subgroups (Lenzenweger, Clarkin, Yeomans, Kernberg, & Levy, 2008).

## BORDERLINE PATHOLOGY IN CHILDHOOD

Although research on childhood borderline pathology (BP) evolved in parallel with the adult literature, existing research with youth remains extremely limited in scope. Similar to research on BPD in adults, exploration of BP among children began with clinical descriptions of those who could not be classified as either psychotic or neurotic (Geleerd, 1958; Weil, 1953). These clinical descriptions were followed by preliminary attempts to identify diagnostic criteria for BP in childhood (e.g., Bemporad, Smith, Hanson, & Cicchetti, 1982; Kernberg, Weiner, & Bardenstein, 2000). Despite these early efforts, no consensus was reached regarding diagnostic criteria and neuropsychological correlates of the disorder (Vela, Gottlieb, & Gottlieb, 1983). Furthermore, prospective studies showed that children with BP developed a wide range of Axis II disorders as adults, the most common being antisocial personality disorder (ASPD) rather than BPD (Lofgren, Bemporad, King, Lindem, & O'Driscoll, 1991). To date, there is still no evidence to suggest that BPD can be diagnosed reliably and validly among children.

Nevertheless, there is great interest in delineating possible developmental trajectories to BPD (Beauchaine et al., 2009; Gratz et al., 2009; Lenzenweger & Cicchetti, 2005; Stepp, 2012). This literature is distinct from the downward-extension approach that has been applied successfully to some clinical disorders. Adolescent-onset depression, for example, shows a strong, specific, and direct link to adult depression (Rutter, Kim-Cohen, & Maughan, 2006). In contrast, researchers studying the development of BPD generally describe a developmental pathway characterized by (1) sequential comorbidity (e.g., Fossati, Novella, Donati, Donini, & Maffei, 2002) or (2) heterotypic continuity (e.g., Crowell et al., 2009).

There are differences between these two perspectives that have yet to be tested empirically. The term sequential comorbidity implies that there is a causal link between two disorders in which one reliably precedes the other (i.e., conduct disorder emerges prior to ASPD and increases risk for the disorder directly; see Chapters 13 and 14). Heterotypic continuity means that the longitudinal association between two disorders can be explained by a common set of core traits and/or etiology with different phenotypic expressions across distinct developmental phases (see Beauchaine et al., 2009; Crowell et al., 2009). We hypothesize that SII and BPD represent two points along a heterotypically continuous borderline trajectory (see Crowell et al., in press, for a recent discussion) *and* that SII increases risk for other BPD features (Crowell et al., 2009). Future research could explore whether SII is an early marker of a borderline liability, whether it potentiates risk for BPD, or whether both processes are at work. Clearly, further longitudinal research is needed (Stepp, 2012).

## DIAGNOSTIC, TERMINOLOGICAL, AND CONCEPTUAL ISSUES

Within the current *Diagnostic and Statistical Manual of Mental Disorders* (*DSM-IV-TR*; APA, 2000), self-inflicted injury is included in the criterion lists of major depression (e.g., suicide attempts) and BPD (e.g., recurrent suicidal behavior, gestures, or threats, or self-mutilating behavior). Because BPD is a controversial diagnosis for adolescents (e.g., Stepp, 2012), many clinicians assign one or more Axis I disorders to self-injuring youth, especially major depression (Miller, Rathus, & Linehan, 2007). However, relations between suicidality and psychopathology are more complex than acknowledged within the *DSM-IV*. Suicide risk is elevated in nearly all *DSM* diagnoses, including substance use disorders, externalizing behavior disorders (e.g., oppositional defiant disorder, conduct disorder), anxiety disorders (e.g., generalized anxiety, posttraumatic stress, obsessive-compulsive), eating disorders, other personality disorders (e.g., avoidant, antisocial), and psychotic disorders (APA, 2006). Furthermore, the time-course of suicidality often differs from that of the primary clinical diagnosis—sometimes resolving during the course of a disorder and sometimes extending beyond remission of the psychiatric condition (e.g., Malone, Haas, Sweeney, & Mann, 1995; Mehlum, Friis, Vaglum, & Karterud, 1994).

For these reasons, there have been ongoing efforts to list SII within the *DSM* as a standalone diagnosis (e.g., APA, 2010; Kahan & Pattison, 1984). However, from our perspective, suicidal and nonsuicidal self-injury (NSSI) are better understood by focusing on the stable underlying traits that give rise to SII, rather than by adding a disorder defined primarily by a specific behavior. Developmentally, impulsive and emotionally dysregulated behaviors manifest differently across the lifespan yet they emerge because of coherent vulnerability traits (Beauchaine, Hinshaw, & Pang, 2010). Self-injurious behaviors, for example, appear initially in adolescence or early adulthood, peak during the young adult years, and often remit by later adulthood (CDC, 2008). The current diagnostic system outlines different disorders based on such developmental changes, but this system obscures continuity in risk across disorders that are common etiologically but differ topographically.

There is also debate surrounding the BPD diagnosis, particularly for adolescents. According to current convention, diagnosis of a personality disorder prior to age 18 should occur only when "maladaptive personality traits appear to be pervasive, persistent, and unlikely to be limited to a particular developmental stage or an episode of an Axis I disorder" (APA, 2000, p. 387). As a result, adherents to the *DSM* perspective question the validity of the BPD diagnosis for adolescents (see Griffiths, 2011). For these reasons, researchers examining borderline features among youth often use the construct of "borderline pathology" (BP) to describe their samples (e.g., Guzder, Paris, Zelkowitz, & Marchessault, 1996).

There is increasing evidence that *precursors to* BPD appear well before age 18 (Bradley, Zittel Conklin, & Westen, 2005; Westen & Chang, 2000). Moreover, BPD features do not appear to represent a transitory developmental stage. Rather, the presence of BP in adolescence is a risk factor for negative outcomes in adulthood (Stepp, 2012). In a large, randomly selected community cohort (Winograd, Cohen, & Chen, 2008), adolescent BPD symptoms predicted low academic and occupational attainment, low partner involvement, and relatively few attained developmental milestones 20 years later. Adolescent BP was also associated with adult borderline symptoms, a BPD diagnosis, overall impairment, and service utilization. And, even though BPD features decline during this developmental transition as a general trend (Johnson et al., 2000; Lenzenweger, Johnson, & Willett, 2004), there is high rank-order stability of criteria across time (Bornovalova, Hicks, Iacono, & McGue, 2009; Lenzenweger, 1999).

The BPD diagnosis captures a heterogeneous population (Lenzenweger et al., 2008). As with many *DSM-IV* disorders, BPD is assigned using a polythetic criterion set (APA, 2000). Any five out of nine symptoms merits a diagnosis, which produces 151 different ways to meet criteria for BPD (Skodol, Gunderson et al., 2002). In spite of this potential heterogeneity, not all combinations are equally likely, and there are common features among those with the diagnosis. Affect dysregulation is a core feature of BPD, with one study finding that more than 90% of those with the diagnosis meet this criterion (Zanarini, Frankenburg, Hennen, Reich, & Silk, 2004). In a confirmatory factor analysis of BPD criteria, a three-factor model fit the data well, including behavior dysregulation, affect dysregulation, and disturbed interpersonal relatedness (Sanislow et al., 2002). Among many competing models for understanding BPD, these three dimensions appear to characterize the borderline diagnosis best in terms of both behavioral and biological correlates (Skodol, Siever et al., 2002). However, a recent study with participants from three countries indicated that a four-factor structure fit best, including affective instability, identity problems, negative relationships, and self-harm (De Moor, Distel, Trull, & Boomsma, 2009).

Factor analytic and latent class studies have provided the preliminary empirical corpus for subtyping within the BPD diagnosis. However, these studies are all exploratory and atheoretical in nature. Moreover, neither factor nor cluster analytic procedures are well suited to address the pressing question: "are there different types of BPD patients?" Following from this question, Lenzenweger and colleagues (2008) have applied a model-based taxonomy for studying heterogeneity within the BPD diagnosis. They found three phenotypically distinct groups within the overall BPD category: Group 1 had low levels of antisocial, aggressive, and paranoid features; Group 2 showed elevated paranoid features; and Group 3 had high antisocial and aggressive features. There are almost certainly etiological differences between these three groups. Understanding these differences will be essential for early intervention and prevention efforts (see also Paris, 2007).

## ETIOLOGICAL FORMULATIONS

The following sections are informed by our biosocial developmental model of borderline personality development (Crowell et al., 2009) in which we hypothesize the following:

- Trait impulsivity and emotional sensitivity are early-emerging biological vulnerabilities that confer risk for SII, BPD, and other disorders characterized by poor behavioral control.
- Extreme emotional lability is shaped and maintained within high-risk developmental contexts, which are characterized by intermittent reinforcement of aversive behaviors paired with chronic invalidation of intense expressions of emotion.
- Over time, biological vulnerabilities interact with environmental risks to potentiate more extreme behavioral and emotion dysregulation.
- By adolescence, these Biology × Environment interactions promote a constellation of identifiable problems and maladaptive coping strategies such as SII, which indicates heightened risk for BPD.
- Early features of borderline pathology may further exacerbate risk for BPD by negatively affecting one's abilities to navigate stage-salient developmental tasks,

form appropriate interpersonal relationships, and develop healthy strategies for coping with distress.

We adhere to a developmental psychopathology perspective in which BPD and SII can be viewed as outcomes of multiple interacting risk factors, causal events, and transactional processes. This framework is particularly well suited for understanding the emergence of problems during adolescence and the continuity of these problems throughout development (Beauchaine et al., 2009; Cicchetti & Rogosch, 2002). The concepts of multifinality and equifinality are particularly useful for understanding the development of BPD (Beauchaine et al., 2009). Specifically, some youth with borderline features or SII may not develop BPD (i.e., multifinality), whereas those who develop BPD as adults may have distinct developmental trajectories that do not necessarily include borderline features or SII (i.e., equifinality). Each of the following sections is guided by our etiological theory (for other models see Fonagy, Target, & Gergely, 2000; Judd & McGlashan, 2003; Kernberg, 1967, 1975).

## FAMILIALITY AND HERITABILITY

Research on the development of BPD and SII suggests strong biological under-pinnings for both conditions. This is not surprising given that impulsivity has a heritability of approximately .80, has established neuroanatomical correlates, and predisposes to several psychiatric disorders—including SII and BPD (Beauchaine et al., 2009; Beauchaine & Neuhaus, 2008). Family and twin studies provide evidence in favor of our developmental hypothesis that trait impulsivity and emotional labil-ity are vulnerabilities for BPD and SII. These traits co-aggregate in family members of those with BPD and/or SII and are associated with dysfunction in specific yet interdependent neural systems (Crowell et al., 2009; White, Gunderson, Zanarini, & Hudson, 2003). Importantly, even though trait impulsivity and emotion dysreg-ulation have clear genetic and biological correlates, the phenotypic expression of these traits is a function of environmental risk exposure, a point to which we return below.

SII also aggregates in families and includes a clinical phenotype characterized by both suicide and suicide attempts (e.g., Brent & Mann, 2005). Family, twin, and adoption studies suggest that between 17% and 45% of the heritability of suicide is due to additive genetic effects. Across nearly every study, familial risk persists even following statistical control of psychiatric disorders. Following such adjustments, researchers have found a 2- to 12-fold elevation in rates of suicidality for first degree relatives of suicide victims (Mann et al., 2009). Although the source of familial risk for suicide is unknown, there is consistent evidence that impulsive aggressive traits and mood disorders co-aggregate in suicide pedigrees (Brent & Mann, 2005; McGirr et al., 2008; Soloff, Lynch, Kelly, Malone, & Mann, 2000; Spirito & Esposito-Smythers, 2006). Moreover, impulsive aggression appears to mediate the relation between familial risk and individual suicide outcomes (McGirr et al., 2009). In other words, impulsive aggression may be an intermediate phenotype for suicide (see also Mann et al., 2009).

The construct of impulsive aggression can be parsed into traits such as impulsivity, hostility, and aggression. At the diagnostic level, such behaviors often manifest as Cluster B personality disorders (antisocial, borderline, histrionic, and narcissistic). These disorders share a common behavioral profile of emotion and behavior dysregulation, high rates of psychiatric comorbidity, poor interpersonal relationships, high health care utilization, and elevated risk for suicide. Findings from one study suggest that familial aggregation of suicide may be explained primarily by transmission of Cluster B traits (McGirr et al., 2009).

Similarly, researchers examining BPD in twin samples report heritability coefficients between .37 and .69, with no evidence of shared environmental effects (Bornovalova, et al., 2009; Distel et al., 2008; Kendler et al., 2008; Torgersen et al., 2000). Family studies of those with BPD reveal significant familial aggregation of mood and impulse control disorders (see White et al., 2003, for a review). Recently, Zanarini, Barison, Frankenburg, Reich, and Hudson (2009) examined psychopathology in 1,580 first-degree relatives of BPD participants and 472 relatives of those with other Axis II diagnoses. They found that BPD co-aggregates with mood and anxiety disorders, alcohol and drug abuse/dependence, pain disorder, and several personality disorders (antisocial, histrionic, narcissistic, and sadistic).

Because BPD captures a highly heterogeneous population, some researchers have also examined familiality of the core features of BPD—affective, behavioral, cognitive, and interpersonal instability. These studies find that impulsivity and emotion dysregulation aggregate at higher rates within family members of BPD probands than in the relatives of those with other diagnoses (Silverman et al., 1991; Zanarini et al., 2004). In the few studies that have evaluated heritability of the component features, approximately 31% to 49% of the heritability of BPD can be attributed to additive genetic effects (Distel et al., 2010; Jang, Livesley, Vernon, & Jackson, 1996; Livesley, Jang, & Vernon, 1998).

A recent family study found that first-degree relatives of those with BPD show a three- to fourfold increase in risk for the disorder (Gunderson et al., 2011). Gunderson and colleagues also sought to evaluate whether familiality of BPD is transmitted via (1) a single latent psychopathological construct from which the core features of BPD emerge (a common pathway model) or (2) co-aggregation of separate BPD features leading to the disorder only when a sufficient number of traits reach critical levels of severity (an independent pathway model). They found modest support for the common over-the-independent-pathway model. However, other biological and familial evidence would suggest that core BPD features emerge due to distinct, albeit highly correlated, vulnerability factors (see later).

Family-level research is essential and will improve our understanding of both SII and BPD. Specifically, family designs are a powerful means of identifying trait-based vulnerabilities for disorders, even if there is phenotypic variability in the family (e.g., Beauchaine, 2009; Lahey & D'Onofrio, 2010). This phenomenon has been discussed extensively in an emerging literature on endophenotypes, or vulnerabilities that fall intermediate to the genotype-phenotype relation (Gottesman & Gould, 2003; Mann et al., 2009). Historically, twin studies have been considered the gold standard for evaluating the relative strength of heritable, shared environmental, and nonshared environmental contributions to disease and disorder. Although this model has proved reasonably useful for applying a numerical coefficient to the "heritable" risk for psychopathology, the translation of these findings into specific genetic alleles has been quite limited (see Chapter 3). Because there are few brain disorders that arise from a single genetic cause, research on the heritability of SII and BPD will benefit from further exploration of endophenotypic markers of risk.

## GENETICS AND NEUROTRANSMITTER DYSFUNCTION

Over the past decade, genetic and other biological research on SII and BPD has increased exponentially. A majority of studies focus on genes and neurotransmitters that are presumed to underlie impulsivity and affective instability—underlying vulnerabilities to both SII and BPD. Thus, we focus our discussion on the two relevant monamine neurotransmitter systems that have received the most attention: serotonin (5HT) and dopamine (DA). Although our review is circumscribed, other biological systems have also received attention in the literature. Functional magnetic resonance imaging (fMRI) studies have identified dysfunctional activation patterns and reduced functional connectivity within fronto-limbic regions of the brain (see Hughes, Crowell, Uyeji, & Coan, 2012, for a review). Measures of peripheral psychophysiology have revealed differences among those with BPD and SII versus controls across the biological systems that govern behavioral inhibition and emotion regulation abilities (Crowell, Beauchaine et al., in press; Crowell et al., 2005; Kuo & Linehan, 2009; Thorell, 2009). Finally, theoretical and empirical work highlights possible dysregulation of acetylcholine, norepinephrine, endogenous opioids, and the limbic-hypothalamic-pituitary-adrenal axis (LHPA; Bandelow, Schmahl, Falkai, & Wedekind, 2010; Coryell & Schlesser, 2001). Readers are referred to Depue and Lenzenweger (2001, 2005) for integrative reviews of neurotransmitter dysfunction (see also Beauchaine et al., 2009; Crowell et al., 2009; Depue, 2009; Gurvits, Koenigsberg, & Siever, 2000).

Relations between behavior and dysregulated neurotransmitter activity are extremely complex (see Bandelow et al., 2010; Beauchaine, Neuhaus, Zalewski, Crowell, & Potapova, 2011). However, across both animal and human studies, 5HT activity is associated with impulsive aggression, trait and state anxiety, and mood regulation (see, e.g., Christianson et al., 2010; Silva et al., 2010; van Goozen, Fairchild, Snoek, & Harold, 2007), whereas DA activity is linked to novelty-seeking, reward dependence, impulsivity, and aggression (Beauchaine et al., 2010; Beauchaine & Neuhaus, 2008; Buckholtz et al., 2010; Castellanos & Tannock, 2002; Cloninger, 1986, 1987; Depue & Collins, 1999; Sagvolden, Aase, Johansen, & Russell, 2005). However, it is important to note that these distinctions oversimplify the functional role that neurotransmitters play in shaping behavior. For example, DA contributes to at least some aspects of both mood and emotion regulation (e.g., Ashby, Isen, & Turken, 1999; Dremencov, el Mansari, & Blier, 2009; Forbes & Dahl, 2012), and 5HT modulates mesolimbic dopamine activity (Adell & Artigas, 2004). Thus, these neurotransmitter systems are interdependent in their effects on behavior. We review each in turn below.

## DOPAMINE

As with all biological systems, DA networks are sensitive to environmental input. This sensitivity can confer risk or benefit, depending upon contextual factors, child temperament, and the age at which a stressor is encountered (Cicchetti & Valentino, 2006; see also Chapter 8). In some cases, adaptations within these systems can also confer risk for psychopathology (e.g., prenatal insults, abuse or neglect, or recreational drug use; Beauchaine et al., 2011; Gatzke-Kopp, 2011; Mead, Beauchaine, & Shannon, 2010). Specific effects on the DA system vary, depending on the nature and timing of environmental events.

There is consensus that DA dysfunction contributes to some of the behavioral traits seen in BPD, including SII (Osuch & Payne, 2009; Sher & Stanley, 2009). Several researchers hypothesize *hyper*-activation in one or more of the DA systems (Friedel, 2004; Skodol, Siever et al., 2002). These researchers suggest that psychotic-like symptoms in BPD may emerge due to an excess of dopamine, drawing upon the limited evidence in favor of antipsychotic treatment for these BPD features (e.g., Lieb, Völlm, Rücker, Timmer, & Stoffers, 2010). In one small study (Grootens et al., 2008), BPD patients with psychotic-like symptoms performed similar to those with schizophrenia on an eye-saccade task, whereas BPD participants without psychotic symptoms performed similar to typical controls. However, the few fMRI and PET studies to date are largely inconsistent with the *hyper*-activation hypothesis. In a recent review, O'Neill & Frodl (in press) evaluated the literature on fMRI and PET studies of BPD. They report volume reductions across several dopaminergically innervated structures that are implicated in reward processing and motivated behavior, including the anterior cingulate cortex (ACC) and the dorsolateral prefrontal cortex (DLPFC). Moreover, across most of these studies, BPD participants showed hypometabolism across these and other dopaminergically innervated areas, such as the caudate nucleus. Taken together, these studies present a picture where BPD is characterized by dopaminergic deficiencies, similar to other impulse control disorders.

Indeed, even though up to 40% of those with BPD report transient, psychotic-like experiences (Zanarini, Gunderson, & Frankenburg, 1990), symptoms of anger, impulsivity, and affective instability are far more common (affecting 80% to 90% of those with the diagnosis) and more stable (McGlashan et al., 2005). Empirical research with depressed adults (e.g., Epstein et al., 2006), adolescents (Forbes & Dahl, 2012), and impulsive children and adolescents (e.g., Beauchaine et al., 2010; Bush et al., 1999; Vaidya et al., 1998) suggests that anger, impulsivity, and affective instability are attributable to *attenuated* mesolimbic DA functioning. There is also evidence of DA dysfunction among individuals at risk for suicide. For example, the authors of one study (Roy, Karoum, & Pollack, 1992) found that depressed suicide attempters had significantly reduced peripheral markers of DA (homovanillic acid, dihydroxy-phenylacetic acid, and total body output of DA) compared with depressed patients who had never attempted suicide. Moreover, patients who reattempted suicide during a 5-year follow-up had significantly smaller urinary outputs of homovanillic acid and total DA than patients who did not reattempt suicide, who had never attempted suicide, and typical controls. This study confirmed earlier studies (Roy, Dejong, &

Linnoila, 1989), suggesting that decreased DA neurotransmission may contribute to suicidal behavior. Another study found evidence of reduced DA turnover in the basal ganglia of depressed suicide victims (Bowden et al., 1997). Finally, data from challenge tests using apomorphine (a DA agonist) have indicated that compared with controls, a smaller response is observed among depressed (Pitchot, Hansenne, Moreno, & Ansseau, 1992) and nondepressed (Pitchot, Hansenne, & Ansseau, 2001) suicide attempters and also suicide victims (Pitchot, Reggers et al., 2001). In sum, findings suggest reduced DA among suicidal individuals.

Studies of DA among those with BPD are more limited. In a small sample of adults with BPD with or without nonsuicidal self-injury, there were no differences between the NSSI and no-NSSI groups in their cerebrospinal fluid levels of DA or 5HT (Stanley et al., 2010). Unfortunately, the authors did not include a non-BPD group for comparison. In a genetic association study of depressed adults, BPD symptoms were associated with differences on the 9-repeat allele of the dopamine transporter gene (DAT1, SLC6A3), even when childhood abuse and neglect were included in the statistical models (Joyce et al., 2006). In another study conducted with two independent samples of young adults, the DRD4–616 C/G promoter variant was associated with BPD. In these same samples, two DRD2 polymorphisms (Taq1A and Taq1B) were related to impulsive, self-damaging behaviors (Nemoda et al., 2010). Again, these findings are consistent with a *hypo*dopaminergic model of BPD. However, given the heterogeneity of the BPD diagnosis, further research with well-defined samples is essential. Moreover, small-scale genetic association studies should be interpreted with caution until the findings are replicated in studies that test Gene × Gene *and* Gene × Environment interactions.

## Serotonin

Evidence suggests that impulsive aggression and mood dysregulation are linked to specific genetic polymorphisms and functional impairments within the 5HT system. Deficits in central 5HT have been associated consistently with mood disorders, suicidal behaviors, and aggression (Kamali, Oquendo, & Mann, 2002). Across numerous studies, individuals with personality disorders, including BPD, show a blunted prolactin response to fenfluramine challenge, suggesting reduced central 5HT activity (e.g., Soloff, 2000). Genetic studies have focused on several 5HT candidate genes including those that code for tryptophan hydroxylase (TPH; a rate limiting enzyme in the biosynthesis of 5HT); the promoter region of the serotonin transporter (5HTTlpr); the 5HT1b, 5HT1a, and 5HT2a receptors; and others (Ni, Chan, Chan, McMain, & Kennedy, 2009; Skodol, Siever et al., 2002).

Several studies of 5HT function among both adolescents and adults have supported a role for this neurotransmitter in SII (Mann, 2003; Osuch & Payne, 2009; Zalsman et al., 2011). A postmortem study of suicide victims found higher levels of 5HT2A receptors, 5HT2A proteins, and mRNA expression in the prefrontal and hippocampal areas of adolescent suicide victims (Pandey et al., 2002). Research on the genetics of 5HT in SII has focused on several candidate genes (e.g., 5HTR1A, 5HTR1B) and the serotonin transporter (5HTT). The 5HTR1A gene has been of interest in genetics studies based on findings of deficient 5HT1A receptors in the midbrain and ventral PFC of depressed suicide victims (Arango, Huang, Underwood, & Mann, 2003).

Similarly, research on the 5HTR1B gene emerged following findings that $5HT_{1B}$-knockout mice are impulsive, aggressive, and more likely to self-administer drugs and alcohol (Zhuang et al., 1999). Brezo and colleagues (2010) followed over 1,200 individuals for 22 years, and found that three variants of the $5HTR_{2A}$ gene interacted with physical and/or sexual abuse histories to predict later suicidal behavior. Moreover, these genes differed from those that interacted with stress to predict depression, suggesting that depression and suicidality may have partially independent etiological pathways. However, genetic research to date has produced conflicting results, with the gene coding for the serotonin transporter (5HTT) being the most promising link between 5HT and self-inflicted injury (Zalsman, 2010).

Several studies indicate that individuals with the short allele (i.e., *s/s* or *s/l* genotypes) are more likely than *l/l* individuals to engage in suicidal behavior (Anguelova, Benkelfat, & Turecki, 2003) or to have committed suicide by violent means (Lin & Tsai, 2004). Although further work is needed, evidence suggests that individuals with BPD also have fewer platelet serotonin transporter binding sites and that this variability is likely due to polymorphisms of the 5HTT gene (Greenberg et al., 1999; however see Pascual et al., 2008 for an alternative finding). Across a majority of studies, the short allele of the 5HTTLPR is associated with increased risk for psychopathology, particularly among those exposed to environmental adversity. For example, the interaction between short allele status (*s/s* or *s/l*) and stressful life events predicted higher impulsivity scores among adults with BPD (Wagner, Baskaya, Lieb, Dahmen, & Tadifa, 2009). In a high-risk sample of young adults followed from infancy, Lyons-Ruth (e.g., 2008) found that each short allele of the 5HTTLPR conferred a twofold increased risk for borderline or antisocial features, such that those with the *s/s* polymorphism were at fourfold greater risk.

Another prospective study assessed variation in the 5HTTLPR gene and suicide ideation among maltreated and control children from low-SES backgrounds (Cicchetti, Rogosch, Sturge-Apple, & Toth, 2010). As predicted, maltreated children were at highest risk for suicidal ideation, regardless of the number of *s* alleles. Similarly, *s* allele status did not predict suicidal ideation for youth who experienced multiple forms of abuse. However, when risk exposure was lower (1 to 2 types of abuse versus 3 to 4) *s*-allele carriers (*s/s, s/l*) demonstrated higher levels of suicidal ideation than *l/l*-allele carriers. This finding converges with other reports in the literature (see McGuffin et al., 2010; Uher & McGuffin, 2009).

## OTHER BIOLOGICAL VULNERABILITIES

In addition to affecting neurotransmitter systems, chronic stress also leads to elevated LHPA axis responses. Furthermore, there is increasing evidence that the LHPA axis is involved in suicidal behavior. This evidence comes from studies using the dexamethasone suppression test (DST), a challenge of LHPA axis reactivity. Although the DST is not a useful indicator of depression because many who are depressed do not exhibit abnormal LHPA axis functioning (see Beauchaine & Marsh, 2006), nonsuppression of cortisol in response to the DST among depressed individuals predicts heightened risk for future suicide. Coryell and Schlesser (2001) followed a group of depressed patients over 15 years and found that nonsuppressors were at 14-fold greater risk of death by suicide than those who suppressed cortisol in response to the DST. This finding is supported by meta-analytic results indicating that cortisol nonsuppression is predictive of later death by suicide (Lester, 1992). Although studies of the DST among individuals with BPD are limited, findings suggest that cortisol nonsuppression may be related to SII, PTSD, and/or a history of abuse, rather than a diagnosis of BPD or depression (Krishnan, Davidson, Rayasam, & Shope, 1984; Wingenfeld, Spitzer, Rullkötter, & Löwe, 2010).

There is also emerging interest in the neurobiological correlates of affiliation and the role of this trait in personality disorders, including BPD (Depue & Lenzenweger, 2005). High affiliation is a measurable personality trait characterized by warmth, affection, and the tendency to enjoy/value close interpersonal bonds. The biological systems involved in affiliation include norepinephrine, oxytocin, vasopressin, and endogenous opiate activity (Heinrichs & Domes, 2008; Lenzenweger, 2010). Stanley and Siever (2010) propose that individuals with BPD have a vulnerability for low basal opioid levels in limbic circuitry such as the cingulate cortex and the amygdale, paired with a compensatory supersensitivity of $\mu$-opioid receptors. The opioid system plays a key mediating role in self-soothing, separation distress, and pain associated with social exclusion. The $\mu$-opioid receptors are implicated in social and affect regulation. Stanley and Siever argue that transient increases in opioid activity may lead to exaggerated responses to painful stimuli and to negative experiences or emotions.

Furthermore, Stanley and Siever (2010) hypothesize that oxytocin dysregulation may contribute to the difficulty those with BPD experience in establishing trust, reading social cues, and forming appropriate attachments, whereas vasopressin dysregulation may affect the regulation of aggression within intimate relationships. Disruptions to these systems could result in the low affiliative capacity often observed among those with BPD. Dysregulation of the opioid system could emerge via several developmental pathways (genetic vulnerabilities, chronic stress, acute separation, variability in parent-child attachments, etc.).

Other neuroanatomical studies of suicide risk and BPD have focused on the prefrontal cortex (PFC), particularly the ventromedial PFC and its connections with the amygdale (see Hughes et al., 2012, for a recent review). One theory (see Mann, 2003) is that the PFC inhibits impulsive behavior by providing insight into consequences of future actions. Thus, deficits within the PFC may contribute to suicidal and other impulsive behaviors through a diminished capacity to inhibit strong impulses. The ventromedial PFC is rich in both DA- and 5-HT-modulated neurons and is densely connected with the basolateral amygdala, a limbic structure involved in processing emotional and social cues (Le Doux, 1992; Shaw et al., 2005). Changes in amygdala and PFC activation can be measured reliably in fMRI studies where individuals are instructed to regulate emotional responses (e.g., Schaefer et al., 2002). Theories outlining the relation between frontolimbic dysfunction and

BPD suggest that dysfunction of the neural circuitry of emotion regulation leads to impulsive aggression (e.g., Davidson, Putnam, & Larson, 2000). Thus, functional or structural abnormalities within these regions or their interconnections could lead to some of the core deficits seen in BPD.

There is also a rich theoretical literature linking autonomic nervous system (ANS) measures to the central nervous system substrates of various behavioral traits and psychopathological conditions (e.g., Beauchaine, 2001). Of particular relevance to the development of BPD may be the functioning of the parasympathetic nervous system (PNS). PNS activity can be indexed by respiratory sinus arrhythmia (RSA), a marker of vagal influence on cardiac function (see Berntson et al., 1997). Both theoretical and empirical findings suggest that individual differences in RSA are associated with emotion regulation and social affiliative behaviors, with reduced RSA conferring risk for psychopathology and heightened RSA buffering against such risk (Beauchaine, 2001; Katz & Gottman, 1997). Thus, individuals at risk for BPD may also show reduced RSA under emotionally evocative stimulus conditions. In support of this hypothesis, self-injuring adolescents exhibit reduced RSA, both at baseline and during emotion evocation, compared with typical controls (Crowell et al., 2005). Several physiological studies also indicate that BPD and SII are characterized by attenuated electrodermal responding (EDR)—a peripheral biomarker of trait impulsivity (Crowell, Beauchaine et al., 2012; Ebner-Priemer et al., 2005; Herpertz, Kunert, Schwenger, & Sass, 1999; Schmahl et al., 2004; Thorell, 2009). Indeed, reduced EDR is common to many disorders characterized by poor behavioral inhibition (e.g., ADHD, conduct disorder, antisocial personality disorder). Future studies could examine whether attenuated EDR and/or low RSA interact with contextual stressors to heighten risk for BPD.

## CONTEXTUAL AND FAMILY RISK FACTORS

Extant research suggests that two core features of BPD, poor impulse control and emotion dysregulation, have identifiable biological correlates. However, as noted previously, the ways in which these traits manifest are a product of environmental risk exposure. For example, impulsive youth raised in high-risk neighborhoods are at increased risk for substance use, teen pregnancy, and involvement with the juvenile justice system relative to impulsive youth raised in protective neighborhood contexts (Lynam et al., 2000). Furthermore, biometric models of twin data indicate that all externalizing disorders can be traced to a single, highly heritable latent trait. However, at the level of each individual disorder, there is significant variance attributable to environmental effects (Krueger et al., 2002). The implication is that contextual risk contributes to diagnostic heterogeneity observed in family studies, even when vulnerability traits are highly heritable.

There are a number of accounts of family-level risk factors for BPD (Barnow, Spitzer, Grabe, Kessler, & Freyberger, 2006). However, we draw from the extensive literature on the emergence of mood lability among impulsive youth (see Beauchaine et al., 2009; Snyder, Edwards, McGraw, & Kilgore, 1994; Snyder, Schrepferman, & St. Peter, 1997). Family processes that shape emotion dysregulation have been well delineated in such samples and may translate well to youth at risk for BPD (Beauchaine et al., 2009). In fact, we have suggested that extreme emotional lability observed among those with BPD is shaped and maintained in high-risk developmental contexts characterized by intermittent reinforcement of emotionally labile behaviors *and* chronic invalidation of intense emotional experience (Crowell et al., 2009). Because our model is transactional and ecological, we acknowledge that (a) children play an active role in shaping their environment and (b) the family system is affected by variables other than parenting (e.g., financial strain, isolation). Still, we briefly review the literature on parenting and parent-child interactions, which provide a rich target for intervention.

Researchers studying the development of externalizing behavior problems have found that repeated escalating exchanges between children and their parents function as a training ground for emotionally labile behavior patterns, contributing to the emergence oppositional defiant disorder, conduct disorder, and ASPD (Beauchaine, Gatzke-Kopp, & Mead, 2007; Patterson, Chamberlain, & Reid, 1982; Patterson, DeBaryshe, & Ramsey, 1989; Patterson, Dishion, & Bank, 1984). These interactions often involve negative reinforcement of emotional outbursts (e.g., a tantrum is negatively reinforced when the parent withdraws the request to tidy up), excessive verbosity and nagging (e.g., prolonged debates following requests), and excessive threats of punishment that are often not followed through.

Although developed independently, Linehan's (1993) developmental model of BPD proposes that the disorder emerges, in part, due to an invalidating caregiving environment. Within this context, a child's expressions of emotion are often rejected, invalidated, or disregarded. As a consequence, the child learns to inhibit his/her emotions, especially those that are negative and unpleasant, or she/he learns to escalate emotions to a level needed to generate a response from caregivers. Thus, invalidating environments haphazardly punish emotional expressions, while intermittently reinforcing extreme emotional displays.

Common to both of these models is the theory that emotional lability is shaped within families via operant conditioning. The theories differ, however, in their hypotheses regarding when and why emotional outbursts occur. In Patterson's coercion model, aversive behaviors emerge as a means of avoiding demands, whereas Linehan suggests that negative affect increases when the child has unmet emotional needs. Both processes may occur in youth at risk for BPD (see Beauchaine et al., 2009), but it is also possible that distinct operant conditioning patterns contribute to multifinality in the development of ASPD and BPD. Children at risk for BPD may also evoke different parenting strategies than children on an antisocial trajectory. Importantly, boys with ASPD and girls with BPD often come from the same families (Goldman, D'Angelo, & DeMaso, 1993), suggesting that there are common vulnerabilities and risks for the two disorders.

To our knowledge, there are no longitudinal studies examining parenting practices as a prospective marker of risk for BPD or SII. However, several lines of research suggest that family processes may contribute to psychopathology, especially among youth who are vulnerable biologically (Beauchaine et al., 2009; Crowell et al., 2009). For example, a recent study examined the role of "proximal processes" in the development of schizoid personality disorder (Lenzenweger, 2010). Proximal processes are parenting behaviors that facilitate development (e.g., problem solving, doing creative activities, or developing and pursuing mutual goals), which is consistent with Vygotsky's (1978) theory on the *zone of proximal development*. In this study, there was an absence of recalled proximal processes among adults with schizoid personality disorder. This introduces a potential direction for future prospective studies of personality development and borderline pathology.

Given the complex interplay between biological and psychosocial risks, research on borderline personality development would benefit from studies that examine both. Although cross-sectional, in a study of self-injuring adolescents and their mothers, dyads in the SII group expressed higher levels of negative affect and lower levels of positive affect and cohesiveness during a conflict task (Crowell et al., 2008b). Furthermore, adolescent serotonin levels interacted with dyadic negativity and conflict, accounting for 64% of the variance in self-injury. Unfortunately, many studies of SII and BPD do not assess these Biology × Environment interactions, which may explain the contradictory findings on family risk factors and the development of clinical problems.

For example, research examining neglect and abuse has produced conflicting results, possibly because biological vulnerabilities were not assessed. Although several studies have reported increased risk for SII among victims of abuse (see Lang & Sharma-Patel, 2011, for a recent review), a recent meta-analysis reported that the relationship between childhood sexual abuse (CSA) and SII is relatively small (Klonsky & Moyer, 2008). The authors concluded that CSA is not causal in the development of SII and instead believe that the two are modestly related due to their correlation with the same psychiatric risk factors. However, the studies included in this meta-analysis did not assess biological factors, such as the short allele of the 5HTTLPR.

Similarly, the relation between childhood abuse and BPD has also been debated extensively. Many individuals with BPD describe a history of neglect, broadly defined (92%), physical abuse (25% to 73%), and/or sexual abuse (40% to 76%; Zanarini, 2000). Thus, researchers have examined trauma as one etiological factor in the development of BPD (Gratz, Latzman, Tull, Reynolds, & Lejuez, 2011; Soloff, Lynch, & Kelly, 2002). Recently, Zanarini and colleagues examined retrospective reports of childhood sexual abuse among the BPD participants enrolled in their 10-year longitudinal study (2011). They reported six predictors of self-injury: (1) female sex, (2) dysphoric cognitions, (3) dissociative symptoms, (4) depression, (5) history of childhood sexual abuse, and (6) sexual assaults as an adult. Thus, traumatic experiences may increase risk for SII among those with BPD. Again, the authors did not assess biological or potentially heritable vulnerability factors.

The retrospective nature of these studies is a significant limitation. However, several recent studies have evaluated abuse and borderline pathology in children and adolescents or in prospective studies. For example, Gratz and colleagues (2011) examined BP features in a sample of 225 8- to 11-year-old children. In their sample, impulsivity, affective instability, and emotional abuse each accounted for a significant amount of the variance in childhood BP features. They also examined the interaction between affective dysfunction and emotional abuse and found that emotional abuse predicated BP features for youth who were high on affect dysregulation, but not for those who scored low on this trait. In a prospective longitudinal study, Widom, Czaja, and Paris (2009) followed 500 children with a documented history of abuse or neglect and a matched, nonvictimized comparison group. Not surprisingly, abuse/neglect predicted several clinical problems in adulthood, including BPD. Although there appears to be a relation between BPD and childhood maltreatment, researchers highlight the importance of viewing no single event as causal in the pathogenesis of BPD (Zanarini et al., 1998). The current consensus is that even though histories of abuse are common among individuals with BPD, they are neither necessary nor sufficient for the development of the disorder (Zanarini et al., 1997).

## THEORETICAL SYNTHESIS AND FUTURE DIRECTIONS

In sum, BPD and SII likely emerge due to repeated, complex interactions between biological vulnerabilities and contextual stressors. The relative weights of these vulnerabilities and risk factors are likely to vary widely across individuals and developmental stages. Thus, it is not surprising that different studies have identified distinct constellations of vulnerability and risk. In this review, we have presented our biosocial developmental model of BPD and presented evidence in favor of our first three developmental hypotheses.

We also suggest that by adolescence, there are a constellation of identifiable problems and maladaptive coping strategies, such as SII, that indicate heightened risk for BPD (Hypothesis 4). To test this hypothesis, self-injuring adolescents will need to be followed into adulthood. A short-term longitudinal study may be effective (e.g., 5- to 10-year follow-up), as BPD typically emerges by early adulthood. There is preliminary evidence to suggest that adolescent self-injurers differ from depressed teens (the diagnostic group to which most self-injuring adolescents are assigned) in ways that may be relevant for the development of BPD. In a recent study, SII adolescents scored higher than depressed participants on concurrent measures of externalizing psychopathology, emotion dysregulation, and BPD features (Crowell, Derbidge et al., in press). SII participants also exhibited attenuated electrodermal responding, a peripheral biomarker of trait impulsivity. Thus, SII participants evidence a pattern of risk and vulnerability factors that may predispose a subset of these adolescents to later BPD.

Finally, we theorize that BP features may further exacerbate risk for BPD by affecting a person's ability to navigate stage-salient developmental tasks, form appropriate interpersonal relationships, and develop healthy strategies for coping with distress. Although longitudinal studies following youth with BP features are only beginning to emerge (e.g., Bernstein, Cohen, Skodol, Bezirganian, & Brook, 1996; Burke & Stepp, 2012; Crick, Murray-Close, & Woods, 2005; Stepp, Burke, Hipwell, & Loeber, 2012), there can be little doubt that borderline traits contribute to significant functional impairment, interpersonal distress, difficulties with identity and self-image, and risk for suicide. Unfortunately, the BPD diagnosis is highly stigmatized, which has contributed to a broad unwillingness to identify and treat adolescents for borderline features. However, providing early intervention, even for those youth who meet only one or two diagnostic criteria, could fundamentally alter a child's developmental trajectory away from BPD and toward healthier and more adaptive outcomes.

## REFERENCES

Adell, A., & Artigas, F. (2004). The somatodendritic release of dopamine in the ventral tegmental area and its regulation by afferent transmitter systems. *Neuroscience and Biobehavioral Reviews, 28*, 415–431.

American Psychiatric Association. (1980). *Diagnostic and statistical manual of mental disorders* (3rd ed.). Washington, DC: Author.

American Psychiatric Association. (2000). *Diagnostic and statistical manual of mental disorders* (4th ed., text rev.). Washington, DC: Author.

American Psychiatric Association. (2006). *Practice guidelines for the treatment of psychiatric disorders: Compendium.* Arlington, VA: Author.

American Psychiatric Association. (2010). DSM-5 development: Non-suicidal self-injury. Retrieved from http://www.dsm5.org/ProposedRevisions/Pages/proposedrevision.aspx?rid=443

Anguelova, M., Benkelfat, C., & Turecki, G. (2003). A systematic review of association studies investigating genes coding for serotonin receptors and the serotonin transporter: II. Suicidal behavior. *Molecular Psychiatry, 8*, 646–653.

Arango, V., Huang, Y.-Y., Underwood, M. D., & Mann, J. J. (2003). Genetics of the serotonergic system in suicidal behavior. *Journal of Psychiatric Research, Brain Imaging, and Post-Mortem Studies in Affective Disorders, 37*, 375–386.

Ashby, G., Isen, A., & Turken, A. (1999). A neuropsychological theory of positive affect and its influence on cognition. *Psychological Review, 106*, 529–550.

Bandelow, B., Schmahl, C., Falkai, P., & Wedekind, D. (2010). Borderline personality disorder: A dysregulation of the endogenous opioid system? *Psychological Review, 117*, 623–636.

Barnow, S., Spitzer, C., Grabe, H. J., Kessler, C., & Freyberger, H. J. (2006). Individual characteristics, familial experience, and psychopathology in children of mothers with borderline personality disorder. *Journal of the American Academy of Child and Adolescent Psychiatry, 45*, 965–972.

Beauchaine, T. P. (2001). Vagal tone, development, and Gray's motivational theory: Toward an integrated model of autonomic nervous system functioning in psychopathology. *Development and Psychopathology, 13*, 183–214.

Beauchaine, T. P. (2009). Role of biomarkers and endophenotypes in prevention and treatment of psychopathological disorders. *Biomarkers in Medicine, 3*, 1–3.

Beauchaine, T. P., Gatzke-Kopp, L., & Mead, H. K. (2007). Polyvagal theory and developmental psychopathology: Emotion dysregulation and conduct problems from preschool to adolescence. *Biological Psychology, 74*, 174–184.

Beauchaine, T. P., Hinshaw, S. P., & Pang, K. L. (2010). Comorbidity of attention-deficit/hyperactivity disorder and early-onset conduct disorder: Biological, environmental, and developmental mechanisms. *Clinical Psychology: Science and Practice, 17,* 327–336.

Beauchaine, T. P., Klein, D. N., Crowell, S. E., Derbidge, C., & Gatzke-Kopp, L. (2009). Multifinality in the development of personality disorders: A biology × sex × environment interaction model of antisocial and borderline traits. *Development and Psychopathology, 21,* 735–770.

Beauchaine, T. P., & Marsh, P. (2006). Taxometric methods: Enhancing early detection and prevention of psychopathology by identifying latent vulnerability traits. In D. Cicchetti & D. Cohen (Eds.), *Developmental psychopathology* (2nd ed., pp. 931–967). Hoboken, NJ: Wiley.

Beauchaine, T. P., & Neuhaus, E. (2008). Impulsivity and vulnerability to psychopathology. In T. P. Beauchaine & S. P. Hinshaw (Eds.), *Child and adolescent psychopathology* (pp. 129–156). Hoboken, NJ: Wiley.

Beauchaine, T. P., Neuhaus, E., Brenner, S., & Gatzke-Kopp, L. (2008). Ten good reasons to consider biological processes in prevention and intervention research. *Development and Psychopathology, 20,* 745–774.

Beauchaine, T. P., Neuhaus, E., Zalewski, M., Crowell, S. E., & Potapova, N. (2011). The effects of allostatic load on neural systems subserving motivation, mood regulation, and social affiliation. *Development and Psychopathology, 23,* 975–999.

Bemporad, J. R., Smith, H. F., Hanson, G., & Cicchetti, D. (1982). Borderline syndromes in childhood: Criteria for diagnosis. *American Journal of Psychiatry, 139,* 596–602.

Berman, A. L., Jobes, D. A., & Silverman, M. M. (2006). *Adolescent suicide: Assessment and intervention* (2nd ed.). Washington, DC: American Psychological Association.

Bernstein, D. P., Cohen, P., Skodol, A., Bezirganian, S., & Brook, J. S. (1996). Childhood antecedents of adolescent personality disorders. *American Journal of Psychiatry, 153,* 907–913.

Berntson, G. G., Bigger, T. J., Eckberg, D. L., Grossman, P., Kaufmann, P. G., Malik, M., . . . van der Molen, M. W. (1997). Heart rate variability: Origins, methods, and interpretive caveats. *Psychophysiology, 34,* 623–648.

Bornovalova, M. A., Hicks, B. M., Iacono, W. G., & McGue, M. (2009). Stability, change, and heritability of borderline personality disorder traits from adolescence to adulthood: A longitudinal twin study. *Development and Psychopathology, 21,* 1335–1353.

Bowden, C., Cheetham, S. C., Lowther, S., Katona, C. L. E., Crompton, M. R., & Horton, R. W. (1997). Reduced dopamine turnover in the basal ganglia of depressed suicides. *Brain Research, 769,* 135–140.

Bradley, R., Zittel Conklin, C., & Westen, D. (2005). The borderline personality diagnosis in adolescents: Gender differences and subtypes. *Journal of Child Psychology and Psychiatry, 46,* 1006–1019.

Brent, D. A., & Mann, J. J. (2005). Family genetic studies, suicide, and suicidal behavior. *American Journal of Medical Genetics Part C: Seminars in Medical Genetics, 133C,* 13–24.

Brezo, J., Bureau, A., Merette, C., Jomphe, V., Barker, E. D., Vitaro, F., & Turecki, G. (2010). Differences and similarities in the serotonergic diathesis for suicide attempts and mood disorders: A 22-year longitudinal gene-environment study. *Molecular Psychiatry, 15,* 831–843.

Buckholtz, J. W., Treadway, M. T., Cowan, R. L., Woodward, N. D., Li, R., Ansari, M. S., . . . Zald, D. H. (2010). Dopaminergic network differences in human impulsivity. *Science, 329,* 532–532.

Burke, J. D., & Stepp, S. D. (2012). Adolescent disruptive behavior and borderline personality disorder symptoms in young adult men. *Journal of Abnormal Child Psychology, 40,* 35–44.

Bush, G., Frazier, J. A., Rauch, S. L., Seidman, L. J., Whalen, P. J., Jenike, M. A., . . . Biederman, J. (1999). Anterior cingulate cortex dysfunction in attention-deficit/hyperactivity disorder revealed by fMRI and the counting stroop. *Biological Psychiatry, 45,* 1542–1552.

Castellanos, F. X., & Tannock, R. (2002). Neuroscience of attention-deficit/hyperactivity disorder: The search for endophenotypes. *Nature Reviews. Neuroscience, 3,* 617–628.

Centers for Disease Control and Prevention. (2009). Injury prevention & control: Violence prevention. Retrieved from http://www.cdc.gov/ViolencePrevention/pub/youth_suicide.html

Centers for Disease Control and Prevention. (2008). *National hospital ambulatory medical care survey: 2008 emergency department summary tables.* 1–32. Retrieved from http://www.cdc.gov/nchs/fastats/suicide.htm

Christianson, J. P., Ragole, T., Amat, J., Greenwood, B. N., Strong, P. V., Paul, E. D., . . . Maier, S. F. (2010). 5-Hydroxytryptamine 2C receptors in the basolateral amygdala are involved in the expression of anxiety after uncontrollable traumatic stress. *Biological Psychiatry, 67,* 339–345.

Cicchetti, D., & Rogosch, F. A. (1996). Equifinality and multifinality in developmental psychopathology. *Development and Psychopathology, 8,* 597–600.

Cicchetti, D., & Rogosch, F. A. (2002). A developmental psychopathology perspective on adolescence. *Journal of Consulting and Clinical Psychology, 70,* 6–20.

Cicchetti, D., Rogosch, F. A., Sturge-Apple, M., & Toth, S. L. (2010). Interaction of child maltreatment and 5-HTT polymorphisms: Suicidal ideation among children from low-SES backgrounds. *Journal of Pediatric Psychology, 35,* 536–546.

Cicchetti, D., & Valentino, K. (2006). An ecological-transactional perspective on child maltreatment: Failure of the average expectable environment and its influence on child development. In D. Cicchetti & D. J. Cohen (Eds.), *Developmental psychopathology, Vol. 3: Risk, disorder, and adaptation* (2nd ed., pp. 129–201). Hoboken, NJ: Wiley.

Clark, L. A. (2005). Temperament as a unifying basis for personality and psychopathology. *Journal of Abnormal Psychology, 114,* 505–521.

Cloninger, C. R. (1986). A unified biosocial theory of personality and its role in the development of anxiety states. *Psychiatric Developments, 4,* 167–226.

Cloninger, C. R. (1987). A systematic method for clinical description and classification of personality variants. A proposal. *Archives of General Psychiatry, 44,* 573–588.

Coryell, W., & Schlesser, M. (2001). The dexamethasone suppression test and suicide prediction. *American Journal of Psychiatry, 158,* 748–753.

Crick, N. R., Murray-Close, D., & Woods, K. (2005). Borderline personality features in childhood: A short-term longitudinal study. *Development and Psychopathology, 17*, 1051–1070.

Crowell, S. E., Beauchaine, T. P., Hsiao, R. C., Vasilev, C. A., Yaptangco, M., Linehan, M. M., McCauley, E. (2012). Differentiating adolescent self-injury from adolescent depression: Possible implications for borderline personality development. *Journal of Abnormal Child Psychology, 40*, 45–57.

Crowell, S. E., Beauchaine, T. P., & Linehan, M. M. (2009). A biosocial developmental model of borderline personality: Elaborating and extending Linehan's theory. *Psychological Bulletin, 135*, 495–510.

Crowell, S. E., Beauchaine, T. P., McCauley, E., Smith, C., Stevens, A. L., & Sylvers, P. D. (2005). Psychological, physiological, and serotonergic correlates of para-suicidal behavior among adolescent girls. *Development and Psychopathology, 17*, 1105–1127.

Crowell, S. E., Beauchaine, T. P., McCauley, E., Smith, C. J., Vasilev, C. A., & Stevens, A. L. (2008). Parent-child interactions, peripheral serotonin, and self-inflicted injury in adolescents. *Journal of Consulting and Clinical Psychology, 76*, 15–21.

Crowell, S. E., Derbidge, C. M., & Beauchaine, T. P. (in press). Developmental approaches to understanding suicidal and self-injurious behaviors. In M. K. Nock (Ed.), *Oxford handbook of suicide and self-injury*. Oxford, United Kingdom: Oxford University Press.

Davidson, R. J., Putnam, K. M., & Larson, C. L. (2000). Dysfunction in the neural circuitry of emotion regulation—A possible prelude to violence. *Science, 289*, 591–594.

De La Fuente, J. M., & Bobes, J. (2009). Editorial: Issues for DSM-V: I, including biological variables to objectively comfort the clinical diagnosis of borderline personality disorder; and II, proposing a new subcategory to be included in the criteria sets for further study. *International Journal of Social Psychiatry, 55*, 195–197.

De Moor, M. H. M., Distel, M. A., Trull, T. J., & Boomsma, D. I. (2009). Assessment of borderline personality features in population samples: Is the personality assessment inventory–borderline features scale measurement invariant across sex and age? *Psychological Assessment, 21*, 125–130.

Depue, R. A. (2009). Genetic, environmental, and epigenetic factors in the development of personality disturbance. *Development and Psychopathology, 21*, 1031–1061.

Depue, R. A., & Collins, P. F. (1999). Neurobiology of the structure of personality: Dopamine, facilitation of incentive motivation, and extraversion. *Behavioral and Brain Sciences, 22*, 491–517.

Depue, R. A., & Lenzenweger, M. F. (2001). A neurobehavioral dimensional model. In W. J. Livesley (Ed.), *Handbook of personality disorders. Theory, research, and treatment* (pp. 136–176). New York, NY: Guilford Press.

Depue, R. A., & Lenzenweger, M. F. (2005). A neurobehavioral dimensional model of personality disturbance. In M. F. Lenzenweger & J. F. Clarkin (Eds.), *Major theories of personality disorder* (2nd ed., pp. 391–454). New York, NY: Guilford Press.

Distel, M. A., Trull, T. J., Derom, C. A., Thiery, E. W., Grimmer, M. A., Martin, N. G., . . . Boomsma, D. I. (2008). Heritability of borderline personality disorder features is similar across three countries. *Psychological Medicine, 38*, 1219–1229.

Distel, M. A., Willemsen, G., Ligthart, L., Derom, C. A., Martin, N. G., Neale, M. C., . . . Boomsma, D. I. (2010). Genetic covariance structure of the four main features of borderline personality disorder. *Journal of Personality Disorders, 24,* 427–444.

Dremencov, E., el Mansari, M., & Blier, P. (2009). Brain norepinephrine system as a target for antidepressant and mood stabilizing medications. *Current Drug Targets, 10,* 1061–1068.

Ebner-Priemer, U. W., Badeck, S., Beckmann, C., Wagner, A., Feige, B., Weiss, I., . . . Bohus, M. (2005). Affective dysregulation and dissociative experience in female patients with borderline personality disorder: A startle response study. *Journal of Psychiatric Research, 39,* 85–92.

Epstein, J., Pan, H., Kocsis, J. H., Yang, Y., Butler, T., Chusid, J., . . . Silbersweig, D. A. (2006). Lack of ventral striatal response to positive stimuli in depressed versus normal subjects. *American Journal of Psychiatry, 163,* 1784–1790.

Flood, R. A., & Seager, C. P. (1968). A retrospective examination of psychiatric case records of patients who subsequently committed suicide. *British Journal of Psychiatry, 114,* 443–450.

Fonagy, P., Target, M., & Gergely, G. (2000). Attachment and borderline personality disorder: A theory and some evidence. *Psychiatric Clinics of North America, 23,* 103–122.

Forbes, E. E., & Dahl, R. E. (2012). Research Review: Altered reward function in adolescent depression: What, when and how? *Journal of Child Psychology and Psychiatry, 53,* 3–15.

Fossati, A., Novella, L., Donati, D., Donini, M., & Maffei, C. (2002). History of childhood attention deficit/hyperactivity disorder symptoms and borderline personality disorder: A controlled study. *Comprehensive Psychiatry, 43,* 369–377.

Friedel, R. O. (2004). Dopamine dysfunction in borderline personality disorder: A hypothesis. *Neuropsychopharmacology, 29,* 1029–1039.

Gatzke-Kopp, L. M. (2011). The canary in the coalmine: The sensitivity of mesolimbic dopamine to environmental adversity during development. *Neuroscience and Biobehavioral Reviews, 35,* 794–803.

Geleerd, E. R. (1958). Borderline states in childhood and adolescence. *Psychoanalytic Study of the Child, 13,* 279–295.

Goldman, S. J., D'Angelo, E. J., & DeMaso, D. R. (1993). Psychopathology in the families of children and adolescents with Borderline Personality Disorder. *American Journal of Psychiatry, 150,* 1832–1835.

Gottesman, I. I., & Gould, T. D. (2003). The endophenotype concept in psychiatry: Etymology and strategic intentions. *American Journal of Psychiatry, 160,* 636–645.

Grant, B. F., Chou, S. P., Goldstein, R. B., Huang, B., Stinson, F. S., Saha, T. D., Ruan, W. J. (2008). Prevalence, correlates, disability, and comorbidity of DSM-IV borderline personality disorder: Results from the wave 2 national epidemiologic survey on alcohol and related conditions. *Journal of Clinical Psychiatry, 69,* 533–545.

Gratz, K. L. (2003). Risk factors for and functions of deliberate self-harm: An empirical and conceptual review. *Clinical Psychology: Science and Practice, 10,* 192–205.

Gratz, K. L., Latzman, R. D., Tull, M. T., Reynolds, E. K., & Lejuez, C. W. (2011). Exploring the association between emotional abuse and childhood borderline personality features: The moderating role of personality traits. *Behavior Therapy*, *42*, 493–508.

Gratz, K. L., Tull, M. T., Reynolds, E. K., Bagge, C. L., Latzman, R. D., Daughters, S. B., & Lejuez, C. W. (2009). Extending extant models of the pathogenesis of borderline personality disorder to childhood borderline personality symptoms: The roles of affective dysfunction, disinhibition, and self- and emotion-regulation deficits. *Development and Psychopathology*, *21*, 1263–1291.

Greenberg, B. D., Tolliver, T. J., Huang, S.-J., Li, Q., Bengel, D., & Murphy, D. L. (1999). Genetic variation in the serotonin transporter promoter region affects serotonin uptake in human blood platelets. *American Journal of Medical Genetics*, *88*, 83–87.

Griffiths, M. (2011). Validity, utility and acceptability of borderline personality disorder diagnosis in childhood and adolescence: Survey of psychiatrists. *Psychiatrist*, *35*, 19–22.

Grootens, K. P., van Luijtelaar, G., Buitelaar, J. K., van der Laan, A., Hummelen, J. W., & Verkes, R. J. (2008). Inhibition errors in borderline personality disorder with psychotic-like symptoms. *Progress in Neuro-Psychopharmacology and Biological Psychiatry*, *32*, 267–273.

Gunderson, J. G. (2010). Revising the borderline diagnosis for DSM-V: An alternative proposal. *Journal of Personality Disorders*, *24*, 694–708.

Gunderson, J. G., & Singer, M. T. (1975). Defining borderline patients: An overview. *American Journal of Psychiatry*, *132*, 1–10.

Gunderson, J. G., Zanarini, M. C., Choi-Kain, L. W., Mitchell, K. S., Jang, K. L., & Hudson, J. I. (2011). Family study of borderline personality disorder and its sectors of psychopathology. *Archives of General Psychiatry*, *68*, 753–762.

Gurvits, I. G., Koenigsberg, H. W., & Siever, L. J. (2000). Neurotransmitter dysfunction in patients with borderline personality disorder. *Psychiatric Clinics of North America*, *23*, 27.

Guzder, J., Paris, J., Zelkowitz, P., & Marchessault, K. (1996). Risk factors for borderline pathology in children. *Journal of the American Academy of Child and Adolescent Psychiatry*, *35*, 26–33.

Heath, N. L., Baxter, A. L., Toste, J. R., & McLouth, R. (2010). Adolescents' willingness to access school-based support for nonsuicidal self-injury. *Canadian Journal of School Psychology*, *25*, 260–276.

Heinrichs, M., & Domes, G. (2008). Neuropeptides and social behaviour: Effects of oxytocin and vasopressin in humans. *Progress in Brain Research*, *170*, 337–350.

Heisel, M. J., Conwell, Y., Pisani, A. R., & Duberstein, P. R. (2011). Concordance of self- and proxy-reported suicide ideation in depressed adults 50 years of age or older. *Canadian Journal of Psychiatry*, *56*, 219–226.

Herpertz, S. C., Kunert, H. J., Schwenger, U. B., & Sass, H. (1999). Affective responsiveness in borderline personality disorder: A psychophysiological approach. *American Journal of Psychiatry*, *156*, 1550–1556.

Hilt, L. M., Cha, C. B., & Nolen-Hoeksema, S. (2008). Nonsuicidal self-injury in young adolescent girls: Moderators of the distress-function relationship. *Journal of Consulting and Clinical Psychology*, *76*, 63–71.

Hughes, A. E., Crowell, S. E., Uyeji, L., & Coan, J. A. (2012). A developmental neuroscience of borderline pathology: Emotion dysregulation and social baseline theory. *Journal of Abnormal Child Psychology, 40*, 21–33.

Jang, K. L., Livesley, W. J., Vernon, P. A., & Jackson, D. N. (1996). Heritability of personality disorder traits: A twin study. *Acta Psychiatrica Scandinavica, 94*, 438–444.

Johnson, J. G., Cohen, P., Kasen, S., Skodol, A. E., Hamagami, F., & Brook, J. S. (2000). Age-related change in personality disorder trait levels between early adolescence and adulthood: A community-based longitudinal investigation. *Acta Psychiatrica Scandinavica, 102*, 265–275.

Joyce, P. R., McHugh, P. C., McKenzie, J. M., Sullivan, P. F., Mulder, R. T., Luty, S. E., ... Kennedy, M. A. (2006). A dopamine transporter polymorphism is a risk factor for borderline personality disorder in depressed patients. *Psychological Medicine: A Journal of Research in Psychiatry and the Allied Sciences, 36*, 807–813.

Judd, P. H., & McGlashan, T. H. (2003). *A developmental model of BPD: Understanding variations in course and outcome*. Arlington, VA: American Psychiatric Press.

Kahan, J., & Pattison, E. M. (1984). Proposal for a distinctive diagnosis: The deliberate self-harm syndrome (DSH). *Suicide and Life-Threatening Behavior, 14*, 17–35.

Kamali, M., Oquendo, M. A., & Mann, J. J. (2002). Understanding the neurobiology of suicidal behavior. *Depression and Anxiety, 14*, 164–176.

Katz, L. F., & Gottman, J. M. (1997). Buffering children from marital conflict and dissolution. *Journal of Clinical Child Psychology, 26*, 157–171.

Kendler, K. S., Aggen, S. H., Czajkowski, N., Roysamb, E., Tambs, K., Torgersen, S., ... Reichborn-Kjennerud, T. (2008). The structure of genetic and environmental risk factors for DSM-IV personality disorders: A multivariate twin study. *Archives of General Psychiatry, 65*, 1438–1446.

Kernberg, O. (1967). Borderline personality organization. *Journal of American Psychoanalytic Association, 15*, 641–685.

Kernberg, O. (1975). *Borderline conditions and pathological narcissism*. New York, NY: Jason Aronson.

Kernberg, P. F., Weiner, A. S., & Bardenstein, K. K. (2000). *Personality disorders in children and adolescents*. New York, NY: Basic Books.

Klonsky, E. D., & Moyer, A. (2008). Childhood sexual abuse and non-suicidal self-injury: Meta-analysis. *British Journal of Psychiatry, 192*, 166–170.

Knight, R. P. (1953). Borderline states. *Bulletin of the Menninger Clinics, 17*, 1–12.

Koenigsberg, H. W., Siever, L. J., Lee, H., Pizzarello, S., New, A. S., Goodman, M., ... Prohovnik, I. (2009). Neural correlates of emotion processing in borderline personality disorder. *Psychiatry Research, 172*, 192–199.

Krishnan, K. R., Davidson, J. R., Rayasam, K., & Shope, F. (1984). The dexamethasone suppression test in borderline personality disorder. *Biological Psychiatry, 19*, 1149–1153.

Krueger, R. F., Hicks, B. M., Patrick, C. J., Carlson, S. R., Iacono, W. G., & McGue, M. (2002). Etiologic connections among substance dependence, antisocial behavior, and personality: Modeling the externalizing spectrum. *Journal of Abnormal Psychology, 111*, 411–424.

Krueger, R. F., Markon, K. E., Patrick, C. J., Benning, S. D., & Kramer, M. D. (2007). Linking antisocial behavior, substance use, and personality: An integrative quantitative model of the adult externalizing spectrum. *Journal of Abnormal Psychology*, *116*, 645–666.

Kuo, J. R., & Linehan, M. M. (2009). Disentangling emotion processes in borderline personality disorder: Physiological and self-reported assessment of biological vulnerability, baseline intensity, and reactivity to emotionally evocative stimuli. *Journal of Abnormal Psychology*, *118*, 531–544.

Lahey, B. B., & D'Onofrio, B. M. (2010). All in the family: Comparing siblings to test causal hypotheses regarding environmental influences on behavior. *Current Directions in Psychological Science*, *19*, 319–323.

Lamph, G. (2011). Raising awareness of borderline personality disorder and self-injury. *Nursing Standard 26*, 35–40.

Lang, C. M., & Sharma-Patel, K. (2011). The relation between childhood maltreatment and self-injury: A review of the literature on conceptualization and intervention. *Trauma, Violence & Abuse*, *12*, 23–37.

Le Doux, J. E. (1992). Emotion in the amygdala. In J. P. Aggleton (Ed.), *The amygdala: Neurobiological aspects of emotion, memory, and mental dysfunction* (pp. 339–351). New York, NY: Wiley-Liss.

Lenzenweger, M. F. (1999). Stability and change in personality disorder features: The longitudinal study of personality disorders. *Archives of General Psychiatry*, *56*, 1009–1015.

Lenzenweger, M. F. (2010). A source, a cascade, a schizoid: A heuristic proposal from the longitudinal study of personality disorders. *Development and Psychopathology*, *22*, 867–881.

Lenzenweger, M. F., & Cicchetti, D. (2005). Toward a developmental psychopathology approach to borderline personality disorder. *Development and Psychopathology*, *17*, 893–898.

Lenzenweger, M. F., Clarkin, J. F., Yeomans, F. E., Kernberg, O. F., & Levy, K. N. (2008). Refining the borderline personality disorder phenotype through finite mixture modeling: Implications for classification. *Journal of Personality Disorders*, *22*, 313–331.

Lenzenweger, M. F., Johnson, M. D., & Willett, J. B. (2004). Individual growth curve analysis illuminates stability and change in personality disorder features: The longitudinal study of personality disorders. *Archives of General Psychiatry*, *61*, 1015–1024.

Lenzenweger, M. F., Lane, M. C., Loranger, A. W., & Kessler, R. C. (2007). DSM-IV personality disorders in the national comorbidity survey replication. *Biological Psychiatry*, *62*, 553–564.

Lester, D. (1992). The dexamethasone suppression test as an indicator of suicide: A meta-analysis. *Pharmacopsychiatry*, *25*, 265–270.

Lieb, K., Völlm, B., Rücker, G., Timmer, A., & Stoffers, J. M. (2010). Pharmacotherapy for borderline personality disorder: Cochrane systematic review of randomised trials. *British Journal of Psychiatry*, *196*, 4–12.

Lin, P.-Y., & Tsai, G. (2004). Association between serotonin transporter gene promoter polymorphism and suicide: Results of a meta-analysis. *Biological Psychiatry, 55,* 1023–1030.

Linehan, M. M. (1993). *Cognitive-behavioral treatment of borderline personality disorder.* New York, NY: Guilford Press.

Linehan, M. M. (1997). Behavioral treatments of suicidal behaviors. *Definitional obfuscation and treatment outcomes. Annals New York Academy of Sciences, 836,* 302–328.

Livesley, W. J., Jang, K. L., & Vernon, P. A. (1998). Phenotypic and genetic structure of traits delineating personality disorder. *Archives of General Psychiatry, 55,* 941–948.

Lofgren, D. P., Bemporad, J. R., King, J., Lindem, K., & O'Driscoll, G. (1991). A prospective follow-up study of so-called borderline children. *American Journal of Psychiatry, 148,* 1541–1547.

Loranger, A. W. (1999). *International personality disorder examination: DSM-IV and ICD-10 interviews.* Odessa, FL: Psychological Assessment Resources.

Loranger, A. W., Oldham, J. M., & Tulis, E. H. (1982). Familial transmission of DSM-III borderline personality disorder. *Archives of General Psychiatry, 39,* 795–799.

Loranger, A. W., Susman, V. L., Oldham, J. M., & Russakoff, M. (1988). *The personality disorder examination (PDE) Manual.* Yonkers, NY: DV Communications.

Lynam, D., Caspi, A., Moffitt, T. E., Wikström, P. O. H., Loeber, R., & Novak, S. (2000). The interaction between impulsivity and neighborhood context on offending: The effects of impulsivity are stronger in poorer neighborhoods. *Journal of Abnormal Psychology, 109,* 563–574.

Lyons-Ruth, K. (2008). Contributions of the mother-infant relationship to dissociative, borderline, and conduct symptoms in young adulthood. *Infant Mental Health Journal, 29,* 203–218.

Malone, K. M., Haas, G. L., Sweeney, J. A., & Mann, J. J. (1995). Major depression and the risk of attempted suicide. *Journal of Affective Disorders, 34,* 173–185.

Mann, J. J. (2003). Neurobiology of suicidal behaviour. *Nature Reviews Neuroscience, 4,* 819–828.

Mann, J. J., Arango, V. A., Avenevoli, S., Brent, D. A., Champagne, F. A., Clayton, P., . . . Wenzel, A. (2009). Candidate endophenotypes for genetic studies of suicidal behavior. *Biological Psychiatry, 65,* 556–563.

Mason, P. (1954). Suicide in adolescents. *Psychoanalytic Review, 41,* 48–54.

McGirr, A., Alda, M., Seguin, M., Cabot, S., Lesage, A., & Turecki, G. (2009). Familial aggregation of suicide explained by cluster B traits: A three-group family study of suicide controlling for major depressive disorder. *American Journal of Psychiatry, 166,* 1124–1134.

McGirr, A., Renaud, J., Bureau, A., Seguin, M., Lesage, A., & Turecki, G. (2008). Impulsive-aggressive behaviours and completed suicide across the life cycle: A predisposition for younger age of suicide. *Psychological Medicine, 38,* 407–417.

McGlashan, T. H., Grilo, C. M., Sanislow, C. A., Ralevski, E., Morey, L. C., Gunderson, J. G., . . . Pagano, M. (2005). Two-year prevalence and stability of individual DSM-IV criteria for schizotypal, borderline, avoidant, and obsessive-compulsive personality disorders: Toward a hybrid model of Axis II disorders. *American Journal of Psychiatry, 162*, 883–889.

McGuffin, P., Perroud, N., Uher, R., Butler, A., Aitchison, K. J., Craig, I., . . . Farmer, A. (2010). The genetics of affective disorder and suicide. *European Psychiatry, 25*, 275–277.

Mead, H. K., Beauchaine, T. P., & Shannon, K. E. (2010). Neurobiological adaptations to violence across development. *Development and Psychopathology, 22*, 1–22.

Mehlum, L., Friis, S., Vaglum, P., & Karterud, S. (1994). The longitudinal pattern of suicidal behaviour in borderline personality disorder: A prospective follow-up study. *Acta Psychiatrica Scandinavica, 90*, 124–130.

Miller, A. L., Rathus, J. H., & Linehan, M. M. (2007). *Dialectical behavior therapy with suicidal adolescents*. New York, NY: Guilford Press.

Millon, T. (1983). *Millon clinical multiaxial inventory manual*. Minneapolis, MN: National Computer Systems.

Muehlenkamp, J. J., Ertelt, T. W., Miller, A. L., & Claes, L. (2011). Borderline personality symptoms differentiate non-suicidal and suicidal self-injury in ethnically diverse adolescent outpatients. *Journal of Child Psychology and Psychiatry, 52*, 148–155.

Muehlenkamp, J. J., & Gurierrez, P. M. (2004). An investigation of differences between self-injurious behavior and suicide attempts in a sample of adolescents. *Suicide and Life-Threatening Behavior, 34*, 12–23.

Nemoda, Z., Lyons-Ruth, K., Szekely, A., Bertha, E., Faludi, G., & Sasvari-Szekely, M. (2010). Association between dopaminergic polymorphisms and borderline personality traits among at-risk young adults and psychiatric inpatients. *Behavioral and Brain Functions, 6*, 4–4.

Ni, X., Chan, D., Chan, K., McMain, S., & Kennedy, J. L. (2009). Serotonin genes and gene-gene interactions in borderline personality disorder in a matched case-control study. *Progress in neuro-psychopharmacology and biological psychiatry, 33*, 128–133.

Niedtfeld, I., Schulze, L., Kirsch, P., Herpertz, S. C., Bohus, M., & Schmahl, C. (2010). Affect regulation and pain in borderline personality disorder: A possible link to the understanding of self-injury. *Biological Psychiatry, 68*, 383–391.

Nock, M. K., Guilherme, B., Bromet, E. J., Cha, C. B., Kessler, R. C., & Lee, S. (2008). Suicide and suicidal behavior. *Epidemiologic Reviews, 30*, 133–154.

Offer, D., & Barglow, P. (1960). Adolescent and young adult self-mutilation incidents in a general psychiatric hospital. *Archives of General Psychiatry, 3*, 194–204.

O'Neill, A. O., & Frodl, T. (in press). Brain structure and function in borderline personality disorder. *Brain Structure and Function*.

Osuch, E. A., & Payne, G. W. (2009). Neurobiological perspectives on self-injury. In M. K. Nixon & N. L. Heath (Eds.), *Self-injury in youth: The essential guide to assessment and intervention*. (pp. 79–110). New York, NY: Taylor & Francis.

Pandey, G. N., Dwivedi, Y., Rizavi, H. S., Ren, X., Pandey, S. C., Pesold, C., . . . Tamminga, C. A. (2002). Higher expression of serotonin 5-HT 2a receptors in the postmortem brains of teenage suicide victims. *American Journal of Psychiatry, 159*, 419–429.

Paris, J. (2007). The nature of borderline personality disorder: Multiple dimensions, multiple symptoms, but one category. *Journal of Personality Disorders, 21,* 457–473.

Paris, J., Zweig-Frank, H., Ng Ying Kin, N. M. K., Schwartz, G., Steiger, H., & Nair, N. P. V. (2004). Neurobiological correlates of diagnosis and underlying traits in patients with borderline personality disorder compared with normal controls. *Psychiatry Research, 121,* 239–252.

Pascual, J. C., Soler, J., Barrachina, J., Campins, M. J., Alvarez, E., Pérez, V., . . . Baiget, M. (2008). Failure to detect an association between the serotonin transporter gene and borderline personality disorder. *Journal of Psychiatric Research, 42,* 87–88.

Patterson, G. R., Chamberlain, P., & Reid, J. B. (1982). A comparative evaluation of a parent-training program. *Behavior Therapy, 13,* 638–650.

Patterson, G. R., DeBaryshe, B. D., & Ramsey, E. (1989). A developmental perspective on antisocial behavior. *American Psychologist, 44,* 329–335.

Patterson, G. R., Dishion, T. J., & Bank, L. (1984). Family interaction: A process model of deviancy training. *Aggressive Behavior, 10,* 253–267.

Pitchot, W., Hansenne, M., & Ansseau, M. (2001). Role of dopamine in non-depressed patients with a history of suicide attempts. *European Psychiatry, 16,* 424–427.

Pitchot, W., Hansenne, M., Moreno, A. G., & Ansseau, M. (1992). Suicidal behavior and growth hormone response to apomorphine test. *Biological Psychiatry, 15,* 1213–1219.

Pitchot, W., Reggers, J., Pinto, E., Hansenne, M., Fuchs, S., Pirard, S., & Ansseau, M. (2001). Reduced dopaminergic activity in depressed suicides. *Psychoneuroendocrinology, 26,* 331–335.

Reutfors, J., Bahmanyar, S., Jönsson, E. G., Ekbom, A., Nordström, P., Brandt, L., & Ösby, U. (2010). Diagnostic profile and suicide risk in schizophrenia spectrum disorder. *Schizophrenia Research, 123,* 251–256.

Roy, A., Dejong, J., & Linnoila, M. (1989). Cerebrospinal-fluid monoamine metabolites and suicidal behavior in depressed patients—A 5-year follow-up-study. *Archives of General Psychiatry, 46,* 609–612.

Roy, A., Karoum, F., & Pollack, S. (1992). Marked reduction in indexes of dopamine metabolism among patients with depression who attempt suicide. *Archives of General Psychiatry, 49,* 447–450.

Rutter, M., Kim-Cohen, J., & Maughan, B. (2006). Continuities and discontinuities in psychopathology between childhood and adult life. *Journal of Child Psychology and Psychiatry, 47,* 276–295.

Sagvolden, T., Aase, H., Johansen, E. B., & Russell, V. A. (2005). A dynamic developmental theory of attention-deficit/hyperactivity disorder (ADHD) predominantly hyperactive/impulsive and combined subtypes. *Behavioral and Brain Sciences, 28,* 397–468.

Sanislow, C. A., Grilo, C. M., Morey, L. C., Bender, D. S., Skodol, A. E., Gunderson, J. G., & McGlashan, T. H. (2002). Confirmatory factor analysis of DSM-IV criteria for borderline personality disorder: Findings from the collaborative longitudinal personality disorders study. *American Journal of Psychiatry, 159,* 284–290.

Schaefer, S. M., Jackson, D. C., Davidson, R. J., Aguirre, G. K., Kimberg, D. Y., & Thompson-Schill, S. L. (2002). Modulation of amygdalar activity by the conscious regulation of negative emotion. *Journal of Cognitive Neuroscience, 15,* 913–921.

Schmahl, C. G., Elzinga, B. M., Ebner, U. W., Simms, T., Sanislow, C., Vermetten, E., . . . Douglas Bremner, J. (2004). Psychophysiological reactivity to traumatic and abandonment scripts in borderline personality and posttraumatic stress disorders: A preliminary report. *Psychiatry Research, 126,* 33–42.

Seiden, R. H. (1978). Where are they now? A follow-up study of suicide attempters from the Golden Gate Bridge. *Suicide and Life-Threatening Behavior, 8,* 1–13.

Shaw, P., Bramham, J., Lawrence, E. J., Morris, R., Baron-Cohen, S., & David, A. S. (2005). Differential effects of lesions of the amygdala and prefrontal cortex on recognizing facial expressions of complex emotions. *Journal of Cognitive Neuroscience, 17,* 1410–1419.

Sher, L., & Stanley, B. (2009). Biological models of nonsuicidal self-injury. In M. K. Nock (Ed.), *Understanding nonsuicidal self-injury: Origins, assessment, and treatment* (pp. 99–116). Washington, DC: American Psychological Association.

Shneidman, E. S. (1991). The commonalities of suicide across the life span. In A. A. Leenaars (Ed.), *Life span perspectives of suicide: Time-lines in the suicide process* (pp. 39–52). New York, NY: Plenum Press.

Silva, H., Iturra, P., Solari, A., Villarroel, J., Jerez, S., Jiménez, M., . . . Bustamante, M. L. (2010). Fluoxetine response in impulsive-aggressive behavior and serotonin transporter polymorphism in personality disorder. *Psychiatric Genetics, 20,* 25–30.

Silverman, J., Pinkham, L., Horvath, T., Coccaro, E., Klar, H., Schear, S., . . . Siever, L. J. (1991). Affective and impulsive personality disorder traits in the relatives of patients with borderline personality disorder. *American Journal of Psychiatry, 148,* 1378–1385.

Simpson, G. (1950). Methodological problems in determining the aetiology of suicide. *American Sociological Review, 15,* 658–663.

Simpson, M. A. (1975). The phenomenology of self-mutilation in a general hospital setting. *Canadian Psychiatric Association Journal, 20,* 429–434.

Skodol, A. E., Gunderson, J. G., Pfohl, B., Widiger, T. A., Livesley, W. J., & Siever, L. J. (2002). The borderline diagnosis I: Psychopathology, comorbidity, and personality structure. *Biological Psychiatry, 51,* 936–950.

Skodol, A. E., Siever, L. J., Livesley, W. J., Gunderson, J. G., Pfohl, B., & Widiger, T. A. (2002). The borderline diagnosis II: Biology, genetics, and clinical course. *Biological Psychiatry, 51,* 951–963.

Snyder, J., Edwards, P., McGraw, K., & Kilgore, K. (1994). Escalation and reinforcement in mother-child conflict: Social processes associated with the development of physical aggression. *Development and Psychopathology, 6,* 305–321.

Snyder, J., Schrepferman, L., & St. Peter, C. (1997). Origins of antisocial behavior: Negative reinforcement and affect dysregulation of behavior as socialization mechanisms in family interaction. *Behavior Modification, 21,* 187–215.

Soloff, P. H. (2000). Psychopharmacology of borderline personality disorder. *Psychiatric Clinics of North America, 23,* 169–192.

Soloff, P. H., Lynch, K. G., & Kelly, T. M. (2002). Childhood abuse as a risk factor for suicidal behavior in borderline personality disorder. *Journal of Personality Disorders, 16*, 201–214.

Soloff, P. H., Lynch, K. G., Kelly, T. M., Malone, K. M., & Mann, J. J. (2000). Characteristics of suicide attempts of patients with major depressive episode and borderline personality disorder: A comparative study. *American Journal of Psychiatry, 157*, 601–608.

Spirito, A., & Esposito-Smythers, C. (2006). Attempted and completed suicide in adolescence. *Annual Review of Clinical Psychology, 2*, 237–266.

Spitzer, R. L., Endicott, J., & Gibbon, M. (1979). Crossing the border into borderline personality and borderline schizophrenia. The development of criteria. *Archives of General Psychiatry, 36*, 17–24.

Stanley, B., Sher, L., Wilson, S., Ekman, R., Huang, Y.-y., & Mann, J. J. (2010). Non-suicidal self-injurious behavior, endogenous opioids and monoamine neurotransmitters. *Journal of Affective Disorders, 124*, 134–140.

Stanley, B., & Siever, L. J. (2010). The interpersonal dimension of borderline personality disorder: Toward a neuropeptide model. *American Journal of Psychiatry, 167*, 24–39.

Stepp, S. D. (2012). Development of borderline personality disorder in adolescence and young adulthood: Introduction to the special section. *Journal of Abnormal Child Psychology, 40*, 1–5.

Stepp, S. D., Burke, J. D., Hipwell, A. E., & Loeber, R. (2012). Trajectories of attention deficit hyperactivity disorder and oppositional defiant disorder symptoms as precursors of borderline personality disorder symptoms in adolescent girls. *Journal of Abnormal Child Psychology, 40*, 7–20.

Stern, A. (1938). Psychoanalytic investigation of and therapy in the border line group of neuroses. *Psychoanalytic Quarterly, 7*, 467–489.

Thombs, B. D., & Bresnick, M. G. (2008). Mortality risk and length of stay associated with self-inflicted burn injury: Evidence from a national sample of 30,382 adult patients. *Critical Care Medicine, 36*, 118–125.

Thorell, L. H. (2009). Valid electrodermal hyporeactivity for depressive suicidal propensity offers links to cognitive theory. *Acta Psychiatrica Scandinavica, 119*, 338–349.

Torgersen, S., Lygren, S., Oien, P. A., Skre, I., Onstad, S., Edvardsen, J., & Kringlen, E. (2000). A twin study of personality disorders. *Comprehensive Psychiatry, 41*, 416–425.

Trull, T. J., Jahng, S., Tomko, R. L., Wood, P. K., & Sher, K. J. (2010). Revised NESARC personality disorder diagnoses: Gender, prevalence, and comorbidity with substance dependence disorders. *Journal of Personality Disorders, 24*, 412–426.

Uher, R., & McGuffin, P. (2009). The moderation by the serotonin transporter gene of environmental adversity in the etiology of depression: 2009 update. *Molecular Psychiatry, 15*, 18–22.

Vaidya, C. J., Austin, G., Kirkorian, G., Ridlehuber, H. W., Desmond, J. E., Glover, G. H., & Gabrieli, J. D. E. (1998). Selective effects of methylphenidate in attention deficit hyperactivity disorders: A functional magnetic resonance study. *Proceedings of the National Academy of Sciences, 95,* 14494–14499.

van Goozen, S. H. M., Fairchild, G., Snoek, H., & Harold, G. T. (2007). The evidence for a neurobiological model of childhood antisocial behavior. *Psychological Bulletin, 133,* 149–182.

Van Orden, K. A., Witte, T. K., Holm-Denoma, J., Gordon, K. H., & Joiner, T. E. Jr., (2011). Suicidal behavior on Axis VI: Clinical data supporting a sixth Axis for DSM-V. *Crisis, 32,* 110–113.

Vela, R. M., Gottlieb, E. H., & Gottlieb, H. P. (1983). Borderline syndromes in childhood: A critical review. In K. S. Robson (Ed.), *The borderline child: Approaches to etiology, diagnosis, and treatment* (pp. 31–48). New York, NY: McGraw-Hill.

Vygotsky, L. S. (1978). *Mind and society: The development of higher psychological processes.* Cambridge, MA: Harvard University Press.

Wagner, S., Baskaya, O. R., Lieb, K., Dahmen, N., & Tadifa, A. (2009). The 5-HTTLPR polymorphism modulates the association of serious life events and impulsivity in patients with borderline personality disorder. *Journal of Psychiatric Research, 43,* 1067–1072.

Weil, A. P. (1953). Certain severe disturbances of ego development in childhood. *Psychoanalytic Study of the Child, 8,* 271–287.

Westen, D., & Chang, C. M. (2000). Adolescent personality pathology: A review. *Adolescent Psychiatry, 25,* 61–100.

White, C. N., Gunderson, J. G., Zanarini, M. C., & Hudson, J. I. (2003). Family studies of borderline personality disorder: A review. *Harvard Review of Psychiatry, 11,* 8–19.

Widiger, T. A., & Trull, T. J. (1993). Borderline and narcissistic personality disorders. In P. B. Sutker & H. E. Adams (Eds.), *Comprehensive handbook of psychopathology* (2nd ed., pp. 371–394). New York, NY: Plenum Press.

Widom, C. S., Czaja, S. J., & Paris, J. (2009). A prospective investigation of borderline personality disorder in abused and neglected children followed up into adulthood. *Journal of Personality Disorders, 23,* 433–446.

Wingenfeld, K., Spitzer, C., Rullkötter, N., & Löwe, B. (2010). Borderline personality disorder: Hypothalamus pituitary adrenal axis and findings from neuroimaging studies. *Psychoneuroendocrinology, 35,* 154–170.

Winograd, G., Cohen, P., & Chen, H. (2008). Adolescent borderline symptoms in the community: Prognosis for functioning over 20 years. *Journal of Child Psychology and Psychiatry, 49,* 933–941.

Zalsman, G. (2010). Timing is critical: Gene, environment and timing interactions in genetics of suicide in children and adolescents. *European Psychiatry: The Journal of the Association of European Psychiatrists, 25,* 284–286.

Zalsman, G., Patya, M., Frisch, A., Ofek, H., Schapir, L., Blum, I., ... Tyano, S. (2011). Association of polymorphisms of the serotonergic pathways with clinical traits of impulsive-aggression and suicidality in adolescents: A multi-center study. *World Journal of Biological Psychiatry, 12,* 33–41.

Zanarini, M. C. (2000). Childhood experiences associated with the development of borderline personality disorder. *Psychiatric Clinics of North America, 23,* 89–101.

Zanarini, M. C., Barison, L. K., Frankenburg, F. R., Reich, D. B., & Hudson, J. I. (2009). Family history study of the familial coaggregation of borderline personality disorder with axis I and nonborderline dramatic cluster axis II disorders. *Journal of Personality Disorders, 23,* 357–369.

Zanarini, M. C., Frankenburg, F. R., Dubo, E. D., Sickel, A. E., Trikha, A., Levin, A., & Reynolds, V. (1998). Axis I comorbidity of borderline personality disorder. *American Journal of Psychiatry, 155,* 1733–1739.

Zanarini, M. C., Frankenburg, F. R., Dubo, E. D., Sickel, A. E., Trikha, A., Levin, A., & Reynolds, V. (1998). Axis II comorbidity of borderline personality disorder. *Comprehensive Psychiatry, 39,* 296–302.

Zanarini, M. C., Frankenburg, F. R., Hennen, J., Reich, D. B., & Silk, K. R. (2004). Axis I comorbidity in patients with borderline personality disorder: 6-year follow-up and prediction of time to remission. *American Journal of Psychiatry, 161,* 2108–2114.

Zanarini, M. C., Frankenburg, F. R., Yong, L., Raviola, G., Reich, D. B., Hennen, J., . . . Gunderson, J. G. (2004). Borderline psychopathology in the first-degree relatives of borderline and axis II comparison probands. *Journal of Personality Disorders, 18,* 449–447.

Zanarini, M. C., Gunderson, J. G., & Frankenburg, F. R. (1990). Cognitive features of borderline personality disorder. *American Journal of Psychiatry, 147,* 57–63.

Zanarini, M. C., Horwood, J., Wolke, D., Waylen, A., Fitzmaurice, G., & Grant, B. F. (2011). Prevalence of DSM-IV borderline personality disorder in two community samples: 6,330 English 11-year-olds and 34,653 American adults. *Journal of Personality Disorders, 25,* 607–619.

Zanarini, M. C., Laudate, C. S., Frankenburg, F. R., Reich, D. B., & Fitzmaurice, G. (2011). Predictors of self-mutilation in patients with borderline personality disorder: A 10-year follow-up study. *Journal of Psychiatric Research, 45,* 823–828.

Zanarini, M. C., Williams, A. A., Lewis, R. E., Reich, R. B., Vera, S. C., Marino, M. F., . . . Frankenburg, F. R.. (1997). Reported pathological childhood experiences associated with the development of borderline personality disorder. *American Journal of Psychiatry, 154,* 1101–1106.

Zhuang, X., Gross, C., Santarelli, L., Compan, V., Trillat, A. C., & Hen, R. (1999). Altered emotional states in knockout mice lacking 5-HT1A or 5-HT1B receptors. *Neuropsychopharmacology, 21,* 52S-60S.

Zilboorg, G. (1936). Differential diagnostic types of suicide. *Archives of General Psychiatry, 35,* 270–291.

Zlotnick, C., Donaldson, D., Spirito, A., & Pearlstein, T. (1997). Affect regulation and suicide attempts in adolescent inpatients. *Journal of the American Academy of Child and Adolescent Psychiatry, 36,* 793–798.

Zlotnick, C., Mattia, J. I., & Zimmerman, M. (1999). Clinical correlates of self-mutilation in a sample of general psychiatric patients. *Journal of Nervous and Mental Disease, 187,* 296–301.

# PART V

## OTHER DISORDERS

# CHAPTER 19

# Bipolar Disorder

JOSEPH C. BLADER AND GABRIELLE A. CARLSON

## PHENOMENOLOGY AND IMPACT

**B**IPOLAR DISORDER (BPD) DESCRIBES a pattern of cyclic major mood disturbance over an extended period of time that usually crystallizes by early adulthood. Severity and course vary among affected individuals, but overall it is a grave psychiatric illness that heightens risk for early mortality (Khalsa, 2008, Dutta, 2007) and is a leading cause of disability worldwide (World Health Organization, 2002).

Criteria established for the diagnosis of BPD are anchored primarily in data and clinical experience derived from affected adults. Nevertheless, onset of BPD in adolescence is common (Kessler et al., 2005), and it is vital that clinicians caring for adolescents be familiar with the disorder.

Very few preadolescents fulfill diagnostic criteria for BPD. However, many children seen in clinical settings experience frequent, intermittent, and severe emotional upsets with minimal provocation that lead to dyscontrolled and harmful behaviors. The possibility that these youngsters' difficulties represent a form of BPD has been a significant and controversial area of debate over the past 20 years.

Some research suggests that during adolescence or preadolescence, individuals who go on to develop BPD exhibit premorbid signs or symptoms that do not yet meet full diagnostic criteria (viz., they are *subsyndromal*). Symptoms that are changes from a person's ordinary functioning may gradually emerge months or even years before the onset of the full disorder; such a period is a *prodromal phase*. Premorbid signs and prodromal phases are notable in other serious disorders, for example, in unipolar depression (Chapter 17) and schizophrenia (Chapter 21). One may also show lifelong characteristics that resemble symptoms (i.e., they are part of a person's *premorbid functioning* and do not represent changes in behavior), but nonetheless increase the risk for later development of a disorder. Reliably distinguishing youth whose behavior signals a prodromal phase or who have traits that increase risk for an illness from others who display the same features but who will not proceed to develop the syndrome (i.e., multifinality, see Chapter 1) is important for early intervention and family education. The capacity to make these prognoses relies on understanding of the disorder's progression over developmental periods and therefore poses a key concern for developmental psychopathologists.

These issues about onset, continuity, and differential diagnosis all hinge on a shared understanding of BPD. The adult presentation of BPD, in which patients experience mania or mixed episodes called *bipolar I disorder*, is best characterized and therefore serves as its prototype. It is therefore useful to start our discussion by describing the history and phenomenology of BPD by focusing on its appearance in mature individuals, and then proceed to discuss conceptual and clinical issues in how its manifestations may differ among youth.

## HISTORICAL CONTEXT

The existence of a disturbance in which the same individual oscillates between extremes of excitement and melancholy was articulated early in Western medical writings. Aretaeus of Cappadocia, in present-day Turkey, a major figure in the history of medicine thought to have practiced in Alexandria and Rome during the 1st to 2nd centuries C.E., often receives credit for the first linkage of these episodes to a single underlying illness (Angst & Marneros, 2001; Sedler, 1983). In modern times, Baillarger's (1809–1891) and Falret's (1794–1870) descriptions of a cyclical disturbance of depression and manic excitement established the entity in the emerging discipline of psychiatry. Emil Kraepelin (1856–1926) elaborated on these accounts, providing the designation *manic-depressive insanity* (Kraepelin, 1921). His goal was to distinguish forms of manic-depression, which were fundamentally disturbances of mood, from *dementia praecox*, which he regarded as involving fundamental disturbances of thought. The latter idea, as amended by Eugen Bleuler (1857–1939), was the forerunner of today's concept of schizophrenia.

Our understanding of BPD in youth began with attempts to identify young people who exhibited versions of the manic-depressive condition Kraepelin described. Child psychiatrists in the 1920s and 1930s concluded that Kraepelin's description of manic-depression occurred among youth but was rare, appearing mostly in adolescents. In the 1950s, papers on youth manic-depression reported that the condition was indeed rare, with depression predominating, although an *alternate form* with more typical childhood behavioral (i.e., disruptive and externalizing) psychopathology was proposed. A review from that time (Anthony & Scott, 1960) also concluded that it was exceptionally rare before age 11 (see Carlson & Glovinsky, 2009, for a review).

Lithium's efficacy for the treatment of acute mania was established in the early 1950s, and its value as prophylaxis in preventing relapse was confirmed later. These developments motivated a search for a symptom constellation in younger children that lithium treatment might alleviate. A review of 211 published studies and case reports (Youngerman & Canino, 1978) of the use of lithium in youth found 46 reports with enough detail to adequately characterize the patients and their responses. Of the 22 cases of children, only two had manic-depression and two had "atypical mood disorder." Twenty-four cases involving adolescents included nine with manic-depression and 13 with atypical mood disorder (the remaining two had other conditions). Response to lithium was poor in those without classic BPD, and interest diminished accordingly.

Over the past 20 years or so, however, BPD among children and adolescents has reemerged as a topic of considerable interest, importance, and debate (Biederman, Klein, Pine, & Klein, 1998). The rate of BPD diagnoses among youth in clinical settings has risen dramatically (Blader & Carlson, 2007; Moreno et al., 2007). One contributing factor is recognition of frequent onset of BPD in mid- to late adolescence, with possible prodromal signs evident even earlier. In addition, volatile, explosive, and labile affect is prominent among many children typically diagnosed with externalizing disorders (e.g., severe ODD and many instances of chronic conduct disorder), comorbid with long-standing attention-deficit/hyperactivity disorder (ADHD). Traditionally, these problems have come under the rubric of disruptive behavior disorders, a classification approach that many felt gave insufficient weight to children's affective storms, whose presence usually signals greater impairments than uncomplicated ADHD or ODD. Thinking of them as manifestations of bipolar illness had some appeal as a means to focus on the affective disturbance of these very troubled youngsters, which might also subsume the high activity levels hitherto regarded as ADHD. This way of thinking, however, requires significant shifts in traditional concepts of bipolar disorder to incorporate the important differences in symptoms and course that typify the clinical presentation of most preadolescents.

As a result, today's literature on preadolescent BPD imposes on readers the burden of critically evaluating patient selection criteria. Bipolar diagnoses for children have become, to a large degree, in the "eye of the beholder." For instance, discrete episodes of illness are integral to the definition of BPD, but some clinicians contend that an early-onset form of the disorder may be chronic and not show demarcated periods of illness and remission. Patient selection criteria are also important in case–control studies. Research cited in support of a more expansive approach to BPD often shows much greater impairment between those diagnosed with BPD (i.e., "cases") and those with ADHD (used as "controls"). Critics contend that the more appropriate comparator group would be youngsters with ADHD and a disruptive disorder who show behavioral volatility but who do not fulfill criteria for a major mood disorder, because that is the real distinction at issue (Carlson, 1998, 2007; Carlson & Glovinsky, 2009).

With this context in mind, in the next section we detail BPD's diagnostic criteria before moving into issues, many of them controversial, that arise in their application among youth.

## DIAGNOSTIC CRITERIA AND CLINICAL PRESENTATION

In most formal definitions, BPD comprises: (1) episodes of *depression*; interspersed to greater or lesser degree with (2) episodes of *manic (or mixed) symptoms*; (3) intervals between episodes, during which mood state and functioning may vary widely both across patients and for the same person over time; and (4) an overall course of illness that is *chronic* (American Psychiatric Association [APA], 2000; Goodwin & Jamison, 2007; World Health Organization, 2010).

## BIPOLAR I DISORDER

Bipolar I disorder (BPDI) is the diagnosis applied to either (1) a person experiencing an *episode of mania* or a *mixed episode* (described later), or (2) one who is experiencing an episode of major depressive disorder or of hypomania but has had a manic or mixed episode in the past. Thus, if a manic or mixed episode has ever occurred, a diagnosis of BPDI supersedes a diagnosis of unipolar depression, even if the current episode includes only depressive symptoms. A manic episode must last at least one week, or less if hospitalization is necessary. In the *DSM-IV*, *specifiers* accompany the diagnosis to describe the episode's type ("most recent episode manic," "most recent episode depressed," etc.), severity (e.g., "severe, with psychotic features"), and course (e.g., "rapid cycling," "with full interepisode recovery") (APA, 2000).

Within BPDI, major depressive episodes conform to the conventional signs and symptoms of major depressive disorder (MDD) that develop among those with no history of bipolar illness (unipolar depression; see Chapter 17), and are no less painful. In contrast, a person seldom experiences the cardinal mood disturbances of mania as problematic. Instead, most seem to have near-boundless energy, enthusiasm, high self-regard, confidence, and not infrequently, creativity, charisma, and generosity that may be uncharacteristic of the person at other times. However, in mania, euphoric exuberance and misguided convictions about one's insights, abilities, entitlements, and infallibility usually lead to severely disinhibited behavior with high likelihood of negative consequences. This combination of strong motivation to pursue unrealistic aims incautiously, of drive toward immediate intense pleasures, and of diminished self-restraint is the essence of mania.

Accordingly, the conduct that ensues during manic episodes may harm the individual, those close to him or her, or the broader community. Common harmful behaviors include belligerence, drug abuse, promiscuity, plundering one's financial resources, gambling, and impulsive unannounced journeys that leave others worried about the person's whereabouts. Poor judgment and irresponsibility endanger occupational and family roles, and thus the well-being of dependents and co-workers. When people interacting with the patient seem perplexed or do not reciprocate enthusiasm, they risk being perceived as obstructionist or ungrateful. Social strife and rage are common results. Impatience with others' shortcomings or uncooperativeness, and inevitable frustration with unattained goals and desires, often manifest as irritability and embitterment.

A significant subgroup of patients experience psychotic features during manic episodes (Kennedy et al., 2005; Müller-Oerlinghausen, Berghöfer, & Bauer, 2002). These often arise as delusions that aggrandize one's abilities or even identity (e.g., of being an important official or historical person, spiritual messenger, of royal heritage). Hallucinations may occur that reinforce one's elevated status (e.g., special messages from powerful or famous people or spirits). Paranoid or persecutory delusions focus on dangers associated with having a special mission, such as being the target of the envious or "the enemy" (Keck et al., 2003). Generally, the ideas expressed are intelligible, even if absurd and too rapid to follow easily. That is, they lack the incoherence or apparent meaninglessness (*formal thought disorder*) common in other psychotic illnesses such as schizophrenia and schizoaffective disorder.

Psychotic features during a manic episode that emphasize one's importance or powers are called *mood-congruent* psychotic features. Those that do not have such a clear relationship to inflated worth (e.g., belief that one really deserves punishment, that one's mind is being controlled by others) are considered *mood-incongruent*.

In the *DSM-IV* a *mixed episode* occurs when an individual fulfills simultaneously the criteria for a manic episode and for a major depressive episode. This turns out to be a rather stringent requirement, and change seems likely (*DSM-5* Task Force, 2012b). Concern that current mixed-episode criteria are too restrictive derives from the fact that many patients display an admixture of negative affect along with the heightened behavioral or cognitive activation seen in mania, yet they do not meet criteria for major depression and mania simultaneously (Bauer, Simon, Ludman, & Unützer, 2005; Dilsaver, Benazzi, & Akiskal, 2005; Goldberg et al., 2009; Maj, Pirozzi, Magliano, & Bartoli, 2003; Sato, Bottlender, Kleindienst, & Möller, 2002). For instance, a severely depressed person may experience racing thoughts about his or her worthlessness and exhibit agitated reckless behavior. Or a person with the high activity and "drive" of mania may simultaneously express despair and suicidal ideation. It is also not uncommon to observe dramatic changes in mood state within a brief period of time (*mood lability*). For instance, a person may, even during the same interview, appear exuberant and elated at first, but then despondent and tearful. However, other symptoms of MDD (e.g., changes in appetite, sleep, psychomotor retardation) cannot be seen in this short time. Moreover, this commingling of mania and MDD symptoms may occur as a person transitions from one type of episode to another, such as from a manic to a depressive episode. The current proposal, therefore, is to replace the mixed-episode type with a mixed-episode *specifier* that one might append to any type of BPD episode (*DSM-5* Task Force, 2012b). A "mixed episode," as currently defined, would be diagnosed as a manic episode with mixed features.

Correctly identifying manic episodes, mixed episodes, agitated depression, or severe mood lability is far more than a semantic exercise. For example, antidepressant medications can induce mania or hypomania among individuals susceptible to BPD (Goldberg & Truman, 2003). On the other hand, most antimanic agents are either not effective for the acute treatment of nonbipolar depression or have a much larger side effect burden than modern antidepressants (Ketter, Citrome, Wang, Culver, & Srivastava, 2011; Nelson & Papakostas, 2009).

## OTHER FORMS OF BPD: BIPOLAR II DISORDER AND CYCLOTHYMIC DISORDER

Bipolar II disorder (BPDII) and cyclothymia involve episodes of *hypomania*. Hypomania differs from mania chiefly in terms of severity and level of impairment. That is, one can observe changes in activity level, impulse control, cognition, and mood that do not have the same adverse effects on role functioning and personal safety as a manic episode. In fact, these periods may be fruitful in some respects, such as greater work productivity or creativity (Judd & Akiskal, 2003). Nevertheless, such episodes are not entirely benign, and the consequences of poor judgment and impulsivity may be significant. Just as in mania, hypomania represents a marked, episodic change from the person's ordinary mood and functioning (i.e., it is not a personality trait). As noted earlier, such episodes may occur among individuals with histories of mania (e.g., BPDI, most recent episode hypomanic); indeed, it is a great relief when their hypomanic episodes remit without escalation into full-blown mania. By the same token, among individuals who have been depressed for a long time, the distinction between onset of a hypomanic episode and fairly rapid remission from their depression is not always easy for clinicians who have not known the person in his or her disorder-free (or *premorbid*) state.

Bipolar II disorder is the diagnosis applied for an individual who is experiencing either (1) an episode of hypomania, or (2) an episode of major depression but who also had a prior episode of hypomania yet *never* had a full manic episode. In effect, any prior history of a full manic episode supersedes a diagnosis of BPDII.

Cyclothymic disorder is a still milder form of BPD. The diagnosis is used to characterize individuals who have frequent distinct periods of hypomanic symptoms and depressive symptoms over a 2-year period (one for children and adolescents), none of which is ever quite severe enough to constitute a manic, mixed, or major depressive episode.

Some data indicate that hypomania is associated with rapid intense mood shifts and more episodes. When the total number of episodes in a year exceeds four, it is called *rapid cycling* (Kupka et al., 2005; Papadimitriou, Calabrese, Dikeos, & Christodoulou, 2005). Some studies have examined the proportion of time patients spend in manic/hypomanic versus depressive moods, or the proportion of manic/hypomanic versus depressive episodes or symptoms (Nierenberg et al., 2010). This research shows marked variability between individuals in the "tilting" of their illness toward depressive versus manic symptoms. Nonetheless, current conceptualizations view all such mood cycling as manifestations of a single fundamental illness, namely BPD (Benazzi, 2006). This approach is essentially the descendant of Kraepelin's view that nearly all mood disorders are expressions of a single overarching illness, what he termed manic-depressive insanity. In addition, the concept of a *bipolar spectrum* is often used today, although definitions vary considerably (see review by Youngstrom et al., 2010).

## PREVALENCE

The single-point prevalence of BPD among adults in the United States is generally agreed to be about 1% to 1.5%, with lifetime prevalence of disorders in the BPD spectrum around 4.5% (Kessler et al., 2006; Merikangas et al., 2007).

Recent epidemiological estimates in the United States show lifetime prevalence among adolescents for bipolar I or II disorder combined of 2.9%. Prevalence increases with age during adolescence. Fully 89.7% of adolescents with these disorders were classified as manifesting "severe" impairment.

Despite increased use of BPD diagnoses for young people in U.S. clinical settings (Blader & Carlson, 2007; Harpaz-Rotem, Leslie, Martin, & Rosenheck, 2005; Moreno et al., 2007), there is no conclusive evidence that the rate of affected individuals, when applying the same diagnostic criteria, is rising over time (Van Meter, Moreira, & Youngstrom, 2011). Rates of epidemiologically determined BPD among youth in the United States are similar to those in other countries (Van Meter et al., 2011). However, non-U.S. health providers do not show the same increase in the *clinical use* of these diagnoses as their U.S. counterparts (Meyer, Koßmann-Böhm, & Schlottke, 2004; Soutullo et al., 2005).

## DEVELOPMENTAL PROGRESSION

Adolescent-onset BPD seems to show, unfortunately, the course of a particularly severe illness (Lewinsohn, Seeley, & Klein, 2003; Merikangas et al., 2010), with high rates of serial hospitalizations, substance abuse, attempted and completed suicides, less robust response to lithium and divalproex, and worse interepisode functioning than adult-onset BPD (Birmaher et al., 2006; Goldstein et al., 2005; Wilcox & Anthony, 2004). In the short term, many youth seem to recover from the functional nadir of their index episode, but subsequent exacerbations and relapse are common (Birmaher et al., 2006). In addition, 20% to 25% of adolescents diagnosed with bipolar II or bipolar NOS progress to fulfill criteria for a more severe form of BPD (i.e., bipolar I) (Axelson, Birmaher, Strober, et al., 2011). Risk for adverse outcomes rises with earlier onset, presence of psychotic features, mixed manic and depressive features, and low socioeconomic resources (Birmaher et al., 2006).

Results from longitudinal clinical studies with children show continuity of impairments, whereas specific diagnoses at follow-up are more variable. Among 15 boys with ADHD who also met criteria for mania, only 1 was diagnosed with mania 6 years later (Hazell, Carr, Lewin, & Sly, 2003), although all continued to display marked functional impairments. Other longitudinal studies (Biederman et al., 2004; Geller, Tillman, Bolhofner, & Zimerman, 2008) continue to show high rates of ADHD and mania from 4 to 8 years after baseline assessments.

## COURSE AND OUTCOMES OF BIPOLAR DISORDER IN ADULTHOOD

Most information on the course and outcomes of BPD comes from clinical groups, and indicate that it is a chronic condition. However, analyses of community epidemiological surveys raise the prospect that a number of individuals may achieve syndromal remission by middle adulthood (Cicero, Epler, & Sher, 2009). Still, this finding awaits clarification in extended longitudinal studies.

In clinical samples, the overall trend with age is for depressive episodes to become more frequent and longer (Kupka et al., 2005; Suppes, Brown, Schuh, Baker, & Tohen, 2005). In the best of cases, functioning between episodes of mood disturbance can be quite good (*full interepisode recovery*) and one enjoys social and occupational success. The likelihood of good outcomes increases with a stable, tolerant family and a social milieu that buffers a person from the consequences of illness and from stresses that would otherwise aggravate it. At the same time, this interpersonal environment must be firm about treatment adherence and lifestyle practices that may forestall relapse (Alloy et al., 2005; Johnson, Lundströem, Åberg-Wistedt, & Mathé, 2003).

Less fortunate individuals experience an unstable, often unremitting course. Although depression may come to predominate the clinical presentation, outcomes for those with BPD are more often worse than for unipolar depression (Goldberg & Harrow, 2011). They may drift downward socially as interpersonal and occupational functioning become increasingly erratic and inadequate. Interepisode recovery is incomplete in such cases. Sources of social support may become either alienated or actively rejected by the increasingly irascible patient. Legal entanglements are common complications. Civil liabilities arise from failure to meet financial or family obligations. Criminal activity may stem from explosiveness, belligerence, and violence, sometimes impelled by psychotic delusions but often also from impatience and anger with others who act to thwart the person's immediate attainment of some, often peculiar, objective.

Alcohol and drug abuse are strongly related to BPD, and when present, course of illness is worse and risk of death from external causes is higher (Blader, 2011; Cardoso et al., 2008; Friedman et al., 2005; Goldberg, 2010; Goldberg, Garno, Leon, Kocsis, & Portera, 1999; Grant et al., 2005; Keck et al., 1998). Over time, a sizable proportion of individuals become permanently disabled (Judd & Akiskal, 2003; Judd et al., 2005; Morgan, Mitchell, & Jablensky, 2005). Social marginalization and loneliness are common outcomes that exacerbate the illness. The risk for suicide and age-adjusted mortality from all causes is high, particularly among those with earlier onset and impulsivity (Dilsaver et al., 1997; Fiedorowicz et al., 2009; Garno, Goldberg, Ramirez, & Ritzler, 2005; Novick, Swartz, & Frank, 2010; Östby, Brandt, Correia, Ekbom, & Sparén, 2001).

## CONCEPTUAL AND PRACTICAL ISSUES IN THE DIAGNOSIS OF BIPOLAR DISORDER AMONG YOUTH

Bipolar disorder epitomizes the difficulties encountered when one takes a psychopathological entity defined by *symptom descriptions* cultivated within one population—in this case early- to midlife adults—and transplants it to another population—in this case children. The same underlying disturbance that produces observed symptoms among mature individuals might produce different behavioral manifestations among youth. Conversely, similar behavioral abnormalities may reflect different underlying causes even within the same age group—otherwise there would be no need for differential diagnosis. But similar behaviors *across* age groups may have different likelihoods of signifying a particular disorder (i.e., for which the symptoms are *pathognomonic*). We consider the symptoms and course of BPD in the light of these developmental considerations.

### Symptom Differences and Confounding Comorbidities

A manic episode is defined by persistence of a cardinal mood abnormality (becoming highly elated, euphoric, expansive, or irritable) lasting (as noted earlier) at least one week or less if hospitalization is needed. In addition, there are behaviors that signify an "activated" state, and current criteria require at least three of these behaviors (or four if the mood disturbance is irritability): grandiosity, talkativeness, flight of ideas, distractibility, increased activity or psychomotor agitation, and excessive involvement in pleasurable activities that risk adverse consequences.

An *elevated or euphoric* mood is an exaggerated feeling of well-being that the person may describe as feeling "high," "ecstatic," or "on top of the world" (APA, 2000, p. 825). *Expansiveness* means "lack of restraint in expressing one's feelings, frequently with an overvaluation of one's significance or importance." Adolescents are better equipped linguistically and experientially to articulate feelings of euphoria/elation than children. Among children, however, mood is usually inferred from behavior. Hence, terms such as *silly* and *giddy* are used to describe a child's euphoria. However, it is difficult to determine when and if such behaviors indicate elation. Children may seek attention with silly antics for a variety of nonmanic reasons, or may be susceptible to extreme emotional displays in high stimulation situations, such as parties or family gatherings (Carlson & Meyer, 2006). Therefore, although an abrupt and sustained change in demeanor from sullen or reserved to euphoric or expansive may suggest mania, it is less clear when one observes elevated mood in a typically excitable person.

Euphoria and elation were thought to be fairly specific to mania (Geller et al., 2002). However, recent epidemiological research indicates high prevalence of brief periods of such mood states among adolescents, based on both parent report (12.7%) and youth self-report (28%) (Stringaris et al., 2010; Stringaris, Stahl, Santosh, & Goodman, 2011). Importantly, endorsement of such mood changes correlates with higher risk for psychopathology but not bipolar disorder specifically (see also Lewinsohn, Klein, & Seeley, 1995).

Extreme *irritability* (i.e., being easily annoyed or angered with minimal provocation) is also an affective disturbance seen in mania. However, irritability manifests in a number of other disorders, including unipolar depression. Recognizing that irritability is less specific to mania, the *DSM-IV* requires 4 rather than 3 of the other manic symptoms to define a manic episode. There is some evidence, however, that adolescents are indeed susceptible to a normative, developmentally specific form of hyperemotionality, which may magnify periods of irritability (Arnett, 1999; Casey, Getz, & Galvan, 2008; Casey, Jones, & Somerville, 2011). In addition, half the symptoms for oppositional defiant disorder (ODD), which is highly prevalent among children comorbid with ADHD, also involve displays of irritability or hostile affect. Longitudinal studies of young people with high ratings of irritability show heightened risk for anxiety and mood disorders but not BPD specifically (Stringaris et al., 2011).

*Grandiosity*, or inflated appraisal of one's worth, power, knowledge, importance, or identity, is easily identified in adults with mania. Naturally, adolescents' grandiose claims or delusions reflect age-typical values. One girl, who believed she was a pop music idol, spent an hour picking out items in a clothing boutique. When it was her turn in line to pay, she was content to step aside and let others ahead because, she explained, she was waiting for her manager to come and complete the purchase. In children, inflated self-esteem may be hard to differentiate from excessive bragging to peers or just cognitive immaturity. For instance, a child may interpret a compliment "you swim like a fish" to mean that he can swim across the ocean (Carlson & Meyer, 2006). Even in adolescents, who may feel that they can achieve greatness without finishing high school or are popular without evidence to substantiate it, distinguishing truly inflated self-esteem from a defensive stance requires real clinical skill (Harrington & Myatt, 2003).

*Decreased need for sleep* is relatively straightforward when sleep time is replaced with energetic pursuit of activities and daytime fatigue is absent. Among children, one has to distinguish true decreased *need* for sleep from (a) highly prevalent bedtime struggles, especially among children with behavioral difficulties; and (b) true insomnia and night waking that typically occur among those with anxieties (Blader, Koplewicz, Abikoff, & Foley, 1997). This distinction can be accomplished by asking how tired the child is during the day, whether he or she is difficult to rouse after late sleep onset, and tends to wake up later on nonschool days.

*Increased talkativeness* and its close relative, *flight of ideas*, are pathognomonic when the person is ordinarily reserved and shy outside of manic/hypomanic episodes. *DSM-IV* symptoms for ADHD include *talks excessively* and *is distractible*, both ingredients for chattiness with lots of digressions. Given the high comorbidity with ADHD consistently reported in clinical samples of children identified with BPD, using these criteria to identify a manic episode superimposed on preexisting ADHD is typically futile. Clinicians should take heed, though, of the occasional instance when a child, usually a more expressive one, spontaneously reports that his or her brain is on "overdrive" to a degree that is uncomfortable (e.g., Goodwin & Jamison, 2007, p. 189).

Similarly, *distractibility* as a symptom of mania is also a symptom or feature of numerous disorders, some of which designate the problem as "impaired ability to concentrate." It is particularly troublesome, though, that distractibility is not only central to the inattentive subtype of ADHD but also to depression. Practically speaking, then, unless it is clear that one's focus and attention has undergone marked changes, distractibility contributes little to differential diagnosis.

*Increases in goal-directed activity* in older individuals with BPD generally have a focus and purpose, albeit of a rather grandiose or quixotic nature, as noted earlier. A few children with BPD do get excited about a project they intend to start or an invention they claim will reap millions of dollars. Many children, of course, ruminate or talk about such big plans, but *acting* on these ideas may be more suggestive of BPD. One youngster sneaked out of his home to spend most of the night in the 24-hour photocopying store preparing brochures for a business he was planning to launch. This type of activity must be differentiated from the more aimless but energetic high-activity level intrinsic to ADHD, or the intense, even obsessional interests, of some children on the high-functioning autistic spectrum.

The term *psychomotor agitation* has been rightly criticized for its ambiguities (Day, 1999), but nonetheless conveys *discomfort* (pacing, hang-wringing, repositioning, or frantically distraught inability to settle) that should be distinguished from the restlessness of children with ADHD. The former persists and is, clearly, unpleasant; the latter is relieved as soon as the child is permitted to resume enjoyment of his or her frenetic activity level.

*Excessive involvement in pleasurable activities* better conveys a BPD-specific abnormality for people who in the past have shown normal self-restraint and a characteristically cautious, even avoidant, approach to new ventures. Among the majority of children considered for a BPD diagnosis, however, impulse-control deficits have been present early in life. Rushing headlong into something that offers the promise of excitement or fun with little concern for consequences will therefore often be present well in advance of symptoms more specific to BPD. Hypersexuality among children and adolescents may include frequent masturbation, often with little regard for privacy, unusual sexual inquisitiveness and preoccupation, or grabbing for others' genitals or breasts. However, these behaviors among children always require further consideration of possible sexual abuse and inappropriate exposure to pornography or others' sexual behavior. Intense sexual behavior or interest may be a manifestation of mania, but mania certainly does not rule out maltreatment. Moreover, histories of sexual abuse portend worse outcomes among those with BPD (Leverich et al., 2002).

*Psychotic symptoms* among children can be difficult to differentiate from the magical or unrealistic thinking, active imagination, cognitive immaturity, exaggeration, and imaginary friends common to this age group. In some controversial instances, behavior that would not be intrinsically psychotic among adults is interpreted as such among children. For instance, in one clinical trial for BPDI, 77.1% of 6- to 15-year-olds reported psychotic features (Geller et al., 2012). Psychotic grandiosity was inferred when, in one example, a youngster wrote to his principal demanding the dismissal of a specific teacher. Although perhaps insolent, there was no indication the child believed he was, say, a government official with such powers. Unfortunately, such misinterpretations of psychosis may contribute to the problems extrapolating the diagnosis of mania from adults to children.

## Onset of Mood Disturbance

When a behavioral abnormality first appears as a clear departure from one's usual self, it is easy to conclude that an untoward change is underway. BPD traditionally emphasizes such change. Imagine that a 25-year-old reserved and timid woman rapidly turns gregarious, uses coarse language, adopts an unconventional appearance, invades others' personal space, seems sexually preoccupied, suddenly gets on a bus to New York to start her modeling career, and is hospitalized because she grew belligerent at a modeling agency where she showed up insisting she had an appointment. Chances are good she had a manic episode. Now, suppose that for most of her life and possibly worsening with adolescence she had been highly extroverted, had poor boundaries, was impulsive, a bit irresponsible, flamboyant in appearance, known to be demanding, argumentative and sulky at times, but was generally likeable and never had mental health care. Her sudden departure, combativeness, and possible delusions still need psychiatric attention, but when should we deduce that her difficulties first began? Were the preceding years a sort of prodromal phase? Or did personality traits that gelled during adolescence establish *higher risk* for bipolar illness, but not an inexorable progression toward it? There are no clear answers to these questions, despite their importance for a developmental perspective on psychopathology.

For children, the situation is further complicated because, as we have seen, many behavioral disturbances that might otherwise signify possible BPD in a more mature person, such as irritability, talkativeness, and distractibility, are frequent early in life. That is, there may be no acute *break* or onset characteristic of psychopathology first developing among older individuals. When symptoms comprise only those that are nonspecific to BPD (irritability, impulsiveness, poor judgment in fulfillment of one's desires), it is particularly controversial whether BPD without a clear onset is a valid characterization of the problem.

### EPISODES OF MOOD DISTURBANCE

The concept of an episode for a major mood disorder has two elements. One is that these recurring periods of disturbance should be distinguishable from a person's usual self. The other is that *during* this time of illness, problems with mood and associated behavior are observable or experienced most of the time. In other words, during the episode they are persistent rather than transient phenomena.

### DISTINCT PERIODS OF MOOD SYMPTOMS OR EXACERBATION

In BPD, major depressive episodes or mania typically last on the order of weeks, sometimes more, and are generally longer for depression than mania. Recovery may not necessarily be complete, in which case periods of serious exacerbation represent "episodes." A *rapid cycling* course of illness is defined by at least four episodes in a year. However the clinical significance of this pattern, when controlling for duration of illness overall, remains uncertain and, in any event, is often not a stable year-after-year phenomenon (Bauer, Beaulieu, Dunner, Lafer, & Kupka, 2008).

In this framework, episodicity implies an onset with a significant change from ordinary functioning. When observed among children, it increases suspicion that bipolar disorder may be present. However, when symptoms chiefly involve those less specific to mania, such as irritability, and there is no evidence that the child shows a qualitative departure from his or her regular self, the standard criteria for BPD are not met. One corollary is that if a child has shown lifelong disturbances of this type the disorder is clearly not episodic. Relatedly, periods of remission that occur spontaneously are uncommon among children, which is yet another deviation from BPD's episodic nature. Some children may function and feel better during school breaks when they do not have to contend with the rigors of daily routine and academic demands, but one should not confuse this offset of an 'episode'.

### PERSISTENCE VERSUS TRANSIENCE OF MOOD DISTURBANCE

One of the hallmarks of MDD is persistent negative affect that largely quashes both the capacity to experience pleasure (*anhedonia*) and the motivation to pursue experiences ordinarily found enjoyable (*apathy*). Likewise, when irritability is the dominant mood state in MDD or BPD, one feels irritable most of the time regardless of situational context. This touchiness comes across as an effort to repel most any stimulation and is impervious to positive events. In fact, brightening up when something good happens (or *mood reactivity*) is considered part of *atypical depression*. Similarly, a striking characteristic of classic elated mania is one's imperviousness to things that go badly. Of course, stressful or intensely stimulating situations may precipitate depression or mania. But the point here is that persistence of the mood disturbance in circumstances no longer congruent with it is an important characteristic of major mood disorders.

A number of children do show persistent negative mood that changes only minimally with positive events. Caregivers are both baffled and frustrated because their efforts to cheer or soothe the child are not successful and interactions with the child are therefore unrewarding. For young children who also have symptoms of ADHD, differential diagnosis between depression superimposed on ADHD versus possible BPD can be difficult.

It is far more common, however, that children who manifest with significant irritability are, in fact, highly *overreactive* to events. They show heightened emotional reactivity when provoked, mild as that provocation may seem to others. When things are going their way they are euthymic. Their brittle frustration tolerance, in order words, leads to frequent but relatively short-lived upsets, even meltdowns, followed by return to a normal mood state. Similarly, momentary elation may be brought on by exciting or stimulating events, so the reaction is not qualitatively inappropriate although its expression may be too intense for the context.

Some clinicians, however, do infer mood cycles from such relatively brief periods of behavioral dyscontrol. Those who regard these incidents as manifestations of BPD often refer to this form of affective oscillation as *ultradian* cycling, meaning that cycles appear many times within a single day (e.g., Geller, Tillman, & Bolhofner, 2007; Kramlinger & Post, 1996). This notion is controversial because others find it too improbable that these transient, frequent bouts of hyperemotionality, typically anchored in some provocation, equal a major mood episode or cycle in the conventional diagnostic sense (e.g., Leibenluft, 2011).

The important conceptual issue, presently unresolved, is whether such transient incidents of affective and behavior dyscontrol share any underlying perturbations with BPD or, for that matter, unipolar depression. Several deviations in development are related to momentary emotion dysregulation (see Chapter 11). For instance, temperament studies often find both an *affective tone* factor that is distinct from *negative reactivity* (Muris & Ollendick, 2005; Sanson & Prior, 1999). The latter is common in ADHD (Melnick & Hinshaw, 2000), especially with comorbid ODD/CD, and in fact often remits with treatment primarily directed toward ADHD (Blader, Pliszka, Jensen, Schooler, & Kafantaris, 2010).

## ALTERNATIVE APPROACHES TO EMOTIONAL VOLATILITY IN YOUTH

We have seen that most children with clinically significant disturbances of affect and impulse control do not fulfill current criteria for bipolar I or II disorders. This section summarizes some recent proposals to distinguish their difficulties from both adult-derived criteria for major mood disorders and from other existing diagnoses that emphasize chiefly disruptive behaviors.

### DISTINGUISHING "NARROW," "INTERMEDIATE," AND "BROAD" PHENOTYPES

Leibenluft and colleagues (2011; Leibenluft, Charney, Towbin, Bhangoo, & Pine, 2003) offered a classification scheme that acknowledges the diverse clinical presentations (*phenotypes*) of children for which the appropriateness of bipolar diagnosis has been considered. The four categories they propose reflect how far a phenotype departs from the current *DSM-IV* criteria.

1. First, a *narrow phenotype* has a symptom presentation, course, and episodicity fully aligned with current criteria for (adult) BPD, with the additional requirement that the mood abnormality be *euphoria* or that there be other signs of pathological grandiosity.
   They define two intermediate phenotypes.
2. One intermediate phenotype encompasses manic episodes that last from 1 to 3 days, instead of the *DSM*-stipulated 4 (hypomania) to 7 (mania). Current nomenclature would classify a number of these situations as bipolar disorder not otherwise specified (NOS).
3. The other allows irritability to be the main mood aberration, so long as there is also evidence of well-demarcated episodes.
4. Their final category is a *broad phenotype* denoted as severely disturbed behavior and mood dysregulation, which essentially describes chronic negative emotional reactivity and impulsivity. This group has sometimes been branded as having severe mood dysregulation (see later). Criteria for the broad phenotype also require rather pervasive and persistent negative mood (at least half the time).

Whether these phenotypes will come to meaningfully distinguish discrete forms of psychopathology remains uncertain. But as a provisional means to reduce heterogeneity in research samples it may prove useful.

### DISRUPTIVE MOOD DYSREGULATION DISORDER

Another proposal detaches from the BPD realm the rageful irritability, common among children, that lacks other key symptoms of BPD. Disruptive mood dysregulation disorder (DMDD) would be a new mood disorder diagnosis with onset before 10 years that is under consideration for *DSM-5* (*DSM-5* Task Force, 2012a). In effect, it would characterize a subgroup of individuals in the "broad phenotype" category discussed earlier who have a persistently negative mood that is punctuated by frequent, episodic, and severe temper outbursts in reaction to stressors. It would be distinguishable from DBDs by emphasis on chronically negative mood (sadness, irritability, or anger) even in the absence of acute provocation. By contrast, as we have noted, most children with severe behavioral disturbances do not display persistently negative mood and appear euthymic when there is no provocation to elicit their upsets. DMDD would not subsume ODD/CD, which, along with ADHD, may be diagnosed concurrently. Such "trimorbidity" is expected to be high (Brotman et al., 2006; Carlson, 2007; Dickstein et al., 2009). If the individual's symptoms meet full syndromal criteria for another mood disorder (e.g., MDD, dysthymic disorder, BPD), then that other disorder would supersede DMDD.

DMDD advocates seek to provide a classification for children whose explosive outbursts seem underrecognized in current nomenclature, while avoiding the perils of an overly elastic redefinition of bipolar disorder that others have proposed. Still, premature adoption of DMDD may introduce another set of difficulties. These include a limited evidence base to distinguish it reliably from other disorders, uncertainty about its potential prevalence, and strong reliance on essentially one symptom (viz., irritability that both "smolders" and "flares") to make a diagnosis (see Axelson, Birmaher, Findling, et al., 2011).

## RISK FACTORS AND ETIOLOGICAL FORMULATIONS

### CLINICAL RISK FACTORS

*Clinical risk factors* are disorders or symptoms whose presence raises the likelihood that one will develop the target disorder later.

*Depression.* Patients who develop BPD often experience depression as their first episode (Beesdo et al., 2009; Chengappa et al., 2003; Nadkarni & Fristad, 2010). Predicting who among depressed young people will develop a bipolar course becomes important in deciding treatment.

Among adolescents with MDD, there are some factors that may increase the likelihood that BPD will evolve. These factors include precipitous onset of the depressive episode, psychotic features, manic symptoms below threshold for BPD diagnosis, family history, and susceptibility to hypomania with antidepressant treatment (Beesdo et al., 2009; Fiedorowicz et al., 2011; Strober & Carlson, 1982; Zimmermann et al., 2008; Zimmermann et al., 2009).

The conversion rate of unipolar MDD to BPD (*switching*) varies across studies partly as a function, not surprisingly, of recruitment strategy and length of follow-up. For example, a community epidemiological sample reported a switch rate of 4% over 7 years for those identified at baseline with MDD (Beesdo et al., 2009). The incidence of switching rose to 20% in clinical samples (Fiedorowicz et al., 2011), and 40.5% with long-term follow-up of an inpatient cohort (Goldberg, Harrow, & Whiteside, 2001). Clinical samples show a switch rate from childhood MDD to bipolar I or II disorder of 6% of child outpatients over 10 years (Weissman et al., 1999), 19% of adolescent outpatients over 7 years (Rao et al., 1995), and 20% of adolescent inpatients over 3 to 4 years (Strober & Carlson, 1982).

*Bipolar disorder NOS.* BPD NOS has been frequently used to diagnose those who do not present with either symptoms or duration of illness sufficient to fulfill criteria for a specific BPD diagnosis, especially children (Blader & Carlson, 2007).

In one sense, it may function in clinical settings to enable less-restrictive use of BPD diagnosis to convey the severity of a child's behavioral symptoms. However, there is mounting evidence that some young patients who warrant the BPD NOS diagnosis because they experience manic symptoms for fewer than the four days required for hypomania are indeed at higher risk for later development of bipolar I or II disorders (Axelson, Birmaher, Strober, et al., 2011). This group corresponds to one of the "intermediate" phonotypes mentioned earlier (Leibenluft et al., 2003). Conversion to BPD I or BPD II disorder occurred among 45% of 7- to 17-year-olds within 5 years, with median time to conversion from study entry of 58 weeks *across* disorders (Axelson, Birmaher, Strober, et al., 2011). Other samples corroborate the high impairment of young people who meet manic episode criteria except for duration (Stringaris, Santosh, Leibenluft, & Goodman, 2010). In community samples, moreover, brief but memorable and distinct periods of elation were associated with higher risk for psychopathology though not BPD specifically (Stringaris et al., 2011).

## BIOLOGICAL SUSCEPTIBILITY FACTORS

*Heritability and genetic markers.* Liability for development of BPD increases among those who have affected biological relatives. In the case of classic (narrow phenotype) BPD, heritability estimates are as high as 80% (Craddock & Sklar, 2009; Nurnberger et al., 2011), and early-onset BPD may be even more firmly grounded in genetic risk (a phenonemon observed across many psychiatric disorders; see Chapter 21). Bipolar disorder heritability estimates exceed those for unipolar MDD (Craddock & Forty, 2006), often considerably. In addition, many characteristics associated with the postulated "broad phenotype" of BPD (affective instability, deficient impulse control) are highly heritable as well (Bartels et al., 2004; Doyle et al., 2010; Rujescu et al., 2002; Todd et al., 2001).

Efforts to determine the specific genes underlying familial risk have accounted for only a small portion of heritability (Schulze, 2010; Sklar et al., 2008)—a problem that pervades psychiatric genetics (see Chapter 3). It may turn out that BPD with psychotic features has a different genetic basis than other forms of BPD. Family association and molecular studies are converging on this possibility (International Schizophrenia Consortium et al., 2009; Lichtenstein et al., 2009; MacQueen, Hajek, & Alda, 2005), and comports with cluster-analytic studies that find high correlations between schizophrenia and manic episodes (Kotov et al., 2011; see Chapter 21).

*Neurodevelopmental antecedents.* Some findings suggest that perinatal events are associated with BPD in childhood. For instance, obstetrical complications are more prevalent among children diagnosed with BPD than controls, 54% versus 16% respectively (Pavuluri, Henry, Nadimpalli, O'Connor, & Sweeney, 2006). Studies involving adults do not indicate a major influence of perinatal problems, though wide variation in the definitions of such complications precludes a firm conclusion (Scott, McNeill, Cavanagh, Cannon, & Murray, 2006).

A study of 11- to 18-year-old psychiatric inpatients compared the neurodevelopmental status of youth who had BPD or unipolar depression with psychotic features (per ICD-10) to patients diagnosed with nonpsychotic unipolar depressive disorder

(Sigurdsson, Fombonne, Sayal, & Checkley, 1999). The former group had higher rates of premorbid language, motor, and social developmental problems, leading the authors to conclude they predispose more strongly to BPD than to depression. There were no differences in perinatal complications.

*Disturbances of the sleep-wake cycle.* There are some data to suggest that circadian rhythms governing the sleep-wake cycle may be relevant to the development of BPD and its exacerbations. It has been known for many years that sleep deprivation in some individuals with MDD provides temporary symptomatic relief but in a number of cases elicits hypomania (Giedke & Schwarzler, 2002). Regularizing sleep and wake times is widely seen as important to avoiding relapse of BPD (Frank et al., 2008; Fristad, 2006; Harvey, 2008; Miklowitz et al., 2011). Some authors have therefore posited that vulnerability toward circadian irregularity may have etiological significance for BPD (Harvey, Mullin, & Hinshaw, 2006; Jones, 2001; Nievergelt et al., 2006).

## COGNITIVE FACTORS AND OTHER POTENTIAL MARKERS

It is usually impractical to assemble a large cohort of people, measure potential genetically determined markers of risk, and wait to see who develops the disorder. An alternative is to compare the unaffected relatives of people with a disorder to controls who do not have affected relatives. The premise is that if a marker is heritable, it will be more prevalent in the former group.

In BPD research, this approach has suggested cognitive markers involving impaired response inhibitions and other executive functions (Bora, Yucel, & Pantelis, 2009; Hasler, Drevets, Gould, Gottesman, & Manji, 2006). However, in other studies problems with attention were found among patients themselves but not preferentially among their relatives (Clark, Kempton, Scarna, Grasby, & Goodwin, 2005; Clark, Sarna, & Goodwin, 2005).

Functional deficits related to attention and inhibitory controls often implicate the dorsolateral prefontal cortex (DLPFC) and the ventrolateral prefrontal cortex (VLPFC) in ADHD (Halperin & Schulz, 2006; Pliszka et al., 2006). Some research suggests that functions subserved by VLPFC but *not* DLFPC are specifically deficient in patients with BPD and their relatives (Frangou, Haldane, Roddy, & Kumari, 2005).

Well-known cognitive features of depression include a tendency to exaggerate and dwell on misfortunes or one's perceived shortcomings and to face the future with hopelessness and dread (Beck, 2008). However, an analogue of such cognitive biases for mania has yet to be confirmed (Alloy et al., 2005). Current efforts to evaluate overly positive self-related cognitions along with the individual's attributions for them may advance this area (Jones, Mansell, & Waller, 2006).

## NEUROANATOMICAL AND NEUROPHYSIOLOGICAL FACTORS

The amygdala is a distinct structure in the medial anterior portion of each temporal lobe that adjoins the hippocampus. Its role in motivation, emotion encoding, and response to threat has been thoroughly described, and it is a natural focus of interest for mood and anxiety disorders. Reduced amygdala volumes have been reported among the first-degree relatives, including children, of adults with BPD (Chang et al., 2005; Hajek, Carrey, & Alda, 2005). Among patients themselves, reduced amygdala volumes have been reported in BPD, but also in other disorders of affective instability (Blumberg et al., 2005; Rosso et al., 2005; Szeszko et al., 1999). Recent work suggests that patients with BPD receiving pharmacotherapy may display amygdala *enlargement*, whereas untreated patients show decreased volumes relative to healthy controls (Savitz et al., 2010).

Functional neuroimaging studies show increased amygdala activity elicited by emotion-relevant stimuli among adults with BPD compared with controls (Altshuler et al., 2005). Moreover, prefrontal cortical areas may be relatively underactive, contributing to less "top-down" control over emotional reactivity in those with BPD (Chepenik et al., 2010; Foland et al., 2008). However, among children in a similar paradigm, those with ADHD (but no mood disturbance) showed amygdala hyperactivation, while children with DMDD showed hypoactivation. Interpretation is complicated by the findings that children with strictly-defined BPD showed no difference from controls (Brotman et al., 2010).

Another brain region of interest for BPD is the cingulate gyrus, a long rostral-caudal band of cortex that integrates several components of the limbic system. The anterior cingulate cortex in particular is involved in regulating affect, self-monitoring, and evaluating changes in external reward contingencies. Reductions in volume of the anterior cingulate have been reported in BPD patients and their unaffected close relatives. Cortical thickness specifically, rather than overall regional volume, was shown to be less in patients than controls, and this distinction may be important in future work (Fornito et al., 2008). However, similar findings also apply to ADHD (e.g., Beauchaine, Sauder, Gatzke-Kopp, Shannon, & Aylward, in press).

Scalp electroencephalographic (EEG) recordings taken while participants make simple responses to infrequent stimuli ordinarily show a large positive spike about 300 ms after stimulus presentation. This event-related potential (ERP), called the *P300*, is thought to reflect attentional and response organizing activities. Patients with a number of psychiatric disorders that have a common denominator of behavioral disinhibition (but also including schizophrenia) show reduced amplitude and longer latency of P300 than nonaffected individuals. There is some evidence that right-lateralized P300 abnormalities might be a biomarker of adult BPD (Lahera et al., 2009; Pierson, Jouvent, Quintin, Perez-Diaz, & Leboyer, 2000). In comparing children diagnosed with BPD to nondiagnosed control participants, the former exhibited reduced and delayed P300 only when response errors were penalized, suggesting that frustration disrupts attentional allocation in this disorder (Rich et al., 2005).

## EXPERIENTIAL AND ENVIRONMENTAL SUSCEPTIBILITY FACTORS

It is difficult to judge to what extent stressful life experiences contribute to the onset of BPD because (a) retrospective reports carry potential biases toward overidentification of events, as patients and families strive to make attributions; (b) many stressful events can arise as a consequence of behavior changes caused by the incipient disorder (i.e., gene-environment correlation; see Chapter 3); and (c) few studies include comparison groups. In any case, there are more data on the association of life events with the course of BPD than with its onset. Some have proposed models that address the potential for stressful events to exert different effects over time (Bender & Alloy, 2011).

Among youth-onset BPD, efforts have been made to distinguish stressful life events that are independent of the patients' behavior. One investigation revealed higher rates of such independent stressful events in the families of youth with BPD than those with uncomplicated ADHD and no other diagnosis (Tillman et al., 2003). Retrospective self-reports of child maltreatment are markedly elevated among adults with mood and personality disorders, especially women (MacMillan et al., 2001). Among adults with BPD, several studies report high prevalence of severe childhood trauma, which is associated with a more pernicious course of illness (e.g., early onset, fewer remissions, suicidality) (Garno, Goldberg, Ramirez, & Ritzler, 2005; Neria, Bromet, Carlson, & Naz, 2005).

Psychotropic medications in therapeutic doses can elicit a manic-like episode in some individuals. Manic symptoms that first emerge during treatment with antidepressants are sometimes referred to as *medication-induced switching*. Currently, although medication-induced mania does not "count" toward a diagnosis of BPD, some contend that those who do *switch* have vulnerability toward BPD and that exposure to the offending drugs may hasten progression of the illness. This important issue remains unsettled (Bauer et al., 2006). In children, it is known that exposure to selective serotonin reuptake inhibitors (SSRIs) can produce behavioral disinhibition, but there is no evidence that this is related to BPD vulnerability (Safer & Zito, 2006; Walkup & Labellarte, 2001). Another concern is that children with ADHD whose explosive, aggressive behavior might lie in the 'bipolar spectrum' will worsen when treated with stimulant medications. Treatment and observational studies do not support this notion (Blader et al., 2010; Carlson & Mick, 2003).

## PATHOGENESIS

Despite hints about potentially contributory factors in the development of BPD, its exact etiology and pathophysiology remain unknown.

When structurally diverse pharmacological agents affect an illness, one approach is to examine the functional properties (e.g., receptor binding) these compounds may share to infer clues about underlying pathogenesis. However, in BPD as in most other psychiatric conditions, treatments are chiefly "symptom-modifying" rather than "disease-modifying." Therapies that help to subdue symptom expression but do not reverse the underlying illness process may exert their effects through pathways unrelated to etiology. With this caveat in mind, three potential mechanisms of action for antimanic drugs illustrate recent work on the pathogenesis of BPD.

Arachidonic acid (AA) is an abundant fatty acid in the brain, and a building block of neuronal membranes, which are phospholipid bilayers. Phospholipases (PLAs) contribute to the turnover of AA from membrane back into the cytosol, and

AA and its metabolites have significant roles in neuronal function and protection. Depolarization increases PLA activity, and thus the cascade of AA metabolism and signaling. The "arachidonic cascade hypothesis" for BPD stems from findings that effective medications for the disorder alter enzymatic activity or downstream metabolites of AA (Rapoport, Basselin, Kim, & Rao, 2009).

Inositol is a constituent of phospholipase C, a complex on the interior surface of neuron membranes that breaks down when the synapse-facing G-protein-coupled receptor to which it is attached receives adequate neurotransmitter binding. The breakdown of phospholipase C constitutes a key component of the neuron's response to neurotransmission, setting in motion a number of cellular events. Lithium and other antimanic drugs share the capacity to inhibit free inositol, thereby down-regulating receptor production (Williams, Cheng, Mudge, & Harwood, 2002), which leads to the *inositol-depletion hypothesis* for their mechanism. It has been debated whether these inositol-related intracellular cascades may be dysregulated in BPD (Harwood, 2005; Silverstone et al., 2002).

It has also been known for some time that lithium inhibits glycogen synthase kinase-$3\beta$ (GSK3-b), an enzyme that regulates some intraneuronal signaling pathways. Evidence that valproic acid, an anticonvulsant effective in treating mania, also shares this property (Eickholt et al., 2005) has spurred interest in pathways that involve GSK3-b as perhaps influential in BPD (Einat & Manji, 2006).

## COMORBIDITY

ADHD is the leading comorbidity reported among children diagnosed with BPD (e.g., Arnold et al., 2011; Biederman et al., 2005; Carlson, 1998; Pavuluri, Birmaher, & Naylor, 2005). Among adolescents, rates of comorbid ADHD drop as precipitous onset of bipolar symptoms becomes more prevalent with age (e.g., Kafantaris, Coletti, Dicker, Padula, & Pollack, 1998). Retrospective studies of adults with BPD suggest lower, but not negligible, rates of premorbid ADHD: 15% among males, but only 5% among women (Nierenberg et al., 2005). Childhood behavioral problems were more prevalent among adults with earlier onset of bipolarity (<21 years of age) (Carlson, Bromet, & Sievers, 2000).

Substance abuse is common among adolescents and adults with BPD, and it is the most prevalent secondary diagnosis among inpatients with the disorder (Blader, 2011). Community and clinical outpatient studies also show elevated rates of substance abuse, especially among younger individuals (Kessler, Berglund, et al., 2005; Kessler, Chiu, Demler, Merikangas, & Walters, 2005). This onset in turn further increases risk for self-injurious behaviors (Goldstein et al., 2005; Lewinsohn et al., 2003). The link between BPD and substance abuse may in part be mediated by conduct disorder in adolescence (Carlson, Bromet, & Jandorf, 1998).

Prevalence estimates of comorbid anxiety disorders vary considerably in child BPD. One research group (Dickstein et al., 2005) found that 77% of children who met *narrow* criteria for bipolar I or II disorder had at least one comorbid anxiety disorder. However, children showing signs of mania culled from psychiatric clinic attendees did not have increased rates of anxiety disorder relative to other patients, although when present they were more severe (Findling et al., 2010).

## SEX DIFFERENCES

Epidemiological studies of bipolar illness in adult populations have shown similar rates for both sexes (Grant et al., 2005; Merikangas et al., 2007), which also seems to be the case among adolescents (Johnson, Cohen, & Brook, 2000; Lewinsohn et al., 2003).

Males are often more prevalent in research samples of children diagnosed with BPD (Biederman et al., 2005; Findling et al., 2010; Geller, Tillman, Craney, & Bolhofner, 2004), as well as those admitted to inpatient care (Blader & Carlson, 2007). On recent treatment study, though, had no gender difference (Geller et al., 2012).

## CULTURAL FACTORS

Mood disorders may be more prevalent among Hispanic adolescents compared with non-Hispanic white adolescents in the United States (Merikangas et al., 2010), but differences for bipolar disorder specifically are uncertain.

However, there may be differences in the use of diagnoses in clinical settings, which, given no epidemiological evidence for differences in prevalence, could indicate bias in practices. Specifically, African American individuals, especially men, have been less likely to receive a diagnosis of BPD and more likely to receive a diagnosis of schizophrenia or schizoaffective disorder than white patients (Kilbourne et al., 2005; Strakowski et al., 2003). Similar findings have emerged among adolescents (DelBello, Lopez-Larson, Soutullo, & Strakowski, 2001). There may be a trend to impute higher rates of psychotic features to African American patients, both adults and adolescents, the accuracy of which is uncertain (Patel, DelBello, & Strakowski, 2006).

The extent to which nonracial cultural factors affect symptom expression in BPD is an interesting issue about which there is little empirical literature.

## THEORETICAL SYNTHESIS AND FUTURE DIRECTIONS

Severe behavioral dyscontrol occasioned by affective instability, regardless of specific diagnosis, most often has a chronic course and confers risk for impairments that entail grave personal and familial misfortune. The challenge for developmental psychopathology is to better elucidate the myriad ways these difficulties can develop early in life, which would enable the development of appropriate interventions.

Current understanding of mental illness remains grounded principally in a descriptive approach to symptom co-occurrence and patterns of onsets and course. Improved grasp of the underlying mechanisms of disorder has a core goal for decades, but difficulties in observing the brain in action and the ephemeral nature of behavior itself make progress reliant on incremental advances in technology and conceptual approaches.

The signature features and course of BPD are well characterized, and the fact that it develops frequently during middle to late adolescence makes it an important focus for developmental psychopathologists. Their perspective on multiple interactions over time among biological susceptibilities, other developmental factors, and social/environmental influences is essential for considering BPD in youth. Beside *classic* BPD, which represents a qualitative change in behavior that occurs with well-delineated episodes, other forms of early-onset, chronic, and unremitting affective and behavioral volatility have been postulated to constitute a variant of BPD among youth. At this time, it remains uncertain whether these forms of impairment are (a) developmental versions of the same disease processes that underlie later-onset BPD, (b) separate types of illness that might involve perturbations of the same mechanisms of self-control and mood that are implicated in BPD, or (c) fundamentally different problems, such as severe ADHD with ODD, that demonstrate some phenotypic overlap with BPD. A better detailed account of the underpinnings of impulse control, emotional states, affective regulation, and social adaptation, as well as the diverse ways that these areas can incur dysfunction, will be pivotal to advancement of the science. It is also imperative that a developmental framework inform the evolution of this knowledge.

# REFERENCES

Alloy, L. B., Abramson, L. Y., Urosevic, S., Walshaw, P. D., Nusslock, R., & Neeren, A. M. (2005). The psychosocial context of bipolar disorder: Environmental, cognitive, and developmental risk factors. *Clinical Psychology Review, 25*, 1043–1075. doi: 10.1016/j.cpr.2005.06.006

Altshuler, L., Bookheimer, S., Proenza, M. A., Townsend, J., Sabb, F., Firestine, A.,...Cohen, M. S. (2005). Increased amygdala activation during mania: A functional magnetic resonance imaging study. *American Journal of Psychiatry, 162*, 1211–1213. doi: 10.1176/appi.ajp.162.6.1211

American Psychiatric Association. (2000). *Diagnostic and statistical manual of mental disorders* (4th ed.). Washington, DC: American Psychiatric Press.

Angst, J., & Marneros, A. (2001). Bipolarity from ancient to modern times: Conception, birth and rebirth. *Journal of Affective Disorders, 67*, 3–19.

Anthony, E. J., & Scott, P. (1960). Manic-depressive psychosis in childhood. *Journal of Child Psychology and Psychiatry, 1*, 53–72.

Arnett, J. J. (1999). Adolescent storm and stress, reconsidered. *American Psychologist, 54*, 317–326.

Arnold, L. E., Demeter, C., Mount, K., Frazier, T. W., Youngstrom, E. A., Fristad, M.,...Axelson, D. A. (2011). Pediatric bipolar spectrum disorder and ADHD: Comparison and comorbidity in the LAMS clinical sample. *Bipolar Disorders, 13*, 509–521. doi: 10.1111/j.1399–5618.2011.00948.x

Axelson, D. A., Birmaher, B., Findling, R. L., Fristad, M. A., Kowatch, R. A., Youngstrom, E. A.,...Diler, R. S. (2011). Concerns regarding the inclusion of temper dysregulation disorder with dysphoria in the Diagnostic and Statistical Manual of Mental Disorders, 5th Edition. [Commentary]. *Journal of Clinical Psychiatry, 72,* 1257–1262. doi: 10.4088/jcp.10com06220

Axelson, D. A., Birmaher, B., Strober, M. A., Goldstein, B. I., Ha, W., Gill, M. K., . . . Keller, M. B. (2011). Course of subthreshold bipolar disorder in youth: Diagnostic progression from bipolar disorder not otherwise specified. *Journal of the American Academy of Child and Adolescent Psychiatry, 50,* 1001–1016. doi: 10.1016/j.jaac.2011.07.005

Bartels, M., van den Oord, E. J., Hudziak, J. J., Rietveld, M. J., van Beijsterveldt, C. E., & Boomsma, D. I. (2004). Genetic and environmental mechanisms underlying stability and change in problem behaviors at ages 3, 7, 10, and 12. *Developmental Psychology, 40,* 852–867. doi: 10.1037/0012–1649.40.5.852

Bauer, M., Beaulieu, S., Dunner, D. L., Lafer, B., & Kupka, R. (2008). Rapid cycling bipolar disorder: Diagnostic concepts. *Bipolar Disorders, 10* (1, Pt 2), 153–162. doi: 10.1111/j.1399–5618.2007.00560.x

Bauer, M., Rasgon, N., Grof, P., Glenn, T., Lapp, M., Marsh, W., . . . Whybrow, P. C. (2006). Do antidepressants influence mood patterns? A naturalistic study in bipolar disorder. *European Psychiatry, 21,* 262–269. doi: 10.1016/j.eurpsy.2006.04.009

Bauer, M. S., Simon, G. E., Ludman, E., & Unützer, J. (2005). "Bipolarity" in bipolar disorder: Distribution of manic and depressive symptoms in a treated population. *British Journal of Psychiatry, 187,* 87–88.

Beck, A. T. (2008). The evolution of the cognitive model of depression and its neurobiological correlates. *American Journal of Psychiatry, 165,* 969–977. doi: 10.1176/appi.ajp.2008.08050721

Beauchaine, T. P., Sauder, C., Gatzke-Kopp, L. M., Shannon, K. E., & Aylward, E. (in press). Neuroanatomical correlates of heterotypic comorbidity in externalizing youth. *Journal of Clinical Child and Adolescent Psychology.*

Beesdo, K., Hofler, M., Leibenluft, E., Lieb, R., Bauer, M., & Pfennig, A. (2009). Mood episodes and mood disorders: Patterns of incidence and conversion in the first three decades of life. *Bipolar Disorders, 11,* 637–649. doi: 10.1111/j.1399–5618.2009.00738.x

Benazzi, F. (2006). Mood patterns and classification in bipolar disorder. *Current Opinion in Psychiatry, 19,* 1–8.

Bender, R. E., & Alloy, L. B. (2011). Life stress and kindling in bipolar disorder: Review of the evidence and integration with emerging biopsychosocial theories. *Clinical Psychology Review, 31,* 383–398. doi: 10.1016/j.cpr.2011.01.004

Biederman, J., Faraone, S. V., Wozniak, J., Mick, E., Kwon, A., & Aleardi, M. (2004). Further evidence of unique developmental phenotypic correlates of pediatric bipolar disorder: Findings from a large sample of clinically referred preadolescent children assessed over the last 7 years. *Journal of Affective Disorders, 82*(Suppl. 1), 45–58.

Biederman, J., Faraone, S. V., Wozniak, J., Mick, E., Kwon, A., Cayton, G. A., & Clark, S. V. (2005). Clinical correlates of bipolar disorder in a large, referred sample of children and adolescents. *Journal of Psychiatric Research, 39,* 611–622.

Biederman, J., Klein, R. G., Pine, D. S., & Klein, D. F. (1998). Resolved: Mania is mistaken for ADHD in prepubertal children [Debate Forum]. *Journal of the American Academy of Child and Adolescent Psychiatry, 37,* 1091–1099.

Birmaher, B., Axelson, D., Strober, M., Gill, M. K., Valeri, S., Chiappetta, L., . . . Keller, M. (2006). Clinical course of children and adolescents with bipolar spectrum disorders. *Archives of General Psychiatry, 63,* 175–183.

Blader, J. C. (2011). Acute inpatient care for psychiatric disorders in the United States, 1996 through 2007. *Archives of General Psychiatry, 68,* 1276–1283. doi: 10.1001/archgenpsychiatry.2011.84

Blader, J. C., & Carlson, G. A. (2007). Increased rates of bipolar disorder diagnoses among U.S. child, adolescent, and adult inpatients, 1996–2004. *Biological Psychiatry, 62,* 107–114. doi: 10.1016/j.biopsych.2006.11.006

Blader, J. C., Koplewicz, H. S., Abikoff, H., & Foley, C. (1997). Sleep problems of elementary school children. A community survey. *Archives of Pediatrics and Adolescent Medicine, 151,* 473–480.

Blader, J. C., Pliszka, S. R., Jensen, P. S., Schooler, N. R., & Kafantaris, V. (2010). Stimulant-responsive and stimulant-refractory aggressive behavior among children with ADHD. *Pediatrics, 126,* e796–e806. doi: 10.1542/peds.2010–0086

Blumberg, H. P., Fredericks, C., Wang, F., Kalmar, J. H., Spencer, L., Papademetris, X., . . . Krystal, J. H. (2005). Preliminary evidence for persistent abnormalities in amygdala volumes in adolescents and young adults with bipolar disorder. *Bipolar Disorders, 7,* 570–576. doi: 10.1111/j.1399–5618.2005.00264.x

Bora, E., Yucel, M., & Pantelis, C. (2009). Cognitive endophenotypes of bipolar disorder: A meta-analysis of neuropsychological deficits in euthymic patients and their first-degree relatives. *Journal of Affective Disorders, 113,* 1–20. doi: 10.1016/j.jad.2008.06.009

Brotman, M. A., Rich, B. A., Guyer, A. E., Lunsford, J. R., Horsey, S. E., Reising, M. M., . . . Leibenluft, E. (2010). Amygdala activation during emotion processing of neutral faces in children with severe mood dysregulation versus ADHD or bipolar disorder. *American Journal of Psychiatry, 167,* 61–69. doi: 10.1176/appi.ajp.2009.09010043

Brotman, M. A., Schmajuk, M., Rich, B. A., Dickstein, D. P., Guyer, A. E., Costello, E. J., . . . Leibenluft, E. (2006). Prevalence, clinical correlates, and longitudinal course of severe mood dysregulation in children. *Biological Psychiatry, 60,* 991–997. doi: 10.1016/j.biopsych.2006.08.042

Cardoso, B. M., Kauer Sant'Anna, M., Dias, V. V., Andreazza, A. C., Cereser, K. M., & Kapczinski, F. (2008). The impact of co-morbid alcohol use disorder in bipolar patients. *Alcohol, 42,* 451–457. doi: 10.1016/j.alcohol.2008.05.003

Carlson, G. A. (1998). Mania and ADHD: Comorbidity or confusion. *Journal of Affective Disorders, 51,* 177–187.

Carlson, G. A. (2007). Who are the children with severe mood dysregulation, a.k.a. "rages"? [Editorial]. *American Journal of Psychiatry, 164,* 1140–1142. doi: 10.1176/appi.ajp.2007.07050830

Carlson, G. A., Bromet, E. J., & Jandorf, L. (1998). Conduct disorder and mania: What does it mean in adults. *Journal of Affective Disorders, 48,* 199–205.

Carlson, G. A., Bromet, E. J., & Sievers, S. (2000). Phenomenology and outcome of subjects with early- and adult-onset psychotic mania. *American Journal of Psychiatry, 157*, 213–219. doi: 10.1176/appi.ajp.157.2.213

Carlson, G. A., & Glovinsky, I. (2009). The concept of bipolar disorder in children: A history of the bipolar controversy. *Child and Adolescent Psychiatric Clinics of North America, 18*, 257–271. doi: 10.1016/j.chc.2008.11.003

Carlson, G. A., & Meyer, S. E. (2006). Phenomenology and diagnosis of bipolar disorder in children, adolescents, and adults: Complexities and developmental issues. *Development and Psychopathology, 18*, 939–969. doi: 10.1017/S0954579406060470

Carlson, G. A., & Mick, E. (2003). Drug-induced disinhibition in psychiatrically hospitalized children. *Journal of Child and Adolescent Psychopharmacology, 13*, 153–163. doi: 10.1089/104454603322163871

Casey, B. J., Getz, S., & Galvan, A. (2008). The adolescent brain. *Developmental Review, 28*, 62–77. doi: 10.1016/j.dr.2007.08.003

Casey, B. J., Jones, R. M., & Somerville, L. H. (2011). Braking and accelerating of the adolescent brain. *Journal of Research on Adolescence, 21*, 21–33. doi: 10.1111/j.1532–7795.2010.00712.x

Chang, K., Karchemskiy, A., Barnea-Goraly, N., Garrett, A., Simeonova, D. I., & Reiss, A. (2005). Reduced amygdalar gray matter volume in familial pediatric bipolar disorder. *Journal of the American Academy of Child and Adolescent Psychiatry, 44*, 565–573. doi: 10.1097/01.chi.0000159948.75136.0d

Chengappa, K. N., Kupfer, D. J., Frank, E., Houck, P. R., Grochocinski, V. J., Cluss, P. A., & Stapf, D. A. (2003). Relationship of birth cohort and early age at onset of illness in a bipolar disorder case registry. *American Journal of Psychiatry, 160*, 1636–1642.

Chepenik, L. G., Raffo, M., Hampson, M., Lacadie, C., Wang, F., Jones, M. M., . . . Blumberg, H. P. (2010). Functional connectivity between ventral prefrontal cortex and amygdala at low frequency in the resting state in bipolar disorder. *Psychiatry Research: Neuroimaging, 182*, 207–210. doi: 10.1016/j.pscychresns.2010.04.002

Cicero, D. C., Epler, A. J., & Sher, K. J. (2009). Are there developmentally limited forms of bipolar disorder? *Journal of Abnormal Psychology, 118*, 431–447. doi: 10.1037/a0015919

Clark, L., Kempton, M. J., Scarna, A., Grasby, P. M., & Goodwin, G. M. (2005). Sustained attention-deficit confirmed in euthymic bipolar disorder but not in first-degree relatives of bipolar patients or euthymic unipolar depression. *Biological Psychiatry 57*, 183–187. doi: 10.1016/j.biopsych.2004.11.007

Clark, L., Sarna, A., & Goodwin, G. M. (2005). Impairment of executive function but not memory in first-degree relatives of patients with bipolar I disorder and in euthymic patients with unipolar depression. *American Journal of Psychiatry, 162*, 1980–1982. doi: 10.1176/appi.ajp.162.10.1980

Craddock, N., & Forty, L. (2006). Genetics of affective (mood) disorders. *European Journal of Human Genetics, 14*, 660–668. doi: 10.1038/sj.ejhg.5201549.

Craddock, N., & Sklar, P. (2009). Genetics of bipolar disorder: Successful start to a long journey. *Trends in Genetics, 25*, 99–105. doi: 10.1016/j.tig.2008.12.002

Day, R. K. (1999). Psychomotor agitation: Poorly defined and badly measured. *Journal of Affective Disorders, 55*(2–3), 89–98.

DelBello, M. P., Lopez-Larson, M. P., Soutullo, C. A., & Strakowski, S. M. (2001). Effects of race on psychiatric diagnosis of hospitalized adolescents: A retrospective chart review. *Journal of Child and Adolescent Psychopharmacology, 11*, 85–103.

Dickstein, D. P., Rich, B. A., Binstock, A. B., Pradella, A. G., Towbin, K. E., Pine, D. S., & Leibenluft, E. (2005). Comorbid anxiety in phenotypes of pediatric bipolar disorder. *Journal of Child and Adolescent Psychopharmacology, 15*, 534–548. doi: 10.1089/cap.2005.15.534

Dickstein, D. P., Towbin, K. E., Van Der Veen, J. W., Rich, B. A., Brotman, M. A., Knopf, L., ... Leibenluft, E. (2009). Randomized double-blind placebo-controlled trial of lithium in youths with severe mood dysregulation. *Journal of Child and Adolescent Psychopharmacology, 19*, 61–73. doi: 10.1089/cap.2008.044

Dilsaver, S. C., Benazzi, F., & Akiskal, H. S. (2005). Mixed states: The most common outpatient presentation of bipolar depressed adolescents? *Psychopathology, 38*, 268–272.

Dilsaver, S. C., Chen, Y.-W., Swann, A. C., Shoaib, A. M., Tsai-Dilsaver, Y., & Krajewski, K. J. (1997). Suicidality, panic disorder and psychosis in bipolar depression, depressive-mania and pure-mania. *Psychiatry Research, 73*, 47–56.

Doyle, A. E., Biederman, J., Ferreira, M. A., Wong, P., Smoller, J. W., & Faraone, S. V. (2010). Suggestive linkage of the child behavior checklist juvenile bipolar disorder phenotype to 1p21, 6p21, and 8q21. *Journal of the American Academy of Child and Adolescent Psychiatry, 49*, 378–387. doi: 10.1016/j.jaac.2010.01.008

*DSM-5* Task Force. (2012a). D 00: Disruptive mood dysregulation disorder [Web page]. *DSM-5 Development/Proposed Revisions.* Arlington, VA: American Psychiatric Association. Retrieved from http://www.dsm5.org/ProposedRevision/Pages/proposedrevision.aspx?rid=397

*DSM-5* Task Force. (2012b). Mixed features specifier [Web page]. *DSM-5 Development/Proposed Revisions/Mood Disorders.* Arlington, VA: American Psychiatric Association. Retrieved from http://www.dsm5.org/ProposedRevisions/Pages/proposedrevision.aspx?rid=483

Eickholt, B. J., Towers, G. J., Ryves, W. J., Eikel, D., Adley, K., Ylinen, L. M. J., ... Williams, R. S. B. (2005). Effects of valproic acid derivatives on inositol trisphosphate depletion, teratogenicity, glycogen synthase kinase-3$\beta$ inhibition, and viral replication: A screening approach for new bipolar disorder drugs derived from the valproic acid core structure. *Molecular Pharmacology, 67*, 1426–1433. doi: 10.1124/mol.104.009308

Einat, H., & Manji, H. K. (2006). Cellular plasticity cascades: Genes-to-behavior pathways in animal models of bipolar disorder. *Biological Psychiatry, 59*, 1160–1171.

Fiedorowicz, J. G., Endicott, J., Leon, A. C., Solomon, D. A., Keller, M. B., & Coryell, W. H. (2011). Subthreshold hypomanic symptoms in progression from unipolar major depression to bipolar disorder. *American Journal of Psychiatry, 168*, 40–48. doi: 10.1176/appi.ajp.2010.10030328

Fiedorowicz, J. G., Leon, A. C., Keller, M. B., Solomon, D. A., Rice, J. P., & Coryell, W. H. (2009). Do risk factors for suicidal behavior differ by affective disorder polarity? *Psychological Medicine, 39,* 763–771. doi: 10.1017/S0033291708004078

Findling, R. L., Youngstrom, E. A., Fristad, M. A., Birmaher, B., Kowatch, R. A., Arnold, L. E., . . . Horwitz, S. M. (2010). Characteristics of children with elevated symptoms of mania: The longitudinal assessment of manic symptoms (LAMS) study. *Journal of Clinical Psychiatry, 71*(12), 1664–1672. doi: 10.4088/jcp.09m05859yel

Foland, L. C., Altshuler, L. L., Bookheimer, S. Y., Eisenberger, N., Townsend, J., & Thompson, P. M. (2008). Evidence for deficient modulation of amygdala response by prefrontal cortex in bipolar mania. *Psychiatry Research, 162,* 27–37. doi: 10.1016/j.pscychresns.2007.04.007

Fornito, A., Malhi, G. S., Lagopoulos, J., Ivanovski, B., Wood, S. J., Saling, M. M., . . . Yucel, M. (2008). Anatomical abnormalities of the anterior cingulate and paracingulate cortex in patients with bipolar I disorder. *Psychiatry Research: Neuroimaging, 162,* 123–132. doi: 10.1016/j.pscychresns.2007.06.004

Frangou, S., Haldane, M., Roddy, D., & Kumari, V. (2005). Evidence for deficit in tasks of ventral, but not dorsal, prefrontal executive function as an endophenotypic marker for bipolar disorder. *Biological Psychiatry, 58,* 838–839. doi: 10.1016/j.biopsych.2005.05.020

Frank, E., Soreca, I., Swartz, H. A., Fagiolini, A. M., Mallinger, A. G., Thase, M. E., . . . Kupfer, D. J. (2008). The role of interpersonal and social rhythm therapy in improving occupational functioning in patients with bipolar I disorder. *American Journal of Psychiatry, 165,* 1559–1565. doi: 10.1176/appi.ajp.2008.07121953

Friedman, S. H., Shelton, M. D., Elhaj, O., Youngstrom, E. A., Rapport, D. J., Packer, K. A., . . . Calabrese, J. R. (2005). Gender differences in criminality: Bipolar disorder with co-occurring substance abuse. *Journal of the American Academy of Psychiatry and the Law, 33,* 188–195.

Fristad, M. A. (2006). Psychoeducational treatment for school-aged children with bipolar disorder. *Development and Psychopathology, 18,* 1289–1306. doi: 10.1017/S0954579406060627

Garno, J. L., Goldberg, J. F., Ramirez, P. M., & Ritzler, B. A. (2005). Bipolar disorder with comorbid cluster B personality disorder features: Impact on suicidality. *Journal of Clinical Psychiatry, 66,* 339–345.

Garno, J. L., Goldberg, J. F., Ramirez, P. M., & Ritzler, B. A. (2005). Impact of childhood abuse on the clinical course of bipolar disorder. *British Journal of Psychiatry, 186,* 121–125. doi: 10.1192/bjp.186.2.121

Geller, B., Luby, J. L., Joshi, P., Wagner, K. D., Emslie, G., Walkup, J. T., . . . Lavori, P. (2012). A randomized controlled trial of risperidone, lithium, or divalproex sodium for initial treatment of bipolar I disorder, manic or mixed phase, in children and adolescents. *Archives of General Psychiatry, early online release [January 4]* (issue pending), pages pending. doi: 10.1001/archgenpsychiatry.2011.1508

Geller, B., Tillman, R., & Bolhofner, K. (2007). Proposed definitions of bipolar I disorder episodes and daily rapid cycling phenomena in preschoolers, school-aged children, adolescents, and adults. *Journal of Child and Adolescent Psychopharmacology, 17*, 217–222. doi: 10.1089/cap.2007.0017

Geller, B., Tillman, R., Bolhofner, K., & Zimerman, B. (2008). Child bipolar I disorder: Prospective continuity with adult bipolar I disorder, characteristics of second and third episodes, predictors of 8-year outcome. *Archives of General Psychiatry, 65,* 1125–1133. doi: 10.1001/archpsyc.65.10.1125

Geller, B., Tillman, R., Craney, J. L., & Bolhofner, K. (2004). Four-year prospective outcome and natural history of mania in children with a prepubertal and early adolescent bipolar disorder phenotype. *Archives of General Psychiatry, 61,* 459–467. doi: 10.1001/archpsyc.61.5.459

Geller, B., Zimerman, B., Williams, M., Delbello, M. P., Bolhofner, K., Craney, J. L., . . . Nickelsburg, M. J. (2002). DSM-IV mania symptoms in a prepubertal and early adolescent bipolar disorder phenotype compared to attention-deficit hyperactive and normal controls. *Journal of Child and Adolescent Psychopharmacology, 12,* 11–25. doi: 10.1089/10445460252943533

Giedke, H., & Schwarzler, F. (2002). Therapeutic use of sleep deprivation in depression. *Sleep Medicine Reviews, 6,* 361–377. doi: S1087079202902352 [pii]

Goldberg, J. F. (2010). Substance abuse and switch from depression to mania in bipolar disorder. *American Journal of Psychiatry, 167,* 868–869. doi: 10.1176/appi.ajp.2010.10030367

Goldberg, J. F., Garno, J. L., Leon, A. C., Kocsis, J. H., & Portera, L. (1999). A history of substance abuse complicates remission from acute mania in bipolar disorder. *Journal of Clinical Psychiatry, 60,* 733–740.

Goldberg, J. F., & Harrow, M. (2011). A 15-year prospective follow-up of bipolar affective disorders: Comparisons with unipolar nonpsychotic depression. *Bipolar Disorders, 13,* 155–163. doi: 10.1111/j.1399–5618.2011.00903.x

Goldberg, J. F., Harrow, M., & Whiteside, J. E. (2001). Risk for bipolar illness in patients initially hospitalized for unipolar depression. *American Journal of Psychiatry, 158,* 1265–1270.

Goldberg, J. F., Perlis, R. H., Bowden, C. L., Thase, M. E., Miklowitz, D. J., Marangell, L. B., . . . Sachs, G. S. (2009). Manic symptoms during depressive episodes in 1,380 patients with bipolar disorder: Findings from the STEP-BD. *American Journal of Psychiatry, 166,* 173–181. doi: 10.1176/appi.ajp.2008.08050746

Goldberg, J. F., & Truman, C. J. (2003). Antidepressant-induced mania: An overview of current controversies. *Bipolar Disorders, 5,* 407–420. doi: 10.1046/j.1399–5618.2003.00067.x

Goldstein, T. R., Birmaher, B., Axelson, D., Ryan, N. D., Strober, M. A., Gill, M. K., . . . Keller, M. (2005). History of suicide attempts in pediatric bipolar disorder: Factors associated with increased risk. *Bipolar Disorders, 7,* 525–535.

Goodwin, F. K., & Jamison, K. R. (Eds.). (2007). *Manic-depressive illness: Bipolar and recurrent depression* (2nd ed.). New York, NY: Oxford University Press.

Grant, B. F., Stinson, F. S., Hasin, D. S., Dawson, D. A., Chou, S. P., Ruan, W. J., & Huang, B. (2005). Prevalence, correlates, and comorbidity of bipolar I disorder and axis I and II disorders: Results from the national epidemiologic survey on alcohol and related conditions. *Journal of Clinical Psychiatry, 66,* 1205–1215.

Hajek, T., Carrey, N., & Alda, M. (2005). Neuroanatomical abnormalities as risk factors for bipolar disorder. *Bipolar Disorders, 7,* 393–403. doi: 10.1111/j.1399–5618.2005.00238.x

Halperin, J. M., & Schulz, K. P. (2006). Revisiting the role of the prefrontal cortex in the pathophysiology of attention-deficit/hyperactivity disorder. *Psychological Bulletin, 132,* 560–581. doi: 10.1037/0033–2909.132.4.560

Harpaz-Rotem, I., Leslie, D. L., Martin, A., & Rosenheck, R. A. (2005). Changes in child and adolescent inpatient psychiatric admission diagnoses between 1995 and 2000. *Social Psychiatry and Psychiatric Epidemiology, 40,* 642–647.

Harrington, R., & Myatt, T. (2003). Is preadolescent mania the same condition as adult mania? A British perspective. *Biological Psychiatry, 53,* 961–969.

Harvey, A. G. (2008). Sleep and circadian rhythms in bipolar disorder: Seeking synchrony, harmony, and regulation. *American Journal of Psychiatry, 165,* 820–829. doi: 10.1176/appi.ajp.2008.08010098

Harvey, A. G., Mullin, B. C., & Hinshaw, S. P. (2006). Sleep and circadian rhythms in children and adolescents with bipolar disorder. *Development and Psychopathology, 18,* 1147–1168. doi: 10.1017/S095457940606055X

Harwood, A. J. (2005). Lithium and bipolar mood disorder: The inositol-depletion hypothesis revisited. *Molecular Psychiatry, 10,* 117–126. doi: 10.1038/sj.mp.4001618

Hasler, G., Drevets, W. C., Gould, T. D., Gottesman, I. I., & Manji, H. K. (2006). Toward constructing an endophenotype strategy for bipolar disorders. *Biological Psychiatry, 60,* 93–105. doi: 10.1016/j.biopsych.2005.11.006

Hazell, P. L., Carr, V., Lewin, T. J., & Sly, K. (2003). Manic symptoms in young males with ADHD predict functioning but not diagnosis after 6 years. *Journal of the American Academy of Child and Adolescent Psychiatry, 42,* 552–560. doi: 10.1097/01.CHI.0000046830.95464.33

International Schizophrenia Consortium, Purcell, S. M., Wray, N. R., Stone, J. L., Visscher, P. M., O'Donovan, M. C., . . . Sklar, P. (2009). Common polygenic variation contributes to risk of schizophrenia and bipolar disorder. *Nature, 460,* 748–752. doi: 10.1038/nature08185

Johnson, J. G., Cohen, P., & Brook, J. S. (2000). Associations between bipolar disorder and other psychiatric disorders during adolescence and early adulthood: A community-based longitudinal investigation. *American Journal of Psychiatry, 157,* 1679–1681.

Johnson, L., Lundströem, O., Åberg-Wistedt, A., & Mathé, A. A. (2003). Social support in bipolar disorder: Its relevance to remission and relapse. *Bipolar Disorders, 5,* 129–137.

Jones, S., Mansell, W., & Waller, L. (2006). Appraisal of hypomania-relevant experiences: Development of a questionnaire to assess positive self-dispositional appraisals in bipolar and behavioural high risk samples. *Journal of Affective Disorders, 93,* 19–28. doi: 10.1016/j.jad.2006.01.017

Jones, S. H. (2001). Circadian rhythms, multilevel models of emotion and bipolar disorder—An initial step towards integration? *Clinical Psychology Review, 21,* 1193–1209. doi: 10.1016/S0272–7358(01)00111–8

Judd, L. L., & Akiskal, H. S. (2003). The prevalence and disability of bipolar spectrum disorders in the US population: Re-analysis of the ECA database taking into account subthreshold cases. *Journal of Affective Disorders, 73*, 123–131.

Judd, L. L., Akiskal, H. S., Schettler, P. J., Endicott, J., Leon, A. C., Solomon, D. A., . . . Keller, M. B. (2005). Psychosocial disability in the course of bipolar I and II disorders: A prospective, comparative, longitudinal study. *Archives of General Psychiatry, 62*, 1322–1330.

Kafantaris, V., Coletti, D. J., Dicker, R., Padula, G., & Pollack, S. (1998). Are childhood psychiatric histories of bipolar adolescents associated with family history, psychosis, and response to lithium treatment? *Journal of Affective Disorders, 51*, 153–164.

Keck, P. E. Jr., McElroy, S. L., Havens, J. R., Altshuler, L. L., Nolen, W. A., Frye, M. A., . . . Post, R. M. (2003). Psychosis in bipolar disorder: Phenomenology and impact on morbidity and course of illness. *Comprehensive Psychiatry, 44*, 263–269.

Keck, P. E., Jr., McElroy, S. L., Strakowski, S. M., West, S. A., Sax, K. W., Hawkins, J. M., . . . Haggard, P. (1998). 12-month outcome of patients with bipolar disorder following hospitalization for a manic or mixed episode. *American Journal of Psychiatry, 155*, 646–652.

Kennedy, N., Everitt, B., Boydell, J., van Os, J., Jones, P. B., & Murray, R. M. (2005). Incidence and distribution of first-episode mania by age: Results from a 35-year study. *Psychological Medicine, 35*, 855–863.

Kessler, R. C., Akiskal, H. S., Ames, M., Birnbaum, H., Greenberg, P., Hirschfeld, R. M. A., . . . Wang, P. S. (2006). Prevalence and effects of mood disorders on work performance in a nationally representative sample of U.S. workers. *American Journal of Psychiatry, 163*, 1561–1568. doi: 10.1176/appi.ajp.163.9.1561

Kessler, R. C., Berglund, P., Demler, O., Jin, R., Merikangas, K. R., & Walters, E. E. (2005). Lifetime prevalence and age-of-onset distributions of DSM-IV disorders in the national comorbidity survey replication. *Archives of General Psychiatry, 62*, 593–602. doi: 10.1001/archpsyc.62.6.593

Kessler, R. C., Chiu, W. T., Demler, O., Merikangas, K. R., & Walters, E. E. (2005). Prevalence, severity, and comorbidity of 12-month DSM-IV disorders in the national comorbidity survey replication. *Archives of General Psychiatry, 62*, 617–627. doi: 10.1001/archpsyc.62.6.617

Ketter, T. A., Citrome, L., Wang, P. W., Culver, J. L., & Srivastava, S. (2011). Treatments for bipolar disorder: Can number needed to treat/harm help inform clinical decisions? *Acta Psychiatrica Scandinavica, 123*, 175–189. doi: 10.1111/j.1600-0447.2010.01645.x

Kilbourne, A. M., Bauer, M. S., Han, X., Haas, G. L., Elder, P., Good, C. B., . . . Pincus, H. (2005). Racial differences in the treatment of veterans with bipolar disorder. *Psychiatric Services, 56*, 1549–1555.

Kotov, R., Ruggero, C. J., Krueger, R. F., Watson, D., Yuan, Q., & Zimmerman, M. (2011). New dimensions in the quantitative classification of mental illness. *Archives of General Psychiatry, 68*, 1003–1011. doi: 10.1001/archgenpsychiatry.2011.107

Kraepelin, E. (1921). *Manic-depressive insanity and paranoia* (R. M. Barclay, Trans.). Edinburgh, United Kingdom: E. & S. Livingstone.

Kramlinger, K. G., & Post, R. M. (1996). Ultra-rapid and ultradian cycling in bipolar affective illness. *British Journal of Psychiatry, 168,* 314–323.

Kupka, R. W., Luckenbaugh, D. A., Post, R. M., Suppes, T., Altshuler, L. L., Keck, P. E. Jr., . . . Nolen, W. A. (2005). Comparison of rapid-cycling and non-rapid-cycling bipolar disorder based on prospective mood ratings in 539 outpatients. *American Journal of Psychiatry, 162,* 1273–1280.

Lahera, G., Pedrera, A., Cabanes, L., Fernandez-Lorente, J., Simal, P., Montes, J. M., & Saiz-Ruiz, J. (2009). P300 event-related potential in euthymic patients with bipolar disorder. *Progress in Neuro-Psychopharmacology and Biological Psychiatry, 33,* 16–19. doi: 10.1016/j.pnpbp.2008.09.017

Leibenluft, E. (2011). Severe mood dysregulation, irritability, and the diagnostic boundaries of bipolar disorder in youths. [Research Support, N.I.H., Intramural]. *American Journal of Psychiatry, 168,* 129–142. doi: 10.1176/appi.ajp.2010.10050766

Leibenluft, E., Charney, D. S., Towbin, K. E., Bhangoo, R. K., & Pine, D. S. (2003). Defining clinical phenotypes of juvenile mania. *American Journal of Psychiatry, 160,* 430–437.

Leverich, G. S., McElroy, S. L., Suppes, T., Keck, P. E., Jr., Denicoff, K. D., Nolen, W. A., . . . Post, R. M. (2002). Early physical and sexual abuse associated with an adverse course of bipolar illness. *Biological Psychiatry, 51,* 288–297. doi: 10.1016/S0006–3223(01)01239–2,

Lewinsohn, P. M., Klein, D. N., & Seeley, J. R. (1995). Bipolar disorders in a community sample of older adolescents: Prevalence, phenomenology, comorbidity, and course. *Journal of the American Academy of Child and Adolescent Psychiatry, 34,* 454–463.

Lewinsohn, P. M., Seeley, J. R., & Klein, D. N. (2003). Bipolar disorders during adolescence. *Acta Psychiatrica Scandinavica, 108*(Suppl. 418), 47–50.

Lichtenstein, P., Yip, B. H., Bjork, C., Pawitan, Y., Cannon, T. D., Sullivan, P. F., & Hultman, C. M. (2009). Common genetic determinants of schizophrenia and bipolar disorder in Swedish families: A population-based study. *Lancet, 373,* 234–239. doi: 10.1016/S0140–6736(09)60072–6

MacMillan, H. L., Fleming, J. E., Streiner, D. L., Lin, E., Boyle, M. H., Jamieson, E., . . . Beardslee, W. R. (2001). Childhood abuse and lifetime psychopathology in a community sample. *American Journal of Psychiatry, 158,* 1878–1883. doi: 10.1176/appi.ajp.158.11.1878

MacQueen, G. M., Hajek, T., & Alda, M. (2005). The phenotypes of bipolar disorder: Relevance for genetic investigations. *Molecular Psychiatry, 10,* 811–826. doi: 10.1038/sj.mp.4001701

Maj, M., Pirozzi, R., Magliano, L., & Bartoli, L. (2003). Agitated depression in bipolar I disorder: Prevalence, phenomenology, and outcome. *American Journal of Psychiatry, 160,* 2134–2140. doi: 10.1176/appi.ajp.160.12.2134

Melnick, S. M., & Hinshaw, S. P. (2000). Emotion regulation and parenting in AD/HD and comparison boys: Linkages with social behaviors and peer preference. *Journal of Abnormal Child Psychology, 28,* 73–86.

Merikangas, K. R., Akiskal, H. S., Angst, J., Greenberg, P. E., Hirschfeld, R. M., Petukhova, M., & Kessler, R. C. (2007). Lifetime and 12-month prevalence of bipolar spectrum disorder in the national comorbidity survey replication. *Archives of General Psychiatry, 64,* 543–552. doi: 10.1001/archpsyc.64.5.543

Merikangas, K. R., He, J. P., Burstein, M., Swanson, S. A., Avenevoli, S., Cui, L., . . . Swendsen, J. (2010). Lifetime prevalence of mental disorders in U.S. adolescents: Results from the national comorbidity survey replication—Adolescent Supplement (NCS-A). *Journal of the American Academy of Child and Adolescent Psychiatry, 49,* 980–989. doi: 10.1016/j.jaac.2010.05.017

Meyer, T. D., Koßmann-Böhm, S., & Schlottke, P. F. (2004). Do child psychiatrists in Germany diagnose bipolar disorders in children and adolescents? Results from a survey. *Bipolar Disorders, 6,* 426–431. doi: 10.1111/j.1399–5618.2004.00131.x

Miklowitz, D. J., Chang, K. D., Taylor, D. O., George, E. L., Singh, M. K., Schneck, C. D., . . . Garber, J. (2011). Early psychosocial intervention for youth at risk for bipolar I or II disorder: A one-year treatment development trial. *Bipolar Disorders, 13,* 67–75. doi: 10.1111/j.1399–5618.2011.00890.x

Moreno, C., Laje, G., Blanco, C., Jiang, H., Schmidt, A. B., & Olfson, M. (2007). National trends in the outpatient diagnosis and treatment of bipolar disorder in youth. *Archives of General Psychiatry, 64,* 1032–1039. doi: 10.1001/archpsyc.64.9.1032

Morgan, V. A., Mitchell, P. B., & Jablensky, A. V. (2005). The epidemiology of bipolar disorder: Sociodemographic, disability and service utilization data from the Australian national study of low prevalence (psychotic) disorders. *Bipolar Disorders, 7,* 326–337.

Müller-Oerlinghausen, B., Berghöfer, A., & Bauer, M. (2002). Bipolar disorder. *Lancet, 359,* 241–247.

Muris, P., & Ollendick, T. H. (2005). The role of temperament in the etiology of child psychopathology. *Clinical Child and Family Psychology Review, 8,* 271–289. doi: 10.1007/s10567–005–8809-y

Nadkarni, R. B., & Fristad, M. A. (2010). Clinical course of children with a depressive spectrum disorder and transient manic symptoms. *Bipolar Disorders, 12,* 494–503. doi: 10.1111/j.1399–5618.2010.00847.x

Nelson, J. C., & Papakostas, G. I. (2009). Atypical antipsychotic augmentation in major depressive disorder: A meta-analysis of placebo-controlled randomized trials. [Meta-Analysis]. *American Journal of Psychiatry, 166,* 980–p991. doi: 10.1176/appi.ajp.2009.09030312

Neria, Y., Bromet, E. J., Carlson, G. A., & Naz, B. (2005). Assaultive trauma and illness course in psychotic bipolar disorder: Findings from the Suffolk County Mental Health Project. *Acta Psychiatrica Scandinavica, 111,* 380–383. doi: 10.1111/j.1600–0447.2005.00530.x

Nierenberg, A. A., Akiskal, H. S., Angst, J., Hirschfeld, R. M., Merikangas, K. R., Petukhova, M., & Kessler, R. C. (2010). Bipolar disorder with frequent mood episodes in the national comorbidity survey replication (NCS-R). *Molecular Psychiatry, 15,* 1075–1087. doi: 10.1038/mp.2009.61

Nierenberg, A. A., Miyahara, S., Spencer, T., Wisniewski, S. R., Otto, M. W., Simon, N., . . . STEP-BD Investigators. (2005). Clinical and diagnostic implications of lifetime attention-deficit/hyperactivity disorder comorbidity in adults with bipolar disorder: Data from the first 1000 STEP-BD participants. *Biological Psychiatry, 57,* 1467–1473.

Nievergelt, C. M., Kripke, D. F., Barrett, T. B., Burg, E., Remick, R. A., Sadovnick, A. D., . . . Kelsoe, J. R. (2006). Suggestive evidence for association of the circadian genes PERIOD3 and ARNTL with bipolar disorder. *American Journal of Medical Genetics. Part B: Neuropsychiatric Genetics, 141,* 234–241. doi: 10.1002/ajmg.b.30252

Novick, D. M., Swartz, H. A., & Frank, E. (2010). Suicide attempts in bipolar I and bipolar II disorder: A review and meta-analysis of the evidence. *Bipolar Disorders, 12,* 1–9. doi: 10.1111/j.1399–5618.2009.00786.x

Nurnberger, J. I. Jr., McInnis, M., Reich, W., Kastelic, E., Wilcox, H. C., Glowinski, A., . . . Monahan, P. O. (2011). A high-risk study of bipolar disorder. Childhood clinical phenotypes as precursors of major mood disorders. *Archives of General Psychiatry, 68,* 1012–1020. doi: 10.1001/archgenpsychiatry.2011.126

Ösby, U., Brandt, L., Correia, N., Ekbom, A., & Sparén, P. (2001). Excess mortality in bipolar and unipolar disorder in Sweden. *Archives of General Psychiatry, 58,* 844–850.

Papadimitriou, G. N., Calabrese, J. R., Dikeos, D. G., & Christodoulou, G. N. (2005). Rapid cycling bipolar disorder: Biology and pathogenesis. *International Journal of Neuropsychopharmacology, 8,* 281–292.

Patel, N. C., DelBello, M. P., & Strakowski, S. M. (2006). Ethnic differences in symptom presentation of youths with bipolar disorder. *Bipolar Disorders, 8,* 95–99. doi: 10.1111/j.1399–5618.2006.00279.x

Pavuluri, M. N., Birmaher, B., & Naylor, M. W. (2005). Pediatric bipolar disorder: A review of the past 10 years. *Journal of the American Academy of Child and Adolescent Psychiatry, 44,* 846–871.

Pavuluri, M. N., Henry, D. B., Nadimpalli, S. S., O'Connor, M. M., & Sweeney, J. A. (2006). Biological risk factors in pediatric bipolar disorder. *Biological Psychiatry, 60,* 936–941. doi: 10.1016/j.biopsych.2006.04.002

Pierson, A., Jouvent, R., Quintin, P., Perez-Diaz, F., & Leboyer, M. (2000). Information processing deficits in relatives of manic depressive patients. *Psychological Medicine, 30,* 545–555.

Pliszka, S. R., Glahn, D. C., Semrud-Clikeman, M., Franklin, C., Perez, R., III, Xiong, J., & Liotti, M. (2006). Neuroimaging of inhibitory control areas in children with attention deficit hyperactivity disorder who were treatment naïve or in long-term treatment. *American Journal of Psychiatry, 163,* 1052–1060. doi: 10.1176/appi.ajp.163.6.1052

Rao, U., Ryan, N. D., Birmaher, B., Dahl, R. E., Williamson, D. E., Kaufman, J., . . . Nelson, B. (1995). Unipolar depression in adolescents: Clinical outcome in adulthood. *Journal of the American Academy of Child and Adolescent Psychiatry, 34,* 566–578. doi: 10.1097/00004583–199505000–00009

Rapoport, S. I., Basselin, M., Kim, H. W., & Rao, J. S. (2009). Bipolar disorder and mechanisms of action of mood stabilizers. *Brain Research Reviews, 61,* 185–209. doi: 10.1016/j.brainresrev.2009.06.003

Rich, B. A., Schmajuk, M., Perez-Edgar, K. E., Pine, D. S., Fox, N. A., & Leibenluft, E. (2005). The impact of reward, punishment, and frustration on attention in pediatric bipolar disorder. *Biological Psychiatry, 58,* 532–539. doi: 10.1016/j.biopsych.2005.01.006

Rosso, I. M., Cintron, C. M., Steingard, R. J., Renshaw, P. F., Young, A. D., & Yurgelun-Todd, D. A. (2005). Amygdala and hippocampus volumes in pediatric major depression. *Biological Psychiatry, 57,* 21–26.

Rujescu, D., Giegling, I., Bondy, B., Gietl, A., Zill, P., & Moller, H. J. (2002). Association of anger-related traits with SNPs in the TPH gene. *Molecular Psychiatry, 7,* 1023–1029. doi: 10.1038/sj.mp.4001128

Safer, D. J., & Zito, J. M. (2006). Treatment-emergent adverse events from selective serotonin reuptake inhibitors by age group: Children versus adolescents. *Journal of Child and Adolescent Psychopharmacology, 16,* 159–169. doi: 10.1089/cap.2006.16.159

Sanson, A., & Prior, M. (1999). Temperament and behavioral precursors to oppositional defiant disorder and conduct disorder. In H. C. Quay & A. E. Hogan (Eds.), *Handbook of disruptive behavior disorders* (pp. 397–417). Dordrecht, Netherlands: Kluwer.

Sato, T., Bottlender, R., Kleindienst, N., & Möller, H.-J. (2002). Syndromes and phenomenological subtypes underlying acute mania: A factor analytic study of 576 manic patients. *American Journal of Psychiatry, 159,* 968–974. doi: 10.1176/appi.ajp.159.6.968

Savitz, J., Nugent, A. C., Bogers, W., Liu, A., Sills, R., Luckenbaugh, D. A., . . . Drevets, W. C. (2010). Amygdala volume in depressed patients with bipolar disorder assessed using high resolution 3T MRI: The impact of medication. *NeuroImage, 49,* 2966–2976. doi: 10.1016/j.neuroimage.2009.11.025

Schulze, T. G. (2010). Genetic research into bipolar disorder: The need for a research framework that integrates sophisticated molecular biology and clinically informed phenotype characterization. *Psychiatric Clinics of North America, 33,* 67–82. doi: 10.1016/j.psc.2009.10.005

Scott, J., McNeill, Y., Cavanagh, J., Cannon, M., & Murray, R. (2006). Exposure to obstetric complications and subsequent development of bipolar disorder: Systematic review. *British Journal of Psychiatry, 189,* 3–11. doi: 10.1192/bjp.bp.105.010579

Sedler, M. J. (1983). Falret's discovery: The origin of the concept of bipolar affective illness. *American Journal of Psychiatry, 140,* 1127–1133.

Sigurdsson, E., Fombonne, E., Sayal, K., & Checkley, S. (1999). Neurodevelopmental antecedents of early-onset bipolar affective disorder. *British Journal of Psychiatry, 174,* 121–127.

Silverstone, P. H., Wu, R. H., O'Donnell, T., Ulrich, M., Asghar, S. J., & Hanstock, C. C. (2002). Chronic treatment with both lithium and sodium valproate may normalize phosphoinositol cycle activity in bipolar patients. *Human Psychopharmacology, 17,* 321–327.

Sklar, P., Smoller, J. W., Fan, J., Ferreira, M. A., Perlis, R. H., Chambert, K., . . . Purcell, S. M. (2008). Whole-genome association study of bipolar disorder. *Molecular Psychiatry, 13,* 558–569. doi: 10.1038/sj.mp.4002151

Soutullo, C. A., Chang, K. D., Díez-Suárez, A., Figueroa-Quintana, A., Escamilla-Canales, I., Rapado-Castro, M., & Ortuño, F. (2005). Bipolar disorder in children and adolescents: International perspective on epidemiology and phenomenology. *Bipolar Disorders, 7*, 497–506. doi: 10.1111/j.1399–5618.2005.00262.x

Strakowski, S. M., Keck, P. E., Arnold, L. M., Collins, J., Wilson, R. M., Fleck, D. E., . . . Adebimpe, V. R. (2003). Ethnicity and diagnosis in patients with affective disorders. *Journal of Clinical Psychiatry, 64*, 747–754.

Stringaris, A., Baroni, A., Haimm, C., Brotman, M., Lowe, C. H., Myers, F., . . . Leibenluft, E. (2010). Pediatric bipolar disorder versus severe mood dysregulation: Risk for manic episodes on follow-up. *Journal of the American Academy of Child and Adolescent Psychiatry, 49*, 397–405. doi: 10.1097/00004583–201004000–00014

Stringaris, A., Santosh, P., Leibenluft, E., & Goodman, R. (2010). Youth meeting symptom and impairment criteria for mania-like episodes lasting less than four days: An epidemiological enquiry. *Journal of Child Psychology and Psychiatry, 51*, 31–38. doi: 10.1111/j.1469–7610.2009.02129.x

Stringaris, A., Stahl, D., Santosh, P., & Goodman, R. (2011). Dimensions and latent classes of episodic mania-like symptoms in youth: An empirical enquiry. *Journal of Abnormal Child Psychology, 39*, 925–937. doi: 10.1007/s10802–011–9520–8

Strober, M., & Carlson, G. (1982). Bipolar illness in adolescents with major depression: Clinical, genetic, and psychopharmacologic predictors in a three- to four-year prospective follow-up investigation. *Archives of General Psychiatry, 39*, 549–555.

Strober, M., & Carlson, G. (1982). Predictors of bipolar illness in adolescents with major depression: A follow-up investigation. *Adolescent Psychiatry, 10*, 299–319.

Suppes, T., Brown, E., Schuh, L. M., Baker, R. W., & Tohen, M. (2005). Rapid versus non-rapid cycling as a predictor of response to olanzapine and divalproex sodium for bipolar mania and maintenance of remission: Post hoc analyses of 47-week data. *Journal of Affective Disorders, 89*, 69–77.

Szeszko, P. R., Robinson, D., Alvir, J. M. J., Bilder, R. M., Lencz, T., Ashtari, M., . . . Bogerts, B. (1999). Orbital frontal and amygdala volume reductions in obsessive-compulsive disorder. *Archives of General Psychiatry, 56*, 913–919.

Tillman, R., Geller, B., Nickelsburg, M. J., Bolhofner, K., Craney, J. L., DelBello, M. P., & Wigh, W. (2003). Life events in a prepubertal and early adolescent bipolar disorder phenotype compared to attention-deficit hyperactive and normal controls. *Journal of Child and Adolescent Psychopharmacology, 13*, 243–251. doi: 10.1089/104454603322572570

Todd, R. D., Rasmussen, E. R., Neuman, R. J., Reich, W., Hudziak, J. J., Bucholz, K. K., . . . Heath, A. (2001). Familiality and heritability of subtypes of attention deficit hyperactivity disorder in a population sample of adolescent female twins. *American Journal of Psychiatry, 158*, 1891–1898.

Van Meter, A. R., Moreira, A. L., & Youngstrom, E. A. (2011). Meta-analysis of epidemiologic studies of pediatric bipolar disorder. *Journal of Clinical Psychiatry, 72*, 1250–1256. doi: 10.4088/JCP.10m06290

Walkup, J., & Labellarte, M. (2001). Complications of SSRI treatment. *Journal of Child and Adolescent Psychopharmacology, 11*, 1–4. doi: 10.1089/104454601750143320

Weissman, M. M., Wolk, S., Wickramaratne, P., Goldstein, R. B., Adams, P., Greenwald, S., ... Steinberg, D. (1999). Children with prepubertal-onset major depressive disorder and anxiety grown up. *Archives of General Psychiatry, 56,* 794–801.

Wilcox, H. C., & Anthony, J. C. (2004). Child and adolescent clinical features as forerunners of adult-onset major depressive disorder: Retrospective evidence from an epidemiological sample. *Journal of Affective Disorders, 82,* 9–20.

Williams, R. S., Cheng, L., Mudge, A. W., & Harwood, A. J. (2002). A common mechanism of action for three mood-stabilizing drugs. *Nature, 417,* 292–295.

World Health Organization. (2002). *World health report.* Geneva, Switzerland: WHO Press.

World Health Organization. (2010). Chapter V, mental and behavioural disorders. *International statistical classification of diseases and related health problems.* Geneva, Switzerland: WHO Press.

Youngerman, J., & Canino, I. A. (1978). Lithium carbonate use in children and adolescents. A survey of the literature. *Archives of General Psychiatry, 35,* 216–224.

Youngstrom, E., Van Meter, A., & Algorta, G. P. (2010). The bipolar spectrum: Myth or reality? *Current Psychiatry Reports, 12,* 479–489. doi: 10.1007/s11920–010–0153–3

Zimmermann, P., Bruckl, T., Lieb, R., Nocon, A., Ising, M., Beesdo, K., & Wittchen, H. U. (2008). The interplay of familial depression liability and adverse events in predicting the first onset of depression during a 10-year follow-up. *Biological Psychiatry, 63,* 406–414. doi: 10.1016/j.biopsych.2007.05.020

Zimmermann, P., Bruckl, T., Nocon, A., Pfister, H., Lieb, R., Wittchen, H. U., ... Angst, J. (2009). Heterogeneity of DSM-IV major depressive disorder as a consequence of subthreshold bipolarity. *Archives of General Psychiatry, 66,* 1341–1352. doi: 10.1001/archgenpsychiatry.2009.158

# CHAPTER 20

# Autism Spectrum Disorders

SUSAN FAJA AND GERALDINE DAWSON

A UTISM SPECTRUM DISORDERS (ASD) are a group of developmental disorders characterized by impairments in social and communication behavior, and a restricted range of activities and interests. Recent advances have helped explain the causes of ASD, which include both genetic and environmental risk factors. Effective treatments for reducing core and associated symptoms are being developed. In this chapter, we review current findings regarding genetic and environmental risk and protective factors, early brain and behavioral development, and we provide a perspective that offers hope for improved outcomes for many individuals with ASD.

## HISTORICAL CONTEXT

Leo Kanner (1943) first characterized autism. In his seminal work, he described a variety of behaviors that gave rise to modern diagnostic criteria, including lack of social reciprocity and emotional awareness, delays in communication, atypical use of language, and repetitive interests and behaviors. At the same time in Austria, Hans Asperger described a high-functioning form of autism (Frith, 1991, translation). He characterized children studied as "little professors" with intense interests and the ability to provide lengthy descriptions of their interests.

## TERMINOLOGICAL AND CONCEPTUAL ISSUES

Autism spectrum disorders include autistic disorder, Asperger's disorder, and pervasive developmental disorder not otherwise specified (PDD-NOS). In addition, two rare disorders are included under the current classification of PDDs: Rett's disorder and childhood disintegrative disorder. ASDs are extremely heterogeneous in their presentation. *DSM-IV* diagnostic criteria include four types of impairments in each of three domains: social interaction, communication, and repetitive or restricted behaviors or interests (American Psychiatric Association, 2000). These symptoms typically appear before age 3. A diagnosis of autistic disorder requires at least 6 of 12 symptoms. Asperger's disorder and PDD-NOS require fewer symptoms, or symptoms in only two of three domains. Thus, autism varies in severity, and individuals with different combinations of symptoms may meet diagnostic criteria. The complex array of symptoms associated with ASD present significant challenges to scientists and clinicians, including questions regarding the definition and measurement of symptoms across differing levels of intellect and development.

In many cases, reliable diagnosis may be made as early as 24 months (Lord et al., 2006), and infants at risk for autism are being identified at increasingly younger ages. Yet many children continue to go undiagnosed until preschool (Coonrod & Stone, 2004) or later (Shattuck et al., 2009). Diagnostic criteria focus on behaviors observed in children ages 2 to 3 years and above (Sigman, Dijamco, Gratier, & Rozga, 2004), although screening tools exist for infants (e.g., the First Year Inventory; Reznick, Baranek, Reavis, Watson, & Crais, 2007) and toddlers (e.g., Modified-Checklist for Autism in Toddlers; Robins, Fein, Barton, & Green, 2001). Delays in diagnosis result in late entry into early intervention programs, which improve prognosis.

The proposed *DSM-5* diagnostic criteria for ASD combine social and communication symptoms into a single social communication domain, with restricted and repetitive patterns of behavior and interests comprising the other core domain (Neurodevelopmental Disorders Work Group, 2011). The classifications of autistic disorder, Asperger's disorder, and PDD-NOS will be eliminated and replaced by the classification of autism spectrum disorder. Proposed changes to criteria reflect the need to account for a wider range of developmental levels and to use a dimensional rather than categorical approach to symptoms (Rutter, 2011).

## COMORBIDITIES

ASD is associated with several comorbid conditions. Most commonly, ASD is accompanied by developmental delay or intellectual disability; however, a significant portion of individuals with ASD has average to above average intelligence. Approximately 40% of children with ASD are estimated to have cognitive impairment (IQ ≤ 70; Autism and Developmental Disabilities Monitoring [ADDM], 2009). Higher rates of intellectual disability are found in girls with ASD (Centers for Disease Control [CDC], 2007). Given the large number of children who have both ASD and intellectual disability, it is important to consider a child's developmental level and typical developmental milestones when making a diagnosis.

A wide range of medical comorbidities, including sleep disorders, gastrointestinal disorders, psychiatric conditions, and seizures are associated with ASD. Sleep disruptions are estimated to affect 50% to 80% of children with ASD (see Richdale & Schreck, 2009, for review). The prevalence of gastrointestinal disorders is not completely understood, but is estimated to affect between 9% and 70% of children with ASD (see Buie et al., 2010, for review). Common psychiatric comorbidities include attention-deficit/hyperactivity disorder, anxiety disorders (specific phobia, obsessive compulsive disorder, social anxiety disorder), and depression (Leyfer et al., 2006; Simonoff et al., 2008). Prevalence rates of seizures range from 5% to 39% (Ballaban-Gil & Tuchman, 2000; Tidmarsh & Volkmar, 2003) with an increasing risk for seizures with age.

## Socioeconomic Considerations

Autism is reported throughout the world including Europe (Lauritsen, Pedersen, & Mortensen, 2005) and Asia (Kim et al., 2011). It affects individuals regardless of socioeconomic level (Fombonne, 1999, 2003). Although the gap is narrowing, socioeconomic status, particularly parental education level, continues to be related to age of diagnosis (Fountain, King, & Bearman, 2011). Diagnosis is also delayed for children in the Medicaid system (Mandell et al., 2010). Furthermore, racial and ethnic disparities in identification of ASD, particularly among black and Hispanic children, persist for school age children who are well beyond the age at which ASD may be diagnosed reliably (Mandell et al., 2009).

## PREVALENCE

Once believed to be a rare disorder, it is now estimated that ASD affects approximately 1 in 88 children in the United States (ADDM, 2012), a prevalence rate higher than that of type 1 diabetes, blindness, Down syndrome, childhood cancer, or cystic fibrosis (Kuehn, 2007). Approximately 1 million individuals are affected in the United States, with an annual societal cost of more than $35 billion per year and approximately $3.2 million per individual (Ganz, 2007). Data from a large sample of children ages 3 to 17 years suggest a nearly fourfold increase in the prevalence of autism, which represents the largest relative increase compared to other developmental disabilities between 1997 and 2008 (Boyle et al., 2011). Changes in prevalence result at least in part from broadened diagnostic criteria with revisions to the *DSM*, methodological differences in prevalence research, and increasing awareness and use of ASD diagnoses. The effect of increasing awareness is difficult to quantify. However, epidemiological data from California (Hertz-Picciotto & Delwiche, 2009; King & Bearman, 2009) suggest that historical changes in diagnostic criteria, diagnostic substitution, inclusion of milder cases, and an earlier age at diagnosis do not fully account for the increase in prevalence, leaving a substantial portion of the increased rates unexplained.

Autism affects males more commonly than females, with a ratio of 4.5 to 1, and prevalence for boys is 1 in 54 (ADDM, 2012). However, affected females are more likely than males to have comorbid intellectual disability in the severe range (IQ < 35), which is associated with worse autism symptoms (Volkmar, Szatmari, & Sparrow, 1993). Among a large sample of children and adolescents with higher intelligence, symptom expression was roughly equivalent for boys and girls with the exception of fewer repetitive, stereotyped behaviors among females with ASD, suggesting differences in symptom severity may be due to the presence of comorbid intellectual disability (Mandy et al., 2012).

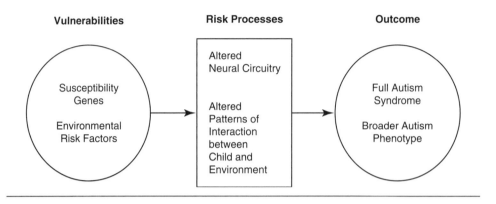

**Figure 20.1**   Experience-based risk processes in autism.

## ETIOLOGICAL FORMULATIONS

ASD is now recognized as a group of multiple conditions with multiple etiologies involving genetic and environmental risk factors. The emergence and severity of autism symptoms can be understood with a developmental framework that considers the combined effects of early genetic and environmental risk factors. The resulting risk processes are atypical early brain development and atypical engagement with the environment. The final outcome of these risk processes is symptom expression, as illustrated in Figure 20.1. Genetic and environmental risk factors lead to abnormalities in brain development that contribute to altered patterns of interaction between the child and his or her environment. Such altered interactions, or risk processes, are hypothesized to disrupt critical input, influencing the development of brain circuitry during early sensitive periods, thus serving as mediators of the effects of early susceptibilities on later outcomes, including the full autism syndrome. As a result, there is not a one-to-one correspondence between genetic or environmental factors and the occurrence of autism. Rather, there are individual differences in developmental pathways that children follow (i.e., equifinality, see Chapter 1), which can be explained in terms of interactions between early risk factors and the context in which children develop. Although changes in developmental pathways are always possible, canalization constrains the magnitude and quality of such changes. Thus, "the longer an individual continues along a maladaptive ontogenetic pathway, the more difficult it is to reclaim a normal developmental trajectory" (Cicchetti & Cohen, 1995, p. 7). The earlier that risk for autism is detected and intervention begins, the greater the chance that intervention will alter abnormal developmental trajectories.

## GENETICS AND HERITABILITY

Twin studies, sibling risk rates, and evidence of subthreshold symptoms in first-degree relatives provide strong evidence for genetic risk factors in autism. Seminal twin studies (e.g., Bailey et al., 1995; Folstein & Rutter, 1977) suggested very high heritabilities for autism (e.g., 90%; Bailey et al., 1995) based on concordance rates for monozygotic (MZ) versus dizygotic (DZ) twin pairs. However, these studies were limited by small sample sizes and possible ascertainment biases. A study using a population-based sample in which diagnosis was confirmed using research-reliable assessment measures found concordance for autism among MZ twin pairs of 58% and 60% for males and females, respectively (Hallmayer et al., 2011). The concordance rate for DZ twins, 21% and 27% for males and females, respectively, was higher than previously reported. When milder cases were included (i.e., autism spectrum versus strict autism), concordance rates were 50% and 77% for male and female MZ pairs and 31% and 36% for male and female DZ pairs. These concordance rates suggest heritability for strict autism is 37%, whereas shared environmental factors contribute 55%, confirming significant genetic heritability for ASD, albeit lower than previously reported. These findings also highlight the role of shared environmental risk factors, such as prenatal conditions. Replication of this finding will be crucial.

Sibling risk, or recurrence, rates are estimated to be 19% based on a large prospective study (Ozonoff et al., 2011), which is higher than previous reports of 3% to 10% (e.g., Constantino, Zhang, Frazier, Abbacchi, & Law, 2010; Lauritsen et al., 2005) and much higher than rates in comparison families. Ozonoff and colleagues (2011) followed infant siblings prospectively until 36 months, when most cases are likely to be detected, yielding recurrence estimates that were more robust to methodological issues including stoppage and overselection of families with concerns about later-born siblings. Recurrence risk for ASD was increased nearly threefold for male than female siblings. Furthermore, recurrence risk was 32% when there are two affected siblings in a family, which is significantly higher than the 14% recurrence rate in families with one affected child (Ozonoff et al., 2011). Current findings of recurrence rates in siblings (Ozonoff et al., 2011) and DZ concordance rates (Hallmayer et al., 2011) are comparable.

Finally, subthreshold symptoms, or a "broader phenotype" of ASD, including difficulties such as severe social dysfunction and isolation, language delays, and atypical (i.e., ASD-like) communication, are found in 4% to 20% of siblings who do not meet criteria for an ASD (Bolton et al., 1994; Constantino et al., 2010; Piven et al., 1990). Some parents also exhibit broader phenotype features of ASD (Bailey et al, 1995; Folstein & Rutter, 1977; Losh et al., 2009).

Although the mode of inheritance in autism is not completely understood, recent research in this area suggests that there may be multiple genetic pathways that confer risk for the autism phenotype. In many cases, rare genetic variations with high probability of affecting the phenotype (i.e., highly penetrant) are involved, whereas in other cases the genetic variations may be more common but with modest impact (Abrahams & Geschwind, 2008). In addition, despite strong evidence of heritability in families, some cases of ASD appear to be a result of rare, highly penetrant de novo mutations (see Chapter 3).

Association and linkage studies indicate some role for common variants, but their effect size is small. Several genome-wide linkage studies of autism have been published (Cantor et al., 2005; Lamb et al., 2005; McCauley et al., 2005; Morrow et al.,

2008; Schellenberg et al., 2006; Szatmari et al., 2007; Wang et al., 2009), though no single region has been consistently associated specifically with autism. Reducing the heterogeneity of the sample based on the presence of certain features of the proband, such as sex or language acquisition, has increased linkage signals (e.g., Schellenberg et al., 2006), a finding common in psychiatric genetics.

More than 100 genes have been tested as candidates for autism susceptibility loci. Some are promising common variants given large sample association studies and independent replications. A positive association between autism and the gene encoding the MET receptor tyrosine kinase, located on Chromosome 7, was examined, and an association between the C allele in the promoter region of the MET gene was shown (Campbell et al., 2006). MET signaling is involved in neocortical and cerebellar development, immune function, and gastrointestinal repair. Also located on Chromosome 7, CNTNAP2 (Contactin-associated protein 2) has been identified via specific endophenotypic markers for language (Alarcón et al., 2008; Arking et al., 2008). CNTNAP2 is known for its role in potassium channels along axons and neuronal migration.

Recent technological advances have permitted the use of genome-wide association studies of single nucleotide polymorphisms (SNP) and their role as common variants in genetic risk for ASD. SNPs are changes at one base pair of DNA. In contrast to linkage studies, genome-wide associations are nontargeted investigations. Three have been conducted in ASD (Anney et al., 2010; Wang et al., 2009; and Weiss et al., 2009) with significant, but nonoverlapping results implicating two different regions of chromosome 5p and a region of 20p, including regions that encode the neural adhesion molecules cadherin 9 and 10 (CDH9 and CDH10). These studies highlight the need for larger samples to resolve conflicting results.

Another recent development in the understanding of autism genetic susceptibility is the likely role of rare mutations. In particular, copy number variations (CNV) are structural gains or losses in the genome of 1 kilobase or greater, which may be either inherited or de novo. CNVs are found in 10% of simplex (1 affected sibling) and 2% of multiplex (2 affected siblings) cases of ASD (Sebat et al., 2007; but see Pinto et al., 2010), which suggests different genetic structural mechanisms for familial versus "sporadic" cases of ASD. CNVs may be highly penetrant, causing ASD alone, or may work in combination with common variants in order to cross the threshold of genetic susceptibility. It should be noted that CNVs are also found in unaffected family members as well as unaffected controls, suggesting that their effects are not always clinically significant. Some CNVs occur more frequently at specific genetic loci. Furthermore, CNVs identified in ASD samples may overlap with regions already associated with ASD or intellectual disability (Cook & Scherer, 2008; Guilmatre et al., 2009; Pinto et al., 2010). In genome-wide studies, CNVs were found at 7q, 15q, 16p, and 22q (Glessner et al., 2009; Sanders et al., 2011), disrupting groups of genes involved in neuronal cell adhesion, proliferation, projection and motility as well as GTPase/Ras signaling (Glessner et al., 2009; Pinto et al., 2010). CNVs have also been implicated in disrupting genes involved in ubiquitination, which alters protein function and targets proteins for degradation (Glessner et al., 2009).

Single gene mutations have also been reported in autism samples, including mutations of the neuroligin 3 and neuroligin 4 genes (Jamain et al., 2003) and SHANK3 (Durand et al., 2007), although these mutations fall within the rare causes of autism. Other single gene disorders are associated with increased risk for autism or expression of an autistic-like phenotype, including Fragile X syndrome, Rett syndrome, Angelman syndrome, and tuberous sclerosis (see Moss & Howlin, 2009; Veenstra-VanderWeele & Cook, 2004, for reviews). One factor underlying this association may be the presence of intellectual disability, although the severity of intellectual impairment is inconsistent across genetic syndromes, suggesting their ASD-like phenotypes may not be accounted for by intellectual disability alone (Moss & Howlin, 2009). Although there appears to be overlap in features, careful clinical examination of cases also suggests subtle differences in the presentation across these syndromes, providing potentially important targets for future research on phenotypes (Moss & Howlin, 2009). Single gene disorders have provided important clues for identifying drug targets. Mouse models of single-gene disorders associated with ASD such as tuberous sclerosis, Fragile X, and Rett syndrome illustrate the use of targeted pharmacological agents to reverse behavioral, biochemical, and electrophysiological phenotypes even in adult animals (Silva & Ehninger, 2009).

One approach to integrating the multiple genetic risk factors for ASD (i.e., rare and de novo variations, and common variants with small effect size) has been to examine the possibility that candidates contribute to a functional network (see Peça, Ting, & Feng, 2011, for an illustration of such a synaptic network). An application of this approach identified clusters of CNVs in a functional network of loci involved in synapse development, axon targeting, and neuron motility (Gilman et al., 2011). In particular, many of the genes implicated were related to cell-adhesion and scaffolding at the synapse as well as regulating protein synthesis.

In summary, there is strong evidence for genetic influences in autism, yet the role of susceptibility genes is complex. Evidence thus far indicates that multiple genes interact to increase susceptibility to ASD by influencing gene expression or encoding functional changes in proteins that are part of complex regulatory networks. As we discuss in more detail below, the expression and effects of many genes are influenced by environmental factors, offering hope that early intervention can alter genetic expression, brain development, and behavioral outcomes.

## ENVIRONMENTAL RISK FACTORS

Concordance rates of less than 100%, along with a 600% increase in prevalence in recent decades (some of which may reflect an "actual" increase), suggest that environmental factors are also involved in the etiology of autism. Recent studies have identified a number of potential environmental risk factors, including advanced parental age, low birth weight, prenatal exposure to pollution and pesticides, maternal infection, and use of certain medications (e.g., SSRIs) during pregnancy (Atladottir et al., 2010; Bilder, Pinborough-Zimmerman, Miller, & McMahon, 2009; Croen, Grether, Yoshida, Odouli, & Hendrick, 2011; Croen, Najjar, Fireman, & Grether, 2007; Pinto-Martin et al., 2011; Roberts et al., 2007; Shelton, Tancredi,

Hertz-Picciotto, 2010; Volk, Hertz-Picciotto, Delwiche, Lurman, & McConnell, 2011). Advanced parental age is consistently associated with increased risk of ASD (Bilder et al., 2009; Croen et al., 2007; Shelton et al., 2010), and may represent a gene-environment interaction resulting in increased risk of spontaneous mutation in older gametes or increased familial genetic risk associated with broader phenotype traits. Involvement of the immune system in neurodevelopment is increasingly understood as one possible mechanism, involving the transfer of maternal immunoglobulin G (IgG) antibodies that bind to fetal brain protein during pregnancy (Braunschweig et al., 2008). An association between maternal IgG reactivity to specific fetal brain proteins and child diagnosis of autism has been reported from a large cohort (Braunschweig et al., 2012). Also, exposure to teratogens such as thalidomide between the 20th and 24th day of pregnancy, and valproic acid (i.e., Depakote), are associated with increased risk of developing autism (Moore et al., 2000; Rasalam et al., 2005; Strömland, Nordin, Miller, Akerstrom, & Gillberg, 1994). A meta-analysis of perinatal and neonatal factors found that uterine bleeding, abnormal presentation, fetal distress, low birth weight, low Apgar scores, feeding difficulties, and hyperbilirubinemia were related with increased ASD risk (Gardener, Spiegelman, & Buka, 2011). It is possible that these perinatal and neonatal conditions may not play a causal role but are instead correlates of fetal abnormalities or genetic factors (Bolton et al., 1997).

Involvement of vaccinations during the first years of life, especially the measles-mumps-rubella (MMR) vaccination, has been hypothesized as an environmental factor. However, a number of epidemiological studies have failed to confirm an association between the MMR vaccine and autism (see Wilson, Mills, Ross, McGowan, & Jadad, 2003, for a review). Thimerosal, a preservative containing ethyl mercury that was added to many vaccines, has also been examined and no evidence of increased risk has been found (Parker, Schwartz, Todd, & Pickering, 2004).

Genes and environmental factors that regulate the expression of other genes without changing the primary DNA sequence, known as epigenetic mechanisms (see Chapter 3), may also be related to the etiology of ASD (Grafodatskaya et al., 2010). For example, examining postmortem brains of individuals with autism and other genetic syndromes in which 15q11–13 GABR genes are implicated (i.e., Prader-Willi, Angelman, and Rett syndromes), revealed expression of GABR genes consistent with epigenetic dysregulation in half of the cases with autism and one case of five with Rett's disorder (Hogart, Nagarajan, Patzel, Yasui, & LaSalle, 2007). A second example is an investigation of H3K4me3, which is dependent on epigenetic methylation for neuronal health (Shulha et al., 2012). Using postmortem tissue from the prefrontal cortex of ASD cases and controls, disruptions were detected in a subset of ASD cases but not controls, particularly at genetic loci involved with connectivity as well as social and cognitive function.

## DEVELOPMENTAL PROGRESSION

The risk processes of atypical behavior and brain development emerge within the first year of life and subsequently impact the course of development for individuals with ASD.

## Behavioral Symptoms Apparent in Infancy

Initial studies of the early course of ASD focused on retrospective parent reports and retrospective videotape analysis. Parents often report having concerns between their child's first and second birthday including difficulties in communication development, social behavior, affective responses, and sensory peculiarities (Dahlgren & Gillberg, 1989; De Giacomo & Fombonne, 1998; Young, Brewer, & Pattison, 2003). More recently, prospective studies of high-risk infant siblings and infants with risk markers identified in population screenings have improved understanding of the earliest autism phenotypic features and symptoms by allowing for direct testing and longitudinal measurement. Extension of these findings to clinical settings provides hope for earlier detection and additional opportunities to follow non-familial infants prospectively. As an example, the first large-scale application of a pediatrician-administered screening checklist targeting social communication and symbolic skills at the 1-year well-baby check up reached 10,479 families (Pierce et al., 2011).

Given the recurrence rates of ASD in families, following infant siblings of children with ASD prospectively allows for examination of children at risk. These infants generally do not exhibit clear symptoms at 6 months, and there is evidence that children later diagnosed with ASD have social function comparable to typically developing children in the first few months of life (Landa & Garrett-Mayer, 2006; Ozonoff et al., 2010; Zwaigenbaum et al., 2005). However, there are clues about possible early markers of the broader autism phenotype. At 4 months, siblings of children with ASD had weaker synchrony during infant-initiated portions of a mother-child interaction, were less upset and displayed more neutral expressions during a still face paradigm, and interestingly, responded *more* when their names were called than did infant siblings of typically developing children (Yirmiya et al., 2006). At 6 months, in a still-face paradigm, siblings of children with ASD looked at their parents' faces for a similar duration as did comparison infants, but smiled less, shifted their gaze less, and looked away from parents' faces longer (Cassel et al., 2007; Ibanez, Messinger, Newell, Lambert, & Sheskin, 2008). High-risk 6-month-old siblings also looked more at objects while learning about them and spent less time spontaneously looking at caregivers than did low risk siblings (Bhat, Galloway, & Landa, 2010). These findings parallel retrospective videotape analysis that found infants who later developed autism had increased interest in objects and reduced vocalizations, looking at faces, smiling at others, and attempts to seek physical contact compared with typically developing 6-month-olds (Maestro et al., 2002). Thus, despite generally similar behavior in the first 6 months including social responses, the earliest markers of the ASD phenotype may include preference for non-social objects, reduced or uncoordinated emotional response, and fewer infant-initiated social behaviors.

Emergence of symptoms among children who later develop an ASD has been documented between 6 and 12 months. First, during this period eye contact declines and by 8 to 10 months infants are less likely to respond to their name (Clifford & Dissanayake, 2008; Nadig et al., 2001; Ozonoff et al., 2010; Werner, Dawson, Osterling, & Dinno, 2000). By 12 months, infants later diagnosed with an ASD are distinguished from typically developing infants by reduced orienting when called by name, less time spent looking at faces, and decreased social interest (Baranek, 1999; Osterling & Dawson, 1994, Osterling, Dawson, & Munson, 2002; Zwaigenbaum et al., 2005). Moreover, looking at people and responding to name best distinguished infants with autism from infants with developmental delay without autism at 9 to 12 months of age (Baranek, 1999; Osterling et al., 2002). Second, directed vocalizations (e.g., babbling or crying while looking at a person) decreased in the second six months of life (Ozonoff et al., 2010). During the same period, differences in the development of prespeech consonant sounds distinguished infant siblings with more severe outcomes (i.e., provisional diagnoses of ASD or broader phenotype characteristics) from those with less severe outcomes (Paul, Fuerst, Ramsay, Chawarska, & Klin, 2011). Third, the rate of growth of visual attention between 6 and 12 months distinguished infants who developed an ASD; they spent longer fixating on a single object and had less active spontaneous visual exploration (Zwaigenbaum et al., 2005). Finally, differences emerged in temperament. Parent ratings suggested that 6-month-olds who later developed ASD had a lower activity level. By 12 months, these children had more frequent and intense reactions to distress (Zwaigenbaum et al., 2005).

In children with ASD, declines in communication, reductions in cognitive and symbolic development, and the emergence of sensory and repetitive behaviors occur between 12 and 24 months. Children who received an ASD diagnosis were distinguished from at-risk siblings at 12 months by their reduced receptive language and gesture use (Zwaigenbaum et al., 2005). Landa and Garrett-Mayer (2006) followed the cognitive development of high-risk infant siblings who later developed an ASD compared with language-delayed and unaffected groups. Although infants did not differ at 6 months, children who received ASD diagnoses differed from the unaffected group in receptive and expressive language and overall intelligence by 14 months. Reduced ability to follow verbal instructions, babble or make complex vocalizations, vocally imitate, and use single words and phrases distinguished the ASD group from comparison children in video analyses (Mars et al., 1998; Werner & Dawson, 2005). Also consistent with these findings are reports of lower cognitive and receptive and expressive language abilities in the broader ASD phenotype. Language and cognitive profiles and gesture use differed among high- and low-risk infant siblings between 12 and 24 months (Stone, McMahon, Yoder, & Walden, 2007; Toth, Dawson, Meltzoff, Greenson, & Fein, 2006). The broader cognitive and language phenotype of ASD was investigated prospectively in high- and low-risk siblings from 4 months to 7 years. Early language ability, but not cognitive ability, was reduced from 14 to 54 months and the rate of development differed for children exhibiting the broader phenotype, suggesting that early differences in the language phenotype are meaningful for later outcome (Gamliel, Yirmiya, Jaffe, Manor, & Sigman, 2009).

Joint attention is the ability to "coordinate attention between interactive social partners with respect to objects or events in order to share an awareness of the objects or events" (Mundy, Sigman, Ungerer & Sherman, 1986). At 14 to 34 months, high-risk siblings who did not develop symptoms were distinguished from those with later symptoms by joint attention skills (Landa, Holman, & Garrett-Mayer, 2007;

Sullivan et al., 2007; Yoder, Stone, Walden, & Malesa, 2009). Children with a later ASD diagnosis and social impairment had reduced response to joint attention, less initiation of joint attention for the purpose of sharing, and poor triadic gaze shifting (Landa et al., 2007; Yoder et al., 2009). Variation in joint attention also predicted future language ability among children who received a diagnosis of autism or its broader phenotype (Sullivan et al., 2007). In general, joint attention ability is diminished in high-risk siblings between 12 and 24 months, suggesting that it is also an aspect of the early broader phenotype. Less initiation of joint attention by 15 months and reduced response to joint attention by 18 months distinguished high- from low-risk siblings (Cassel et al., 2007). Siblings were also less likely to direct the attention of others and had fewer social-communication interactions with parents (Stone et al., 2007).

Stereotyped movements and repetitive behaviors also emerge between 12 and 24 months. When infant siblings of children with ASD and typical development were presented with objects and allowed to play freely for a minute, children with a later diagnosis of ASD exhibited more atypical behavior including spinning, rotating, rolling, and unusual visual examination (Ozonoff, Macari et al., 2008). An investigation of repetitive movements at 12 and 18 months indicated that the subset of high-risk siblings later diagnosed with an ASD also waved their arms more than those who did not receive a diagnosis and low-risk siblings at both time points (Loh et al., 2007). Both high-risk groups also engaged in a "hands to ears" posture more often than low-risk siblings.

In contrast to the *early onset* course, characterized by symptoms by 12 to 14 months, the phenomenon of *regression* is characterized by a loss of skills after more typical development for the first year or two and later development of autism symptoms. It is estimated that 24% of children with ASD exhibit regression by 36 months (Parr et al., 2011). Regression during the second year of life is well documented by parental report (Lord, Shulman, & DiLavore, 2004; Werner & Dawson, 2005), videotape (Werner & Dawson, 2005), and prospective studies (Landa et al., 2007). Of interest, 12-month-olds with later regression were similar and, in some domains, better than typically developing infants in social communication abilities (Landa et al., 2007; Werner & Dawson, 2005). The group with early onset ASD already exhibited clear impairments. By 24 months, both groups of children with ASD had fewer social and communication behaviors than comparison children. Detailed prospective examination of nine infants who received ASD diagnoses also suggests the presence of two subgroups on the basis of the presence or absence of cognitive decline between 12 and 24 months (Bryson et al., 2007). However, as implied above and suggested by Ozonoff, Heung, and colleagues (2008), evidence strongly suggests that autism *emerges* between 6 and 24 months – even in cases of "early onset." These authors suggest there is evidence of two additional courses – *plateau* and *mixed onset* (i.e., with mixed delay and regression), and recommend a dimensional rather than categorical approach to understanding the onset of ASD symptoms (Ozonoff, Heung et al., 2008). Finally, these authors suggest that defining regression broadly to include loss of social engagement would include many more children.

## TODDLER-PRESCHOOL PERIOD

By the toddler-preschool period, in addition to cognitive, language, and behavioral difficulties, at least five key domains of social behavior are affected in autism. These include social orienting, joint attention, attention to emotional cues, motor imitation, and face processing.

First, young children with autism fail to spontaneously orient to naturally occurring social stimuli. Compared to children with intellectual disability without autism and typically developing children, young children with ASD more frequently fail to orient to both social and nonsocial stimuli, but this failure is much more extreme for social stimuli (Dawson, Meltzoff, Osterling, Rinaldi, & Brown, 1998; Dawson, Toth et al., 2004). Mundy and Neal (2001) proposed that the developmental pathway of young children with autism is altered because children are deprived of appropriate social stimulation by failing to orient to it. The ability to anticipate events may contribute to orienting. In a comparison of blink inhibition, which is thought to measure anticipation of important information in a dynamic scene, toddlers with typical development inhibited blinking just before events, whereas toddlers with ASD had the greatest inhibition just after the onset of the event (Shultz, Klin, & Jones, 2011). Consistent with visual attention findings from infancy, toddlers with ASD in this study looked more at physical objects in the scenes. The authors hypothesized that this difference placed the group with autism at a disadvantage in anticipating the behavior of the children in the video.

Second, joint attention continues to distinguish children with autism from those with developmental delay and typical development as toddlers (Adamson, Bakeman, Deckner, & Romski, 2009) and preschoolers (Bacon, Fein, Morris, Waterhouse, & Allen, 1998; Dawson, Meltzoff, Osterling, & Rinaldi, 1998; Mundy et al., 1986; Sigman et al., 1999). Joint attention skills are also a good predictor of both concurrent and future language skills in children with autism (Adamson et al., 2009; Dawson, Meltzoff, Osterling, Rinaldi et al., 1998; Sigman et al., 1999; Sullivan et al., 2007). Additionally, early joint attention is an important predictor of social outcomes such as peer engagement (Sigman et al., 1999).

A third core domain of impairment is failure to attend and respond to others' emotions in a normal manner. Many but not all children with autism demonstrate a lack of sensitivity to emotional states of others. When adults display facial expressions of distress, children with autism look less at the adult and show less concern compared to children with intellectual disability and typical development (Bacon et al., 1998; Dawson, Meltzoff, Osterling, & Rinaldi et al., 1998; Dawson, Toth et al., 2004). Reduced response to an examiner's distress is present by 12 months in children who develop ASD relative to high- and low-risk comparison children, is persistent when measured every 6 months through age 3, and differences remain after controlling for verbal ability and social responsiveness (Hutman et al., 2010).

A fourth domain of impairment is the ability to imitate others. Failure to spontaneously imitate, especially in social play contexts, is a core early impairment in ASD (Dawson & Adams, 1984; Rogers, Bennetto, McEvoy, & Pennington, 1996). Imitation ability discriminates toddlers with autism from those with developmental delay and communication disorders (Stone, Lemanek, Fishel, Fernandez & Altemeier,

1990; Stone, Ousley & Littleford, 1997). Individuals with autism perform poorly in virtually all aspects of imitation (Rogers, Hepburn, Stackhouse & Wehner, 2003), including imitating motor movements (Stone et al., 1997), facial expressions (Loveland et al. 1994), style of tasks (Hobson & Lee, 1999), actions involving imaginary objects (Rogers et al., 1996), and vocalizations (Dawson & Adams, 1984).

Finally, face-processing abilities in individuals with autism are impaired. Toddlers between 18 and 30 months with ASD demonstrate slower habituation to faces than children with developmental delays, typical development or non-ASD infant siblings (Webb et al., 2010). These group differences, thought to measure rate of learning, were not found for objects. Habituation rate for faces correlated with social skills and verbal ability. Children with ASD also have increasingly atypical gaze patterns to faces from 2 to 4 years of age (Chawarska & Shic, 2009). By middle childhood, children with ASD perform worse than mental age- and chronological age-matched peers on face processing tasks, including tests of recognition (Boucher & Lewis, 1992; Klin et al., 1999) and discrimination (Tantam, Monoghan, Nicholson, & Stirling, 1989).

## ABNORMAL NEURAL DEVELOPMENT IN AUTISM

On average individuals with autism exhibit an atypical pattern of growth in head circumference (HC) characterized by small-to-normal head size at birth followed by accelerated growth that appears to begin in the first year of life, most often in the first 6 months (Chawarska et al., 2011; Dawson et al., 2007; Dementieva et al., 2005; Mraz, Green, Dumont-Mathieu, Makin, & Fein, 2007; Redcay & Courchesne, 2005). It is interesting to note that the timing of the onset of accelerated head growth slightly precedes, and then overlaps with, the onset of behavioral symptoms. In comparison, although HC is larger than normal by 12 months of age, its rate of growth after 12 months is not different from normal, suggesting deceleration after 12 months relative to the first year (Dawson et al., 2007). Acceleration in HC during the first year is related to increased symptoms in affected children (Chawarska et al., 2011; Mraz et al., 2007; but see Dementieva et al., 2005) and larger HC at 12 months and deceleration in growth rate after 12 months in high-risk infant siblings predicts autism symptoms (Elder, Dawson, Toth, Fein, & Munson, 2008). Larger HC in older children is also associated with more severe social symptoms and history of language delay (Lainhart et al., 2006). One caveat is that increased HC is associated with generalized growth in height and weight (Mraz et al., 2007; Sacco et al., 2007; but see Lainhart et al., 2006; Webb et al., 2007), suggesting the possible involvement of growth factors that act on both neural and skeletal development. Finally, a connection between larger HC and a history of allergic or immune disorders has been reported (Sacco et al., 2007).

*Structural brain imaging in young children with autism.* Results from magnetic resonance imaging (MRI) studies are consistent with the results of HC studies. For example, 2- to 4-year-olds with ASD have larger total cerebral volumes than controls, including IQ-matched children with developmental delay (Courchesne et al., 2001; Hazlett et al., 2011; Schumann et al., 2010; Sparks et al., 2002), particularly in the frontal and temporal lobes and cingulate cortex (Courchesne, Campbell, & Solso,

2011; Hazlett et al., 2011; Schumann et al., 2010). Larger overall brain volume appears to be meaningful; 2- to 4-year-old children with ASD and regression (i.e., loss of language or social engagement, responsiveness or interest) had larger total cerebral volumes than children with ASD and no regression and typically developing children (Nordahl et al., 2011).

Abnormal brain growth appears to be due to enlargement of both white and gray matter, with an anterior-to-posterior gradient of overgrowth, which may be due to increased cortical surface area, neuronal density, packing abnormalities and/or immune-mediated processes such as reactive gliosis and edema (Carper, Moses, Tigue, & Courchesne, 2002; Casanova, 2004; Hazlett et al., 2011; Schumann et al., 2010; Vargas, Nascimbene, Krishnan, Zimmerman, & Pardo, 2005; see Amaral, Schumann, & Nordahl, 2008, for review). These possibilities are being tested via postmortem and imaging studies. Postmortem investigation of the prefrontal cortex in boys with ASD revealed more neurons in the autism cases than comparison cases (Courchesne, Mouton et al., 2011). This suggests deviations in brain growth during the prenatal period because cortical neurons are not generated postnatally. A magnetic resonance spectroscopy study of 3- to 4-year-olds with ASD revealed regional and global decreases in a marker for neuronal integrity and neuronal-glial homeostasis, distributed predominantly in gray matter (Friedman et al., 2003). Postmortem examination of markers of neuroimmune response in the prefrontal cortex of children with ASD found more frequent and severe differences in the ASD cases, including the majority of the youngest cases (Morgan et al., 2010). Whether these disruptions are causal in the pathogenesis of ASD, are secondary immune responses to disturbances in brain integrity, or reflect genetic and/or environmental influences remains unknown. These findings implicate more than one type of neural alteration very early in development that may account for early brain overgrowth.

Other volumetric abnormalities, especially in medial temporal lobe (MTL) structures such as the amygdala, are found in ASD (e.g., Aylward et al., 1999; Schumann et al., 2004). These structures have been strongly implicated in ASD-related symptom expression, particularly social perception and behavior (see Baron-Cohen et al., 2000; Schultz, 2005, for reviews). Mosconi et al. (2009) reported enlarged amygdala volumes at 2 and 4 years of age, and enlargement was associated with joint attention ability at the second time point. Munson et al. (2006) reported amygdala enlargement (relative to total brain volume) in 3- to 4-year-old children with autism was associated with more severe social and communication impairments at 3, 4, and 6 years.

*Neuroimaging of structural and functional connectivity in children with autism.* Symptoms of ASD involve higher-order social and communication behaviors that rely on networks within the brain to work efficiently and in coordination. Reported differences in white matter (i.e., myelinated axons) (Courchesne et al., 2001; Sparks et al., 2002), abnormal minicolumn width (Casanova, 2004) and cell numbers (Courchesne, Mouton et al., 2011), particularly in regions involved in higher-order behaviors, have led to understanding the neurobiology of autism as a disorder of connectivity (Minshew & Williams, 2007). Diffusion tensor imaging (DTI) is a form of magnetic resonance imaging that measures properties of white matter pathways, including the direction of information flowing along them, and allows for tracing of tracts between brain structures and measurement of the integrity of the tracts (see Thomason & Thompson, 2011, for review). Use of DTI in children and adolescents with ASD has revealed disrupted structural connectivity (Ameis et al., 2011; Cheng et al., 2010; Shukla, Keehn, & Muller, 2011). Recent DTI with infants suggests disrupted connectivity in white matter tracts by 6 months in infants who develop ASD (Wolff et al., 2012). Some investigations suggest that disruptions to connectivity may vary with development, though findings have been somewhat mixed (Ameis et al., 2011; Cheng et al., 2010; Jou et al., 2011; Shukla et al., 2011). Although structural connectivity is generally disrupted in ASD, there appears to be some specificity in certain pathways with long-range (i.e., corticocortical and interhemispheric) connections involved in socioemotional and information processing.

Specifically, Ameis et al. (2011) found differences between children with ASD and controls in a tract (right uncinate fasciculus) thought to be involved in processing novel stimuli and visual learning, decoding emotional content in auditory stimuli, and self-regulation. Increased mean diffusivity was also found in a pathway (inferior longitudinal fasciculus) that mediates connectivity between structures that process biological motion and eye gaze, face identity, and emotional expressions and significance (Ameis et al., 2011). Other groups have reported reduced integrity of the uncinate fasciculus and inferior longitudinal fasciculus pathways in children with ASD (Cheon et al. 2011; Jou et al., 2011; Shukla et al., 2011). Cheon et al. (2011) also reported differences in the integrity of a pathway (anterior thalamic radiation) that is important to information processing. Relative to other tracts, Jou et al. (2011) found the poorest integrity in the inferior frontal-occipital fasciculus, which connects all lobes of the cortex and is thought to be broadly involved in social cognition. Other groups also report disrupted connectivity in the inferior frontal-occipital fasciculus in children with ASD (Cheng et al., 2010; Shukla et al., 2011).

Connectivity may also be examined by measuring the correspondence in functional MRI activation between regions in a brain network during a task or at rest. The examination of connectivity during a passive facial emotion processing task revealed that children and adolescents with ASD had reduced long-range functional connectivity, increased local functional connectivity, and reduced functional segregation (Rudie et al., 2011). A second study investigated synchronization of spontaneous responses in sleeping toddlers and preschoolers (i.e., a resting state paradigm). Reduced interhemispheric synchronization in the superior temporal gyri (associated with language processing) of young children with autism ages 12 to 46 months relative to those with language delay and typical development suggests reduced functional connectivity between hemispheres (Dinstein et al., 2011). Of interest, synchronization strength correlated positively with verbal ability and negatively with symptom severity.

*Electrophysiology in young children with autism.* Electrophysiology is a noninvasive measure of brain function, particularly the timing of brain responses. The electrical brain response may be linked to specific events, yielding event-related potentials (ERPs). Because it is conducive to use with infants and toddlers while they are awake, it provides a means of measuring brain function in very young children with ASD and high-risk siblings.

Several groups have measured the function of social-emotional systems. At 10 months, high-risk infant siblings had faster responses to objects at components involved with face processing (the N290 and P400), relative to comparison siblings (McCleery, Akshoomoff, Dobkins, & Carver, 2009). No group differences were detected in response to faces at the N290 and low-risk infants had faster N400 responses to faces. Also at 10 months, high-risk infants differed from comparison children in their neural response to faces with direct gaze, but not averted gaze (Elsabbagh et al., 2009). In particular, high-risk siblings responded more slowly at a later component (P400) for direct versus indirect gaze, but did not differ for earlier components (P1 and N290). The P400 is sensitive to face processing, particularly top-down attention modulation. Thus, results of both studies are consistent with behavioral findings of disrupted attention to social stimuli as an early phenotype. Furthermore, brain response to *dynamic* stimuli with shifting eye gaze at 6 to 10 months predicted later diagnosis of ASD at 36 months (Elsabbagh et al., 2012). At 18 to 47 months, young children with ASD exhibited similar ERP responses to familiar and unfamiliar faces as 12- to 30-month-old typically developing comparison children suggesting delayed neural development in this social domain (Webb et al., 2011). Similarly by age 3 to 4 years, children with ASD showed the same differential ERP response to familiar versus unfamiliar objects as comparison children, but not for familiar versus unfamiliar faces, paralleling the responses to novel/familiar faces by younger typically developing children (i.e., toddlers) (Dawson, Carver et al., 2002; Webb et al., 2011). Three- to 4-year-olds with ASD also exhibited atypical ERP responses to fearful faces, consistent with slower information processing, and individual differences in ERP latency were associated with performance on behavioral tasks requiring social attention (Dawson, Webb, Carver, Panagiotides, & McPartland, 2004). Together, these studies demonstrate functional impairments in brain response of children with ASD by 6 months for processing eye gaze, and by age 3 for neural differentiation between the face of each child's mother and a stranger and slower processing of emotional content conveyed by faces.

ERP studies have also been used to investigate language processing. Preschoolers with ASD preferred listening to mechanical–sounding auditory signals (signals acoustically matched to speech and referred to as "sine-wave analogs") rather than speech (motherese), a dramatically different listening preference compared with typically developing children (Kuhl et al., 2005). Preference for mechanical sounds correlated with lower language ability, more severe autism symptoms, and abnormal ERPs to speech sounds, whereas children with autism who preferred motherese had a more typical pattern of differential ERPs to contrasting phonemes.

## PROTECTIVE FACTORS

Early intervention may serve to counteract risk processes as the course of ASD unfolds, producing more adaptive processes of interaction with the environment. As a consequence, downstream brain and behavioral development may be more typical, and symptom expression may be reduced. A number of intervention approaches are available.

*Early comprehensive interventions.* Early intensive behavioral intervention initiated during the preschool period and sustained for 2 to 4 years has shown a significant impact on outcome in a large subset of children with autism, including significant gains in IQ, language, and educational placements (see Rogers & Vismara, 2008, for review). Common factors of many such early interventions include a comprehensive curriculum with an intensive delivery of treatment (25 hours/week for at least 2 years), sensitivity to development, highly trained staff, involvement of parents, supervisory and review mechanisms, and behavioral strategies for reducing interfering behaviors (National Research Council, 2001). When these features are present, results are impressive for up to 50% of children. To date, the approach to early behavioral intervention developed by Lovaas (1987) and originally known as the UCLA Young Autism Project (YAP) has the best research support (Rogers & Vismara, 2008) meeting criteria (Chambless & Hollon, 1998) of a *well-established* treatment. The most consistent finding is improved intellectual outcome; some investigations of the YAP model also find behavioral, adaptive, and language gains, and some have reported instances of "recovery." Sallows and Graupner (2005) demonstrated the YAP approach is equally effective when delivered by trained parents or clinicians.

Dawson and Rogers have developed and tested the Early Start Denver Model (ESDM; Rogers & Dawson, 2009), which is a comprehensive early intensive behavioral intervention designed to address the unique needs of toddlers with ASD as young as 12 months. After two years of intervention, toddlers who were randomized to ESDM, rather than treatment as usual, exhibited significantly better cognitive abilities including better expressive and receptive language abilities, steady improvement in adaptive function (rather than a decline observed in the comparison group), and more improvement in diagnostic classifications (i.e., more movement to milder classifications) provided by clinicians naïve to group assignment (Dawson et al., 2010).

*Parent-delivered, targeted interventions.* A more targeted approach to intervention provides training in specific domains for the caregivers of children with ASD. For preschoolers, the two investigations with the strongest empirical support are the Autism Preschool Program (Jocelyn, Casiro, Beattie, Bow, & Kneisz, 1998) and Child's Talk (Aldred, Green, & Adams, 2004). Early parent-delivered interventions targeting social orienting, joint attention, imitation, and other aspects of language and communication, are becoming increasingly available for toddlers with ASD with mixed results. Two types of caregiver-mediated intervention targeting joint attention in toddlers with ASD have yielded positive outcomes including increased response to joint attention, more varied and appropriate play, and improved language ability relative to toddlers randomly assigned to comparison conditions (Drew et al., 2002; Kasari, Gulsrud, Wong, Kwon, & Locke, 2010). Augmenting a comprehensive intervention by targeting caregiver-child synchrony via socially engaged imitation, joint attention and shared affect doubled the frequency of imitation paired with eye contact in the treatment group (Landa, Holman, O'Neill, & Stuart, 2011). Taken together, these findings suggest that environmental influences may change the course of early social communication impairments in toddlers with ASD and that these effects remain at long-term follow-up (Kasari et al., 2010; Landa et al., 2011).

*Interventions for older individuals with ASD.* Social skills training is commonly used with school-aged children, most often in a group format. Social skills interventions improve understanding of social skill concepts and social competence, reduce conflict on play dates, and increase feelings of popularity with fewer feelings of loneliness (DeRosier, Swick, Davis, McMillen, & Matthews, 2010; Frankel et al., 2010; Owens, Granader, Humphrey, & Baron-Cohen, 2008). Social skills groups have also been used with adolescents (Laugeson, Frankel, Mogil, & Dillon, 2009) and adults (Gantman, Kapp, Orenski, & Laugeson, 2012). Outcomes include improved social skills knowledge, more frequent get-togethers with nongroup peers, less loneliness, and increased empathy and social response. These interventions are particularly promising as they suggest the possibility of behavioral changes, including some suggestion of decreased symptom severity, for older children and adults with ASD.

Behavioral interventions are also being developed to address concurrent conditions, such as anxiety. Three recent randomized trials (Sofronoff, Attwood, & Hinton, 2005; Sung et al., 2011; Wood et al., 2009) demonstrated reduction in anxiety symptoms via cognitive behavioral therapy (CBT). To date, the use of medication for individuals with ASD has also focused on mitigating concurrent psychiatric conditions and challenging behaviors rather than core social and communication symptoms and the effects are best understood with older individuals. Atypical neuroleptics, especially risperidone, have received the most research attention for their use in treating maladaptive behaviors in ASD (see Canitano & Scandurra, 2011, for review). Of this class, risperidone and aripiprazole are the only drugs with FDA approval for children and adolescents with ASD. Other psychopharmacological agents include: SSRIs, which have limited benefit; methylphenidate and atomoxetine, which may be useful in some cases but may increase irritability; and antiepileptics, which hold promise but require more research (Canitano & Scandurra, 2011). Work with animals, as described earlier, provides hope for the development of more targeted pharmacological interventions that build on knowledge of the specific genetic risk factors and underlying neurobiology of ASD to address core features of ASD.

## SYNTHESIS AND FUTURE DIRECTIONS

As described earlier, numerous risk factors—genetic and environmental—contribute to varying degrees to the etiology of autism spectrum disorders. These produce early deviations from normal brain development resulting in failure of normal social and communicative development in autism that is apparent early in life. In the first year, brain growth rate is accelerated by 6 months of age. Behavioral divergence appears to follow closely, with earliest correlates including biased attention for objects. However, children who develop ASD do not appear to exhibit clear impairments in social communication until the end of the first year, with some children continuing on a more typical trajectory until later in the second year and then regressing.

Impairments in social orienting, joint attention, response to emotions, imitation, and face processing are evident by toddlerhood and are hallmarks of the disorder. To help explain this wide range of impairments, all of which involve reduced attention to social input, Dawson and others have proposed the social motivation hypothesis (Dawson et al., 2005; Dawson, Carver et al., 2002; Waterhouse, Fein, & Modahl, 1996). According to this hypothesis, some of the social impairments evident in autism, such as impairments in face processing, are not fundamental, but rather are secondary to a primary impairment in social motivation or affective tagging of socially relevant stimuli (Dawson et al., 2005; Grelotti, Gauthier, & Schultz, 2002). That is, reduced social motivation may represent a risk process that alters the pattern of interaction a child has with his or her environment, leading to behavioral and neural outcomes such as those observed in the domain of face processing (Chawarska & Shic, 2009; Dawson, Carver et al., 2002; Webb et al., 2010, 2011). The use of blinking as a "subjective assessment of perceived stimulus salience" among young children during the onset of ASD (Shultz et al., 2011, p. 21270) provides a potential window into the motivation of these children as they experience dynamic events in their environment. Over the course of a short scene, looking preferences may influence access to salient information, illustrating how children with ASD may lag behind and miss key information in their environment. This ongoing interaction between risk factors and the environment can explain further heterogeneity beyond differences in underlying etiology. Understanding these processes also provides opportunities to intervene and shape the input, resulting in a reduction of autism symptoms and neural correlates.

Advances in cognitive and affective developmental neuroscience, developmental psychopathology, neurobiology, and genetics have provided critical information about the causes of ASD and for formulating effective prevention and treatment approaches. At the same time, communication across scientific domains and integration of different types of information at multiple levels of analysis pose new and difficult conceptual and methodological challenges for scientists. Key challenges include understanding how genetic and environmental risk factors interact, which ones play causal roles, how they map to the variety of behaviors observed, and, most importantly, how to map these factors at the individual level. As we learn more about the onset of ASD, it will be critical to distinguish the aspects of the high-risk phenotype that are most predictive of ASD outcome and work backward to better understand their specific underlying biological precursors. In addition, it will be essential to gain more information about the course of development via prospective investigations of low risk samples, where the possibility of de novo genetic disruptions may produce a different constellation of features. Better understanding of the variety of patterns of neural development is needed to determine differences in symptom onset, to understand the potential for plasticity at different points in the lifespan, and to identify specific biological markers of treatment response. In terms of treatment, we have much to learn about which types of ASD best respond to various intervention approaches. In addition, the public health needs are great as the population with ASD ages. It will be vital to understand the heterogeneity of outcomes and the best approaches for intervening.

Animal models provide useful systems for simplifying these complex questions. In addition to the work (described earlier) demonstrating the potential impact of specific pharmacological agents on remediating the underlying neurobiological mechanisms linked to ASD in adult animals, there is good evidence for brain and behavioral plasticity resulting from environmental manipulation (see Nithianan-tharajah & Hannan, 2006, for review). Of particular interest, a strain of mouse pups exhibiting behavioral phenotypes in all three ASD symptom domains (BTBR) reared in the same cage with a highly social strain (B6) exhibited more social approaches as adults compared to those reared with other BTBR mice (Yang, Perry, Weber, Katz, & Crawley, 2011). Early social environment did not affect repetitive self-grooming behavior, suggesting specificity of the environmental influence. Maternal nursing and grooming behavior by rats also influences the behavior of offspring, and evidence suggests the mechanism is epigenetic with maternal behavior directly influencing DNA methylation and chromatin structure (Weaver et al., 2004). These basic research methods provide a way to isolate and manipulate biological and environmental risk and protective factors more directly.

Investigation of intervention at multiple levels of analysis in individuals with ASD may also provide important clues about the effects and limits of the treatment and about predictors of individual treatment response. Building on the developmental picture of face processing and its underlying neurophysiology that suggests a delay in specialization for faces among toddlers and preschoolers with ASD (Webb et al., 2011), we have measured electrophysiological response in children who received intensive intervention (Early Start Denver Model). This work suggests that toddlers randomly assigned to intervention had more normative neural response after intervention than those with ASD in a community control group (Dawson et al., submitted). This model has also been used to measure the effects of targeted face training for adults with ASD (Faja et al., 2011). Those individuals randomly assigned to face training demonstrated both behavioral and neurophysiological changes compared to a group assigned to a control condition (object training).

In conclusion, although the complexity of autism—both in terms of its etiology and heterogeneity of symptom expression—poses significant challenges, research focused on identifying autism susceptibility indices, early identification, and early intervention offer real hope for the future. As early identification and intervention become increasingly effective, the new challenge will be translating these scientific findings into social policy. The considerable funding and effort required to implement large-scale early detection efforts and intensive behavioral intervention programs may cause legislators and insurance companies to pause. Cost-benefit analyses suggest, however, the choice is to pay a lot early or pay a lot more later (Jacobson, Mulick & Green, 1998; Jacobson & Mulick, 2000). Burdening only families with the financial and emotional cost of helping individuals suffering from autism—or simply failing to provide access to interventions we know can substantially change the lives of individuals—is not a choice our society can ethically defend. Thus, research on strategies to translate scientific findings into meaningful and sustainable community-based efforts will be an increasing focus of the future.

# REFERENCES

Abrahams, B. S., & Geschwind, D. H. (2008). Advances in autism genetics: On the threshold of a new neurobiology. *Nature Reviews Genetics, 9*, 341–355.

Adamson, L. B., Bakeman, R., Deckner, D. F., & Romski, M. (2009). Joint engagement and the emergence of language in children with autism and Down syndrome. *Journal of Autism and Developmental Disorders, 39*, 84–96.

Alarcón, M., Abrahams, B. S., Stone, J. L., Duvall, J. A., Perederiy, J. V., Bomar, J. M., . . . Geschwind, D. H. (2008). Linkage, association, and gene-expression analyses identify CNTNAP2 as an autism-susceptibility gene. *American Journal of Human Genetics, 82*, 150–159.

Aldred, C., Green, J., & Adams, C. (2004). A new social communication intervention for children with autism: Pilot randomized controlled treatment study suggesting effectiveness. *Journal of Child Psychology and Psychiatry, 45*, 1420–1430.

Amaral, D. G., Schumann, C. M., & Nordahl, C. W. Neuroanatomy of autism. *Trends in Neuroscience, 31*, 137–145.

Ameis, S. H., Fan, J., Rockel, C., Voineskos, A. N., Lobaugh, N. J., Soorya, L., . . . Anagnostou, E. (2011). Impaired structural connectivity of socio-emotional circuits in autism spectrum disorders: A diffusion tensor imaging study. *PLoS One, 6*, e28044.

American Psychiatric Association. (2000). *Diagnostic and statistical manual of mental disorders* (4th ed., text rev.). Washington, DC: American Psychiatric Association.

Anney, R., Klei, L., Pinto, D., Regan, R., Conroy, J., Magalhaes, T. R., . . . Cook Jr,, E. H. (2010). A genome-wide scan for common alleles affecting risk for autism. *Human Molecular Genetics, 19*, 4072–4082.

Arking, D. E., Cutler, D. J., Brune, C. W., Teslovich, T. M., West, K., Ikeda, M., . . . Chakravarti, A. (2008). A common genetic variant in the neurexin super-family member CNTNAP2 increases familial risk of autism. *American Journal of Human Genetics, 82*, 160–164.

Atladóttir, H. O., Thorson, P., Østergaard, L., Schendel, D. E., Lemcke, S., Abdallah, M., & Parner, E. T. (2010). Maternal infection requiring hospitalization during pregnancy and autism spectrum disorders. *Journal of Autism and Developmental Disorders, 40*, 1423–1430.

Autism and Developmental Disabilities Monitoring (ADDM) Network Surveillance Year 2006 Principal Investigators. (2009). *Prevalence of autism spectrum disorders—Autism and developmental disabilities monitoring network MMWR surveillance summary* (Vol. 58, pp. 1–20). United States, 2006, Centers for Disease Control and Prevention.

Autism and Developmental Disabilities Monitoring (ADDM) Network Surveillance Year 2008 Principal Investigators. (2012). *Prevalence of autism spectrum disorders—Autism and developmental disabilities monitoring network, 14 sites*, United States (Vol. 61, pp. 1–19). Centers for Disease Control and Prevention.

Aylward, E. H., Minshew, N. J., Goldstein, G., Honeycutt, N. A., Augustine, A. M., Yates, K. O., . . . Pearlson, G. D. (1999). MRI volumes of amygdala and hippocampus in non-mentally retarded autistic adolescents and adults. *Neurology, 53*, 2145–2150.

Bacon, A. L., Fein, D., Morris, R., Waterhouse, L., & Allen, D. (1998). The responses of autistic children to the distress of others. *Journal of Autism & Developmental Disorders, 28,* 129–141.

Bailey, A., Le Couteur, A., Gottesman, I., Bolton, P., Simonoff, E., Yuzda, E., & Rutter, M. (1995). Autism as a strongly genetic disorder: Evidence from a British twin study. *Psychological Medicine, 25,* 63–77.

Ballaban-Gil, K., & Tuchman, R. (2000). Epilepsy and epileptiform EEG: Association with autism and language disorders. *Mental Retardation and Developmental Disabilities Research Reviews, 6,* 300–308.

Baranek, G. T. (1999). Autism during infancy: A retrospective video analysis of sensory-motor and social behaviours at 9–12 months of age. *Journal of Autism and Developmental Disorders, 29,* 213–224.

Baron-Cohen, S., Ring, H. A., Bullmore, E. T., Wheelwright, S., Ashwin, C., & Williams, S. C. (2000). The amygdala theory of autism. *Neuroscience and Biobehavioural Reviews, 24,* 355–364.

Bhat, A. N., Galloway, J. C., & Landa, R. J. (2010). Social and non-social visual attention patterns and associative learning in infants at risk for autism. *Journal of Child Psychology and Psychiatry, 51,* 989–997.

Bilder, D., Pinborough-Zimmerman, J., Miller, J., & McMahon, W. (2009). Prenatal, perinatal, and neonatal factors associated with autism spectrum disorders. *Pediatrics, 123,* 1293–300.

Bolton, P., MacDonald, H., Pickles, A., Rios, P., Goode, S., Crowson, M., . . . Rutter, M. (1994). A case–control family history study of autism. *Journal of Child Psychology & Psychiatry, 35,* 877–900.

Bolton, P., Murphy, M., Macdonald, H., Whitlock, B., Pickles, A., & Rutter, M. (1997). Obstetric complications in autism: Consequences or causes of the condition? *Journal of the American Academy of Child and Adolescent Psychiatry, 36,* 272–281.

Boucher, J., & Lewis, V. (1992). Unfamiliar face recognition in relatively able autistic children. *Journal of Child Psychology and Psychiatry and Allied Disciplines, 33,* 843–859.

Boyle, C. A., Boulet, S., Schieve, L. A., Cohen, R. A., Blumberg, S. J., Yeargin-Allsopp, M., . . . Kogan, M. D. (2011). Trends in the prevalence of developmental disabilities in US children, 1997–2008. *Pediatrics, 127,* 1034–1042.

Braunschweig, D., Ashwood, P., Krakowiak, P., Hertz-Picciotto, I., Hansen, R., Croen, L. A., . . . Van de Water, J. (2008). Autism: Maternally derived antibodies specific for fetal brain proteins. *Neurotoxicology, 29,* 226–231.

Braunschweig, D., Duncanson, P., Boyce, R., Hansen, R., Ashwood, P., Pessah, I. N., . . . Van de Water, J. (2012). Behavioral correlates of maternal antibody status among children with autism. *Journal of Autism and Developmental Disorders, 42,* 1435–1445.

Bryson, S. E., Zwaigenbaum, L., Brian, J., Roberts, W., Szatmari, P., Rombough, V., & McDermott, C. (2007). A prospective case series of high-risk infants who developed autism. *Journal of Autism and Developmental Disorders, 37,* 12–24.

Buie, T., Campbell, D. B., Fuchs, G. J. III,, Furuta, G. T., Levy, J., VandeWater, J., ... Winter, H. (2010). Evaluation, diagnosis, and treatment of gastrointestinal disorders in individuals with ASDs: A consensus report. *Pediatrics, 125,* S1–S18.

Campbell, D. B., Sutcliffe, J. S., Ebert, P. J., Militerni, R., Bravaccio, C., Trillo, S., ... Levitt, P. (2006). A genetic variant that disrupts MET transcription is associated with autism. *Proceedings of the National Academy of Sciences, 103,* 16834–16839.

Canitano, R., & Scandurra, V. (2011). Psychopharmacology in autism: An update. *Progress in Neuro-Psychopharmacology & Biological Psychiatry, 35,* 18–28.

Cantor, R. M., Kono, N., Duvall, J. A., Alvarez-Retuerto, A., Stone, J. L., Alarcón, M., ... Geschwind, D. (2005). Replication of autism linkage: fine-mapping peak at 17q21. *American Journal of Human Genetics, 76,* 1050–1056.

Carper, R. A., Moses, P., Tigue, Z. D., & Courchesne, E. (2002). Cerebral lobes in autism: Early hyperplasia and abnormal age effects. *Neuroimage, 16,* 1038–1051.

Casanova, M. F. (2004). White matter volume increase and minicolumns in autism. *Annals of Neurology, 56,* 453.

Cassel, T. D., Messinger, D. S., Ibanez, L. V., Haltigan, J. D., Acosta, S. I., & Buchman, A. C. (2007). Early social and emotional communication in the infant siblings of children with autism spectrum disorders: An examination of the broad phenotype. *Journal of Autism and Developmental Disorders, 37,* 122–32.

Centers for Disease Control and Prevention (2007). *Prevalence of autism spectrum disorders. Surveillance summaries,* February 9. MMWR 2007; 56 (No. SS-1).

Chambless, D. L., & Hollon, S. D. (1998). Defining empirically supported therapies. *Journal of Consulting and Clinical Psychology, 66,* 7–18.

Chawarska, K., Campbell, D., Chen, L., Shic, F., Klin, A., & Chang, J. (2011). Early generalized overgrowth in boys with autism. *Archives of General Psychiatry, 68,* 1021–1031.

Chawarska, K., & Shic, F. (2009). Looking but not seeing: Atypical visual scanning and recognition of faces in 2 and 4-year-old children with autism spectrum disorder. *Journal of Autism and Developmental Disorders, 39,* 1663–1672.

Cheng, Y., Chou, K. H., Chen, I. Y., Fan, Y. T., Decety J., & Lin, C-P. (2010). Atypical development of white matter microstructure in adolescents with autism spectrum disorders. *Neuroimage, 50,* 873–882.

Cheon, K. A., Kim, Y. S., Oh, S. H., Park, S. Y., Yoon, H. W., Herrington J, ... Schultz, R. T. (2011). Involvement of the anterior thalamic radiation in boys with high functioning autism spectrum disorders: A diffusion tensor imaging study. *Brain Research, 1417,* 77–86.

Cicchetti, D., & Cohen, D. J. (1995). Perspectives on developmental psychopathology. In D. Cicchetti & D. J. Cohen (Eds.), *Developmental psychopathology, Vol. I: Theory and methods* (pp. 3–22). New York, NY: Wiley.

Clifford, S. M., & Dissanayake, C. (2008). The early development of joint attention in infants with autistic disorder using home video observations and parental interview. *Journal of Autism and Developmental Disorders, 38,* 791–805.

Cook, E. H. Jr., & Scherer, S. W. (2008). Copy-number variations associated with neuropsychiatric conditions. *Nature, 455,* 919–923.

Coonrod, E. E., & Stone, W. L. (2004). Early concerns of parents of children with autistic and nonautistic disorders. *Infants and Young Children, 17,* 258–268.

Constantino, J. N., Zhang, Y., Frazier, T., & Abbacchi, A. M. (2010). Sibling recurrence and the genetic epidemiology of autism. *American Journal of Psychiatry, 167,* 1349–1356.

Courchesne, E., Campbell, K., & Solso, S. (2011a). Brain growth across the life span in autism: Age-specific changes in anatomical pathology. *Brain Research, 1380,* 138–145.

Courchesne, E., Mouton, P. R., Calhoun, M. E., Semendeferi, K., Ahrens-Barbeau, C., Hallet, M. J., ... Pierce, K. (2011b). Neuron number and size in prefrontal cortex of children with autism. *Journal of the American Medical Association, 306,* 2001–2010.

Courchesne, E., Karns, C., Davis, H. R., Ziccardi, R., Carper, R., Tigue, Z., ... Courchesne, R. Y. (2001). Unusual brain growth patterns in early life in patients with autistic disorder: An MRI study. *Neurology, 57,* 245–254.

Croen, L. A., Grether, J. K., Yoshida, C. K., Odouli, R., & Hendrick, V. (2011). Antidepressant use during pregnancy and childhood autism spectrum disorders. *Archives of General Psychiatry, 68,* 1104–1112.

Croen, L. A., Najjar, D. V., Fireman, B., & Grether, J. K. (2007). Maternal and paternal age and risk of autism spectrum disorders. *Archives of Pediatric and Adolescent Medicine, 161,* 334–340.

Dahlgren, S. O., & Gillberg, C. (1989). Symptoms in the first two years of life. A preliminary population study of infantile autism. *European Archives of Psychiatry and Neurological Sciences, 238,* 169–174.

Dawson, G., & Adams, A. (1984). Imitation and social responsiveness in autistic children. *Journal of Abnormal Child Psychology, 12,* 209–225.

Dawson, G., Carver, L., Meltzoff, A. N., Panagiotides, H., McPartland, J., & Webb, S. J. (2002). Neural correlates of face and object recognition in young children with autism spectrum disorder, developmental delay, and typical development. *Child Development, 73,* 700–717.

Dawson, G., Jones, E., Merkle, K., Venema, K., Lowy, R., Faja, S., ... Webb, S. J. (submitted). *Early behavioral intervention is associated with normalized brain activity in young children with autism.*

Dawson, G., Meltzoff, A. N., Osterling, J., & Rinaldi, J. (1998a). Neuropsychological correlates of early symptoms of autism. *Child Development, 69,* 1276–1285.

Dawson, G., Meltzoff, A. N., Osterling, J., Rinaldi, J., & Brown, E. (1998b). Children with autism fail to orient to naturally occurring social stimuli. *Journal of Autism and Developmental Disorders, 28,* 479–485.

Dawson, G., Munson, J., Webb, S. J., Nalty, T., Abbott, R., & Toth, K. (2007). Rate of head growth decelerates and symptoms worsen in the second year of life in autism. *Biological Psychiatry, 61,* 458–464.

Dawson, G., Rogers, S., Munson, J., Smith, M., Winter, J., Greenson, J., ... Varley, J. (2010). Randomized, controlled trial of an intervention for toddlers with autism: The Early Start Denver Model. *Pediatrics, 125,* e17–e23.

Dawson, G., Toth, K., Abbott, R., Osterling, J., Munson, J., Estes, A., & Liaw, J. (2004a). Early social attention impairments in autism: Social orienting, joint attention, and attention to distress. *Developmental Psychology, 40,* 271–283.

Dawson, G., Webb, S., Carver, L., Panagiotides, H., & McPartland, J. (2004b). Young children with autism show atypical brain responses to fearful versus neutral facial expressions. *Developmental Science, 7,* 340–359.

Dawson, G., Webb, S. J., Wijsman, E., Schellenberg, G., Estes, A., Munson, J., & Faja, S. (2005). Neurocognitive and electrophysiological evidence of altered face processing in parents of children with autism: Implications for a model of abnormal development of social brain circuitry in autism. *Development and Psychopathology, 17,* 679–697.

De Giacomo, A., & Fombonne, E. (1998). Parental recognition of developmental abnormalities in autism. *European Journal of Child and Adolescent Psychiatry, 7,* 131–136.

Dementieva, Y. A., Vance, D. D., Donnelly, S. L., Elston, L. A., Wolpert, C. M., Ravan, S. A., . . . Cuccaro, M. L. (2005). Accelerated head growth in early development of individuals with autism. *Pediatric Neurology, 32,* 102–108.

DeRosier, M. E., Swick, D. C., Davis, N. O., McMillen, J. S., & Matthews, R. (2010). The efficacy of a social skills group intervention for improving social behaviors in children with high functioning autism spectrum disorders. *Journal of Autism Developmental Disorders, 41,* 1033–43.

Dinstein, I., Pierce, K., Eyler, L., Solso, S., Malach. R., Behrmann. M., & Courchesne, E. (2011). Disrupted neural synchronization in toddlers with autism. *Neuron, 70,* 1218–25.

Drew, A., Baird, G., Baron-Cohen, S., Cox, A., Slonims, V., Wheelwright, S., . . . Charman, T. (2002). A pilot randomized control trial of a parent training intervention for pre-school children with autism: Preliminary findings and methodological challenges. *European Child and Adolescent Psychiatry, 11,* 266–272.

Durand, C. M. Betancur, C., Boeckers, T. M., Bockmann, J., Chaste, P., Fauchereau, F., . . . Bourgeron, T. (2007). Mutations in the gene encoding the synaptic scaffolding protein SHANK3 are associated with autism spectrum disorders. *Nature Genetics, 39,* 25–27.

Elder, L. M., Dawson, G., Toth, K., Fein, D., & Munson, J. (2008). Head circumference as an early predictor of autism symptoms in younger siblings of children with autism spectrum disorder. *Journal of Autism and Developmental Disorders, 38,* 1104–1111.

Elsabbagh, M., Mercure, E., Hudry, K., Chandler, S., Pasco, G., Charman, T., . . . BASIS Team. (2012). Infant neural sensitivity to dynamic eye gaze is associated with later emerging autism. *Current Biology, 22,* 1–5.

Elsabbagh, M., Volein, A., Csibra, G., Holmboe, K., Garwood, H., Tucker, L., . . . Johnson, M. J. (2009). Neural correlates of eye gaze processing in the infant broader autism phenotype. *Biological Psychiatry, 65,* 31–38.

Faja, S., Webb, S. J., Jones, E., Merkle, K., Kamara, D., Bavaro, J., . . . Dawson, G. (2011). The effects of face expertise training on the behavioral performance and brain activity of adults with high functioning autism. *Journal of Autism and Developmental Disorders, 42,* 278–293.

Folstein, S., & Rutter, M. (1977). Infantile autism: A genetic study of 21 twin pairs. *Journal of Child Psychology and Psychiatry, 18,* 297–321.

Fombonne, E. (1999). The epidemiology of autism: A review. *Psychological Medicine, 29,* 769–786.

Fombonne, E. (2003). Epidemiology of pervasive developmental disorders. *Trends in Evidence-Based Neuropsychiatry, 5,* 29–36.

Fountain, C., King, M. D., & Bearman, P. S. (2011). Age of diagnosis for autism: Individual and community factors across 10 birth cohorts. *Journal of Epidemiological Community Health, 65,* 503–510.

Frankel, F., Myatt, R., Sugar, C., Whitham, C., Gorospe, C. M., & Laugeson, E. (2010). A randomized controlled study of parent-assisted children's friendship training with children having autism spectrum disorders. *Journal of Autism and Developmental Disorders, 40,* 827–842.

Friedman, S. D., Shaw, D. W., Artru, A. A., Richards, T. L., Gardner, J., Dawson, G.,... Dager, S. R. (2003). Regional brain chemical alterations in young children with autism spectrum disorder. *Neurology, 60,* 100–107.

Frith, U. (1991). *Autism and Asperger syndrome.* Cambridge, United Kingdom: Cambridge University Press.

Gamliel, I., Yirmiya, N., Jaffe, D. H., Manor, O., & Sigman, M. (2009). Developmental trajectories in siblings of children with autism: Cognition and language from 4 months to 7 years. *Journal of Autism and Developmental Disorders, 39,* 1131–1144.

Gantman, A., Kapp, S. K., Orenski, K., & Laugeson, E. A. (2012). Social skills training for young adults with high-functioning autism spectrum disorders: A randomized controlled pilot study. *Journal of Autism and Developmental Disorders, 42,* 1094–1103.

Ganz, M. L. (2007). The lifetime distribution of the incremental societal costs of autism. *Archives of Pediatric and Adolescent Medicine, 161,* 343–349.

Gardener, H., Spiegelman, D., & Buka, S. L. (2011). Perinatal and neonatal risk factors for autism: A comprehensive meta-analysis. *Pediatrics, 128,* 344–355.

Gilman, S. R., Iossifov, I., Levy, D., Ronemus, M., Wigler, M., & Vitkup, D. (2011). Rare de novo variants associated with autism implicate a large functional network of genes involved in formation and function of synapses. *Neuron, 70,* 898–907.

Glessner, J. T., Wang, K., Cai, G., Korvatska, O., Kim, C. E., Wood, S.,... Hakonarson, H. (2009). Autism genome-wide copy number variation reveals ubiquitin and neuronal genes. *Nature, 459,* 569–573.

Grafodatskaya, D., Chung, B., Szatmari, P., & Weksberg, R. (2010). Autism spectrum disorders and epigenetics. *Journal of the American Academy of Child and Adolescent Psychiatry, 49,* 794–809.

Grelotti, D., Gauthier, I., & Schultz, R. (2002). Social interest and the development of cortical face specialization: What autism teaches us about face processing. *Developmental Psychobiology, 40,* 213–225.

Guilmatre, A., Dubourg, C., Mosca, A. L., Legallic, S., Goldenberg, A., Drouin-Garraud, V.,... Campion, D. (2009). Recurrent rearrangements in synaptic and neurodevelopmental genes and shared biologic pathways in schizophrenia, autism, and mental retardation. *Archives of General Psychiatry, 66,* 947–956.

Hallmayer, J., Cleveland, S., Torres, A. Phillips, J., Cohen, B., Torigoe, T., . . . Risch, N. (2011). Genetic heritability and shared environmental factors among twin pairs with autism. *Archives of General Psychiatry, 68,* 1095–1102.

Hazlett, H. C., Poe, M. D., Gerig, G., Styner, M., Chappell, C., Smith, R. G., . . . Piven, J. (2011). Early brain overgrowth in autism associated with an increase in cortical surface area before age 2 years. *Archives of General Psychiatry, 68,* 467–476.

Hertz-Picciotto, I., & Delwiche, L. (2009). The rise in autism and the role of age at diagnosis. *Epidemiology, 20,* 84–90.

Hobson, R. P., & Lee, A. (1999). Imitation and identification in autism. *Journal of Child Psychology and Psychiatry, 40,* 649–659.

Hogart, A., Nagarajan, R. P., Patzel, K. A., Yasui, D. H., & LaSalle, J. M. (2007). 15q11–13 GABA$_A$ receptor genes are normally biallelically expressed in brain yet are subject to epigenetic dysregulation in autism-spectrum disorders. *Human Molecular Genetics, 16,* 691–703.

Hutman, T., Rozga, A., DeLaurentis, A. D., Barnwell, J. M., Sugar, C. A., & Sigman, M. (2010). Response to distress in infants at risk for autism: A prospective longitudinal study. *Journal of Child Psychology and Psychiatry, 51,* 1010–1020.

Ibanez, L. V., Messinger, D. S., Newell, L., Lambert, B., & Sheskin, M. (2008). Visual disengagement in the infant siblings of children with an autism spectrum disorder (ASD). *Autism, 12,* 473–485.

Jacobson, J. W., & Mulick, J. A. (2000). System and cost research issues in treatments for people with autistic disorders. *Journal of Autism and Developmental Disorders, 30,* 585–593.

Jacobson, J. W., Mulick, J. A., & Green, G. (1998). Cost-benefit estimates for early intensive behavioral intervention for young children with autism—general model and single state case. *Behavioral Interventions, 13,* 201–226.

Jamain, S., Quach, H., Betancur, C., Rastam, M., Colineaux, C., Gillberg, I. C., . . . Paris Autism Research International Sibpair Study. (2003). Mutations of the X-linked genes encoding neuroligins NLGN3 and NLGN4 are associated with autism. *Nature Genetics, 34,* 27–29.

Jocelyn, L. J., Casiro, O. G., Beattie, D., Bow, J., & Kneisz, J. (1998). Treatment of children with autism: A randomized controlled trial to evaluate a caregiver-based intervention program in community day-care centers. *Developmental and Behavioral Pediatrics, 19,* 326–334.

Jou, R. J., Mateljevic, N., Kaiser, M. D., Sugrue, D. R., Volkmar, F. R., & Pelphrey, K. A. (2011). Structural neural phenotype of autism: Preliminary evidence from a diffusion tensor imaging study using tract-based spatial statistics. *American Journal of Neuroradiology, 32,* 1607–1613.

Kanner, L. (1943). Autistic disturbances of affective contact. *Nervous Child, 2,* 217–250.

Kasari, C., Gulsrud, A. C., Wong, C., Kwon, S., & Locke, J. (2010). Randomized controlled caregiver mediated joint engagement intervention for toddlers with autism. *Journal of Autism and Developmental Disorders, 40,* 1045–1056.

Kim, Y. S., Leventhal, B. L., Koh, Y-J., Fombonne, E., Laska, E., Lim, E-C., . . . Grinker, R. R. (2011). Prevalence of autism spectrum disorders in a total population sample. *American Journal of Psychiatry, 168*, 904–912.

King, M., & Bearman, P. (2009). Diagnostic change and the increased prevalence of autism. *International Journal of Epidemiology, 38*, 1224–1234.

Klin, A., Sparrow, S. S., deBildt, A., Cicchetti, D. V., Cohen, D. J., & Volkmar, F. R. (1999). A normed study of face recognition in autism and related disorders. *Journal of Autism and Developmental Disorders, 29*, 499–508.

Kuehn, B. M. (2007). CDC: Autism spectrum disorders common. *Journal of the American Medical Association, 297*, 940.

Kuhl, P. K., Coffey-Corina, S., Padden, D., & Dawson, G. (2005). Links between social and linguistic processing of speech in preschool children with autism: Behavioral and electrophysiological measures. *Developmental Science, 7*, 19–30.

Lainhart, J. E., Bigler, E. D., Bocian, M., Coon, H., Dinh, E., Dawson, G., . . . Volkmar, F. (2006). Head circumference and height in autism: A study by the collaborative program of excellence in autism. *American Journal of Medical Genetics A, 140*, 2257–2274.

Lamb, J. A., Barnby, G., Bonora, E., Sykes, N., Bacchelli, E., Blasi, F., . . . International Molecular Genetic Study of Autism Consortium (IMGSAC). (2005). Analysis of IMGSAC autism susceptibility loci: Evidence for sex limited and parent of origin specific effects. *Journal of Medical Genetics, 42*, 132–137.

Landa, R., & Garrett-Mayer, E. (2006). Development in infants with autism spectrum disorders: A prospective study. *Journal of Child Psychology and Psychiatry, 47*, 629–638.

Landa, R. J., Holman, K. C., & Garrett-Mayer, E. (2007). Social and communication development in toddlers with early and later diagnosis of autism spectrum disorders. *Archives of General Psychiatry, 64*, 853–864.

Landa, R. J., Holman, K. C., O'Neill, A. H., & Stuart, E. A. (2011). Intervention targeting development of socially synchronous engagement in toddlers with autism spectrum disorder: A randomized controlled trial. *Journal of Child Psychology and Psychiatry, 52*, 13–21.

Laugeson, E. A., Frankel, F., Mogil, C., & Dillon, A. R. (2009). Parent-assisted social skills training to improve friendships in teens with autism spectrum disorders. *Journal of Autism and Developmental Disorders, 39*, 596–606.

Lauritsen, M. B., Pedersen, C. B. & Mortensen, P. B. (2005). Effects of familial risk factors and place of birth on the risk of autism: A nationwide register-based study. *Journal of Child Psychology and Psychiatry, 46*, 963–971.

Leyfer, O., Folstein, S. E., Bacalman, S., Davis, N. O., Dinh, E., Morgan, J., . . . Lainhart, J. E. (2006). Comorbid psychiatric disorders in children with autism: Interview development and rates of disorders. *Journal of Autism and Developmental Disorders, 36*, 849–861.

Loh, A., Soman, T., Brian, J., Bryson, S. E., Roberts, W., Szatmari, P., . . . Zwaigenbaum, L. (2007). Stereotyped motor behaviors associated with autism in high-risk infants: A pilot videotape analysis of a sibling sample. *Journal of Autism and Developmental Disorders, 37*, 25–36.

Lord, C., Risi, S., DiLavore, P. S., Shulman, C., Thurm, A., & Pickles, A. (2006). Autism from two to nine years of age. *Archives of General Psychiatry, 63*, 694–701.

Lord, C., Shulman, C., & DiLavore, P. (2004). Regression and word loss in autistic spectrum disorders. *Journal of Child Psychology and Psychiatry, 45*, 936–955.

Losh, M., Adolphs, R., Poe, M. D., Couture, S., Penn, D., Baranek, G. T., & Piven, J. (2009). Neuropsychological profile of autism and the broad autism phenotype. *Archives of General Psychiatry, 66*, 518–526.

Lovaas, O. I. (1987). Behavioral treatment and normal educational and intellectual functioning in young autistic children. *Journal of Consulting and Clinical Psychology, 55*, 3–9.

Loveland, K. A., Tunali-Kotoski, B., Pearson, D. A., Bresford, K. A., Ortegon, J., & Chen, C. (1994). Imitation and expression of facial affect in autism. *Development and Psychopathology, 6*, 433–444.

Maestro, S., Muratori, F., Cavallaro, M. C., Pei, F., Stern, D., Golse, B., & Palacio-Espasa, F. (2002). Attentional skills during the first 6 months of age in autism spectrum disorder. *Journal of the American Academy of Child and Adolescent Psychiatry, 41*, 1239–1245.

Mandell, D., Morales, K. H., Xie, M., Lawer, L. J., Stahmer, A. C., & Marcus, S. C. (2010). Age of diagnosis among Medicaid-enrolled children with autism, 2001–2004. *Psychiatric Services, 61*, 822–829.

Mandell, D., Wiggins, L. D., Carpender, L. A., Daniels, J., DiGuiseppi, C., Durkin, M. S., . . . Kirby, R. S. (2009). Racial/ethnic disparities in the identification of children with autism spectrum disorders. *American Journal of Public Health, 99*, 493–498.

Mandy, W., Chilvers, R., Chowdhury, U., Salter, G., Seigal, A., & Skuse, D. (2012). Sex differences in autism spectrum disorder: Evidence from a large sample of children and adolescents. *Journal of Autism and Developmental Disorders, 42*, 1304–1313.

Mars, A. E., Mauk, J. E., & Dowrick, P. W. (1998). Symptoms of pervasive developmental disorders and observed in prediagnostic home videos of infants and toddlers. *Journal of Pediatrics, 132*, 500–504.

McCauley, J. L., Li, C., Jiang, L., Olson, L. M., Crockett, G., Gainer, K., . . . Sutcliffe, J. S. (2005). Genome-wide and ordered-subset linkage analyses provide support for autism loci on 17q and 19p with evidence of phenotypic and interlocus genetic correlates. *BMC Medical Genetics, 6*, 1.

McCleery, J. P., Akshoomoff, N., Dobkins, K. R., & Carver, L. J. (2009). Atypical face versus object processing and hemispheric asymmetries in 10-month-old infants at risk for autism. *Biological Psychiatry, 66*, 950–957.

Minshew, N. J., & Williams, D. L. (2007). The new neurobiology of autism: Cortex, connectivity, and neuronal organization. *Archives of Neurology, 64*, 945–950.

Moore, S., Turnpenny, P., Quinn, A., Glover, S., Lloyd, D., Montgomery, T., & Dean, J. C. (2000). A clinical study of 57 children with fetal anticonvulsant syndromes. *Journal of Medical Genetics, 37*, 489–497.

Morgan, J. T., Chana, G., Pardo, C. A., Achim, C., Semendeferi, K., Buckwalter J, . . . Everall, I. P. (2010). Microglial activation and increased microglial density observed in the dorsolateral prefrontal cortex in autism. *Biological Psychiatry, 68*, 368–376.

Morrow, E. M., Yoo, S. Y., Flavell, S. W., Kim, T. K., Lin, Y., Hill, R. S., . . . Walsh, C. A. (2008). Identifying autism loci and genes by tracing recent shared ancestry. *Science, 321*, 218–223.

Mosconi, M. M., Cody-Hazlett, H., Poe, M. D., Gerig, G., Gimpel-Smith, R., & Piven, J. (2009). Longitudinal study of amygdala volume and joint attention in 2- to 4-year-old children with autism. *Archives of General Psychiatry, 66*, 509–516.

Moss, J., & Howlin, P. (2009). Autism spectrum disorders in genetic syndromes: Implications for diagnosis, intervention and understanding the wider autism spectrum disorder population. *Journal of Intellectual Disability Research, 53*, 852–873.

Mraz, K. D., Green, J., Dumont-Mathieu, T., Makin, S., & Fein, D. (2007). Correlates of head circumference growth in infants later diagnosed with autism spectrum disorders. *Journal of Child Neurology, 22*, 700–713.

Mundy, P., & Neal, R. (2001). *Neural plasticity, joint attention and a transactional social-orienting model of autism* (Vol. 23). San Diego, CA: Academic Press.

Mundy, P., Sigman, M., Ungerer, J., & Sherman, T. (1986). Defining the social deficits of autism: The contribution of nonverbal communication measure. *Journal of Child Psychology and Psychiatry, 27*, 657–669.

Munson, J., Dawson, G., Abbott, R., Faja, S., Webb, S. J., Friedman, S. D., . . . Dager, S. R. (2006). Amygdalar volume and behavioral development in autism. *Archives of General Psychiatry, 63*, 686–693.

Nadig, A. S., Ozonoff, S., Young, G. S., Rozga, A., Sigman, M., & Rogers, S. J. (2001). A prospective study of response to name in infants at risk for autism. *Archives of Pediatric and Adolescent Medicine, 161*, 378–383.

National Research Council. (2001). Educating Children with Autism. National Research Council: Committee on Educational Interventions for Children with Autism. National Academy of Sciences. Washington, DC: National Academy Press.

Neurodevelopmental Disorders Work Group. (2011). *Proposed revisions for neurodevelopmental disorders: Autism spectrum disorder.* Retrieved from http://www.dsm5.org/proposedrevision/Pages/Default.aspx

Nithianantharajah, J., & Hannan, A. J. (2006). Enriched environments, experience-dependent plasticity and disorders of the nervous system. *Nature Reviews Neuroscience, 7*, 697–709.

Nordahl, C. W., Lange, N., Li, D. D., Barnett, L. A., Lee, A., Buonocore, M. H., . . . Amaral, D. G. (2011). Brain enlargement is associated with regression in preschool-age boys with autism spectrum disorders. *Proceedings of the National Academy of Science of the United States of America, 108*, 20195–20200.

Osterling, J., & Dawson, G. (1994). Early recognition of children with autism: A study of first birthday home video tapes. *Journal of Autism and Developmental Disorders, 24*, 247–257.

Osterling, J. A., Dawson, G., & Munson, J. A. (2002). Early recognition of 1-year-old infants with autism spectrum disorder versus mental retardation. *Development and Psychopathology, 14*, 239–251.

Owens, G., Granader, Y., Humphrey, A., & Baron-Cohen, S. (2008). LEGO therapy and the social use of language programme: An evaluation of two social skills interventions for children with high functioning autism and Asperger syndrome. *Journal of Autism and Developmental Disorders, 38*, 1944–1957.

Ozonoff, S., Heung, K., Byrd, R., Hansen, R., & Hertz-Picciotto, I. (2008). The onset of autism: Patterns of symptom emergence in the first years of life. *Autism Research, 1*, 320–328.

Ozonoff, S., Iosif, A.-M., Baguio, F., Cook, I. C., Moore Hill, M., Hutman, T., . . . Young, G. S. (2010). A prospective study of the emergence of early behavioral signs of autism. *Journal of the American Academy of Child and Adolescent Psychiatry, 49*, 256–266.

Ozonoff, S., Macari, S., Young, G. S., Goldring, S., Thompson, M., & Rogers, S. J. (2008). Atypical object exploration at 12 months of age is associated with autism in a prospective sample. *Autism, 12*, 457–472.

Ozonoff, S., Young, G. S., Carter, A., Messinger, D., Yirmiya, N., Zwaigenbaum, L., . . . Stone, W. L. (2011). Recurrence risk for autism spectrum disorders: A baby siblings research consortium study. *Pediatrics, 128*, e488–e495.

Parker, S. K., Schwartz, B., Todd, J., & Pickering, L. K. (2004). Thimerosal-containing vaccines and autistic spectrum disorder: A critical review of published original data. *Pediatrics, 114*, 793–804.

Parr, J. R., Le Couter, A., Baird, G., Rutter, M., Pickles, A., Fombonne, E., . . . International Molecular Genetic Study of Autism Consortium (IMGSAC) Members. (2011). Early developmental regression in autism spectrum disorder: Evidence from an international multiplex sample. *Journal of Autism and Developmental Disorders, 41*, 332–340.

Paul, R., Fuerst, Y., Ramsay, G., Chawarska, K., & Klin, A. (2011). Out of the mouths of babes: Vocal production in infant siblings of children with ASD. *Journal of Child Psychology and Psychiatry, 52*, 588–598.

Peça, J., Ting, J., & Feng, G. (2011). SnapShot: Autism and the synapse. *Cell, 147*, 706–706.e1.

Pierce, K., Carter, C., Weinfeld, M., Desmond, J., Hazin, R., Bjork, R., & Gallagher, B. A. (2011). Detecting, studying, and treating autism early: The one-year well-baby check-up approach. *Journal of Pediatrics, 159*, 458–465.

Pinto, D. Pagnamenta, A. T., Klei, L., Anney, R., Merico, D., Regan, R, . . . Betancur, C. (2010). Functional impact of global rare copy number variation in autism spectrum disorders. *Nature, 466*, 368–372.

Pinto-Martin, J., Levy, S. E., Feldman, J. F., Lorenz, J. M., Paneth, N., & Whitaker, A. H. (2011). Prevalence of autism spectrum disorder in adolescents born weighing <2000 grams. *Pediatrics, 128*, 883–891.

Piven, J., Gayle, J., Chase, G. A., Fink, B., Landa, R., Wzorek, M.M., & Folstein, S. E. (1990). A family history study of neuropsychiatric disorders in the adult siblings of autistic individuals. *Journal of the American Academy of Children and Adolescent Psychiatry, 29*, 177–183.

Rasalam, A. D., Hailey, H., Williams, J. H., Moore, S. J., Turnpenny, P. D., Lloyd, D. J., & Dean, J. C. (2005). Characteristics of fetal anticonvulsant syndrome associated autistic disorder. *Developmental Medicine and Child Neurology, 47*, 551–555.

Redcay, E., & Courchesne, E. (2005). When is the brain enlarged in autism? A meta-analysis of all brain size reports. *Biological Psychiatry, 58*, 1–9.

Reznick, J. S., Baranek, G. T., Reavis, S., Watson, L. R., & Crais, E. R. (2007). A parent-report instrument for identifying one-year-olds at risk for an eventual diagnosis of autism: The first year inventory. *Journal of Autism and Developmental Disorders, 37*, 1691–1710.

Richdale, A. L., & Schreck, K. A. (2009). Sleep problems in autism spectrum disorders: Prevalence, nature, possible biosocial aetiologies. *Sleep Medicine Reviews, 13*, 403–411.

Roberts, E. M., English, P. B., Grether, J. K., Windham, G. C., Somberg, L., & Wolff, C. (2007). Maternal residence near agricultural pesticide applications and autism spectrum disorders among children in the California central valley. *Environmental Health Perspectives, 115*, 1482–1489.

Robins, D. L., Fein, D., Barton, M. L., & Green, J. A. (2001). The modified-checklist for autism in toddlers: An initial study investigating the early detection of autism and pervasive developmental disorders. *Journal of Autism and Developmental Disorders, 31*, 131–144.

Rogers, S. J., & Dawson, G. (2009). *Early start Denver model for young children with autism.* New York, NY: Guilford Press.

Rogers, S. J., Bennetto, L., McEvoy, R., & Pennington, B. F. (1996). Imitation and pantomime in high-functioning adolescents with autism spectrum disorders. *Child Development, 67*, 2060–2073.

Rogers, S. J., Hepburn, S. L., Stackhouse, T., & Wehner, E. (2003). Imitation performance in toddlers with autism and those with other developmental disorders. *Journal of Child Psychology and Psychiatry, 44*, 763–781.

Rogers, S. J., & Vismara, L. A. (2008). Evidence-based comprehensive treatments for early autism. *Journal of Clinical Child and Adolescent Psychology, 37*, 8–38.

Rudie, J. D., Shehzad, Z., Hernandez, L. M., Colich, N. L., Bookheimer, S. Y., Iacoboni, M., & Dapretto, M. (2011). Reduced functional integration and segregation of distributed neural systems underlying social and emotional information processing in autism spectrum disorders. *Cerebral Cortex, Advance Access*, 1–13.

Rutter, M. (2011). Research review: Child psychiatric diagnosis and classification: Concepts, findings, challenges and potential. *Journal of Child Psychology and Psychiatry, 52*, 647–660.

Sacco, R., Militerni, R., Frolli, A., Bravaccio, C., Gritti, A., Elia, M., . . . Persico, A. M. (2007). Clinical, morphological, and biochemical correlates of head circumference in autism. *Biological Psychiatry, 62*, 1038–1047.

Sallows, G. O., & Graupner, T. D. (2005). Intensive behavioral treatment for children with autism: Four-year outcome and predictors. *American Journal on Mental Retardation, 110*, 417–438.

Sanders, S. J., Ercan-Sencicek, A. G., Hus, V., Luo, R., Murtha, M. T., Moreno-De-Luca, D., . . . State, M. W. (2011). Multiple recurrent de novo CNVs, including duplications of the 7q11.23 Williams syndrome region, are strongly associated with autism. *Neuron, 70*, 863–885.

Schellenberg, G., Dawson, G., Sung, Y. J., Estes, A., Munson, J., Rosenthal, E., ... Wijsman, E. M. (2006). Evidence for multiple loci from a genome scan of autism kindreds. *Molecular Psychiatry, 11*, 1049–1060.

Schultz, R. T. (2005). Developmental deficits in social perception in autism: The role of the amygdala and fusiform face area. *International Journal of Developmental Neuroscience, 23*, 125–141.

Schumann, C. M., Bloss, C. S., Barnes, C. C., Wideman, G. M., Carper, R. A., Akshoomoff, N., ... Courchesne, E. (2010). Longitudinal magnetic resonance image study of cortical development through early childhood in autism. *Journal of Neuroscience, 30*, 4419–4427.

Schumann, C. M., Hamstra, J., Goodlin-Jones, B. L., Lotspeich, L. J., Kwon, H., Buonocore, M. H., ... Amaral, D. G. (2004). The amygdala is enlarged in children but not adolescents with autism: The hippocampus is enlarged at all ages. *Journal of Neuroscience, 24*, 6392–6401.

Sebat, J., Lakshmi, B., Malhotra, D., Troge, J., Lese-Martin, C., Walsh, T., ... Wigler, M. (2007). Strong association of de novo copy number mutations with autism. *Science, 316*, 445–449.

Shattuck, P. T., Durkin, M., Maenner, M., Newschaffer, C., Mandell, D. S., Wiggins, L., ... Cuniff, C. (2009). Timing of identification among children with an autism spectrum disorder: Findings from a population-based surveillance study. *Journal of the American Academy of Child and Adolescent Psychiatry, 48*, 474–483.

Shelton, J. F., Tancredi, D. J., & Hertz-Picciotto, I. (2010). Independent and dependent contributions of advanced maternal and paternal ages to autism risk. *Autism Research, 3*, 30–39.

Shukla, D. K., Keehn, B., & Muller, R. A. (2011). Tract-specific analyses of diffusion tensor imaging show widespread white matter compromise in autism spectrum disorder. *Journal of Child Psychology and Psychiatry, 52*, 286–295.

Shulha, H. P., Cheung, I., Whittle, C., Wang, J., Virgil, D., Lin, C. L., ... Weng, Z. (2012). Epigenetic signatures of autism: Trimethylated H3K4 landscapes in prefrontal neurons. *Archives of General Psychiatry, 69*, 314–324.

Shultz, S., Klin, A., & Jones, W. (2011). Inhibition of eye blinking reveals subjective perceptions of stimulus salience. *Proceedings of the National Academy of Sciences of the United States of America, 108*, 21270–21275.

Sigman, M., Dijamco, A., Gratier, M., & Rozga, A. (2004). Early detection of core deficits in autism. *Mental Retardation and Developmental Disabilities Research Reviews, 10*, 221–233.

Sigman, M., Ruskin, E., Arbeile, S., Corona, R., Dissanayake, C., Espinosa, M., ... Zierhut, C. (1999). Continuity and change in the social competence of children with autism, Down syndrome, and developmental delays. *Monographs of the Society for Research in Child Development, 64*, 1–114.

Silva, A. J., & Ehninger, D. (2009). Adult reversal of cognitive phenotypes in neurodevelopmental disorders. *Journal of Neurodevelopmental Disorders, 1*, 150–157.

Simonoff, E., Pickles, A., Charman, T., Chandler, S., Loucas, T., & Baird, G. (2008). Psychiatric disorders in children with autism spectrum disorders: Prevalence, comorbidity, and associated factors in a population-derived sample. *Journal of the American Academy of Child and Adolescent Psychiatry, 47*, 921–929.

Sofronoff, K., Attwood, T., & Hinton, S. (2005). A randomised controlled trial of a CBT intervention for anxiety in children with Asperger syndrome. *Journal of Child Psychology and Psychiatry, 46*, 1152–1160.

Sparks, B. F., Friedman, S. D., Shaw, D. W., Aylward, E. H., Echelard, D., Artru, A. A., . . . Dager, S. R. (2002). Brain structural abnormalities in young children with autism spectrum disorder. *Neurology, 59*, 184–192.

Stone, W., Lemanek, K., Fishel, P., Fernandez, M., & Altemeier, W. (1990). Play and imitation skills in the diagnosis of autism in young children. *Pediatrics, 86*, 267–272.

Stone, W. L., McMahon, C. R., Yoder, P. J., & Walden, T. A. (2007). Early social-communicative and cognitive development of younger siblings of children with autism spectrum disorders. *Archives of Pediatric and Adolescent Medicine, 161*, 384–390.

Stone, W. L., Ousley, O. Y., & Littleford, C. D. (1997). Motor imitation in young children with autism: What's the object? *Journal of Abnormal Child Psychology, 25*, 475–485.

Strömland, K., Nordin, V., Miller, M., Akerstrom, B., & Gillberg, C. (1994). Autism in thalidomide embryopathy: A population study. *Developmental Medicine and Child Neurology, 36*, 351–356.

Sullivan, M., Finelli, J., Marvin, A., Garrett-Mayer, E., Bauman, M., & Landa, R. (2007). Response to joint attention in toddlers at risk for autism spectrum disorder: A prospective study. *Journal of Autism and Developmental Disorders, 37*, 37–48.

Sung, M., Ooi, Y. P., Goh, T. J., Pathy, P., Fung, D. S., Ang, R. P., . . . Lam, C. M. (2011). Effects of cognitive-behavioral therapy on anxiety in children with autism spectrum disorders: A randomized controlled trial. *Child Psychiatry and Human Development, 42*, 634–649.

Szatmari, P., Paterson, A. D., Zwaigenbaum, L., Roberts, W., Brian, J., Liu, X. Q., . . . Meyer, K. J. (2007). Mapping autism risk loci using genetic linkage and chromosomal rearrangements. *Nature Genetics, 39*, 319–328.

Tantam, D., Monaghan, L., Nicholson, J., & Stirling, J. (1989). Autistic children's ability to interpret faces: A research note. *Journal of Child Psychology and Psychiatry, 30*, 623–630.

Thomason, M. E., & Thompson, P. M. (2011). Diffusion imaging, white matter, and psychopathology. *Annual Review of Clinical Psychology, 7*, 63–85.

Tidmarsh, L., & Volkmar, F. R. (2003). Diagnosis and epidemiology of autism spectrum disorders. *Canadian Journal of Psychiatry, 48*, 517–525.

Toth, K., Dawson, G., Meltzoff, A. N., Greenson, J., & Fein, D. (2006). Early social, imitation, play, and language abilities of young non-autistic siblings of children with autism. *Journal of Autism and Developmental Disorders, 37*, 145–157.

Vargas, D. L., Nascimbene, C., Krishnan, C., Zimmerman, A. W., & Pardo, C. A. (2005). Neuroglial activation and neuroinflammation in the brain of patients with autism. *Annals of Neurology, 57*, 67–81.

Veenstra-VanderWeele, J., & Cook Jr.,, E. H. (2004). Molecular genetics of autism spectrum disorder. *Molecular Psychiatry, 9*, 819–832.

Volk, H. E., Hertz-Picciotto, I., Delwiche, L., Lurmann, F., & McConnell, F. (2011). Residential proximity to freeways and autism in the CHARGE study. *Environmental Health Perspectives, 119*, 873–877.

Volkmar, F. R., Szatmari, P., & Sparrow, S. S. (1993). Sex differences in pervasive developmental disorders. *Journal of Autism and Developmental Disorders, 23*, 579–591.

Wang, K., Zhang, H., Ma, D., Bucan, M., Glessner, J. T., Abrahams, B. S., . . . Hakonarson, H. (2009). Common genetic variants on 5p14.1 associate with autism spectrum disorders. *Nature, 459*, 528–33.

Waterhouse, L., Fein, D., & Modahl, C. (1996). Neurofunctional mechanisms in autism. *Psychological Review, 103*, 457–489.

Weaver, I. C. G., Cervoni, N., Champagne, F. A., D'Alessio, A. C., Sharma, S., Seck, J. R., . . . Meaney, M. J. (2004). Epigenetic programming by maternal behavior. *Nature Neuroscience, 7*, 847–854.

Webb, S. J., Jones, E. J. H., Merkle, K., Namkung, J., Toth, K., Greenson, J., . . . Dawson, G. (2010). Toddlers with elevated autism symptoms show slowed habituation to faces. *Child Neuropsychology, 16*, 255–278.

Webb, S. J., Jones, E. J. H., Merkle, K., Venema, K., Greenson, J., Murias, M., & Dawson, G. (2011). Developmental change in the ERP responses to familiar faces in toddlers with autism spectrum disorders versus typical development. *Child Development, 82*, 1868–1886.

Webb, S. J., Nalty, T., Munson, J., Brock, C., Abbott, R., & Dawson, G. (2007). Rate of head circumference growth as a function of autism diagnosis and history of autistic regression. *Journal of Child Neurology, 22*, 1182–1190.

Weiss, L. A., Arking, D. E., Gene Discovery Project of Johns Hopkins & the Autism Consortium, Daly, M. J., & Chakravarti, A. (2009). A genome-wide linkage and association scan reveals novel loci for autism. *Nature, 461*, 802–808.

Werner, E., & Dawson, G. (2005). Validation of the phenomenon of autistic regression using home videotapes. *Archives of General Psychiatry, 62*, 889–895.

Werner, E., Dawson, G., Osterling, J., & Dinno, N. (2000). Brief report: Recognition of autism spectrum disorder before one year of age: A retrospective study based on home videotapes. *Journal of Autism and Developmental Disorders, 30*, 157–162.

Wilson, K., Mills, E., Ross, C., McGowan, J., & Jadad, A. (2003). Association of autistic spectrum disorder and the measles, mumps, and rubella vaccine—A systematic review of current epidemiological evidence. *Archives of Pediatrics and Adolescent Medicine, 157*, 628–634.

Wolff, J., Gu, H., Gerig, G., Elison, J. T., Styner, M., & Gouttard, S. (2012). Differences in white matter fiber tract development present from 6 to 24 months in infants with autism. *American Journal of Psychiatry, 169*, 589–600.

Wood, J. J., Drahota, A., Sze, K., Har, K., Chiu, A., & Langer, D. A. (2009). Cognitive behavioral therapy for anxiety in children with autism spectrum disorders: A randomized, controlled trial. *Journal of Child Psychology and Psychiatry, 50*, 224–234.

Yang, M., Perry, K., Weber, M. D., Katz, A. M., & Crawley, J. N. (2011). Social peers rescue autism-relevant sociability deficits in adolescent mice. *Autism Research, 4,* 17–27.

Yirmiya, N., Gamliel, I., Pilowsky, T., Feldman, R., Baron-Cohen, S., & Sigman, M. (2006). The development of siblings of children with autism at 4 and 14 months: Social engagement, communication, and cognition. *Journal of Child Psychology and Psychiatry, 47,* 511–523.

Yoder, P., Stone, W. L., Walden, T., & Malesa, E. (2009). Predicting social impairment and ASD diagnosis in younger siblings of children with autism spectrum disorder. *Journal of Autism and Developmental Disorders, 39,* 1381–1391.

Young, R. L., Brewer, N., & Pattison, C. (2003). Parental identification of early behavioural abnormalities in children with autistic disorder. *Autism, 7,* 125–143.

Zwaigenbaum, L., Bryson, S., Rogers, T., Roberts, W., Brian, J., & Szatmari, P. (2005). Behavioral manifestations of autism in the first year of life. *International Journal of Developmental Neuroscience, 23,* 143–152.

# CHAPTER 21

# Childhood Schizophrenia

ROBERT F. ASARNOW

## HISTORICAL BACKGROUND AND TERMINOLOGICAL AND CONCEPTUAL ISSUES

C ASES OF CHILDHOOD PSYCHOSIS with no apparent brain disease have been reported for at least 200 years (Fish & Ritvo, 1979), antedating Kraepelin's seminal description of dementia praecox. Kraepelin (1919/1971) observed that dementia praecox could begin during childhood and estimated that 6.2% of cases had their onset prior to age 15. Bleuler (1911/1950), who reconceptualized dementia praecox and renamed it schizophrenia, estimated that 4% of schizophrenic psychoses had their onset prior to age 15. Early child psychiatrists were aware that symptoms of schizophrenia presented somewhat differently in children than in adults; the construct of childhood schizophrenia emerged from attempts to diagnose and classify this broad range of disorders.

Indeed, in the 1930s childhood schizophrenia referred to many different, profound impairments of early onset, paralleling the "numerous expansions and contractions of the concept of schizophrenia" (Kendler et al., 1993, p. 528) in adult psychiatry during the 20th century. For decades, childhood schizophrenia was never operationally defined: "Patients were usually defined in a gross way by either brief case descriptions or a list of major symptoms" (Fish & Ritvo, 1979, p. 249). The construct of childhood schizophrenia included children who today would receive *DSM-IV* (American Psychiatric Association, 2000) diagnoses of autistic disorder, pervasive developmental disorders (PDDs), schizophrenia, or disintegrative psychosis. Furthermore, there were significant variations among clinicians in how childhood schizophrenia was diagnosed. For example, a 30-year follow-up of children diagnosed with Potter's (1933) criteria (that included children who today would be diagnosed with PDD) met *DSM* criteria for schizophrenia (Bennett & Klein, 1966). In contrast, the British working party's (Creak, 1963) criteria for "schizophrenia syndrome of childhood" are quite similar to *DSM-IV* criteria for autism and PDD. To further muddy the waters, Kanner's (1949) descriptions of early infantile autism were similar to other descriptions of childhood schizophrenia.

685

Bender and Grugett (1956) used age of onset to differentiate between two groups of children with schizophrenia. Children with an onset prior to age 2 were similar to children described by Kanner as having infantile autism. In contrast, children with later onsets had more neurotic, paranoid, and sociopathic symptoms, and tended to manifest schizophrenia as adults (Fish & Ritvo, 1979). The *DSM-II* (American Psychiatric Association, 1968) concept of childhood schizophrenia was heavily influenced by Kanner and Bender.

Rutter's (1972) landmark work on the classification of psychiatric disorders and Kolvin's (1971) studies of psychotic children resulted in fundamental changes in the conceptualization and diagnosis of schizophrenia in children. With these newer views, children with schizophrenia had hallucinations, delusions, and formal thought disorder, whereas children with autism had none of these symptoms (Kolvin, 1971). Children with autistic disorder who were followed into adulthood did not have schizophrenia symptoms (Rutter, 1967). Cogently summarizing, Rutter (1972) concluded:

> Childhood schizophrenia has tended to be used as a generic term to include an astonishingly heterogeneous mixture of disorders with little in common, other than their severity, chronicity, and occurrence in childhood. To add to the difficulty, the term has been employed in widely divergent ways by different psychiatrists... We must conclude that the term "childhood schizophrenia" has outlived its usefulness. (p. 315)

Thus, reflecting dissatisfaction with the problems with early constructs, in *DSM-III* (American Psychiatric Association, 1980), *DSM-III-R* (American Psychiatric Association, 1987) and *DSM-IV* (American Psychiatric Association, 1994), diagnostic criteria for schizophrenia in children were identical to those used for adults, with minor allowances made for how specific symptoms may be manifested in childhood. The studies cited in this chapter use either *DSM-III*, *DSM-III-R*, or *DSM-IV* criteria to diagnose schizophrenia in children.

## DIAGNOSTIC ISSUES AND *DSM-IV* CRITERIA

The *DSM-IV* states that the essential symptoms of schizophrenia are "delusions, hallucinations, disorganized speech, grossly disorganized or catatonic behavior, and negative symptoms" (American Psychiatric Association, 1994, p. 285). Schizophrenia has been diagnosed reliably in children older than 7 years using *DSM-III* and *DSM III-R* criteria (J. R. Asarnow, Tompson, & Goldstein, 1994; Russell, Bott, & Sammons, 1989; Spencer & Campbell, 1994). The frequency of core psychotic symptoms in children diagnosed with schizophrenia using *DSM-III-R* criteria is quite similar to the frequency in adults (Russell, 1994). In fact, auditory hallucinations ranged from a prevalence of 80% to 84% of the children investigated in three different studies; delusions were observed in 55% to 63% of the children (Russell, 1994). Note that transient psychotic illness can be misdiagnosed as schizophrenia in children and adults. Most misdiagnosed children have reactive or brief psychotic episodes in the context of chronic affective or behavioral disorders (Stayer et al., 2004), for which the diagnosis of schizophrenia should not be given.

When one applies *DSM-IV* criteria for schizophrenia to children, the child's level of development must be taken into account. It is important to differentiate common childhood phenomena such as imaginary friends, magical thinking, and hypnagogic experiences from true delusions and hallucinations. Hallucinations and delusions in younger children are typically quite simple and unelaborated (Bettes & Walker, 1987; Watkins, Asarnow, & Tanguay, 1988). Children are less likely to experience psychotic symptoms as alien to their experience than are adults, possibly reflecting that (a) the onset of these symptoms is typically quite gradual in children (Russell, 1994) and (b) young children do not have a firm conception as to what normal experiences entail.

The most difficult symptom to diagnose reliably in children and adolescents is "disorganized speech" (Russell, 1994). In the *DSM-IV*, disorganized speech can be manifested in derailment, loose associations, tangentiality, incoherence, and word salad—terms that harken back to Bleuer's descriptions of schizophrenic thought. Applying these criteria to children and adolescents presents special challenges because the cognitive and linguistic processes underlying speech are developing during childhood, with substantial individual differences in the rate of development of these processes. For example, Caplan and associates found that both illogical thinking and loose associations are present in many healthy children younger than 7 years, meaning that overdiagnosing "disorganized speech" in children is a potential problem (Caplan, 1994). Such issues may account for the variation in rates of formal thought disorder in children across studies (R. Asarnow & Karatekin, 1998). In short, without age-appropriate, operational criteria, the diagnosis of formal thought disorder may be unreliable in children.

Social communication has been studied by focusing on the discourse skills used when children organize their sentences during conversations (Caplan, 1994). These are linguistic devices that enable the listener to follow who and what the speaker is referring to. Children with schizophrenia speak less than healthy children and show poorer discourse skills than healthy controls. They are also less likely to show conversational repair, the methods used to self-correct during a conversation in order to clarify messages (Caplan, Guthrie, & Komo, 1996).

## DIFFERENTIAL DIAGNOSTIC ISSUES

Symptoms of schizophrenia can occur in other psychiatric conditions. McClellan and Werry (1994) and Caplan (1994) discuss guidelines for differentiating such conditions from schizophrenia. Making a differential diagnosis involving schizophrenia in children requires ruling out the following psychiatric conditions: mood disorders, schizoaffective disorder, PDDs, communication disorders, obsessive compulsive disorder, posttraumatic stress disorder, dissociative disorders, and medical conditions such as seizure disorders (particularly those involving the temporal lobes), brain tumors, and substance abuse (e.g., PCP, amphetamines, cocaine).

A further differential diagnostic issue is distinguishing between schizophrenia and a recently described form of pediatric psychotic disorder called *multidimensionally impaired disorder* (Gordon et al., 1994; Kumra et al., 1998) that is not included in *DSM-IV*. Children with the latter show poor affect regulation and problems with attention and impulse control. These children typically have an earlier onset of psychotic symptoms as well as behavioral and cognitive problems than do children meeting *DSM-IV* criteria for schizophrenia. When such children were followed up 2 to 8 years after the index diagnosis, two broad patterns of outcome were observed. First, almost half developed a mood disorder (bipolar, major depressive disorder, or schizoaffective disorder). Second, in the remainder psychotic symptoms remitted and disruptive behavior disorders developed. Thus, multidimensionally impaired disorder appears to be a distinct disorder, not strongly related to schizophrenia (Jacobsen & Rapoport, 1998).

PREVALENCE

Schizophrenia with onset in childhood is relatively rare. Very large epidemiological studies are therefore required to give a precise estimate of the prevalence of childhood-onset schizophrenia (COS), and the absence of such investigations has resulted in considerable uncertainty about its prevalence.

It is clear that schizophrenia with onset prior to 12 years of age is an infrequent occurrence. The prevalence rate of such true COS is fewer than 1 in 10,000 (Burd & Kerbeshian, 1987). This figure contrasts with a prevalence of 5 to 7 per 1,000 in the general adult population. In a study of the age distribution of psychotic disorders in 3,280 children in three German counties who sought assistance for psychological problems during a 1-year period, the prevalence of schizophrenia appears to increase dramatically once children reach age 13. These results were replicated in two additional samples of children receiving psychiatric treatment in Germany (Remschmidt, Schulz, Martin, & Warnke, 1994).

DEVELOPMENTAL PROGRESSION AND THE PRODROMAL PHASE

The prodromal phase refers to a transitional period during which symptoms start emerging prior to the onset of frank psychosis. The period prior to the prodrome is commonly referred to as the premorbid phase. As discussed later, in COS the boundaries between the premorbid and prodromal phases are frequently unclear, largely because children with schizophrenia show multiple abnormalities early in their development.

The developmental precursors of COS have been described in a number of retrospective studies, which use archival data and interviews to characterize prepsychotic functioning and symptoms. Children with schizophrenia are likely to have an insidious onset, with fewer than 5% having an acute onset. In a retrospective study (Remschmidt et al., 1994) of consecutive admissions to a child inpatient facility, children with schizophrenia showed both positive and negative symptoms for many years before their first admission. Positive symptoms of schizophrenia involve "excess" behavior patterns, including hallucinations and delusions. Negative symptoms (sometimes termed *deficit* symptoms) include social withdrawal and blunted affect. Premorbid peer relationships, school performance, and general adaptation of children with schizophrenia were worse than those of children who subsequently developed a depressive disorder (J. R. Asarnow & Ben-Meir, 1988).

A number of independent studies have reported that in a substantial number of children who develop schizophrenia, symptoms of PDDs are present prior to the onset of schizophrenia symptoms. The vast majority of children who subsequently develop schizophrenia have early histories of speech and language problems (Jacobsen & Rapoport, 1998; Watkins et al., 1988). Histories of gross impairments in language acquisition prior to 30 months of age were found in 72% of children subsequently diagnosed with schizophrenia. In addition, problems in early motor development were present prior to the onset of psychosis: 28% of the children were hypotonic and 72% had delayed motor milestones or poor coordination (Watkins et al., 1988).

The UCLA COS program (Watkins et al., 1988) identified two somewhat different developmental progressions prior to the first onset of psychotic symptoms. First, children with the most severe speech and language problems prior to 30 months of age often had other autistic or PDD-type symptoms, including a pervasive lack of responsiveness. Subsequently, at ages 6 to 9 years, flat or inappropriate affect, loosening of associations, or incoherence was observed in 71% of this group, but fewer than 10% had developed diagnostically significant hallucinations or delusions. Three years later, however, at ages 9 to 12, 71% had developed diagnostically significant hallucinations or delusions and had their first onset of schizophrenic psychosis.

A second group showed less severe speech and language problems during the first 30 months. They showed fewer psychotic-like symptoms than children with more severe speech and language problems from 6 to 9 years of age. During this age range, 82% were socially impaired and presented with excessive anxiety, constricted or inappropriate affect, magical thinking, suspiciousness, or hypersensitivity to criticism. They also tended to develop overt psychosis by 9 to 12 years. In short, children with more severe speech and language problems had an earlier onset of psychotic symptoms than children with less severe speech and language problems. Yet over time, differences between the two groups decreased, as the frequency of hallucinations and delusions increased in both groups in the 9- to 12-year-old age range (R. F. Asarnow, Brown, & Strandburg, 1995). These two subgroups present an example of equifinality, signaling different developmental pathways to a common outcome (see Chapter 1).

The National Institute of Mental Health (NIMH) study of COS (Jacobsen & Rapoport, 1998) also examined premorbid histories of speech and language problems and PDD symptoms prior to the onset of schizophrenia. They found that 60% of their sample met criteria for a developmental speech and/or language problem, while 34% had transient symptoms of PDD prior to the onset of schizophrenic psychosis (Alaghband-Rad et al., 1995). I discuss later whether these and other findings contradict the current view that autism and schizophrenia are separate disorders.

Early histories of delayed acquisition of speech and language, poor motor functioning, and compromised visual/motor functioning have been observed in children who are at risk for schizophrenia by virtue of having a biological parent with the disorder (J. R. Asarnow & Ben-Meir, 1988; Fish, Marcus, Hans, Auerbach, & Perdue, 1992). Speech and language delays and poor motor functioning were also found in two British birth cohort studies (Done, Crow, Johnstone, & Sacker, 1994; Jones, Murray, Jones, Rodgers, & Marmot, 1994). Motor abnormalities may be associated with genetic liability to schizophrenia because they are found in both medication-free patients and their unaffected first-degree relatives (Rapoport, Addington, & Frangou, 2005).

Clearly, early developmental precursors are present in the vast majority of children who develop schizophrenia prior to late adolescence, as few children with schizophrenia have an acute onset of symptoms. In general, the earlier the onset of schizophrenia, the earlier and more pronounced the presentation of such developmental precursors. Yet such precursors are not diagnostically specific, as they can also be found in the development histories of individuals with bipolar disorder or children with speech and language disorders. The developmental precursors of COS are likely to reflect early manifestations of the disruptions of neural networks that are central to the pathophysiology of the disorder.

The prodromal phase is marked by a continuation of some of the same features present during middle childhood, with gradual emergence of positive and negative symptoms of schizophrenia. Common prodromal features are poor peer relations/social isolation, decline in school functioning, inattention/difficulty concentrating, unusual perceptual experiences (illusions), unusual beliefs and unusual thought process, and blunted and/or depressed affect. Typically, the transition from the prodromal phase to psychosis is relatively gradual. Across three studies the average time from onset of non-psychotic symptoms to a diagnosis of schizophrenia was from 3 to 5 years (Russell, 1994).

## OUTCOME

The essential feature in Kraepelin's concept of dementia praecox was that it was progressive, inevitably eventuating in poor outcomes. Across three follow-up and two retrospective case record studies, most children diagnosed with COS have schizophrenia or schizophrenia-spectrum disorders at follow-up, with longitudinal intervals ranging from 5 to 20 years after initial diagnosis. When outcome is defined as remission of schizophrenia symptoms, the rates of remission range from 3% at an average follow-up of 5 years (Werry, McClellan, & Chard, 1991) to 33% at an average follow-up of 7 years (J. R. Asarnow & Tompson, 1999). At long-term follow-up (about 42 years) only a third of patients continue to suffer from ongoing psychotic symptoms (Eggers, 2002). This latter finding is consistent with reports on the diminution of psychotic symptoms after 60 years of age in patients with adult-onset of schizophrenia (Harding, Brooks, Ashikaga, Strauss, & Breier, 1987).

Whereas symptoms of schizophrenia tend to remit over time, lifetime diagnoses (reflecting the predominant symptom pattern over time) are stable. From adults followed-up more than 42 years after they were diagnosed with schizophrenia during later childhood and early adolescence, only 4 out of 38 had their diagnoses change at follow-up (Eggers, 2002). There does, however, appear to be considerable variation in adaptive, social, and vocational functioning at follow-up. Twenty eight percent of children with schizophrenia have relatively good psychosocial outcomes (J. R. Asarnow & Tompson, 1999). A 10-year follow-up of children and adolescents with schizophrenia revealed that 20% had very good or good outcomes as defined by the global assessment of functioning (GAF), while 42% had a very poor outcome and gross impairment (Fleischhaker et al., 2005). A recent 42-year follow-up of consecutive admissions to a child and adolescent psychiatry service yielded similar results (Remschmidt et al., 2007). Children with schizophrenia are unlikely to be living independently and are highly likely to be in long-term residential care at 15 years postindex diagnosis. They also have low educational attainments and relatively poor work histories (Hollis, 2000).

In general, outcomes in children with schizophrenia, particularly those with onset prior to 14 years of age, are generally worse than when onset is in adulthood (Remschmidt & Theisen, 2005). COS appears to be a severe variant of schizophrenia, which because of early-onset interferes with the acquisition of critical adaptive and social skills, a phenomenon observed in other early-onset forms of psychopathology (see Chapter 1). Consistent with studies of adults with schizophrenia, patients with poorer premorbid adjustment (Eggers, 2002; Fleischhaker et al., 2005; Werry & McClellan, 1992) and negative symptoms (McClellan, McCurry, Snell, & DuBose, 1999) are the most likely to have poor outcomes.

*Family stress.* Stress within the family environment is associated with more negative outcomes in adults with schizophrenia (Kavanagh, 1992). Even though family factors might appear to have potentially more influence on children than adults, there are scant data on the family environments of children with schizophrenia. The extant data "do present a picture of stress and distress" (J. R. Asarnow & Tompson, 1999, p. 10).

Children with schizophrenia show elevated rates of thought disorder during direct interactions, suggesting that these symptoms are expressed in the family environment (Tompson, Asarnow, Hamilton, Newell, & Goldstein, 1997). Parents of children with schizophrenia also show elevated levels of thought disorder during the same interaction task (Tompson et al., 1997) and elevated levels of communication deviance (J. R. Asarnow, Goldstein, & Ben-Meir, 1988), an index of problems establishing and maintaining a shared focus of attention. Distinguishing between the effects of parental behavior on the child with COS versus the effects of the child's behavior on parents is problematic, especially given the strong potential for gene-environment correlation (see Chapter 3). Parents of children with schizophrenia report high levels of burden and disruption (J. R. Asarnow & Horton, 1990). It is unclear the extent to which parental thought disorder reflects parental reactions to a disturbed child, shared genetic vulnerability to schizophrenia, or some other environmental factors (J. R. Asarnow, Tompson, & Goldstein, 2000). What is clear is that the family environment of children with schizophrenia is different from that of children without psychiatric disorders. The functional significance of these differences in family environment has rarely been studied in COS.

Among adults with schizophrenia, returning to homes high in expressed emotion (e.g., hostility, overinvolvement, criticism) is associated with high relapse rates and poor outcomes (Kavanagh, 1992). In contrast to findings with adults, rates of parental expressed emotion in families of children with schizophrenia are comparable to those in families of healthy controls (J. R. Asarnow, Tompson, Hamilton, Goldstein, & Guthrie, 1994). Thus, expressed emotion does not appear to predict outcome in COS. Clinical observation and the relatively scant literature suggest that family environment appears to have a different quality in COS than in adult-onset schizophrenia. The family environment of children with schizophrenia is more similar to that of children with a chronic medical condition or a developmental disability than it is to that of children with a psychiatric disorder with an acute onset, such as depression (J. Asarnow, personal communication). This pattern may reflect the early, insidious onset of the disorder.

## SEX DIFFERENCES

There is an excess of boys to girls when onset of schizophrenia is prior to 12 years of age. However, consistent with findings from adult samples (Hafner & Nowotny, 1995), the sex distribution is nearly equal when onset of schizophrenia is after age 12 (Galdos, Van Os, & Murray, 1993; Werry, McClellan, Andrews, & Ham, 1994).

## COMORBIDITY

In general, children with nearly all psychiatric disorders frequently have comorbid conditions (see Chapter 1), and this is certainly the case with COS. Studies that have used semi-structured diagnostic interviews have reported high rates of comorbidity. Russell et al. (1989) reported that 68% of the children with schizophrenia in the UCLA study met *DSM-III* criteria for another disorder. The most common comorbid diagnoses were conduct/oppositional behaviors (31%) and atypical depression or dysthymic disorder (37%). In children with schizophrenia the boundaries between (a) negative symptoms such as flat affect and (b) depressive symptoms are often unclear. The high rate of depressive disorders, along with reports that a few cases presenting with schizophrenia meet criteria for bipolar or schizoaffective disorder at follow-up, highlights the limitations of cross-sectional diagnoses (J. R. Asarnow, Tompson, & McGrath, 2004).

## OVERLAP BETWEEN AUTISM AND COS

As outlined earlier, a consensus emerged in the 1970s that autism and schizophrenia are separate and distinct disorders at the symptom level. Follow-up studies of patients with autism supported this view by showing that the risk of developing schizophrenia is not elevated in youth with clear autistic disorder (Burd & Kerbeshian, 1987; Volkmar & Cohen, 1991) or their relatives (Rutter, 1967). There is a considerable body of biological research, however, pointing to overlap between autism and COS. As noted earlier, symptoms of autism and PDD frequently occur during infancy and early childhood in children who develop schizophrenia. Forty five genes have been evaluated for positive associations with autism and schizophrenia. Although failures to replicate have been common (see Chapter 3), at least 20 of those genes are positively associated with both autism and schizophrenia, two genes were positive for autism and not schizophrenia, 11 genes were positive for schizophrenia and not autism and schizophrenia, and 12 genes were negatively associated with both disorders (Crespi, Stead, & Elliot, 2010). There are elevated rates of rare copy number variations in both children with autism and children with schizophrenia (Rapoport et al., 2009). In both disorders there is evidence of accelerated rate of brain development paralleling the onset of each of these disorders. "It appears that in autism there is acceleration or excess of early postnatal brain development (1–3 years), whereas in COS there is exaggeration of the brain maturation process of childhood and early adolescence (10–16 years). While autism and COS have been distinguished at the level of clinical symptoms, since DSM III the results of genetic and brain imaging studies indicate that there is overlap in the neurobiological substrates for these disorders" (Rapoport et al., 2009, p.14). It is important to note, however, that molecular genetics findings account for only a few percent of the variance in schizophrenia behaviors, a situation that plagues the entire field of psychiatric genetics (see Chapter 3). Nevertheless, these findings highlight that psychiatric disorders as defined clinically have complex and overlapping pathobiologies.

## RISK FACTORS

This section reviews genetic and nongenetic factors that increase the risk for developing schizophrenia.

### POPULATION-BASED STUDIES

As the ealier discussion suggests, genetic factors are strongly implicated in schizophrenia (Kendler & Diehl, 1993). Every modern controlled study that has used relatively narrow, operationalized criteria for schizophrenia, incorporating personal interviews and diagnoses of family members blind to proband diagnosis, has found that the risk of schizophrenia in first-degree relatives of patients with adult-onset of schizophrenia is greater than in relatives of controls. There is also strong evidence for familial aggregation of schizotypal personality disorder but limited or mixed evidence for aggregation of paranoid, schizoid, and avoidant personality disorders (Kendler, 1997; Kendler & Diehl, 1993; Levinson & Mowry, 1991) in first-degree relatives of patients with adult-onset of schizophrenia. Twin and adoption studies suggest that genetic factors are important in the etiology of schizophrenia (Kendler & Diehl, 1993). Across investigations, the average concordance rates for schizophrenia are 55.8% among monozygotic twins and 13.5% among dizygotic twins, strongly suggesting substantial heritability for this disorder. Still, that 45% of monozygotic twins are discordant for schizophrenia indicates that genes are predisposing factors but not sufficient in many cases to cause schizophrenia, a phenomenon referred to as *incomplete penetrance* (see Chapter 3). In addition, population genetic studies consistently suggest significant genetic heterogeneity. That is, somewhat different sets of susceptibility genes may be found in different groups of individuals with schizophrenia.

The UCLA Family Study (R. F. Asarnow et al., 2001) used modern family methods to compare the aggregation of schizophrenia and schizophrenia spectrum personality disorders in the first-degree relatives of COS, ADHD, and community control probands. There is an increased lifetime morbid risk (a statistic that adjusts for how much of the period of risk an individual has passed through) for schizophrenia and schizotypal personality disorder in parents of the COS probands compared with parents of the ADHD and community control probands. Parents of COS probands diagnosed with schizophrenia had an early age of first onset of schizophrenia (20.8 years). Risk for avoidant personality disorder was also increased in the parents of COS probands compared with parents of community controls. In sum, "The psychiatric disorders that do and do not aggregate in the parents of COS probands are remarkably similar to the disorders that do and do not aggregate in parents of adult-onset schizophrenia probands in modern family studies" (R. F. Asarnow et al., 2001, p. 586). The relative risk (ratio of risk to relatives of COS and community control probands) for schizophrenia in the parents of COS probands is 17, considerably higher than the relative risk of 3 to 6 for schizophrenia observed in parents in adult-onset schizophrenia studies. The strong suggestion is that COS is a more familial and possibly more genetic form of schizophrenia than adult-onset schizophrenia.

The NIMH Child Psychiatry Branch (Nicolson et al., 2003) replicated and extended these findings by comparing the rates of schizophrenia-spectrum disorders in parents of probands with COS with (a) adult-onset schizophrenia and (b) community controls. Parents of COS probands had a significantly higher morbidity risk of schizophrenia spectrum disorders (24.7%) than parents of probands with adult-onset schizophrenia (11.4%). Both of these rates were far higher than those of parents of community comparison probands (1.5%).

SPECIFIC GENES

Until recently it was believed that genetic effects on risk for schizophrenia were due to combinations of a relatively small number (10 to 20) of alleles of moderate effects. As is seen later, rapid developments in genomic scanning technology have resulted in studies that strongly challenge this belief.

Linkage studies have been used to attempt to identify common genes that contribute to risk. Linkage studies employ hundreds of DNA markers spread across the genome to study families containing individuals with schizophrenia, to identify chromosomal regions containing schizophrenia liability genes (see Chapter 3). Once chromosomal regions are identified, fine-mapping positional cloning is used to identify genes contributing to susceptibility to schizophrenia. This approach is entirely empirical and can consequently yield novel findings. The next step after a putative susceptibility gene is identified is to determine the function of that gene, and to elucidate how that function might be involved in the development of symptoms. In studies of adult-onset schizophrenia, a number of potential susceptibility genes have been identified in multiple linkage studies, including dysbindin, neuregulin-1, DISC1, G72, and the alpha 7 nictotinic receptor subunit. A number of these genes have functions that might be related to certain disease mechanisms in schizophrenia. One of the unanticipated results of such linkage studies is the discovery that almost half of the chromosomal locations linked to schizophrenia are also linked to bipolar disorder. Thus, even though these conditions are separable, there may be some common genetic factors for these two psychotic disorders.

A second approach to identifying risk genes for schizophrenia is a candidate gene approach. For example, genes known to have effects in the pathways through which antipsychotic medications act are studied in patients with schizophrenia and in family members. A number of genes, including COMT and GRM3, have been identified. In addition, a number of potential susceptibility genes, including GAD1, have been identified by their altered expression in postmortem studies of the brains of patients with schizophrenia (Risch & Merikangas, 1996).

The NIMH COS study has used family-based association studies to demonstrate that three susceptibility genes identified in studies of adult-onset schizophrenia are present in COS. Each gene had a specific pattern of correlation with aspects of the clinical phenotype (Rapoport et al., 2005). Polymorphisms in the G72 gene are associated with COS, and COS probands with the risk allele associated with schizophrenia had a later age of onset and better premorbid adjustment than COS probands without the risk allele (Addington et al., 2004). Dysbindin is associated with COS, and COS probands with the risk allele have poorer premorbid functioning than COS probands without the risk allele. GAD1 was also associated with COS. GAD1 is believed to be involved in the cortical GABA system, which is thought to be altered in schizophrenia. COS probands with the GAD1 risk allele had an increased rate of loss of frontal gray matter on MRI over time (Addington et al., 2005).

Genome-wide association studies (GWAS) use SNP (single-nucleotide-polymorphisms) arrays, typically in case control studies, to examine the associations between particular alleles and a diagnosis within a population (see Chapter 3). GWAS studies have several advantages over alternative disease gene discovery methods. In contrast to candidate gene studies, which select genes for study based on known or suspected disease mechanisms, GWAS investigations scan the genome in an unbiased fashion and thus have the potential to identify novel risk factors. Compared to family linkage studies approaches, GWAS studies can detect association signals localized to small chromosomal areas containing only a few genes, permitting rapid detection of the actual disease risk gene. Second, GWAS can identify disease genes of modest effects, a severe limitation in linkage studies. The results of GWAS studies of schizophrenia "have indicated that most common disorders (psychiatric and non-psychiatric) are complex, involving large number of genes, each of small effect" (Addington & Rapoport, 2011, p. 1469).

## CYTOGENETIC ABNORMALITIES

Cytogenetic, or chromosomal, mutations can provide information about potential chromosomal locations that are altered in diseases. Common examples detected by karyotyping are Down syndrome and Fragile X. Multiple rare cytogenetic abnormalities have been found in the NIMH COS study. These include one case of Turner's syndrome and four cases of 22q11DS. The 5% rate of 22q11DS in the NIMH-COS study is considerably higher than both the estimated rate of 0.36% in four studies that contained 1,100 adult-onset schizophrenia patients and the rate of 0.025% in the community (Sporn et al., 2004). The 22q11DS deletion syndrome is associated with the velocardialfacial syndrome. 22q11DS is associated with an increased rate of cortical gray matter loss during childhood and adolescence in patients who are not yet psychotic (Sporn et al., 2004).

The use of microarray-based methods permits the detection of much smaller chromosomal mutations. Genome-wide scans of individuals with schizophrenia and ancestry-based controls using microarrays revealed that 15% of adults with schizophrenia compared to 5% of controls have "rare structural variants" that deleted or duplicated one or more genes (Walsh et al., 2008). Twenty-eight percent of an independent sample of children with COS also had copy number variations. Walsh and colleagues (2008) found that most of the rare structural variants were unique and were thought to be de novo mutations. Many of the genes disrupted by structural variants are involved in "signaling networks controlling neurodevelopment" (Walsh et al., 2008). Increased rates of copy number variations, however, are not specific to schizophrenia. In the past several years increased rates of copy number variations, both de novo and inherited, have been reported in individuals with autism, language disorders, OCD and bipolar disorder.

## ENDOPHENOTYPES

Endophenotypes are features that lie intermediate to the phenotype and genotype of schizophrenia (Gottesman & Shields, 1973). In adult-onset schizophrenia, abnormalities in smooth pursuit eye movements, neurocognitive functioning, brain structure, brain electrical activity, and autonomic activity show promise as endophenotypes. These abnormalities are probably closer to the biological effects of schizophrenia genes than are the *DSM-IV* symptoms of schizophrenia themselves (see Chapter 3). In addition, these abnormalities exist as quantitative traits, thereby increasing power in linkage and association studies compared to investigations using *DSM-IV* diagnoses.

A number of endophenotypes identified in first-degree relatives of adults with schizophrenia have also been identified in the first-degree relatives of children with schizophrenia. The performance of parents of COS, ADHD, and community control probands was compared on three neurocognitive tasks: span of apprehension, degraded stimulus-CPT, and trail making test, which have been shown in prior research to detect impairments in patients with adult-onset schizophrenia and ADHD. Parents were excluded from the study if they had diagnoses of psychosis. A combination of scores on the three neurocognitive tests identified 20% of mothers and fathers of COS probands compared to 0% of the mothers or fathers of community control probands. There was diagnostic specificity of the neurocognitive impairments: 12% of mothers of COS probands were identified by a combination of neurocognitive scores compared to 0% of ADHD mothers. A cutoff that identified 2% of the fathers of ADHD probands classified 17% of the fathers of COS probands. In all, endophenotypes related to neurocognitive impairments can produce a level of diagnostic accuracy that may aid in genetic linkage studies (R. F. Asarnow et al., 2002).

Nonpsychotic first-degree relatives of COS patients showed deficits on the Trail Making Test (Gochman et al., 2004) and smooth pursuit eye tracking (Sporn et al., 2005) in the NIMH COS study. In another investigation (Ross, Heinlein, Zerbe, & Radant, 2005), COS patients showed impaired-response inhibition and spatial accuracy on a delayed oculomotor response task. However, children who were not psychotic but had a first-degree relative with schizophrenia did not show abnormalities on this task. In general, adult relatives of patients with schizophrenia show subtle impairments on some of the same tasks identified as potential endophenotypes in studies of adult-onset schizophrenia.

Another potential endophenotype has emerged from brain-imaging studies of COS patients and their siblings. In longitudinal studies COS patients and their nonpsychotic siblings show reduced cortical gray matter in the superior temporal prefrontal areas early in development. In siblings of patients with COS these reductions in gray matter normalize during adolescence, but at younger ages prefrontal and/or temporal gray matter loss may be an endophenotype for COS (Mattai et al., 2011).

## CONCLUSIONS REGARDING GENETIC FINDINGS

The finding that susceptibility genes for adult-onset schizophrenia are associated with COS provides support for the biological continuity of adult- and child-onset schizophrenia (Rapoport et al., 2005). Recent developments in psychiatric genetics point to complex relationships between risk genes and behavioral phenotypes of psychiatric symptoms and disorders (see Chapter 3 for an extended discussion). It appears that in schizophrenia there are both many genes of small effect, which increase risk for schizophrenia and are transmitted within families, as well as some de novo mutations of large effect. There is substantial overlap across disorders in the presence of risk genes. This high-phenotypic variation presents challenges in mapping the pathways from gene to disorder that are required to develop new pharmacological treatments.

There is relatively little known about the normal function of putative susceptibility genes for schizophrenia or how they may affect processes related to the development of schizophrenia. Many of the genes may have multiple functions, which may vary by brain region and developmental stage. The most productive approach to mapping pathways from gene to disease may entail elucidating pathways to endophenotypes that are more proximal to the effects of susceptibility genes than the clinical phenotype of schizophrenia.

## DRUG ABUSE

Drug abuse is widespread in adolescents (see Chapter 15). There is extensive epidemiological evidence that use of cannabis, amphetamines, and cocaine increases risk of developing psychoses (Degenhardt & Hall, 2012). Psychotomimetic drugs such as LSD can also result in psychotic symptoms. Adolescents with a genetic predisposition for schizophrenia are more likely to develop psychotic symptoms and/or show a greater psychotic response to cannabis, amphetamines, cocaine, and psychomimetic drugs than adolescents without a genetic predisposition to schizophrenia (Paparelli et al., 2011). At this point, much work remains in mapping associations between genetic susceptibilities to drug abuse and COS.

## OBSTETRIC COMPLICATIONS

A meta-analysis of 16 case control studies and two historical cohort studies found that the risk (pooled odds ratio) for the development of schizophrenia in adult life was doubled in people with a history of obstetric complications (Geddes & Lawrie, 1995). Patients with schizophrenia with a history of obstetric complications have an earlier age of onset of schizophrenia than patients without a history of obstetric complications. The three types of obstetric complications associated with increased risk for schizophrenia are (a) pregnancy complications (diabetes, bleeding, etc.); (b) abnormal fetal development (e.g., low birth weight); and (c) delivery complications (e.g., asphyxia).

The NIMH and Maudsley Early Onset Schizophrenia studies did not find an increased rate of obstetric complications in COS probands (Rapoport et al., 2005). In contrast, a Japanese study (Matsumoto, Takei, Saito, Kachi, & Mori, 1999) found odds ratios of 6.25 for boys and 2.63 for girls. On balance, obstetric complications do not appear to exert a strong, direct effect on the development of schizophrenia. Moreover, histories of obstetric complications are found in children with a number of neuropsychiatric conditions besides schizophrenia.

Obstetric complications are most likely to constitute one environmental factor that interacts with susceptibility genes for schizophrenia to set in motion a developmental progression eventuating in the disorder. An example of a gene-environment interaction is that fetal hypoxia is associated with reduced gray matter and increased cerebralspinal fluid in patients with schizophrenia and their siblings, but has no effect on brain volumes in individuals at low genetic risk (Cannon et al., 1993). The complexity of gene-environment interactions on brain development is compounded by the fact that certain brain regions may be more susceptible to environmental effects at different developmental periods (Rapoport et al., 2005).

## PARENT AND FAMILY CHARACTERISTICS

Historically, there was considerable interest in the role of parental personality characteristics (e.g., "schizophrenogenic mother") and parent and family communication patterns (e.g., "double bind communications") in the etiology of schizophrenia. This interest was stimulated by psychodynamic theories of personality and psychopathology. There has been scant empirical support for the role of these factors as primary etiological agents in schizophrenia (Hartwell, 1996).

However, there is intriguing evidence (Tienari et al., 2004) that exposure to certain patterns of communication/family environments may interact with a genetic risk for schizophrenia to further increase the risk for schizophrenia-spectrum disorders. In a longitudinal study of children with high-genetic liability to schizophrenia (i.e., those with biological mothers with schizophrenia) who were adopted at an early age, dysfunctional family rearing environments (based on global ratings) and maladaptive parent communication patterns ("communication deviance"—a confusing, unclear communication style that disrupts the focus of attention) interacted with genetic liability in predicting which adoptees developed a schizophrenia-spectrum disorder (Wahlberg et al., 2004; Wynne et al., 2006). Adoptees reared in adoptive families that provided a dysfunctional rearing environment and where parents had high rates of communication deviance were significantly more likely at follow-up to have developed a schizophrenia-spectrum disorder than adoptees reared in adoptive homes that provided more benign psychosocial environments (Wynne et al., 2006). Rearing environment and parental communication patterns in the adoptive homes of children with low genetic liability to schizophrenia had no effect on the rates of schizophrenia spectrum disorders at follow-up.

## INSIGHTS INTO PATHOPHYSIOLOGY

Important insights into disease mechanisms that eventuate in schizophrenia are provided by detailed understanding of brain abnormalities that are central biological features of this disorder. The sections below summarize what is known about brain structure and function in COS.

## BRAIN STRUCTURE

Modern quantitative structural brain imaging methods have made it possible to identify brain abnormalities that are not evident by visual inspection of brain images. Quantitative MRI analysis permits the segmentation of the brain into three compartments: (1) gray matter, somatodendritic tissue of neurons; (2) white matter, myelinated connecting fibers (axons); and (3) cerebrospinal fluid. Gray and white matter segmentation can help determine whether axonal or neuronal loss is primarily responsible for changes in brain volume and organization.

A meta-analysis (Wright et al., 2000) of 58 volumetric MRI studies found that, compared to controls, the mean cerebral volume of adults with schizophrenia was 2% smaller whereas the mean total ventricular volume of those with schizophrenia was greater (126%). Brain regions with the lowest volumes in patients with schizophrenia were the left amygdala (94%), right amygdala (94%), left hippocampus/amygdala (94%), right hippocampus/amygdala (95%), left parahippocampus (93%), right parahippocampus (95%), and left anterior superior temporal gyrus (93%). A recent meta-analysis of voxel-based morphometric studies found that the left superior temporal gyrus and the left medial temporal lobe were key regions of structural difference in patients with schizophrenia, compared to healthy subjects (Honea, Crow, Passingham, & Mackay, 2005). Voxel-based morphometry is a method for detecting group differences in the density or volume of brain matter.

In patients with COS there is a 9.2% reduction in total brain volume (Frazier et al., 1996), a somewhat greater reduction than is observed in patients with adult-onset of schizophrenia. In contrast to studies of adult-onset schizophrenia, four independent cross-sectional studies did not find evidence of hippocampal volume reduction in COS (Rapoport et al., 2005). One study (Taylor et al., 2005) found significant enlargement but another (Matsumoto et al., 2001) found a reduction of the right posterior superior temporal gyrus, an important language center in the brain. Similar to findings in adults, the right anterior cingulate gyrus was larger in COS patients than controls. Anterior cingulate gyrus volumes were relatively smaller in older COS patients than in younger COS patients (Marquardt et al., 2005). In general, COS patients show a greater reduction in brain volumes than adults with schizophrenia.

Longitudinal data from the NIMH COS study (Thompson et al., 2001) provide dramatic evidence of progressive changes in brain structure. Over a follow-up period of up to 5 years, healthy control children showed subtle losses of gray matter, at a rate 1% to 2% per year in the parietal lobes, with almost no detectable change in the rest of the brain. In contrast, COS patients showed a progressive loss of brain tissue starting from the back of the brain and spreading forward. There was a loss of up to 3% to 4% per year in some regions of the brain for these patients. Early deficits in parietal lobe regions that support language extended forward into the temporal lobes, sensorimotor and dorsolateral prefrontal cortices, and frontal eye fields. The trajectory of changes in brain structure in COS appears to represent an exaggeration of processes found in normal brain development (Rapoport et al., 2005). These findings highlight the importance of understanding changes in brain structure and function in a developmental context.

## Neurocognition

Starting with Bleuler's seminal descriptions of associative disturbances in patients with schizophrenia, there has been recognition that cognitive impairments are central deficits in schizophrenia. Conceptual models and experimental methods from what are now called *cognitive psychology* and *behavioral neuroscience* have been used to elucidate the core cognitive impairments in adults with schizophrenia. Early studies focused on higher-order cognitive processes such as attention and memory, with the goal of isolating specific stages of information processing and/or subprocesses impaired in schizophrenia. More recent studies have tended to focus on more elementary cognitive processes that tap circumscribed neural networks. Inferences about the brain systems underlying impaired performance on cognitive tasks draw upon studies of patients with neurological disease and functional brain imaging studies of patients and controls performing cognitive tasks.

Meta-analyses confirm the centrality of cognitive impairments in schizophrenia. The presence of cognitive impairments is the most robust finding when schizophrenia patients are compared to healthy controls. The average effect sizes for common clinical tests of attention, memory, language, and reasoning are twice as large as for structural magnetic resonance imaging and positron emission tomography (Heinrichs, 2004). Although the majority of patients with schizophrenia show impairments on cognitive tests, there is substantial heterogeneity in their performance. A meta-analysis of data on IQ, memory, language, executive function, and attention from 113 studies (4,365 patients and 3,429 controls) found a consistent trend for adult schizophrenia patients to perform more poorly than healthy controls in five cognitive domains: IQ, memory, language, executive function, and attention (Fioravanti, Carlone, Vitale, Cinti, & Clare, 2005).

Attempts to isolate specific brain systems that are impaired in schizophrenia by examining patterns of performance are complicated by the presence of a generalized cognitive impairment. Adults with schizophrenia perform 1.0 to 1.5 standard deviations below healthy controls on most neurocognitive tests (Bilder et al., 2000). Attempts to identify a circumscribed, specific cognitive deficit must be conducted against this background of generalized deficit. Investigators attempt to identify differential deficits (also referred to as *dissociations*) to identify specific cognitive deficits under these conditions. An important methodological issue is that apparent differential deficits observed in patients with schizophrenia frequently reflect the relative psychometric discriminating power of tasks rather than true differences between cognitive abilities (L. Chapman & J. Chapman, 2001). Demonstrating a differential performance deficit requires proving that the control task (the one predicted not to produce deficits in patients) has adequate distributional properties (e.g., no attenuated range) and reliability, comparable to the task hypothesized to detect performance deficits in patients. In the many studies of cognitive functioning in schizophrenia, there are relatively few that have identified differential deficits not explainable by psychometric explanations.

Like adults with schizophrenia, COS patients show a generalized cognitive deficit. This is reflected in Full Scale IQ scores (around 85) about one standard deviation below that of healthy controls (R. F. Asarnow, Tanguay, Bott, & Freeman, 1987; Rhinewine et al., 2005). Longitudinal analyses reveal that there is an initial steep decline in IQ, from about 2 years prior to 2 years after onset of psychotic symptoms. As with adult-onset schizophrenia, there does not appear to be a progressive generalized loss of cognitive function after this initial decline. This stability of general cognitive functioning in COS, for periods up to 13 years, is noteworthy given chronic illness and related long-term exposure to antipsychotic medications and the concomitant, progressive loss of cortical gray matter (Gochman et al., 2005).

As would be expected given the magnitude of the generalized deficit, COS patients perform poorly on a wide variety of cognitive tasks including tests of attention (R. F. Asarnow, Asamen, Granholm, & Sherman, 1994; Rhinewine et al., 2005; Thaden et al., 2006), serial visual search (R. F. Asarnow & Sherman, 1984; Karatekin & Asarnow, 1998); visual and spatial working memory (Karatekin & Asarnow, 1998), verbal learning and memory (Rhinewine et al., 2005), and executive functioning (R. F. Asarnow et al., 1994; Karatekin & Asarnow, 1999; Rhinewine et al., 2005). The challenge in cognitive studies of COS is not so much identifying tasks that differentiate patients from controls but rather in identifying underlying cognitive processes that can produce such a wide range of performance deficits.

Investigators manipulate both stimulus and processing demands of tasks to isolate the specific cognitive processes underlying impaired performance, providing a basis for making inferences about the brain systems underlying impaired cognition in COS. An example of this approach is a study by Karetekin and Asarnow (1998a), who found that COS patients could deploy their attention broadly and engage in parallel visual search at the same rate as healthy controls, but had a slower search rate when they had to focus their attention and search displays serially. These results were interpreted as suggesting that patients with COS had difficulty with executive control of selective attention in the service of self-guided behavior.

## PSYCHOPHYSIOLOGY

Psychophysiology is the study of how psychological activities produce physiological responses. Historically, most psychophysiologists focused on the physiological responses and organ systems innervated by the autonomic nervous system. Starting in the 70s psychophysiologists have focused on the central nervous system, exploring cortical brain potentials such as the many types of event related potentials (ERPs) and functional neuroimaging (fMRI, PET, and MEG). ERPs use averaging techniques to measure the brain's electrical response recorded from the scalp to sensory stimuli and specific cognitive processing demands. Brain activity is reflected in either positive or negative waves (components) that are typically identified by reference to when the peaks occur relative to stimulus onset. Investigators have attempted to capitalize upon the superior temporal resolution of ERPs to identify the precise stage in cognitive processing where impairments first appear in schizophrenia.

One of the earliest ERP differences between adult-onset patients and controls is in the P50 component, a positive wave that occurs about 50 ms after stimulus onset in a sensory gating paradigm. Patients with schizophrenia show less reduction in P50 after a second stimulus, believed to reflect impaired sensory gating (a preattentive sensory habituation mechanism to filter out irrelevant stimuli) (Freedman, Adler, Waldo, Pachtman, & Franks, 1983). Mismatch negativity is a negative wave that occurs about 200 ms postonset of infrequent sounds presented within a sequence of repetitive sounds. Mismatch negativity is reduced in adult-onset patients with chronic schizophrenia and appears to tap sensory memory. The P300 is a positive wave that occurs about 300 ms poststimulus onset when a low-probability event is detected and consciously processed. Patients with adult-onset schizophrenia show reduced P300 amplitudes at midline sites and over the left, but not the right temporal lobe.

The UCLA COS program (R. F. Asarnow et al., 1995; Strandburg et al., 1994) examined ERP components while participants performed tests (e.g., span of apprehension and continuous performance test) that detect cognitive impairments. A consistent finding was the absence of right-lateralized P1/N1 amplitude in COS patients. Healthy controls typically have larger visual P1/N1 components over the right hemisphere. The absence of this lateralization in COS patients could reflect either differences in the strategic utilization of processing capacity of the hemispheres or right hemisphere processing dysfunction. Across investigations, processing negativity was reduced in COS patients compared to healthy controls or children with ADHD. Processing negativity is a family of negative waves that occur within 400 ms of stimulus onset, thought to measure the degree to which attentional and perceptual resources are allocated to cognitive processing. Reduced processing negativity is the earliest component in which cognitive processing abnormalities were detected in COS. COS patients also showed reduced P300 amplitude. Such later components may be the "downstream product of the uncertainty in stimulus recognition created by previous discriminative difficulties, or may be additional neurocognitive deficits" (R. F. Asarnow et al., 1995).

## Neural Networks in Schizophrenia

Neuroanatomic and cognitive data in adult-onset schizophrenia implicate multiple cortical and subcortical structures, and multiple cognitive processes. What is quite clear is that adult-onset schizophrenia is *not* a condition where a focal brain lesion results in tightly circumscribed cognitive impairments. Rather, there is a consensus that at least two neural circuits are central to the pathophysiology of schizophrenia. The first is a front-temporal circuit. As noted above, the frontal and temporal lobes are sites of some of the greatest anatomic differences between patients with schizophrenia and healthy controls. These brain regions support working and secondary memory and executive functions, which are both impaired in patients with schizophrenia. Note that reductions in processing negativities may result from impairments in certain executive functions supported by the frontal lobes that are responsible for the maintenance of an attentional trace (Knight, Hillyard, Woods, & Neville, 1981; Michie, Fox, Ward, Catts, & McConaghy, 1990).

The second is a prefrontal cortical-striatal circuit. This network is the target of almost all antipsychotic medications. Antipsychotic drugs block dopamine receptors in the neocortex and the striatum. The prefrontal cortex partially controls the dopamine reward system that reinforces contextually appropriate stimuli. Abnormalities in reward and motivation (which are key negative symptoms of schizophrenia) may result when this circuit is compromised. There are a number of recent studies (e.g., Foerde et al., 2008) showing that discrete corticostriatal loops are dysfunctional in schizophrenia.

COS patients show the same general pattern of neuroanatomic and cognitive findings as patients with adult-onset of schizophrenia. With the exception of the hippocampus, the volume reductions and degree of cognitive impairment appear to be greater in COS than adult-onset schizophrenia patients.

## TREATMENT

The same antipsychotic medications that are used to treat adults with schizophrenia are used to treat children and adolescents with schizophrenia. In a placebo-controlled study aripiprazole, olanzapine, quetiapine, paliperidone, and risperidone all resulted in greater reductions in the Positive and Negative Symptom Scale (PANNS) total score than placebo in children and adolescents with psychotic symptoms. Across seven head-to-head trials in children and adolescents with psychosis or schizophrenia there was no difference in the efficacy of antipsychotics. These trials did not include clozapine. In contrast, in small studies of limited duration, clozapine resulted in significantly greater reduction of psychotic symptoms than haloperidol and olanzapine (Correll, Kratochvil, & March, 2011). Because of serious side effects, some of which require having to do blood tests continually while patients are being treated with this drug, clozapine is usually used only when patients have not responded to other antipsychotic treatments.

## THEORETICAL SYNTHESIS AND FUTURE DIRECTIONS

For the past 2 decades neurodevelopmental models have provided a useful framework to begin to understand the complex pathways from brain abnormalities to the symptoms of schizophrenia. Neurodevelopmental models of schizophrenia were stimulated by data suggesting that abnormalities in brain development start from very early in life, and typically antedate the first onset of psychotic symptoms by many years. An influential neurodevelopmental model by Weinberger (1987) posits that schizophrenia is "a neurodevelopmental disorder in which a fixed brain lesion from early in life interacts with certain normal maturational events that occur much later" to trigger the onset of psychosis (p. 660). The neurodevelopmental processes that eventuate in schizophrenia are a result of the interaction of genetic and environmental factors.

The results of the studies of COS reviewed above are broadly consistent with neurodevelopmental models of schizophrenia. Total brain and gray matter volumes are reduced and ventricles are enlarged in COS (Rapoport et al., 2005). As with adult-onset schizophrenia, these brain abnormalities are thought to reflect processes beginning during fetal development. Genetic liability to schizophrenia is expressed behaviorally not only as schizophrenia, but in subtle neurocognitive impairments that occur in nonpsychotic relatives of patients and that may be reflected in early language problems. Retrospective studies indicate that well in advance of the onset of psychotic symptoms, COS patients manifest certain neurobehavioral impairments. In infancy and early childhood acquisition of expressive and receptive language is slow and gross motor functioning is impaired. Somewhat later there are impairments in fine motor coordination. These neurobehavioral impairments may be manifestations of the early brain lesions posited by neurodevelopmental models.

It is interesting to note that during middle childhood and adolescence expressive and receptive language skills are among the least impaired functions in patients with COS. This finding suggests that early impairments in language functioning may be developmental delays rather than static, fixed neuropsychological deficits. Children who will develop COS are most likely to be delayed in acquiring skills during infancy and childhood that are at the cusp of development (R. F. Asarnow et al., 1995). This constellation of findings highlights the importance of viewing schizophrenia as resulting from a dynamic developmental process in which the effects of subtle, early biological insults influence how the child responds to normal developmental transitions. The dramatic progressive changes in brain structure in COS described above may be exaggerations of normal cortical development (Rapoport et al., 2005).

## CONTINUITY BETWEEN COS AND ADULT-ONSET SCHIZOPHRENIA

When the same *DSM* criteria used to diagnose adult-onset schizophrenia are applied to children and adolescents, there is overwhelming evidence of continuity of COS and the more typical adult-onset schizophrenia. Children with schizophrenia show the same familial aggregation of psychiatric disorders, structural brain abnormalities (with the exception of the temporal lobe), neurocognitive impairments, and psychophysiological abnormalities that are present in adult-onset schizophrenia. Although the data are quite limited, COS patients appear to respond to the antipsychotic medications used to treat adults with schizophrenia (R. Asarnow & Karatekin, 1998), although they may be less tolerant of these agents than adults (Baldessarini & Teicher, 1995).

The current data suggest that there is an increased familial aggregation of schizophrenia and schizophrenia spectrum disorders, and a greater familial aggregation of neuroanatomical and neurocognitive abnormalities, in COS than in adult-onset schizophrenia. COS may represent a severe, highly genetic, and biologically homogeneous form of schizophrenia in which the biological substrate is more clearly discernable than in adult-onset schizophrenia. This framework sets the stage for challenging questions. What causes a small number of children to develop schizophrenia very early in life? What triggers the onset of psychotic symptoms: An exaggeration of normal developmental processes such as pruning, or the failure of protective processes that normally forestall the emergence of psychotic symptoms? Studying COS may provide invaluable insights into the complex neurodevelopmental pathways that eventuate in schizophrenia.

## REFERENCES

Addington, A. M., Gornick, M., Duckworth, J., Sporn, A., Gogtay, N., Bobb, A., . . . Straub, R. E. (2005). GAD1 (2q31.1), which encodes glutamic acid decarboxylase (GAD-sub-6-sub-7), is associated with childhood-onset schizophrenia and cortical gray matter volume loss. *Molecular Psychiatry, 10*, 581–588.

Addington, A. M., Gornick, M., Sporn, A. L., Gogtay, N., Greenstein, D., Lenane, M., . . . Rapoprt, J. L. (2004). Polymorphisms in the 13q33.2 gene G72/G30 are associated with childhood-onset schizophrenia and psychosis not otherwise specified. *Biological Psychiatry, 55*, 976–980.

Addington, A. M., & Rapoport, J. L. (2011). Annual research review: Impact of advances in genetics in understanding developmental psychopathology. *Journal of Child Psychology and Psychiatry, 10,* 1469–7610.

Alaghband-Rad, J., McKenna, K., Gordon, C. T., Albus, K. E., Hamburger, S. D., Rumsey, J. M., ... Rapoport, J. L. (1995). Childhood-onset schizophrenia: The severity of premorbid course. *Journal of the American Academy of Child and Adolescent Psychiatry, 34,* 1273–1283.

American Psychiatric Association. (1968). *Diagnostic and statistical manual of mental disorders* (2nd ed.). Washington, DC: Author.

American Psychiatric Association. (1980). *Diagnostic and statistical manual of mental disorders* (3rd ed.). Washington, DC: Author.

American Psychiatric Association. (1987). *Diagnostic and statistical manual of mental disorders* (3rd ed., rev.). Washington, DC: Author.

American Psychiatric Association. (1994). *Diagnostic and statistical manual of mental disorders* (4th ed.). Washington, DC: Author.

American Psychiatric Association. (2000). *Diagnostic and statistical manual of mental disorders* (4th ed., text rev.). Washington, DC: Author.

Asarnow, J. R., & Ben-Meir, S. (1988). Children with schizophrenia spectrum and depressive disorders: A comparative study of premorbid adjustment, onset pattern and severity of impairment. *Journal of Child Psychology and Psychiatry, 29,* 477–488.

Asarnow, J. R., Goldstein, M. J., & Ben-Meir, S. (1988). Parental communication deviance in childhood onset schizophrenia spectrum and depressive disorders. *Journal of Child Psychology and Psychiatry, 29,* 825–838.

Asarnow, J. R., & Horton, A. A. (1990). Coping and stress in families of child psychiatric inpatients: Parents of children with depressive and schizophrenia spectrum disorders. *Child Psychiatry & Human Development, 21,* 145–157.

Asarnow, R., & Karatekin, C. (1998). Childhood-onset schizophrenia. In C. E. Coffey & R. A. Brumback (Eds.), *Textbook of pediatric neuropsychiatry* (pp. 617–646). Washington, DC: American Psychiatric Press.

Asarnow, J. R., Tompson, M., Hamilton, E. B., Goldstein, M. J., & Guthrie, D. (1994). Family expressed emotion, childhood-onset depression, and childhood-onset schizophrenia spectrum disorders: Is expressed emotion a nonspecific correlate of child psychopathology or a specific risk factor for depression? *Journal of Abnormal Child Psychology, 22,* 129–146.

Asarnow, J. R., & Tompson, M. C. (1999). Childhood-onset schizophrenia: A follow-up study. *European Child & Adolescent Psychiatry, 8*(Suppl. 1), 9–12.

Asarnow, J. R., Tompson, M. C., & Goldstein, M. J. (2000). Psychosocial factors: The social context of child and adolescent onset schizophrenia. In H. Helmut (Ed.), *Schizophrenia in children and adolescents* (pp. 168–191). New York, NY: Cambridge University Press.

Asarnow, J. R., Tompson, M. C., & McGrath, E. P. (2004). Annotation: Childhood-onset schizophrenia: Clinical and treatment issues. *Journal of Child Psychology and Psychiatry, 45,* 180–194.

Asarnow, R. F., Asamen, J., Granholm, E., & Sherman, T. (1994). Cognitive/neuropsychological studies of children with a schizophrenic disorder. *Schizophrenia Bulletin, 20,* 647–669.

Asarnow, R. F., Brown, W., & Strandburg, R. (1995). Children with a schizophrenic disorder: Neurobehavioral studies. *European Archives of Psychiatry and Clinical Neuroscience. Special Issue: Schizophrenia in childhood and adolescence, 245,* 70–79.

Asarnow, R. F., Nuechterlein, K. H., Fogelson, D., Subotnik, K. L., Payne, D. A., Russell, A. T., . . . Kendler, K. S. (2001). Schizophrenia and schizophrenia-spectrum personality disorders in the first-degree relatives of children with schizophrenia: The UCLA family study. *Archives of General Psychiatry, 58,* 581–588.

Asarnow, R. F., Nuechterlein, K. H., Subotnik, K. L., Fogelson, D. L., Torquato, R. D., Payne, D. L., . . . Guthrie, D. (2002). Neurocognitive impairments in nonpsychotic parents of children with schizophrenia and attention-deficit/hyperactivity disorder: The University of California, Los Angeles family study. *Archives of General Psychiatry, 59,* 1053–1060.

Asarnow, R. F., & Sherman, T. (1984). Studies of visual information processing in schizophrenic children. *Child Development, 55,* 249–261.

Asarnow, R. F., Tanguay, P. E., Bott, L., & Freeman, B. J. (1987). Patterns of intellectual functioning in non-retarded autistic and schizophrenic children. *Journal of Child Psychology and Psychiatry, 28,* 273–280.

Baldessarini, R. J., & Teicher, M. H. (1995). Dosing of antipsychotic agents in pediatric populations. *Journal of Child and Adolescent Psychopharmacology, 5,* 1–4.

Bender, L., & Grugett, A. E. Jr., (1956). A study of certain epidemiological factors in a group of children with childhood schizophrenia. *American Journal of Orthopsychiatry, 26,* 131–145.

Bennett, S., & Klein, H. R. (1966). Childhood schizophrenia: 30 years later. *American Journal of Psychiatry, 122,* 1121–1124.

Bettes, B. A., & Walker, E. (1987). Positive and negative symptoms in psychotic and other psychiatrically disturbed children. *Journal of Child Psychology and Psychiatry, 28,* 555–568.

Bilder, R. M., Goldman, R. S., Robinson, D., Reiter, G., Bell, L., Bates, J. A., . . . Lieberman, J. A. (2000). Neuropsychology of first-episode schizophrenia: Initial characterization and clinical correlates. *American Journal of Psychiatry, 157,* 549–559.

Bleuler, E. (1911/1950). *Dementia praecox, or the group of schizophrenias.* (J. Zinkin, Trans.). New York, NY: International Universities Press.

Burd, L., & Kerbeshian, J. (1987). A North Dakota prevalence study of schizophrenia presenting in childhood. *Journal of the American Academy of Child & Adolescent Psychiatry, 26,* 347–350.

Cannon, T. D., Mednick, S. A., Parnas, J., Schulsinger, F., Praestholm, J, & Vestergaard, A. (1993). Developmental brain abnormalities in the offspring of schizophrenic mothers: I. Contributions of genetic and perinatal factors. *Archives of General Psychiatry, 50,* 551–564.

Caplan, R. (1994a). Communication deficits in childhood schizophrenia spectrum disorders. *Schizophrenia Bulletin, 20,* 671–683.

Caplan, R. (1994b). Thought disorder in childhood. *Journal of the American Academy of Child and Adolescent Psychiatry, 33,* 605–615.

Caplan, R., Guthrie, D., & Komo, S. (1996). Conversational repair in schizophrenic and normal children. *Journal of the American Academy of Child & Adolescent Psychiatry, 35,* 950–958.

Chapman, L. J., & Chapman, J. P. (2001). Commentary on two articles concerning generalized and specific cognitive deficits. *Journal of Abnormal Psychology, 110,* 31–39.

Correll, C. U., Kratochvil, C. J., & March, J. S. (2011). Developments in pediatric psychopharmacology: Focus on stimulants, antidepressants and antipsychotics. *Journal of Clinical Psychiatry, 72,* 655–670.

Creak, E. M. (1963). Childhood psychosis: A review of 100 cases. *British Journal of Psychiatry, 109* (Whole No. 458), 84–89.

Crespi, B., Stead, P. & Elliott, M. (2010). Comparative genomics of autism and schizophrenia. *Proceedings of the National Academy of Sciences, 107,* 1736–1741.

Degenhardt, L., & Hall, W. (2012). Extent of illicit drug use and dependence and their contribution to global burden of disease. *Lancet, 379,* 55–70.

Done, D. J., Crow, T. J., Johnstone, E. C., & Sacker, A. (1994). Childhood antecedents of schizophrenia and affective illness: Social adjustment at ages 7 and 11. *British Medical Journal, 309,* 699–703.

Eggers, C. (2002). Schizophrenia in childhood and adolescence. Symptomatology, clinical course, etiological and therapeutic aspects. *Z Arztl Fortbild Qualitatssich, 96,* 567–577.

Fioravanti, M., Carlone, O., Vitale, B., Cinti, M. E., & Clare, L. (2005). A meta-analysis of cognitive deficits in adults with a diagnosis of schizophrenia. *Neuropsychology Review, 15,* 73–95.

Fish, B., Marcus, J., Hans, S. L., Auerbach, J. G., & Perdue, S. (1992). Infants at risk for schizophrenia: Sequelae of a genetic neurointegrative defect: A review and replication analysis of pandysmaturation in the Jerusalem infant development study. *Archives of General Psychiatry, 49,* 221–235.

Fish, B., & Ritvo, E. R. (1979). Psychoses of childhood. In J. D. Noshpitz (Ed.), *Basic handbook of child psychiatry* (pp. 249–304). New York, NY: Basic Books.

Fleischhaker, C., Schulz, E., Tepper, K., Martin, M., Hennighausen, K., & Remschmidt, H. (2005). Long-term course of adolescent schizophrenia. *Schizophrenia Bulletin, 31,* 769–780.

Foerde, K., Poldrack, R. A., Knowlton, B. J. W., Sabb, F., Bookheimer, S. Y., Bilder, R. M., . . . Asarnow, R. F. (2008). Selective corticostriatal dysfunction in schizophrenia: Examination of motor and cognitive skill learning. *Journal of Abnormal Psychology, 22,* 100–109.

Frazier, J. A., Giedd, J. N., Hamburger, S. D., Albus, K. E., Kaysen D, Vaituzis A. C., . . . Rapoport, J. L. (1996). Brain anatomic magnetic resonance imaging in childhood-onset schizophrenia. *Archives of General Psychiatry, 53,* 617–624.

Freedman, R., Adler, L. E., Waldo, M. C., Pachtman, E., & Franks, R. D. (1983). Neurophysiological evidence for a defect in inhibitory pathways in schizophrenia: Comparison of medicated and drug-free patients. *Biological Psychiatry, 18*, 537–551.

Galdos, P. M., Van Os, J. J., & Murray, R. M. (1993). Puberty and the onset of psychosis. *Schizophrenia Research, 10*, 7–14.

Geddes, J. R., & Lawrie, S. (1995). Obstetric complications and schizophrenia: A meta-analysis. *British Journal of Psychiatry, 167*, 786–793.

Gochman, P. A., Greenstein, D., Sporn, A., Gogtay, N., Keller, B., Shaw, P., . . . Rapoport, J. L. (2005). IQ stabilization in childhood-onset schizophrenia. *Schizophrenia Research, 77*, 271–277.

Gochman, P. A., Greenstein, D., Sporn, A., Gogtay, N., Nicolson, R., Keller, A., . . . Rapoport, J. L. (2004). Childhood onset schizophrenia: Familial neurocognitive measures. *Schizophrenia Research, 71*, 43–47.

Gordon, C. T., Frazier, J. A., McKenna, K., Giedd, J., Zametkin, A., Kaysen, D., . . . Hommer, D. (1994). Childhood-onset schizophrenia: An NIMH study in progress. *Schizophrenia Bulletin, 20*, 697–712.

Gottesman, I. I., & Shields, J. (1973). Genetic theorizing and schizophrenia. *British Journal of Psychiatry. 122*, 15–30.

Hafner, H., & Nowotny, B. (1995). Epidemiology of early-onset schizophrenia. *European Archives of Psychiatry and Clinical Neuroscience. Special Issue: Schizophrenia in childhood and adolescence, 245*, 80–92.

Harding, C. M., Brooks, G. W., Ashikaga, T., Strauss, J. S., & Breier, A. (1987). The Vermont longitudinal study of persons with severe mental illness: II. Long-term outcome of subjects who retrospectively met DSM-III criteria for schizophrenia. *American Journal of Psychiatry, 144*, 727–735.

Hartwell, C. E. (1996). The schizophrenogenic mother concept in American psychiatry. *Psychiatry: Interpersonal and Biological Processes, 59*, 274–297.

Heinrichs, R. W. (2004). Meta-analysis and the science of schizophrenia: Variant evidence or evidence of variants? *Neuroscience and Biobehavioral Reviews, 28*, 379–394.

Hollis, C. (2000). Adult outcomes of child- and adolescent-onset schizophrenia: Diagnostic stability and predictive validity. *American Journal of Psychiatry, 157*, 1652–1659.

Honea, R., Crow, T. J., Passingham, D., & Mackay, C. E. (2005). Regional deficits in brain volume in schizophrenia: A meta-analysis of voxel-based morphometry studies. *American Journal of Psychiatry, 162*, 2233–2245.

Jacobsen, L. K., & Rapoport, J. L. (1998). Research update: Childhood-onset schizophrenia: Implications of clinical and neurobiological research. *Journal of Child Psychology and Psychiatry, 39*, 101–113.

Jones, P., Murray, R., Jones, P., Rodgers, B., & Marmot, M. (1994). Child developmental risk factors for adult schizophrenia in the British 1946 birth cohort. *Lancet, 344*, 1398–1402.

Kanner, L. (1949). Problems of nosology and psychodynamics of early infantile autism. *American Journal of Orthopsychiatry, 19*, 416–426.

Karatekin, C., & Asarnow, R. F. (1998a). Components of visual search in childhood-onset schizophrenia and attention-deficit/hyperactivity disorder. *Journal of Abnormal Child Psychology, 26*, 367–380.

Karatekin, C., & Asarnow, R. F. (1998b). Working memory in childhood-onset schizophrenia and attention-deficit/hyperactivity disorder. *Psychiatry Research, 80*(2), 165–176.

Karatekin, C., & Asarnow, R. F. (1999). Exploratory eye movements to pictures in childhood-onset schizophrenia and attention-deficit/hyperactivity disorder (ADHD). *Journal of Abnormal Child Psychology, 27*, 35–49.

Kavanagh, D. J. (1992). Recent developments in expressed emotion and schizophrenia. *British Journal of Psychiatry, 160*, 601–620.

Kendler, K. S. (1997). The genetic epidemiology of psychiatric disorders: A current perspective. *Social Psychiatry and Psychiatric Epidemiology, 32*, 5–11.

Kendler, K. S., & Diehl, S. R. (1993). The genetics of schizophrenia: A current, genetic-epidemioiogic perspective. *Schizophrenia Bulletin, 19*, 261–285.

Kendler, K. S., McGuire, M., Gruenberg, A. M., O'Hare, A., Spellman, M., & Walsh, D. (1993). The Roscommon family study: I. Methods, diagnosis of probands, and risk of schizophrenia in relatives. *Archives of General Psychiatry, 50*, 527–540.

Knight, R. T., Hillyard, S. A., Woods, D. L., & Neville, H. J. (1981). The effects of frontal cortex lesions on event-related potentials during auditory selective attention. *Electroencephalography and Clinical Neurophysiology, 52*, 571–582.

Kolvin, I. (1971). Studies in the childhood psychoses: I. Diagnostic criteria and classification. *British Journal of Psychiatry, 118*, 381–384.

Kraepelin, E. (1971). *Dementia praecox and paraphrenia* (R. M. Barclay, Trans.). Huntington, NY: Krieger. (Original work published 1919)

Kumra, S., Jacobsen, L. K., Lenane, M., Zahn, T. P., Wiggs, E., Alaghband-Rad, J., . . . Rapoport, J. L. (1998). "Multidimensionally impaired disorder": Is it a variant of very early-onset schizophrenia? *Journal of the American Academy of Child and Adolescent Psychiatry, 37*, 91–99.

Levinson, D. F., & Mowry, B. J. (1991). Defining the schizophrenia spectrum: Issues for genetic linkage studies. *Schizophrenia Bulletin, 17*, 491–514.

Marquardt, R. E. K., Levitt, J. G., Blanton, R. E., Caplan, R., Asarnow, R., Siddarth, P., . . . Toga, A. W. (2005). Abnormal development of the anterior cingulate in childhood-onset schizophrenia: A preliminary quantitative MRI study. *Psychiatry Research: Neuroimaging, 138*, 221–233.

Matsumoto, H., Simmons, A., Williams, S., Hadjulis, M., Pipe, R., Murray, R., & Franqou, S. (2001). Superior temporal gyrus abnormalities in early-onset schizophrenia: Similarities and differences with adult-onset schizophrenia. *American Journal of Psychiatry, 158*, 1299–1304.

Matsumoto, H., Takei, N., Saito, H., Kachi, K., & Mori, N. (1999). Childhood-onset schizophrenia and obstetric complications: A case–control study. *Schizophrenia Research, 38*, 93–99.

Mattai, A. M., Weisinger, B., Greenstein, D., Stidd, R., Clasen, L., Miller, R., . . . Gogtay, N. (2011). Normalization of cortical gray matter deficits in nonpsychotic siblings of patients with childhood-onset schizophrenia. *Journal of the Academy of Child and Adolescent Psychiatry, 50,* 697–704.

McClellan, J., McCurry, C., Snell, J., & DuBose, A. (1999). Early-onset psychotic disorders: Course and outcome over a 2-year period. *Journal of the American Academy of Child and Adolescent Psychiatry, 38,* 1380–1388.

McClellan, J., & Werry, J. (1994). Practice parameters for the assessment and treatment of children and adolescents with schizophrenia. *Journal of the American Academy of Child and Adolescent Psychiatry, 33,* 616–635.

Michie, P. T., Fox, A. M., Ward, P. B., Catts, S. V., & McConaghy, N. (1990). Event-related potential indices of selective attention and cortical lateralization in schizophrenia. *Psychophysiology, 27,* 209–227.

Nicolson, R., Brookner, F. B., Lenane, M., Gochman, P., Ingraham, L. J., Egan, M. F., ... Rapoport, J. L. (2003). Parental schizophrenia spectrum disorders in childhood-onset and adult-onset schizophrenia. *American Journal of Psychiatry, 160,* 490–495.

Paparelli, A., Di Forti, M., Morrison, P. D., & Murray, R. M. (2011) Drug-induced psychosis: How to avoid star gazing in schizophrenia research by looking at more obvious sources of light. *Frontiers in Behavioral Neuroscience, 5,* 1–9.

Potter, H. W. (1933). Schizophrenia in children. *American Journal of Psychiatry, 12,* 1254–1270.

Rapoport, J. C., Addington, A. M., & Frangou, S. (2005). "The neurodevelopmental model of schizophrenia: Update 2005": Corrigendum. *Molecular Psychiatry, 10,* 614.

Rapoport, J., Chavez, A., Greenstein, D., Addington, A., & Gogtay, N. (2009). Autism-spectrum disorders and childhood schizophrenia: Clinical and biological contributions to a relationship revisited. *Journal of the Academy of Child and Adolescent Psychiatry, 48,* 10–18.

Remschmidt, H., Martin, M., Fleischhaker, C., Theisen, F. M., Hennighausen, K., Gutenbrunner, C., & Schultz, E. (2007). Forty-two years later: The outcome of childhood-onset schizophrenia. *Journal of Neural Transmission, 114,* 505–512.

Remschmidt, H. E., Schulz, E., Martin, M., & Warnke, A. (1994). Childhood-onset schizophrenia: History of the concept and recent studies. *Schizophrenia Bulletin, 20,* 727–745.

Remschmidt, H., & Theisen, F. (2005). Schizophrenia and related disorders in children and adolescents. *Journal of Neural Transmission Supplement, 69,* 121–141.

Rhinewine, J. P., Lencz, T., Thaden, E. P., Cervellione, K. L., Burdick, K. E., Henderson, I., ... Kumra, S. (2005). Neurocognitive profile in adolescents with early-onset schizophrenia: Clinical correlates. *Biological Psychiatry, 58,* 705–712.

Risch, N., & Merikangas, K. (1996) The future of genetic studies of complex human disease. *Science, 273,* 1516–1517.

Ross, R. G., Heinlein, S., Zerbe, G. O., & Radant, A. (2005). Saccadic eye movement task identifies cognitive deficits in children with schizophrenia, but not in unaffected child relatives. *Journal of Child Psychology and Psychiatry, 46,* 1354–1362.

Russell, A. T. (1994). The clinical presentation of childhood-onset schizophrenia. *Schizophrenia Bulletin, 20,* 631–646.

Russell, A. T., Bott, L., & Sammons, C. (1989). The phenomenology of schizophrenia occurring in childhood. *Journal of the American Academy of Child and Adolescent Psychiatry, 28,* 399–407.

Rutter, M. (1967). Classification and categorization in child psychiatry. *International Journal of Psychiatry, 3,* 161–187.

Rutter, M. (1972). Childhood schizophrenia reconsidered. *Journal of Autism and Childhood Schizophrenia, 2,* 315–337.

Spencer, E. K., & Campbell, M. (1994). Children with schizophrenia: Diagnosis, phenomenology, and pharmacotherapy. *Schizophrenia Bulletin, 20,* 713–725.

Sporn, A., Greenstein, D., Gogtay, N., Sailer, F., Hommer, D. W., Rawlings, R., . . . Rapoport, J. L. (2005). Childhood-onset schizophrenia: Smooth pursuit eye-tracking dysfunction in family members. *Schizophrenia Research, 73,* 243–252.

Sporn, A. L., Addington, A. M., Gogtay, N., Ordo Altez, A. E., Gornick, M., Clasen, L., . . . Rapoport, J. L. (2004). Pervasive developmental disorder and childhood-onset schizophrenia: Comorbid disorder or a phenotypic variant of a very early onset illness? *Biological Psychiatry, 55,* 989–994.

Stayer, C., Sporn, A., Gogtay, N., Tossell, J., Lenane, M., Gochman, P., & Rapoport, J. L. (2004). Looking for childhood schizophrenia: Case series of false positives. *Journal of the American Academy of Child and Adolescent Psychiatry, 43,* 1026–1029.

Strandburg, R. J., Marsh, J. T., Brown, W. S., Asarnow, R. F., Higa, J., & Guthrie, D. (1994). Continuous-processing related ERPs in schizophrenic and normal children. *Biological Psychiatry, 35,* 525–538.

Taylor, J. L., Blanton, R. E., Levitt, J. G., Caplan, R., Nobel, D., & Toga, A. W. (2005). Superior temporal gyrus differences in childhood-onset schizophrenia. *Schizophrenia Research, 73,* 235–241.

Thaden, E., Rhinewine, J. P., Lencz, T., Kester, H., Cervellione, K. L., Henderson, I., . . . Kumra, S. (2006). Early-onset schizophrenia is associated with impaired adolescent development of attentional capacity using the identical pairs continuous performance test. *Schizophrenia Research, 81,* 157–166.

Thompson, P. M., Vidal, C., Giedd, J. N., Gochman, P., Blumenthal, J., Nicolson, R., . . . Rapoport, J. L. (2001). Mapping adolescent brain change reveals dynamic wave of accelerated gray matter loss in very early-onset schizophrenia. *Proceedings of the National Academy of Sciences, 98,* 11650–11655.

Tienari, P., Wynne, L. C., Sorri, A., Lahti, I., Laksy, K., Moring, J., . . . Wahlberg, K. E. (2004). Genotype-environment interaction in schizophrenia-spectrum disorder: Long-term follow-up study of Finnish adoptees. *British Journal of Psychiatry, 184,* 216–222.

Tompson, M. C., Asarnow, J. R., Hamilton, E. B., Newell, L. E., & Goldstein, M. J. (1997). Children with schizophrenia-spectrum disorders: Thought disorder and communication problems in a family interactional context. *Journal of Child Psychology and Psychiatry, 38,* 421–429.

Volkmar, F. R., & Cohen, D. J. (1991). Comorbid association of autism and schizophrenia. *American Journal of Psychiatry, 148,* 1705–1707.

Wahlberg, K.-E., Wynne, L. C., Hakko, H., Laksy, K., Moring, J., Miettunen, J., & Tienari, P. (2004). Interaction of genetic risk and adoptive parent communication deviance: Longitudinal prediction of adoptee psychiatric disorders. *Psychological Medicine, 34,* 1531–1541.

Walsh, T., McClellan, J. M., McCarthy, S. E., Addington, A. M., Pierce, S. B., Cooper, G. M., . . . Sebat, J. (2008). Rare structural variants disrupt multiple genes in neurodevelopmental pathways in schizophrenia. *Science, 320,* 539–543.

Watkins, J. M., Asarnow, R. F., & Tanguay, P. E. (1988). Symptom development in childhood onset schizophrenia. *Journal of Child Psychology and Psychiatry, 29,* 865–878.

Weinberger, D. R. (1987). Implications of normal brain development for the pathogenesis of schizophrenia. *Archives of General Psychiatry, 44*(7), 660–669.

Werry, J. S., & McClellan, J. M. (1992). Predicting outcome in child and adolescent (early onset) schizophrenia and bipolar disorder. *Journal of the American Academy of Child and Adolescent Psychiatry, 31,* 147–150.

Werry, J. S., McClellan, J. M., Andrews, L. K., & Ham, M. (1994). Clinical features and outcome of child and adolescent schizophrenia. *Schizophrenia Bulletin, 20,* 619–630.

Werry, J. S., McClellan, J. M., & Chard, L. (1991). Childhood and adolescent schizophrenic, bipolar, and schizoaffective disorders: A clinical and outcome study. *Journal of the American Academy of Child and Adolescent Psychiatry, 30,* 457–465.

Wright, I. C., Rabe-Hesketh, S., Woodruff, P. W. R., David, A. S., Murray, R. M., & Bullmore, E. T. (2000). Meta-analysis of regional brain volumes in schizophrenia. *American Journal of Psychiatry, 157,* 16–25.

Wynne, L. C., Tienari, P., Nieminen, P., Sorri, A., Lahti, I., Moring, J., . . . Miettunen, L. (2006). I. Genotype-environment interaction in the schizophrenia spectrum: Genetic liability and global family ratings in the Finnish adoption study. *Family Process, 45,* 419–434.

# CHAPTER 22

# Eating Disorders

ERIC STICE AND CARA BOHON

## HISTORICAL CONTEXT

E ATING DISORDERS ARE PSYCHIATRIC disturbances involving abnormal eating behaviors, maladaptive efforts to control shape or weight, and disturbances in perceived body shape or size. Three eating disorder syndromes are recognized in the literature: anorexia nervosa, bulimia nervosa, and binge eating disorder. Anorexia nervosa was first recognized as a psychiatric disorder more than a century ago, whereas the first published account of bulimia appeared in the late 1970s. Although the prevalence of anorexia nervosa appears to have remained relatively stable over time, the prevalence of bulimia nervosa increased toward the end of the 20th century (Wilson, Becker, & Heffernan, 2003). Stunkard (1959) first described binge eating disorder half a century ago among overweight individuals. This eating disorder has not yet been recognized as a diagnostic entity (American Psychiatric Association [APA], 2000), but considerable research since the early 1990s has led to the likely inclusion of the disorder in the next edition of the *DSM*.

Evidence that the prevalence of anorexia nervosa has been relatively stable over time might be interpreted as suggesting that biological processes play a more prominent role in the etiology of this eating disorder relative to sociocultural factors. In contrast, evidence that the prevalence of bulimia nervosa and binge eating disorder has increased over time might be taken to imply that sociocultural factors, such as an increasing abundance of palatable foods and cultural valuation of thinness for girls and women, play a more pronounced role in the etiology of eating disorders.

## DIAGNOSTIC ISSUES AND *DSM-IV* CRITERIA

### ANOREXIA NERVOSA

Diagnostic criteria for anorexia nervosa include weight loss or failure to gain weight (with weight less than 85% of what would be expected for height, age, and developmental level), intense fear of gaining weight or of becoming fat despite a low body weight, disturbed perception of weight and shape, an undue influence of weight or shape on self-evaluation or a denial of the seriousness of the illness, and amenorrhea in postmenarcheal females (APA, 2000). A distinction is made between a restricting type of anorexia nervosa, in which the person does not engage regularly in binge eating or purging (self-induced vomiting or laxative/diuretic use), and a binge eating/purging type.

Although the diagnostic criteria for anorexia nervosa appear straightforward, this condition can be challenging to assess. In children and adolescents, age- and sex-adjusted norms must be applied. Weight is also adjusted for height using the Body Mass Index (BMI = kg/m$^2$). Furthermore, younger individuals and/or those who are not motivated for treatment may deny fear of weight gain, despite engaging in behaviors that suggest its presence. To address this issue, a proposal for the *DSM-5* allows assessors to use the presence of behaviors that interfere with weight gain as presumptive evidence for this fear. Amenorrhea is also controversial, as individuals with and without this symptom often do not differ on measures of impairment (Bulik, Sullivan, & Kendler, 2000). Moreover, the common yet ill-advised practice of placing amenorrheic individuals on birth control pills to reinstate cycles can obscure this symptom. For these reasons, the current proposal for *DSM-5* eliminate amenorrhea from the diagnostic criteria.

Additional features of anorexia nervosa include a relentless pursuit of thinness and overvaluation of body shape, which usually results in extreme dietary restriction and excessive physical activity (Fairburn & Harrison, 2003). Consequent to semi-starvation, individuals become preoccupied with food and exhibit ritualistic and stereotyped eating, such as cutting food into small pieces, moving food around on the plate, and eating foods in a certain order (Wilson et al., 2003). The 11-year mortality rate is 2.8% for anorexia nervosa, with causes of death including complications of starvation and suicide (Arcelus, Mitchell, Wales, & Nielsen, 2011; Keel & Brown, 2010).

Common physical symptoms associated with anorexia nervosa include yellowish skin (hypercarotenemia), lanugo (fine, downy hair), hypersensitivity to cold, hypotension (low blood pressure), bradycardia (slow heart rate), and other cardiovascular problems. Purging behaviors may cause enlargement of salivary glands and erosion of dental enamel. Dehydration and electrolyte imbalances from chronic purging may lead to serum potassium depletion and consequent hypokalemia, which increases risk of renal failure and cardiac arrhythmia, which sometimes result in death. Osteopenia may also result from malnutrition and decreased estrogen secretion.

## BULIMIA NERVOSA

Bulimia nervosa is marked by recurrent episodes (at least twice weekly for 3 months) of consumption of unusually large amounts of food (coupled with a sense that the eating is out of control), recurrent (at least twice weekly for 3 months) compensatory behaviors to prevent weight gain (e.g., self-induced vomiting, laxative/diuretic abuse, fasting, or excessive exercise), and undue influence of weight and shape on self-evaluation (APA, 2000). If symptoms occur exclusively during a period of anorexia nervosa, the latter diagnosis prevails. During binge episodes, these individuals (and those with binge eating disorder) typically consume between 1,000 and 2,000 calories, often from easily ingestible foods high in fat and sugar content. Bulimia nervosa is associated with guilt and shame regarding eating behaviors (Wilson et al., 2003), which may contribute to the fact that individuals suffer from bulimia nervosa for an average of 6 years before seeking treatment (Fairburn & Harrison, 2003).

Bulimia nervosa can also be challenging to assess, partly as a result of problematic diagnostic criteria. Binge eating specifies the amount of food typically consumed during a binge episode ("larger than most people would eat"), the duration of the binge episode ("in a discrete period of time"), and subjective experience of the episode ("a sense of a lack of control over eating"), but each of these can be ambiguous. For example, some people may endorse uncontrollable binge eating in a discrete period of time yet still report eating a quantity of food that is not larger than what most people eat. Others, particularly males, may endorse eating an amount of food that is larger than what most people eat, but deny a loss of control. Compensatory behaviors, such as fasting and excessive exercise, can also be difficult to assess. The frequency and duration criteria (twice weekly for 3 months) have questionable empirical support (LeGrange et al., 2006; Spoor, Stice, Burton, & Bohon, 2007) and are likely to be reduced to once weekly for 3 months in the *DSM-5*. Finally, undue influence of self-evaluation by weight and shape is endorsed by a large portion of adolescent girls and can be difficult to separate from general body dissatisfaction. These ambiguities suggest that it might be beneficial to use behavioral criteria for bulimia nervosa or that clearer algorithms should be developed.

A common clinical feature of bulimia nervosa includes secrecy about the behavior, related to shame and guilt. Often parents and peers are unaware of the disordered eating. Individuals with bulimia nervosa are typically in the average weight range. Some reports have shown increased mortality in bulimia nervosa (Crow et al., 2009; Fichter, Quadflieg, & Hedlund, 2008). Additional physical complaints include fatigue, headaches, enlarged salivary glands secondary from recurrent vomiting, and erosion of dental enamel and dentin from gastric fluids. Electrolyte abnormalities (hypokalemia and hypochloremia), a result of frequent purging, can result in cardiac arrhythmias and arrest. Laxative abuse can lead to dependence and withdrawal and lead to lasting colon damage. These medical disturbances most typically occur among individuals who are engaging in frequent binge eating and compensatory behaviors; many may resolve with discontinuation of these behaviors.

## Binge Eating Disorder

Binge eating disorder is listed in the *DSM-IV* (APA, 2000) as a provisional eating disorder requiring further study, exemplifying an eating disorder not otherwise specified (EDNOS)—a residual category for eating disorders that are not captured by the categories of anorexia or bulimia nervosa. This eating disorder involves

(a) repeated episodes (at least 2 days per week for 6 months) of uncontrollable binge eating characterized by certain features (e.g., rapid eating, eating until uncomfortably full, eating large amounts of food when not physically hungry, eating alone because of embarrassment, and feeling guilty or depressed after overeating); (b) marked distress regarding binge eating; and (c) the absence of regular compensatory behaviors (e.g., monthly vomiting for weight control). If symptoms occur exclusively during episodes of anorexia or bulimia nervosa, these diagnoses take precedence.

As with bulimia nervosa, the definition of binge eating is unclear; the frequency and duration requirements are unsupported empirically. It is likely that binge eating disorder will be a recognized diagnosis in *DSM-5*, and the frequency and duration requirements will match those of bulimia nervosa. Patterns of eating also vary, such as overeating continuously throughout the day (i.e., grazing) rather than in discrete time periods, underscoring the importance of recording binge eating days in addition to binge eating episodes.

Binge eating disorder is commonly associated with obesity and related medical complications, including hypertension, adverse lipoprotein profiles, diabetes mellitus, atherosclerotic cerebrovascular disease, coronary heart disease, colorectal cancer, reduced life span, and death from a wide range of causes (Fontaine, Redden, Wang, Westfall, & Allison, 2003). Independent of body weight, binge eating confers additional psychiatric and medical risks such as insomnia, specific phobias, daily smoking, alcohol use, and physical pain (Reichborn-Kjennerud, Bulik, Sullivan, Tambs, & Harris, 2004b). There is evidence that many patients with binge eating disorder also have overvaluation of shape and weight (Grilo et al., 2008).

## EATING DISORDER NOT OTHERWISE SPECIFIED (ED-NOS)

The *DSM-IV* currently describes five symptom presentations in addition to binge eating disorder as examples of Eating Disorder Not Otherwise Specified (ED-NOS). These presentations include anorexia nervosa with menses present, anorexia nervosa with normal weight, low-binge frequency bulimia nervosa, chewing and spitting food repeatedly, and purging disorder (the regular use of inappropriate compensatory behavior after eating food that would not be considered a binge episode).

Bespeaking the earlier noted problems with the *DSM-IV* diagnostic criteria for anorexia nervosa and bulimia nervosa, between 40% and 90% of patients presenting for treatment for an eating disorder are diagnosed with ED-NOS (Rockert, Kaplan, & Olmsted, 2007; Zimmerman, Francione-Witt, Chelminski, Young, & Tortolani, 2008). Research on ED-NOS has been difficult because of the heterogeneity of symptoms in the group, but advances have been made in the various domains, particularly purging disorder. Studies have shown similar levels of general psychopathology and health care problems in ED-NOS as in full threshold eating disorder diagnoses (e.g., Peebles, Hardy, Wilson, & Lock, 2010; Santonastaso et al., 2009; Spoor et al., 2007). Furthermore, there is minimal diagnostic crossover between bulimia nervosa and purging disorder (Stice, Marti, Shaw, & Jaconis, 2009), suggesting that purging disorder is distinct from subthreshold bulimia.

## PREVALENCE

Epidemiologic studies using diagnostic interviews suggest that between 0.9% and 2.0% of girls and women and between 0.1% and 0.3% of boys and men experience anorexia nervosa during their lifetimes (Hudson, Hiripi, Pope, & Kessler, 2007; Lewinsohn, Striegel-Moore, & Seeley, 2000; Woodside et al., 2001). Subthreshold anorexia nervosa occurs in 1.1% to 3.0% of adolescent girls (Lewinsohn et al., 2000; Stice et al., 2009). Bulimia nervosa afflicts between 1.1% and 4.6% of girls and women and between 0.1% and 0.5% of boys and men during their lifetimes (Garfinkel et al., 1995; Hudson et al., 2007; Lewinsohn et al., 2000; Woodside et al., 2001). The prevalence of subthreshold bulimia nervosa is more common and ranges from 2.0% to 5.4% (Lewinsohn et al., 2000; Stice et al., 2009). Despite the sex discrepancies, male athletes may be at elevated risk for eating disorders (Wilson et al., 2003). Binge eating disorder afflicts between 0.2% and 3.5% of girls and between 0.9% and 2.0% of boys and men during their lifetimes (Hoek & van Hoeken, 2003; Hudson et al., 2007; Kjelsas, Bjornstrom, & Gotestam, 2004). Community-recruited samples indicate that the prevalence of subthreshold binge eating disorder for adolescent females is 1.6% (Lewinsohn et al., 2000; Stice et al., 2009).

## RISK FACTORS, PROTECTIVE FACTORS, AND ETIOLOGIC FORMULATIONS

### ANOREXIA NERVOSA

Although there are numerous theories regarding etiologic processes involved in the development of anorexia nervosa, few prospective studies have investigated factors that predict onset of anorexia, and no prospective tests of multivariate etiologic models exist. Prospective studies are essential to determine whether a putative risk factor is a precursor, concomitant, or consequence of eating pathology. Several prospective studies have examined particular risk factors for anorexia nervosa. Marchi and Cohen (1990) found that picky eating and digestive problems in early childhood predicted subsequent symptoms of anorexia. Cnattingius, Hultman, Dahl, and Sparen (1999) found that two obstetric complications, premature birth (small for gestational age) and cephalhematoma (a collection of blood under the scalp), were associated with elevated risk for the subsequent development of anorexia nervosa. These obstetric complications were relatively specific to anorexia nervosa, as they did not predict the onset of psychosis or schizophrenia. Bulik and associates (2006) found that premorbid neuroticism predicted the onset of anorexia nervosa among twins. Stice, Presnell, and Bearman (2006) showed that girls with the lowest weight and low scores on a dietary restraint at age 13 were at increased risk for future onset of threshold or subthreshold anorexia nervosa over a 5-year period. Early puberty, perceived pressure to be thin from family, peers, and the media, thin-ideal internalization, body dissatisfaction, depressive symptoms, and low parental and peer support did not predict anorexic pathology onset. Nicholls and Viner (2009) found that infant feeding problems, maternal depressive symptoms, and a history of undereating predicted lifetime anorexia nervosa by age 30. High self-esteem and maternal body mass index were protective factors.

Several studies have investigated predictors of the development of any eating disorder, including anorexia and bulimia nervosa (e.g., McKnight Investigators, 2003; Santonastaso, Friederici, & Favaro, 1999; Stice, Marti, & Durant, 2011). Elevated perceived pressure to be thin, thin-ideal internalization, body dissatisfaction, dieting, depressive symptoms, and psychological disturbances all predict future onset of any eating disorder, suggesting that these may be general risk factors for eating pathology.

## BULIMIA NERVOSA

According to the sociocultural model of bulimia nervosa, internalization of the socially sanctioned thin-ideal for females combines with direct pressures for female thinness (e.g., media portrayed images of the thin ideal) to promote body dissatisfaction, which in turn increases risk for both the initiation of dieting and negative affect, contributing to bulimic pathology (Cattarin & Thompson, 1994; Stice, 2001). Body dissatisfaction, in part based on elevated body mass, is thought to lead vulnerable females to engage in dietary restraint in an effort to conform to this thin-ideal. Dietary restriction enhances the reward value of food by increasing hunger, elevating risk for binge eating. Body dissatisfaction may also contribute to negative affect, which increases the risk of turning to binge eating to provide comfort and distraction from negative emotional states. An important feature of this general model is that contextual factors, such as preoccupation with thinness by family members and peers, play a role in the development of this eating disorder.

Prospective studies that predict onset of future eating disorder symptoms or disorders are better suited to evaluate risk factors than are cross-sectional studies. Consistent with the sociocultural model, prospective studies indicate that thin-ideal internalization, perceived pressure to be thin, body dissatisfaction, dietary restraint, and negative affect increase risk for future onset of bulimic symptoms and bulimic pathology (Field, Camargo, Taylor, Berkey, & Colditz, 1999; Killen et al., 1996; Stice, 2002; Stice et al., 2011). However, prospective studies are vulnerable to third variable alternative explanations, wherein an omitted variable explains the relation between the putative risk factor and future onset of eating pathology. Randomized trials that manipulate a potential risk factor and confirm a subsequent change in symptoms or risk for eating disorder onset permit much firmer inferences. For example, random assignment of adolescent girls to an intervention that reduces thin-ideal internalization through dissonance-induction procedures resulted in reduced eating disorder symptoms and risk for onset of eating disorders relative to assessment-only controls and alternative-intervention controls over 3-year follow-up (Stice et al., 2006; Stice, Marti, Spoor, Presnell, & Shaw, 2008). Other randomized trials have found that interventions that produce reductions in body dissatisfaction, body mass, and negative affect decrease bulimic symptoms (reviewed in Stice, 2002). Interestingly, randomized trials have found that assignment to a weight-loss diet results in decreases in binge eating and bulimic symptoms (Burton & Stice, 2006; Klem, Wing, Simkin-Silverman, & Kuller, 1997; Presnell & Stice, 2003). On the other hand, fasting was a stronger predictor than dietary restraint for the onset of recurrent binge eating and bulimia nervosa over 1- to 5-year follow-up (Stice et al., 2008). Other risk factors have received support in select prospective studies, such as deficits in social support, substance abuse, and elevated body mass; but other hypothesized risk factors have not received support in prospective studies, including early menarche and temperamental impulsivity (Stice, 2002).

Early feeding problems may also increase risk for bulimic symptoms. Marchi and Cohen (1990) found that digestive problems and pica (eating of nonfood substances) in childhood predicted future bulimic symptoms during adolescence. Initial elevations in body mass and longer duration of feeding episodes during infancy predicted emergence of overeating and vomiting during middle childhood (Stice, Agras, & Hammer, 1999).

## Binge Eating Disorder

The few theories regarding etiologic processes that promote binge eating disorder overlap conceptually with etiologic theories for bulimic pathology (Vogeltanz-Holm et al., 2000). Prospective studies show that initial elevations in body mass, perceived pressure for thinness, body dissatisfaction, dietary restraint, negative affect, and a tendency to eat in response to negative emotions (emotional eating) increase the risk for subsequent onset of binge eating (Stice, Killen, Hayward, & Taylor, 1998; Stice, Marti, & Durant, 2011; Stice, Presnell, & Spangler, 2002; Vogeltanz-Holm et al., 2000).

Certain patterns emerge from the risk factor literature. First, the fact that multiple risk factors have been implicated in the development of these disorders provides evidence of equifinality, which posits that multiple pathways may lead to a given psychiatric disorder (von Bertalanffy, 1968; see Chapter 1). For example, at least three different models of bulimia nervosa have been forwarded: binge eating emerges as a response to dysregulated affect; binge eating emerges secondary to extreme dietary restriction, which increases the reinforcing value of food; and binge eating emerges as part of an array of behaviors (e.g., alcohol use, shoplifting, sexual promiscuity) in individuals high in impulsivity (Stice, 2001; Wonderlich & Mitchell, 1997). A recent 8-year prospective study using classification tree analyses suggested that body dissatisfaction, depressive symptoms, and self-reported dieting constitute distinct vulnerability pathways to eating disorder onset (Stice et al., 2011). Second, certain risk factors that have been identified for eating disorders also predict the onset of other psychiatric conditions. For instance, birth complications predict schizophrenia and ADHD; neuroticism and childhood anxiety increase risk for mood and anxiety disorders. Such results are consonant with the notion of multifinality, which posits that the effects of a particular risk factor are qualified by other risk factors operating within the system. Combinations of common and specific risk factors may interact or accumulate, resulting in the final pathway to disease or diseases. For example, an individual with temperamentally high neuroticism could be exposed to an environment that values the thin ideal and supports dieting behavior and exercise to achieve low body weight. Engaging in these behaviors at critical developmental periods could trigger an underlying genetic predisposition to anorexia nervosa. Yet a similarly neurotically predisposed individual who never diets might later, after experiencing a triggering event, develop an anxiety disorder.

## GENETIC AND OTHER BIOLOGICAL FACTORS

*Heritability.* Family studies indicate that relatives of individuals with eating disorders are at elevated risk for eating pathology (e.g., Strober, Freeman, Lampert, Diamond, & Kaye, 2000), though these types of studies cannot determine the effects of genes relative to environmental influences, which are theoretically better addressed by twin and adoption studies (see Chapter 3). Heritability coefficients ($h^2$) from twin studies range widely for anorexia nervosa (.33 to .84) and for bulimia nervosa (.28 to .83), with a smaller range for binge eating disorder (.39 to .41) (Bulik et al., 2006; Bulik, Sullivan, Wade, & Kendler, 2000; Javaras et al., 2008; Klump, Miller, Keel, McGue, & Iacono, 2001; Reichborn-Kjennerud, Bulik, Tambs, & Harris, 2004; Wade, Bulik, Neale, & Kendler, 2000). The remaining variance is accounted for by nonshared environmental factors, with negligible effects of shared environment. One adoption study indicated 59% to 82% genetic influence on all forms of disordered eating, with nonshared environmental factors accounting for the remaining variance and no variance attributed to shared environment (Klump, Suisman, Burt, McGue, & Iacono, 2009). The broad range of estimates is likely to reflect the relatively low prevalence of the traits under study, unreliability in diagnoses, small sample sizes, and/or faulty assumptions in biometric models.

*Genetic studies.* Further evidence suggesting a genetic basis for anorexia and bulimia nervosa has emerged from molecular genetics studies. Association studies compare individuals who display a trait to those who do not display the trait with respect to a candidate gene (or genes) hypothesized to influence the phenotype (eating-disordered behavior). In linkage studies, genetic markers scattered across the genome are used to identify chromosomal regions that may contain genes influencing the trait of interest; specific genes located under the linkage peaks can be further explored using association approaches. Whole genome association (WGA) studies use a data-driven exploratory approach to compare hundreds of thousands to millions of single nucleotide polymorphisms (SNPs) across cases and controls (see Chapter 3). Association studies have focused on genes that are known to affect appetite, weight regulation, and mood—with particular emphasis on the serotonin system. Despite efforts to identify associations between candidate genes and eating disorders, genetic research has yielded only sporadic findings, as a result of small samples (yielding inadequate statistical power) and a tendency to report on only one gene or allele while not disclosing the number of tests performed. For example, linkage studies have not produced replicable findings for anorexia nervosa (Bacanu et al., 2005; Devlin et al., 2002; Grice et al., 2002). Linkage studies of bulimia nervosa have implicated chromosome 10p and 14, with some replication (Bacanu et al., 2005; Bulik et al., 2003; Bulik et al., 2005). The one GWA study found that no SNP reached genome-wide significance (Wang et al., 2011). Thus, almost no reliable findings have emerged from genetic research on eating disorders—a situation not uncommon in psychiatric genetics.

*Neuroendocrine and neurohormonal factors.* Several neurotransmitter systems have been implicated in regulating feeding behavior, including serotonergic (cholinergic), histamergic, and various peptidergic systems (e.g., neuropeptide Y, melanocortin, leptin, orexin and other peptidergic systems; Roth, 2006). Although hundreds of molecular targets have been implicated in regulating feeding behavior, a smaller number (mostly in the serotonergic and dopaminergic systems) have been linked to psychological and behavioral features of eating disorders such as impulsivity and obessionality (Simansky, 2005). The serotonin pathway has been implicated directly in the expression of eating disorders (Jimerson et al., 1997). In long-term weight recovered patients with anorexia or bulimia nervosa, levels of 5-hydroxyindolacetic acid (5-HIAA), a metabolite of serotonin, were elevated in cerebrospinal fluid compared to those of healthy controls (Kaye et al., 1998; Kaye, Gwirtsman, George, & Ebert, 1991). Kaye hypothesized that dysregulated brain serotonin activity could predispose to the development of eating disorders and may contribute to the features of eating disorders such as perfectionism, rigidity, and obsessionality. It is unclear, however, whether sustained abnormalities in serotonin functioning after weight recovery reflects a premorbid trait or a scar, as there is some (although not complete) recovery of abnormal serotonin and transporter content in platelets (Ehrlich et al., 2010).

*Brain structure and functioning studies.* Several structural brain abnormalities have been reported in anorexia nervosa, including gray and white matter loss, increased ventricular size, increased cerebrospinal fluid volume, and enlarged sulci (e.g., Swayze et al., 2003). Although many of these abnormalities normalize after weight restoration, the gray matter loss may persist (Lambe, Katzman, Mikulis, Kennedy, & Zipursky, 1997). Some studies show improvement in gray matter volume, but not full normalization (e.g., Wagner et al., 2006), whereas other studies show normalization (e.g., Castro-Fornieles et al., 2009). Wagner et al. (2006) found no differences in CSF volume or gray and white matter volume in individuals with anorexia and bulimia nervosa who had recovered compared with controls. White matter integrity may be abnormal in underweight individuals with anorexia in some regions, but it is unknown whether this problem resolves with weight restoration, although higher BMI is associated with greater integrity in anorexia (Kazlouski et al., 2011). Structural brain changes in bulimia nervosa are less pronounced than in anorexia nervosa. However, cerebral atrophy has been observed in normal weight individuals with bulimia nervosa (Hoffman et al., 1989), and volumetric differences in particular brain structures have been observed, such as enlarged medial orbitofrontal cortex in bulimia and binge eating disorder (Schäfer, Vaitl, & Schienle, 2010).

In terms of functional differences, individuals with anorexia and bulimia nervosa have globally decreased brain glucose metabolism in the resting state (Frank, Bailer,

Henry, Wagner, & Kaye, 2004). Brain-imaging studies of individuals with anorexia and bulimia nervosa in both the ill and recovered state show elevated activity of the 5-HT$_{1A}$ receptor in frontal-limbic brain regions (Kaye, Bailer, Frank, Wagner, & Henry, 2005). This receptor activity is linked negatively to measures of impulse control and behavioral inhibition, leading Kaye to speculate that an increase in 5-HT$_{1A}$ receptor activity may contribute to the rigid, inflexible, over-controlled, inhibited behavior found in anorexia nervosa and some forms of bulimia nervosa. However, the fact none of these factors, such as impulsivity, have been shown to predict future onset of anorexia nervosa or bulimia nervosa casts some doubt on this speculation.

Overall, neuroimaging studies have found dysfunction in the parietal lobe in individuals with anorexia (Pietrini et al., 2011), which may relate to deficits in self-perception of body weight and shape. The parietal lobe is sexually dimorphic, with decreased volume and surface area in women than men (Kennedy et al., 1998; Koscik, O'Leary, Moser, Andreasen, & Nopoulos, 2008), which may account for the large sex difference in anorexia nervosa. There is evidence of anterior cingulate cortex (ACC) abnormalities in both anorexia and bulimia nervosa (Pietrini et al., 2011). The ACC is implicated in attention and monitoring external contingencies to adapt one's behavior, among other functions. Dysfunction in this region is also present in obsessive-compulsive disorder, other anxiety disorders, and depression—conditions commonly comorbid with eating disorders. Finally, there is evidence of heightened sensitivity of the emotion-related regions such as the medial prefrontal cortex to food stimuli in anorexia and bulimia (Uher et al., 2004), which likely relates to the symptoms of fear and distress related to food.

Individuals with binge eating disorder show greater orbitofrontal cortex activation compared to controls in response to food images, whereas those with bulimia nervosa show greater ACC and insula activation (Schienle, Schäfer, Hermann, & Vaitl, 2009). In response to actual taste receipt, however, individuals recovered from bulimia show reduced ACC activation (Frank et al., 2006), and those with current bulimia showed reduced insula, thalamus, precentral gyrus, and frontal gyrus activation (Bohon & Stice, 2011). This differential response to food cues/images versus actual taste may suggest a mechanism for subsequent binge eating; individuals who experience less reward than anticipated from palatable food intake may compensate by consuming greater amounts of the palatable food.

## DEVELOPMENTAL PROGRESSION

### ANOREXIA NERVOSA

Retrospective data suggest that there are two peak periods of risk for anorexia nervosa onset: around ages 14 and 18 (APA, 2000). These periods correspond to developmental transitions from middle school to high school and from high school to post–high school, which may suggest that developmental stressors can precipitate anorexia among vulnerable individuals. The fact that eating disorders more broadly tend to emerge after puberty also suggests that hormonal changes or concomitant increases in female gender role internalization may increase risk for eating pathology, although the mechanisms are unclear.

Among adolescents with anorexia nervosa, 50% to 70% will recover, 20% will show improvement but will exhibit residual symptoms, and 10% to 20% will develop a chronic course (Berkman et al., 2006; Wilson et al., 2003). Course of illness is on average 10 years (Strober, Freeman, & Morrell, 1997). Residual symptoms include low weight and disturbances in eating, body image, menstrual, and psychosocial functioning. Relapse is common after discharge from inpatient treatment, occurring in one third of cases (Strober et al., 1997). More than one third of patients with the restricting subtype subsequently develop bulimia nervosa and one fourth of individuals with bulimia nervosa subsequently develop anorexia (Tozzi et al., 2005).

Anorexia nervosa has one of the highest mortality rates of any psychiatric disorder. Approximately 6% of patients diagnosed with this disorder die per decade of illness and these patients are 11 times more likely to die than other women of a similar age (Arcelus et al., 2011; Birmingham et al., 2005). The most common causes of death are acute starvation and suicide. The suicide rate for anorexia nervosa is 57 times higher than in the general population (Keel, Fulkerson, & Leon, 1997).

## BULIMIA NERVOSA

The peak period of risk for onset for bulimia nervosa is between 14 and 19 years of age for females (Lewinsohn et al., 2000; Stice et al., 2009). Community-recruited samples suggest that bulimia nervosa typically shows a chronic course characterized by periods of recovery and relapse, whereas subthreshold bulimic pathology shows less chronicity (Bohon, Stice, & Burton, 2009; Fairburn, Cooper, Doll, Norman, & O'Connor, 2000; Stice et al., 2009). In one large study a community-recruited cohort of 102 young women with bulimia nervosa were followed for 5 years (Fairburn et al., 2000). Afflicted individuals often showed marked initial improvement, followed by gradual improvement. By the end of this study, 15% of participants still met diagnostic criteria for bulimia nervosa, 2% met criteria for anorexia nervosa, and 34% met criteria for ED-NOS. This cohort displayed a fluctuating course; each year approximately 33% showed symptom remission and 33% showed relapse. A second study that followed 96 community-recruited adolescent girls with full or subthreshold bulimia nervosa indicated that 38% of the participants with bulimia nervosa recovered over the 1-year follow-up, and 63% of participants with subthreshold bulimia nervosa recovered (Bohon et al., 2009). Another community-recruited study indicated that 40% of women with bulimia nervosa recovered over a 1-year follow-up (Grilo et al., 2003). Even after recovery, however, residual symptoms often remain, including continued impairments in physical and psychosocial functioning (Fairburn et al., 2000). The mortality rate for bulimia nervosa is less than 1% (Keel, Mitchell, Miller, Davis, & Crow, 1999).

Prospective studies have suggested that both diagnosable and subthreshold bulimia nervosa are associated with future onset of depression, suicide attempts, anxiety disorders, substance abuse, obesity, and health problems (Johnson, Cohen,

Kasen, & Brook, 2002; Stice, Cameron, Killen, Hayward, & Taylor, 1999; Stice, Hayward, Cameron, Killen, & Taylor, 2000; Striegel-Moore, Seeley, & Lewinsohn, 2003; Fairburn et al., 2000).

## Binge Eating Disorder

Prospective data suggest that the peak period of risk for onset of binge eating disorder is around age 19 (Stice et al., 2009), though studies have not followed individuals through adulthood. Binge eating typically emerges between 16 and 18 years of age (Stice et al., 1998).

Community-recruited natural history studies suggest that binge eating disorder shows a high remission rate over time, with nearly 50% of cases recovering by 6-month follow-up (Cachelin et al., 1999) and 80% of cases recovering by 3- to 5-year follow-up (Fairburn et al., 2000; Wilson et al., 2003). Retrospective data suggest that the mean duration in years that people suffer from binge eating disorder rivals that of bulimia nervosa (8.1 years). Both durations are substantially longer than that of anorexia nervosa (Hudson et al., 2007). A 12-year prospective study of clinical cases found similar recovery rates for binge eating disorder and bulimia nervosa (Fichter et al., 2008). In addition, binge eating disorder often resolves into a presentation more accurately captured by an ED-NOS diagnosis, with individuals continuing to display some residual symptoms.

Little is known about the course and outcome of young adult binge eating disorder. However, one community-recruited natural history study found that the rate of obesity increased from 20% to 39% over this 5-year study (Fairburn et al., 2000). These findings converge with evidence indicating that binge eating is a risk factor for obesity onset (Stice et al., 2002). Furthermore, low self-confidence, diminished energy level, and discrimination displayed by teachers and peers present significant obstacles to achievement in school and other pursuits among overweight adolescents.

## COMORBIDITY

### Anorexia Nervosa

Although considerable research exists on comorbidity linked to eating disorders, few studies focus on children and adolescents and even fewer on males (see next section for more information on sex differences). However, one study that collapsed across the various eating disorders suggested that men with eating disorders show similar psychiatric comorbidity relative to women with eating disorders (Woodside et al., 2001). Many studies examining comorbidity have used treatment-seeking samples, which are typically biased toward finding elevated comorbidity relative to population levels because each psychiatric condition that an individual has increases the odds of treatment seeking. Nonetheless, these investigations accurately prepare clinicians for comorbid patterns they will encounter. One should also be attentive to whether studies report lifetime comorbidity or concurrent comorbidity.

Studies of community-recruited samples of adolescents indicate that anorexia nervosa shows statistically significant comorbidity with current dysthymia, bipolar disorder, agoraphobia, simple phobia, marijuana dependence, and oppositional defiant disorder, but not with current bulimia nervosa, major depression, conduct disorder, attention-deficit/ hyperactivity disorder, other substance use disorders, social phobia, posttraumatic stress disorder, panic disorder, obsessive-compulsive disorder, or generalized anxiety disorder (Stice & Peterson, 2007). Although there appear to be no comparable data from treatment-seeking samples of adolescents with anorexia nervosa, one large study of adults seeking treatment for this disorder also suggested that the current rates of several disorders were elevated relative to prevalence data available from epidemiologic studies of similarly aged participants (e.g., Garfinkel et al., 1995). Herzog, Keller, Sacks, Yeh, and Lavori (1992) found that the rates of current major depression, obsessive-compulsive disorder, panic disorder, and phobic disorder were substantially higher than the lifetime prevalence rates observed in epidemiologic studies. However, Herzog and associates (1992) showed that the rates of alcohol and drug use disorders among treatment-seeking adults were lower than the lifetime prevalence rates observed in epidemiologic studies. In terms of lifetime comorbidity, the most common comorbid conditions in adults with anorexia nervosa are major depression and anxiety disorders (Kaye et al., 2004; Walters & Kendler, 1995). Anxiety disorders often predate the eating disorder, and depression often persists postrecovery (Kaye et al., 2004; Sullivan, Bulik, Fear, & Pickering, 1998).

## Bulimia Nervosa

Research with community-recruited samples of adolescents indicate that bulimia nervosa shows statistically significant comorbidity with current major depression, dysthymia, bipolar disorder, agoraphobia, social phobia, alcohol dependence, marijuana dependence, and conduct disorder, but not with current simple phobia, overanxious disorder, panic disorder, posttraumatic stress disorder, generalized anxiety disorder, obsessive-compulsive disorder, oppositional defiant disorder, attention deficit hyperactivity disorder, or other substance use disorders (Stice & Peterson, 2007). One large community-recruited sample of adolescents and adults suggested that, relative to those without bulimia nervosa, those with current bulimia nervosa have much higher current prevalence of major depression, any anxiety disorder, social phobia, simple phobia, agoraphobia, panic disorder, generalized anxiety disorder, and alcohol dependence (Garfinkel et al., 1995). Although there appear to be no comparable data from treatment-seeking samples of adolescents with bulimia nervosa, one large study of adults seeking treatment for this eating disorder also suggested that the current rates of several disorders were elevated relative to prevalence data available from epidemiologic studies of similarly aged participants (e.g., Garfinkel et al., 1995). Specifically, Herzog et al. (1992) found that the rates of current major depression and substance use disorders were substantially higher than the lifetime prevalence observed in epidemiologic studies. However, the prevalence of obsessive-compulsive disorder, panic disorder, and phobic disorder were similar to those observed in epidemiologic studies. Common lifetime comorbid psychiatric conditions among adults with bulimia nervosa include anxiety disorders, major depression, dysthymia, substance use, and personality disorders (Wilson et al., 2003).

## BINGE EATING DISORDER

One study of nontreatment seeking adults found that women with binge eating disorder did not show significantly higher rates of major depression, bipolar disorder, dysthymia, substance abuse or dependence, panic disorder, agoraphobia, social phobia, or obsessive-compulsive disorder, relative to weight-matched comparison women (Telch & Stice, 1998). The National Comorbidity Survey Replication found that 78.9% of respondents with binge eating disorder met criteria for at least one *DSM-IV* disorder, although no particular disorder stood out as being more common than others among those with binge eating disorder (Hudson et al., 2007). A study of individuals seeking weight-loss treatment indicated that women with binge eating disorder reported significantly higher rates of current major depression relative to weight-matched comparison participants but that the two groups did not differ in terms of current bipolar disorder, dysthymic disorder, posttraumatic stress disorder, agoraphobia, panic disorder, social phobia, specific phobia, or generalized anxiety disorder (Fontenelle et al., 2003). Similar findings emerged from a second study of treatment-seeking individuals with binge eating disorder (Wilfley et al., 2000). The higher rates of comorbidity from the treatment-seeking sample, relative to the nontreatment-seeking sample, probably emerged because treatment-seeking samples are biased toward finding elevated comorbidity (see earlier). These findings should be generalized to adolescents with caution because all of these estimates emanate from samples of adults.

## SEX DIFFERENCES

Female to male sex ratios of the prevalence of anorexia nervosa and bulimia nervosa are approximately 10:1 (APA, 2000). For anorexia nervosa the amenorrhea criterion applies only to women. Although the *DSM-IV* provides no male equivalent, the International Classification of Diseases-10 notes loss of sexual interest and potency as a criterion for anorexia nervosa in males. Although binge eating disorder shows a similar sex ratio during adolescence, the distribution across sexes seems to become balanced by adulthood (Kjelsas et al., 2004). That both anorexia and bulimia nervosa are more prevalent among females versus males implies that some key difference(s) between the sexes, such as biological factors (e.g., hormonal differences), psychopathology-related factors (e.g., differences in affective disturbances), or developmental experiences (e.g., greater physical objectification of girls and women) play a role in the etiology of these two eating disorders.

There is some evidence that gay males and males who participant in sports with weight-limit requirements are at elevated risk for developing eating disorders

(Wilson et al., 2003). However, little is known about sex differences in risk factors for eating disturbances or course of eating pathology, owing in large part to the low base rate of these disorders in males.

## CULTURAL CONSIDERATIONS

Early stereotypes that eating disorders were confined to the upper-middle class women and girls have generally not been supported in several large studies that have used representative community-recruited samples. Striegel-Moore et al. (2003) explored eating disorders in 2,054 young adult African American and Caucasian women and reported lower prevalences among the former; no African American women were detected with anorexia nervosa, compared with 1.5% of Caucasian women. Striegel-Moore et al. (2005) noted different patterns of eating disorder symptoms across ethnic/racial groups, reporting that binge eating in the absence of purging was more common in African American women, whereas purging in the absence of binge eating was more common in Caucasian women. However, several studies have found no racial or ethnic differences in the prevalence of recurrent binge eating, eating disorder symptoms, or risk factors for eating disorders (Shaw, Ramirez, Trost, Randall, & Stice, 2004; Smith, Marcus, Lewis, Fitzgibbon, & Schreiner, 1998; Striegel-Moore et al., 2000; Yanovski et al., 1992). One consistent difference is that African Americans report less body image dissatisfaction than their White counterparts (Kronenfeld, Reba-Harrelson, Von Holle, Reyes, & Bulik, 2010). There is also evidence that youth who participate in sports with weight requirements or with an extreme focus on appearance are at elevated risk for development of eating disorders because of the emphasis placed on weight and shape within these "cultures" (Wilson et al., 2003).

## SYNTHESIS AND FUTURE DIRECTIONS

It is important to note several controversies in the field as well as gaps in the literature. It will be vital to conduct studies of the phenomenology of eating disorders in large representative samples that contain males and females, children, adolescents, and adults, and participants from multiple racial and ethnic groups. Such studies will shed light on sex differences, developmental differences, and ethnic differences in the manifestation of eating pathology. Additionally, our knowledge of the etiologic and developmental processes that give rise to eating disorders is currently incomplete. Although dozens of psychosocial risk factors have been found to predict future onset of eating disordered symptoms, almost none have been identified that predict onset of full syndrome eating disorders, and many are non-specific to eating disorders. There is a particular dearth of studies on the factors that predict onset of anorexia nervosa. In addition, premorbid biological factors and biomarkers have not yet been identified. Perhaps most importantly, almost no studies have tested integrative models of how psychosocial and biological factors operate together to give rise to eating disorders (e.g., gene-environment correlations and interactions; see Chapter 3). Large prospective studies of high-risk individuals may help address these key questions. Without large prospective studies that assess a wide variety of psychosocial and biological factors, our understanding of etiologic processes will not advance. Such studies will also enable documentation of the developmental course of symptom onset of eating disorders and how this relates to the timing of increases in risk factors for eating disorders.

Another key gap in the literature regards maintaining factors—either psychosocial or biological—that perpetuate eating-disordered behaviors once they emerge. An improved understanding of risk factors is essential for the design of more effective prevention programs, and improved understanding of maintenance factors is vital for the development of more effective treatment interventions.

As noted earlier, prospective designs are highly valuable yet are vulnerable to third-variable alternative explanations. Augmenting these approaches with randomized experiments that focus on suspected risk and maintenance factors is a viable complementary strategy. For instance, it is possible to use randomized prevention trials to effect a lasting reduction in a single putative risk factor (e.g., thin-ideal internalization, negative affect, or body dissatisfaction) and test whether there is a consequent reduction in risk for emergence of eating disorder symptoms during the period of peak risk for onset of these behaviors among those who receive the preventive intervention relative to those who receive a control intervention. It is likewise possible to use treatment intervention to effect a lasting reduction in a single suspected maintenance factor (e.g., objectively measured dietary restraint) and test whether there is a significantly greater reduction in symptoms or the prevalence of the disorder among those who receive this treatment relative to those who receive a control intervention. Although a key weakness of experiments involves ecological validity, the convergence of findings from prospective and experimental studies could boost confidence in our etiologic and maintenance models for eating disorders.

Considerable progress has been made with regard to our understanding of the diagnosis, epidemiology, developmental course, and risk factors for eating disturbances, but there are many unanswered questions. We are confident that rigorous and programmatic research that constructively builds upon our current knowledge base will continue to improve our ability to prevent and treat these pernicious psychiatric disturbances.

## REFERENCES

American Psychiatric Association. (2000). *Diagnostic and statistical manual of mental disorders* (4th ed., text rev.). Washington, DC: American Psychiatric Association.

Arcelus, J., Mitchell, A., Wales, J., & Nielsen, S. (2011). Mortality rates in patients with anorexia nervosa and other eating disorders: A meta-analysis of 36 studies. *Archives of General Psychiatry, 68*, 724–731.

Bacanu, S., Bulik, C., Klump, K., Fichter, M., Halmi, K., Keel, P., et al. (2005). Linkage analysis of anorexia and bulimia nervosa cohorts using selected behavioral phenotypes as quantitative traits or covariates. *American Journal of Medical Genetics Part B: Neuropsychiatry Genetics, 139*, 61–68.

Berkman, N. D., Bulik, C. M., Brownley, K. A., Lohr, K. N., Sedway, J. A., Rooks, A., et al. (2006). *Management of eating disorders. Evidence report/technology assessment no. 135*. (Prepared by the RTI International-University of North Carolina Evidence-Based Practice Center under Contract No. 290–02–0016.) AHRQ Publication No. 06-E010. Rockville, MD: Agency for Healthcare Research and Quality.

Birmingham, C., Su, J., Hlynsky, J., Goldner, E., & Gao, M. (2005). The mortality rate from anorexia nervosa. *International Journal of Eating Disorders, 143–146*.

Bohon, C., & Stice, E. (2011). Reward abnormalities among women with full and subthreshold bulimia nervosa: A functional magnetic resonance imaging study. *International Journal of Eating Disorders, 44*, 585–595.

Bohon, C., Stice, E., & Burton, E. (2009). Maintenance factors for persistence of bulimic pathology: A prospective natural history study. *International Journal of Eating Disorders, 42*, 173–178.

Bulik, C., Bacanu, S., Klump, K., Fichter, M., Halmi, K., Keel, P., et al. (2005). Selection of eating disorders phenotypes for linkage analysis. *American Journal of Medical Genetics Part B: Neuropsychiatry Genetics, 139*, 81–87.

Bulik, C. M., Devlin, B., Bacanu, S. A., Thornton, L., Klump, K. L., Fichter, M. M., et al. (2003). Significant linkage on chromosome 10p in families with bulimia nervosa. *American Journal of Human Genetics, 72*, 200–207.

Bulik, C., Sullivan, P., Tozzi, F., Furberg, H., Lichtenstein, P., & Pedersen, N. (2006). Prevalence, heritability and prospective risk factors for anorexia nervosa. *Archives of General Psychiatry, 63*, 305–312.

Bulik, C., Sullivan, P., Wade, T., & Kendler, K. (2000). Twin studies of eating disorders: A review. *International Journal of Eating Disorders, 27*, 1–20.

Burton, E., & Stice, E. (2006). Evaluation of a healthy-weight treatment program for bulimia nervosa: A preliminary randomized trial. *Behaviour Research and Therapy, 44*, 1727–1738.

Cachelin, F. M., Striegel-Moore, R. H., Elder, K. A., Pike, K. M., Wilfley, D. E., & Fairburn, C. G. (1999). Natural course of a community sample of women with binge eating disorder. *International Journal of Eating Disorders, 25*, 45–54.

Castro-Fornieles, J., Bargallo, N., Lazaro, L., Andres, S., Falcon, C., Plana, M. T., & Junque, C. (2009). A cross-sectional and follow-up voxel-based morphometric MRI study in adolescent anorexia nervosa. *Journal of Psychiatric Research, 43*, 331–340.

Cattarin, J. A., & Thompson, J. K. (1994). A 3-year longitudinal study of body image, eating disturbance, and general psychological functioning in adolescent females. *Eating Disorders, 2*, 114–125.

Cnattingius, S., Hultman, C., Dahl, M., & Sparen, P. (1999). Very preterm birth, birth trauma, and the risk of anorexia nervosa among girls. *Archives of General Psychiatry, 56*, 634–638.

Crow, S. J., Peterson, C. B., Swanson, S. A., Raymond, N. C., Specker, S., Eckert, E. D., & Mitchell, J. E. (2009). Increased mortality in bulimia nervosa and other eating disorders. *American Journal of Psychiatry, 166*, 1342–1346.

Devlin, B., Bacanu, S., Klump, K., Bulik, C., Fichter, M., Halmi, K., et al. (2002). Linkage analysis of anorexia nervosa incorporating behavioral covariates. *Human Molecular Genetics, 11*, 689–696.

Ehrlich, S., Franke, L., Scherag, S., Burghardt, R., Schott, R., Schneider, N.,...Lehmkuhl, U. (2010). The 5-HTTLPR polymorphism, platelet serotonin transporter activity and platelet serotonin content in underweight and weight-recovered females with anorexia nervosa. *European Archives of Psychiatry and Clinical Neuroscience, 260,* 483–490.

Fairburn, C. G., Cooper, Z., Doll, H. A., Norman, P. A., & O'Connor, M. E. (2000). The natural course of bulimia nervosa and binge eating disorder in young women. *Archives of General Psychiatry, 57,* 659–665.

Fairburn, C. G., & Harrison, P. J. (2003). Eating disorders. *Lancet, 361,* 407–416.

Fichter, M. M., Quadflieg, N., & Hedlund, S. (2008). Long-term course of binge eating disorder and bulimia nervosa: Relevance for nosology and diagnostic criteria. *International Journal of Eating Disorders, 41,* 577–586.

Field, A. E., Camargo, C. A., Taylor, C. B., Berkey, C. S., & Colditz, G. A. (1999). Relation of peer and media influences to the development of purging behaviors among preadolescent and adolescent girls. *Archives of Pediatric Adolescent Medicine, 153,* 1184–1189.

Fontaine, K. R., Redden, D. T., Wang, C., Westfall, A. O., & Allison, D. B. (2003). Years of life lost due to obesity. *Journal of the American Medical Association, 289,* 187–193.

Fontenelle, L. F., Mendlowicz, M. V., Menezes, G. B., Papelbaum, M., Freitas, W. R., Godoy-Matos, et al., (2003). Psychiatric comorbidity in a Brazilian sample of patients with binge eating disorder. *Psychiatric Research, 119,* 189–194.

Frank, G. K., Bailer, U. F., Henry, S., Wagner, A., & Kaye, W. H. (2004). Neuroimaging studies in eating disorders. *CNS Spectr, 9,* 539–48.

Frank, G. K., Wagner, A., Achenbach, S., McConaha, C., Skovira, K., Aizenstein, H., et al., (2006). Altered brain activity in women recovered from bulimic-type eating disorders after a glucose challenge: A pilot study. *International Journal of Eating Disorders, 39,* 76–79.

Garfinkel, P. E., Lin, E., Goering, P., Spegg, C., Goldbloom, D. S., Kennedy, S., et al., (1995). Bulimia nervosa in a Canadian community sample: Prevalence and comparison of subgroups. *American Journal of Psychiatry, 152,* 1052–1058.

Grice, D. E., Halmi, K. A., Fichter, M. M., Strober, M., Woodside, D. B., Treasure, J. T., et al. (2002). Evidence for a susceptibility gene for anorexia nervosa on chromosome 1. *American Journal of Human Genetics, 70,* 787–792.

Grilo, C. M., Hrabosky, J. I., White, M. A., Allison, K. C., Stunkard, A. J., & Masheb, R. M. (2008). Overvaluation of shape and weight in binge eating disorder and overweight controls: Refinement of a diagnostic contruct. *Journal of Abnormal Psychology, 117,* 414–419.

Grilo, C. M., Sanislow, C. A., Shea, M. T., Skodol, A. E., Stout, R. L., Pagano, M. E. et al., (2003). The natural course of bulimia nervosa and eating disorder not otherwise specified is not influenced by personality disorders. *International Journal of Eating Disorders, 34,* 319–330.

Herzog, D. B., Keller, M. B., Sacks, N. R., Yeh, C. J., & Lavori, P. W. (1992). Psychiatric comorbidity in treatment-seeking anorexics and bulimics. *Journal of the American Academy of Child and Adolescent Psychiatry, 31,* 810–818.

Hoek, H. W., & van Hoeken, D. (2003). Review of the prevalence and incidence of eating disorders. *International Journal of Eating Disorders, 34,* 383–396.

Hoffman, G. W., Ellinwood, E. H. Jr., Rockwell, W. J., Herfkens, R. J., Nishita, J. K., & Guthrie, L. F. (1989). Cerebral atrophy in bulimia. *Biological Psychiatry, 25,* 894–902.

Hudson, J., Hiripi, E., Pope, H., & Kessler, R. (2007). Prevalence and correlates of eating disorders in the national comorbidity survey replication. *Biological Psychiatry, 61,* 348–358.

Javaras, K. N., Laird, N. M., Reichborn-Kjennerud, T., Bulik, C. M., Pope Jr., H. G., & Hudson, J. I. (2008). Familiality and heritability of binge eating disorder: Results of a case–control family study and a twin study. *International Journal of Eating Disorders 41,* 174–179.

Jimerson, D. C., Wolfe, B. E., Metzger, E. D., Finkelstein, D. M., Cooper, T. B., & Levine, J. M. (1997). Decreased serotonin function in bulimia nervosa. *Archives of General Psychiatry, 54,* 529–534.

Johnson, J. G., Cohen, P., Kasen, S., & Brook, J. S. (2002). Eating disorders during adolescence and the risk for physical and mental disorders during early adulthood. *Archives of General Psychiatry, 59,* 545–552.

Kazlouski, D., Rollin, M. D., Tregellas, J., Shott, M. E., Jappe, L. M., Hagman, J. O., et al., (2011). Altered fimbria-fornix white matter integrity in anorexia nervosa predicts harm avoidance. *Psychiatry Research: Neuroimaging, 192,* 109–116.

Kaye, W. H., Bailer, U. F., Frank, G. K., Wagner, A., & Henry, S. E. (2005). Brain imaging of serotonin after recovery from anorexia and bulimia nervosa. *Physiology of Behavior, 86,* 15–17.

Kaye, W., Bulik, C., Thornton, L., Barbarich, B. S., Masters, K., & the Price Foundation Collaborative Group. (2004). Comorbidity of anxiety disorders with anorexia and bulimia nervosa. *American of Journal of Psychiatry, 161,* 2215–2221.

Kaye, W. H., Greeno, C. G., Moss, H., Fernstrom, J., Fernstrom, M., Lilenfeld, L. R., et al. (1998). Alterations in serotonin activity and psychiatric symptoms after recovery from bulimia nervosa. *Archives of General Psychiatry, 55,* 927–935.

Kaye, W. H., Gwirtsman, H. E., George, D. T., & Ebert, M. H. (1991). Altered serotonin activity in anorexia nervosa after long-term weight restoration. Does elevated cerebrospinal fluid 5-hydroxyindoleacetic acid level correlate with rigid and obsessive behavior? *Archives of General Psychiatry, 48,* 556–562.

Keel, P. K., & Brown, T. A. (2010). Update on course and outcome in eating disorders. *International Journal of Eating Disorders, 43,* 195–204.

Keel, P. K., Fulkerson, J. A., & Leon, G. R. (1997). Disordered eating precursors in pre- and early adolescent girls and boys. *Journal of Youth and Adolescence, 26,* 203–216.

Keel, P. K., Mitchell, J. E., Miller, K. B., Davis, T. L., & Crow, S. J. (1999). Long-term outcome of bulimia nervosa. *Archives of General Psychiatry, 56,* 63–69.

Kennedy, D. N., Lange, N., Makris, N., Bates, J., Meyer, J., & Caviness, V. S. (1998). Gyri of the human neocortex: an MRI-based analysis of volume and variance. *Cerebral Cortex, 8,* 372–384.

Killen, J. D., Taylor, C. B., Hayward, C., Haydel, K. F., Wilson, D. M., Hammer, L., et al., (1996). Weight concerns influence the development of eating disorders: A 4-year prospective study. *Journal of Consulting and Clinical Psychology, 64*, 936–940.

Kjelsas, E., Bjornstrom, C., & Gotestam, K. G. (2004). Prevalence of eating disorders in female and male adolescents (14–15 years). *Eating Behaviors, 5*, 13–25.

Klem, M. L., Wing, R. R., Simkin-Silverman, L., & Kuller, L. H. (1997). The psychological consequences of weight gain prevention in healthy, premenopausal women. *International Journal of Eating Disorders, 21*, 167–174.

Klump, K. L., Miller, K. B., Keel, P. K., McGue, M., & Iacono, W. G. (2001). Genetic and environmental influences on anorexia nervosa syndromes in a population-based twin sample. *Psychological Medicine, 31*, 737–740.

Klump, K. L., Suisman, J. L., Burt, S. A., McGue, M., & Iacono, W. G. (2009). Genetic and environmental influences on disordered eating: An adoption study. *Journal of Abnormal Psychology, 118*, 797–805.

Koscik, T., O'Leary, D., Moser, D. J., Andreasen, N. C., & Nopoulos, P. (2008). Sex differences in parietal lobe morphology: Relationship to mental rotation performance. *Brain and Cognition, 69*, 451–459.

Kronenfeld, L., Reba-Harrelson, L., Von Holle, A., Reyes, M., & Bulik, C. (2010). Ethnic and racial differences in body size perception and satisfaction. *Body Image, 7*, 131–136.

Lambe, E. K., Katzman, D. K., Mikulis, D. J., Kennedy, S. H., & Zipursky, R. B. (1997). Cerebral gray matter volume deficits after weight recovery from anorexia nervosa. *Archives of General Psychiatry, 54*, 537–542.

LeGrange, D., Binford, R. B., Peterson, C. B., Crow, S. J., Crosby, R. D., Klein, M. H., et al. (2006). DSM-IV threshold versus subthreshold bulimia nervosa. *International Journal of Eating Disorders, 39*, 462–467.

Lewinsohn, P. M., Striegel-Moore, R. H., & Seeley, J. R. (2000). Epidemiology and natural course of eating disorders in young women from adolescence to young adulthood. *Journal of the American Academy of Child and Adolescent Psychiatry, 39*, 1284–1292.

Marchi, M., & Cohen, P. (1990). Early childhood eating behaviors and adolescent eating disorders. *Journal of American Academy of Child and Adolescent Psychiatry, 29*, 112–117.

McKnight Investigators. (2003). Risk factors for onset of eating disorders in adolescent girls: Results of the McKnight longitudinal risk factor study. *American Journal of Psychiatry, 160*, 248–254.

Nicholls, D. E., & Viner, R. M. (2009). Childhood risk factors for lifetime anorexia nervosa by age 30 years in a national birth cohort. *Journal of the American Academy of Child and Adolescent Psychiatry, 48*, 791–799.

Peebles, R., Hardy, K. K., Wilson, J. L., & Lock, J. D. (2010). Are diagnostic criteria for eating disorders markers of medical severity? *Pediatrics, 125*, e1193–e1201.

Pietrini, F., Castellini, G., Ricca, V., Polito, C., Pupi, A., & Faravelli, C. (2011). Functional neuroimaging in anorexia nervosa: A clinical approach. *European Psychiatry, 26*, 176–182.

Presnell, K., & Stice, E. (2003). An experimental test of the effect of weight-loss dieting on bulimic pathology: Tipping the scales in a different direction. *Journal of Abnormal Psychology, 112*, 166–170.

Reichborn-Kjennerud, T., Bulik, C., Tambs, K., & Harris, J. (2004a). Genetic and environmental influences on binge eating in the absence of compensatory behaviours: A population-based twin study. *International Journal of Eating Disorders, 36*, 307–314.

Reichborn-Kjennerud, T., Bulik, C. M., Sullivan, P. F., Tambs, K., & Harris, J. R. (2004b) Medical and psychiatric symptoms associated with binge-eating in the absence of compensatory behaviors. *Obesity Research, 12*, 1445–1454.

Rockert, W., Kaplan, A. S., & Olmsted, M. P. (2007). Eating disorder not otherwise specified: The view from a tertiary care treatment center. *International Journal of Eating Disorders, 40*, S99–S103.

Roth, B. (2006). *The serotonin receptors: From molecular pharmacology to human therapeutics.* Totowa, NJ: Humana Press.

Santonastaso, P., Bosello, R., Schiavone, P., Tenconi, E., Degortes, D., & Favaro, A. (2009). Typical and atypical restrictive anorexia nervosa: Weight history, body image, psychiatric symptoms, and response to outpatient treatment. *International Journal of Eating Disorders, 42*, 464–470.

Santonastaso, P., Friederici, S., & Favaro, A. (1999). Full and partial syndromes in eating disorders: A 1-year prospective study of risk factors among female students. *Psychopathology, 32*, 50–56.

Schäfer, A., Vaitl, D., & Schienle, A. (2010). Regional grey matter volume abnormalities in bulimia nervosa and binge-eating disorder. *NeuroImage, 50*, 639–643.

Schienle, A., Schäfer, A., Hermann, A., & Vaitl, D. (2009). Binge-eating disorder: Reward sensitivity and brain activation to images of food. *Biological Psychiatry, 65*, 654–661.

Shaw, H., Ramirez, L., Trost, A., Randall, P., & Stice, E. (2004). Body image and eating disturbances across ethnic groups: More similarities than differences. *Psychology of Addictive Behaviors, 18*, 12–18.

Simansky, K. J. (2005). NIH symposium series: Ingestive mechanisms in obesity, substance abuse and mental disorders. *Physiology and Behavior, 86*, 1–4.

Smith, D. E., Marcus, M. D., Lewis, C. E., Fitzgibbon, M., & Schreiner, P. (1998). Prevalence of binge eating disorder, obesity, and depression in a biracial cohort of young adults. *Annals of Behavioral Medicine, 20*, 227–32.

Spoor, S. T., Stice, E., Burton, E., & Bohon, C. (2007). Relations of bulimic symptom frequency and intensity to psychosocial impairment and health care utilization: Results from a community-recruited sample. *International Journal of Eating Disorders, 40*, 505–514.

Stice, E. (2001). A prospective test of the dual pathway model of bulimic pathology: Mediating effects of dieting and negative affect. *Journal of Abnormal Psychology, 110*, 124–135.

Stice, E. (2002). Risk and maintenance factors for eating pathology: A meta-analytic review. *Psychological Bulletin, 128*, 825–848.

Stice, E., Agras, W. S., & Hammer, L. (1999a). Factors influencing the onset of childhood eating disturbances: A five-year prospective study. *International Journal of Eating Disorders, 25*, 375–387.

Stice, E., Cameron, R., Killen, J. D., Hayward, C., & Taylor, C. B. (1999b). Naturalistic weight reduction efforts prospectively predict growth in relative weight and onset of obesity among female adolescents. *Journal of Consulting and Clinical Psychology, 67*, 967–974.

Stice, E., Davis, K., Miller, N., & Marti, C. N. (2008). Fasting increases risk for onset of binge eating and bulimic pathology: A 5-year prospective study. *Journal of Abnormal Psychology, 117*, 941–946.

Stice, E., Hayward, C., Cameron, R., Killen, J. D., & Taylor, C. B. (2000). Body image and eating related factors predict onset of depression in female adolescents: A longitudinal study. *Journal of Abnormal Psychology, 109*, 438–444.

Stice, E., Killen, J. D., Hayward, C., & Taylor, C. B. (1998). Age of onset for binge eating and purging during adolescence: A four-year survival analysis. *Journal of Abnormal Psychology, 107*, 671–675.

Stice, E., Marti, C. N., & Durant, S. (2011). Risk factors for onset of eating disorders: Evidence of multiple risk pathways from an 8-year prospective study. *Behaviour Research and Therapy, 49*, 622–627.

Stice, E., Marti, C. N., Shaw, H., & Jaconis, M. (2009). An 8-year longitudinal study of the natural history of threshold, subthreshold, and partial eating disorders from a community sample of adolescents. *Journal of Abnormal Psychology, 118*, 587–597.

Stice, E., Marti, N., Spoor, S., Presnell, K., & Shaw, H. (2008). Dissonance and healthy weight eating disorder prevention programs: Long-term effects from a randomized efficacy trial. *Journal of Consulting and Clinical Psychology, 76*, 329–340.

Stice, E., & Peterson, C. (2007). Assessment of eating disorders. In E. J. Mash & R. A. Barkley (Eds.), *Assessment of childhood disorders* (4th ed., pp. 751–780). New York, NY: Guilford Press.

Stice, E., Presnell, K., & Bearman, S. K. (2006). *Risk factors for onset of threshold and subthreshold bulimia nervosa: A 5-year prospective study of adolescent girls.* Unpublished manuscript.

Stice, E., Presnell, K., & Spangler, D. (2002). Risk factors for binge eating onset: A prospective investigation. *Health Psychology, 21*, 131–138.

Striegel-Moore, R. H., Franko, D. L., Thompson, D., Barton, B., Schreiber, G. B., & Daniels, S. R. (2005). An empirical study of the typology of bulimia nervosa and its spectrum variants. *Psychological Medicine, 35*, 1563–1572.

Striegel-Moore, R. H., Seeley, J. R., & Lewinsohn, P. M. (2003). Psychosocial adjustment in young adulthood of women who experience an eating disorder during adolescence. *American Academy of Child and Adolescent Psychiatry, 42*, 587–593.

Strober, M., Freeman, R., Lampert, C., Diamond, J., & Kaye, W. (2000). Controlled family study of anorexia nervosa and bulimia nervosa: Evidence of shared liability and transmission of partial syndromes. *American Journal of Psychiatry, 157*, 393–401.

Strober, M., Freeman, R., & Morrell, W. (1997). The long-term course of severe anorexia nervosa in adolescents: Survival analysis of recovery, relapse, and outcome predictors over 10–15 years in a prospective study. *International Journal of Eating Disorders, 22,* 339–360.

Stunkard, A. J. (1959). Eating patterns and obesity. *Psychiatric Quarterly, 33,* 284–292.

Sullivan, P. F., Bulik, C. M., Fear, J. L., & Pickering, A. (1998) Outcome of anorexia nervosa. *American Journal of Psychiatry, 155,* 939–946.

Swayze, V. W. 2nd, Andersen, A. E., Andreasen, N. C., Arndt, S., Sato, Y., & Ziebell, S. (2003). Brain tissue volume segmentation in patients with anorexia nervosa before and after weight normalization. *International Journal of Eating Disorders, 33,* 33–44.

Telch, C., & Stice, E. (1998). Psychiatric comorbidity in a non-clinical sample of women with binge eating disorder. *Journal of Consulting and Clinical Psychology, 66,* 768–776.

Tozzi, F., Thornton, L., Klump, K., Bulik, C., Fichter, M., Halmi, K., et al. (2005). Symptom fluctuation in eating disorders: Correlates of diagnostic crossover. *American Journal of Psychiatry, 162,* 732–740.

Uher, R., Murphy, T., Brammer, M. J., Dalgleish, T., Phillips, M. L., Ng, V. W., et al., (2004). Medial prefrontal cortex activity associated with symptom provocation in eating disorders. *American Journal of Psychiatry, 161,* 1238–1246.

Vogeltanz-Holm, N. D., Wonderlich, S. A., Lewis, B. A., Wilsnack, S. C., Harris, T. R., Wilsnack, R. W., et al. (2000). Longitudinal predictors of binge eating, intense dieting, and weight concerns in a national sample of women. *Behavior Therapy, 31,* 221–235.

von Bertalanffy, L. (1968). *General systems theory.* New York, NY: Braziller.

Wade, T. D., Bulik, C. M., Neale, M., & Kendler, K. S. (2000). Anorexia nervosa and major depression: Shared genetic and environmental risk factors. *American Journal of Psychiatry, 157,* 469–471.

Wagner, A., Greer, P., Bailer, U., Frank, G., Henry, S., Putnam, K., et al. (2006). Normal brain tissue volumes after long-term recovery in anorexia and bulimia nervosa. *Biological Psychiatry, 59,* 291–293.

Wang, K., Zhang, H., Bloss, C. S., Duvvuri, V., Kaye, W., Schork, N. J., Berrettini, W., et al. (2011). A genome-wide association study on common SNPs and rare CNVs in anorexia nervosa. *Mol. Psychiatry, 16,* 949–959.

Walters, E. E., & Kendler, K. S. (1995). Anorexia nervosa and anorexia-like syndromes in a population-based female twin sample. *American Journal of Psychiatry, 152,* 64–71.

Wilfley, D. E., Friedman, M., Dounchis, J., Stein, R., Welch, R., & Ball, S. (2000). Comorbid psychopathology in binge eating disorder: Relation to eating disorder severity at baseline and following treatment. *Journal of Consulting and Clinical Psychology, 68,* 641–649.

Wilson, G. T., Becker, C. B., & Heffernan, K. (2003). Eating disorders. In E. J. Mash & R. A. Barkley (Eds.), *Child psychopathology* (2nd ed., pp. 687–715). New York, NY: Guilford Press.

Wonderlich, S. A., & Mitchell, J. E. (1997). Eating disorders and comorbidity: Empirical, conceptual, and clinical implications. *Psychopharmacology Bulletin, 33,* 381–390.

Woodside, D. B., Garfinkel, P. E., Lin, E., Goering, P., Kaplan, A. S., Goldbloom, D. S., & Kennedy, S. H. (2001). Comparison of men with full or partial eating disorders, men without eating disorders, and women with eating disorders in the community. *American Journal of Psychiatry, 158,* 570–574.

Yanovski, S. Z., Leet, M., Yanovski, J. A., Flood, M., Gold, P. W., Kissileff, et al. (1992). Food selection and intake of obese women with binge eating disorder. *American Journal of Clinical Nutrition, 56,* 975–980.

Zimmerman, M., Francione-Witt, C., Chelminski, I., Young, D., & Tortolani, C. (2008). Problems applying the DSM-IV eating disorders diagnostic criteria in general psychiatric outpatient practice. *Journal of Clinical Psychiatry, 69,* 381–384.

# Author Index

# Subject Index